W0080542

IDKD Springer Series

Series Editors

Juerg Hodler
Prof. Emeritus of Radiology
University of Zürich
Zurich, Switzerland

Rahel A. Kubik-Huch
Department of Radiology
Kantonsspital Baden
Baden, Switzerland

Gustav K. von Schulthess
Prof. and Dir. Emeritus Nuclear Medicine
University Hospital
Zurich, Switzerland

The world-renowned International Diagnostic Course in Davos (IDKD) represents a unique learning experience for imaging specialists in training as well as for experienced radiologists and clinicians. IDKD reinforces his role of educator offering to the scientific community tools of both basic knowledge and clinical practice. Aim of this Series, based on the faculty of the Davos Course and now launched as open access publication, is to provide a periodically renewed update on the current state of the art and the latest developments in the field of organ-based imaging (chest, neuro, MSK, and abdominal).

Juerg Hodler · Rahel A. Kubik-Huch
Justus E. Roos · Gustav K. von Schulthess
Editors

Diseases of the Abdomen and Pelvis 2023-2026

Diagnostic Imaging

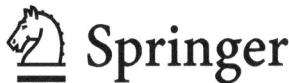
Springer

Editors
Juerg Hodler
Prof. Emeritus of Radiology
University of Zürich
Zurich, Switzerland

Rahel A. Kubik-Huch
Department of Radiology
Kantonsspital Baden
Baden, Aargau, Switzerland

Justus E. Roos
Department of Radiology
Luzerner Kantonsspital
Lucerne, Switzerland

Gustav K. von Schulthess
Prof. and Dir. Emeritus Nuclear Medicine
University Hospital of Zurich
Zurich, Switzerland

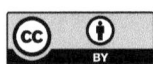

Foundation for the Advancement of Education in Medical Radiology

ISSN 2523-7829   ISSN 2523-7837   (electronic)
IDKD Springer Series
ISBN 978-3-031-27354-4   ISBN 978-3-031-27355-1   (eBook)
https://doi.org/10.1007/978-3-031-27355-1

This Springer imprint is published by the registered company Springer Nature Switzerland AG
The registered company address is: Gewerbestrasse 11, 6330 Cham, Switzerland

Contents

Emergency Radiology of the Abdomen and Pelvis

1

Vincent M. Mellnick and Pierre-Alexandre Poletti

1.1 Trauma Part

Pierre-Alexandre Poletti

> **Learning Objectives**
> - To review the role and limitations of the various imaging modalities in the management of blunt abdominal trauma patients.
> - To review the imaging findings associated with blunt abdominal trauma.
> - To discuss the role of imaging in the grading systems used for the management of blunt abdominal trauma patients.

> **Key Points**
> - Absence of free intraperitoneal fluid at FAST examination does not rule out a major traumatic visceral injury.
> - Abdominal CT protocols must include both arterial and porto-venous phases; they should be completed by delayed series if vascular or urinary tract injuries are seen on initial series.
> - Splenic post-traumatic pseudoaneurysms mandate angiographic embolization; they may develop 24–72 h after trauma.

V. M. Mellnick (✉)
Mallinckrodt Institute of Radiology, Washington University School of Medicine, Saint Louis, MO, USA
e-mail: mellnickv@wustl.edu

P.-A. Poletti
Service of Radiology, University Hospital Geneva, Geneva, Switzerland
e-mail: Pierre-alexandre.poletti@hcuge.ch

1.1.1 Role of Imaging to Assess Blunt Abdominal Polytrauma (BAT) Patients

1.1.1.1 Primary Survey

In a patient admitted with a potential abdominal trauma, a normal clinical examination has been shown insufficient per se to rule out a major intra-abdominal injury [1]. An imaging method should therefore be systematically obtained. Based on the ATLS recommendations [2], a FAST (focused assessment with sonography for trauma) is immediately performed, in addition to pelvic X-Ray, for the initial triage of trauma patients. Six regions are classically examined at FAST: right upper quadrant, hepatorenal fossa (Morison's pouch), left upper quadrant (subphrenic space), splenorenal recess, pelvis (Douglas recess), and pericardium.

Depiction of a large amount of free intraperitoneal fluid in a hemodynamically unstable patient will mandate immediate laparotomy, or CT examination in a stable patient. In a hemodynamically stable patient, a normal FAST examination along with a normal clinical examination are not sufficient to rule out a significant intra-abdominal injury [3]. Indeed, in addition to the well-known limitation of the clinical abdominal examination up to 34% of abdominal injury could be present without associated free fluid, 17% of them would eventually require surgery or angiography embolization [4]. Furthermore, FAST examination can miss a major retroperitoneal bleeding. In isolated minor abdominal trauma, there is no unanimously accepted criteria for systematically performing or not CT in the absence of free intraperitoneal fluid at FAST. It has been suggested that the addition of normal bedside imaging (chest and pelvis X-ray, FAST) normal blood tests and a normal clinical examination could be sufficient to safely discharge an alert patient without further observation or investigation [3]. However, only a minority of patients (<20%) with suspicion of blunt abdominal trauma fulfill these criteria. All other should undergo further investigations.

1.1.1.2 Secondary Survey

Abdominal CT imaging in a hemodynamically stable patient is usually obtained in the frame of a total body CT protocol (secondary survey). In spite of the fact that there is no consensus regarding an optimal CT protocol for polytrauma patients, most authors agree that unenhanced abdominal CT images are not recommended, and that arterial and portal venous phase should be systematically obtained for a better depiction of vascular lesions, using either two acquisitions [5] or one single acquisition with a split contrast bolus. Delayed series should systematically be obtained in case of suspicion of active bleeding on the initial series.

Imaging of Common Abdominal Traumatic Injuries

Intraperitoneal Fluid

Hemoperitoneum is the commonest CT sign to suggest an intra-abdominal organ injury. Rarely, hemoperitoneum can be associated to retroperitoneal organ traumatic lesions, classically kidney injuries (or pancreatic tail injuries) by fluid spreading through the splenorenal ligament. In the absence of active bleeding, hemoperitoneum has a density between 20 and 40 HU. At the direct contact of the lesion, clotted blood achieves a higher density (50–70 HU) which is referred to as the "sentinel clot sign." This sign if often useful to identify the actual site of injury [6]. Free fluid without evident organ injury may be present at CT in 1–5% of trauma patients and does not always herald need for surgery.

Organ Injuries

In a consecutive series of trauma patients with positive CT for at least one intra-abdominal injury [7] the following organ were involved, by order of frequency: spleen (37%), liver (32%), urinary tract (15%), bowel and mesentery (11%), pancreas (3%), diaphragm (<1%).

Spleen Injuries

Spleen is the most frequently encountered organ injury in blunt abdominal trauma patients. Most splenic injuries can be treated conservatively, in the absence of absolute clinical indication for surgery at admission. However, delayed failure of nonsurgical treatment (bleeding) has been formerly reported in 10–31% of cases [8] and may occur up to 10 days (or even later) after trauma. A major improvement in the non-operative management of blunt splenic trauma patients was achieved when two major observations were reported in the scientific literature. Firstly, an association was established between the presence of intrasplenic vascular injuries at CT and an increased risk of delayed bleeding [9]. Secondly, the angiographic embolization of these vascular injuries has been associated with a significant drop in the rate of unsuccessful non-operative management (from 13% to 6%) [10]. Based on these observations, the classical AAST-1994 surgical splenic injury scale classification,

only based on morphological criteria, was completed by a CT-based classification initially proposed by Stuart Mirvis [11] and slightly reshuffled in 2018 [12]. This classification takes into account vascular lesions (pseudoaneurysms, arteriovenous fistula or active bleedings) confined within the spleen (Fig. 1.1) and those extending beyond the spleen (active bleeding). Vascular splenic lesions appear at CT as focal blush of contrast with an attenuation close to arteries and greater than that of the spleen parenchyma. Delayed CT images must be systematically obtained in the presence of a vascular lesion to differentiate those that vanishes (pseudoaneurysms and arteriovenous fistula) from those which stay and expand (active bleeding).

Whether a systematic follow-up imaging patients should be performed in hemodynamically stable blunt splenic trauma patients remains a yet unsolved question. It has been reported that a majority of traumatic splenic pseudoaneuryms (38%–74%) would only be detected on control CT performed within 24–72 h after admission [13]. For practical reasons, most of the trauma associations do not recommend a systematic delayed CT in hemodynamically stable splenic trauma patients. With a reported 75% sensitivity and 100% specificity for detection of delayed splenic pseudoaneurysms (in skilled hands), bedside contrast enhanced sonographic examination has been advocated as a good option in this setting [14].

Liver Injuries

The AAST liver injury classification, as well as its adaptation for CT proposed by Stuart Mirvis in 1989, were based on the anatomic disruption of the liver, including the length and depth of the lacerations, as well as the size of the subcapsular hematoma.

Most of liver injuries, including high AAST grade lesions (III–V), can be managed non-operatively in hemodynami-

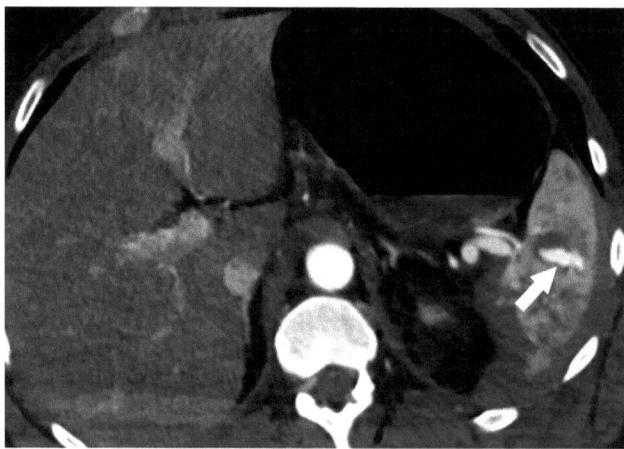

Fig. 1.1 AAST Grade IV splenic injury. A 41-year-old man admitted after a motor vehicle collision. Axial contrast enhanced CT image, arterial phase, shows a blush of contrast media (arrow) within a splenic hypodense laceration, consistent with an arterial pseudoaneurysm

cally stable patients. In 2018, the AAST-based liver grading system has been updated in a new organ injury scaling (OIS). The major change of the 2018 OIS is the inclusion of vascular lesions, confined in the liver parenchyma or freely bleeding into the peritoneum, to define severity. Such lesions are seen in about 20% of blunt liver trauma patients.

The most common ominous CT signs to be considered predictive of failure of non-operative management are the presence of an extracapsular bleeding into the peritoneal cavity, the extension of the laceration into the major hepatic veins or vena cava, and the presence of an important hemoperitoneum [15, 16]. Systematic routine follow-up CT is not recommended in blunt liver trauma patients; repeated imaging should only be guided by a patient's clinical status. Bile duct injuries (biloma, biliary fistula, bile leak) have been reported as a complication in 2–8% of blunt liver trauma patients. MRI with biliary specific contrast agent may be used to identify the involvement of a main bile duct which could mandate surgical management. CT or ultrasound follow-up examination can be recommended in case of clinical suspicion of liver abscess that complicate liver trauma in about 4% of cases.

Urinary Tract Injuries

Urinary tract injuries are usually, but not always, associated with a gross hematuria. CT examination is the reference standard for the evaluation of the urinary tract. Arterial phases are important to demonstrate vascular kidney injuries while portal venous phases will better show parenchymal damage and differentiate an active bleeding from a pseudoaneurysm. The AAST classification for renal injuries has been slightly revised in 2018. Grade I to III renal injuries, the vast majority (75–98%) of renal traumatic lesions, do not involve the collecting system and are managed non-operatively. Any vascular injuries, including active bleeding, confined within the Gerota fascia are still considered grade III. Grade IV injuries extend into the collecting system or involve segmental renal vein or artery injuries (active bleeding or thrombosis) (Fig. 1.2). Grade 5 injuries refer to avulsion of the main renal artery or vein, a devascularized kidney with active bleeding or an extended maceration with loss of identifiable parenchyma. Surgical treatment or angiographic therapeutic management may be indicated in grade IV and V injuries. Any attempt of reperfusion of a devascularized kidney should be performed within 5 h after trauma to avoid irreversible ischemic damages.

Ureteral injury is exceedingly rare in blunt trauma and CT signs may be very subtle, such as mild periureteral fluid or fat stranding. A 3–20 min delayed excretory phase series are required to make the definitive diagnosis of partial or complete ureteral tear.

Bladder injuries are associated with pelvic fractures in 90% of cases, while about 2–11% of pelvic fracture have bladder rupture. Thus, a CT cystography should complete the initial CT series in the presence of a pelvic rim fracture, ideally by instilling at least 250 mL of diluted contrast media into the bladder. This technique has been reported 95% sensitive and 99% specific to detect a bladder rupture. It should not be performed if the patient requires angiography since the extravasated contrast material can obscure the sites of bleeding. Extravasation of vesical contrast material in the extraperitoneal tissues, including the prevesical space of Retzius, is characteristic of extraperitoneal bladder rupture [17]. This is the most frequent type (80%) of bladder rupture in adult patients, which can be treated by transurethral or suprapubic bladder catheterization. Spreading of contrast media into the peritoneal recesses is the hallmark of intraperitoneal bladder rupture, which account for about 20% of cases [17]. They require surgical repair to avoid peritonitis (Fig. 1.3). Rarely, both intra- and extraperitoneal bladder ruptures may coexist.

Bowel and Mesenteric Injuries

CT signs of bowel and mesenteric injuries may be subtle and often require a meticulous analysis for not being overlooked. Delay in assessing the diagnosis of these conditions is associated with a high morbidity due to peritonitis, sepsis, hemorrhage, or bowel ischemia. Most traumatic bowel injuries involve the small bowel, especially the proximal jejunum and the distal ileum. The transverse colon is the most frequent site of large bowel traumatic injuries. Some CT signs of bowel injuries are usually very specific but few sensitive to assess the diagnosis of bowel rupture: discontinuity of the bowel wall (rare), intra- or retroperitoneal air without other reason to explain this air, segmental absence of enhancement (devascularization). Some nonspecific signs, such as segmental bowel thickening or free intraperitoneal fluid, unexplained by a solid organ injury, should alert for a potential bowel perforation.

However, an extended diffuse small bowel circumferential hyper-enhanced wall thickening is more suggestive of a shock bowel syndrome (hypoperfusion complex), especially in the presence of a flat vena cava, enhanced adrenal grands, and delayed nephrograms. A diffuse small bowel wall thickening (without hyperenhancement), along with a dilated vena cava, is classically observed after a vigorous resuscitation (volume overload). An update of the AAST-bowel and mesentery classification, including the recent advances in CT imaging has been recently released [18].

If a bowel injury is clinically suspected in the absence of clear CT signs of bowel rupture, a follow-up CT can be performed 4–6 h later, after admission of i.v. and oral contrast to look for an extravasation of intra-intestinal contrast material.

CT signs suggestive of mesenteric injuries consist in an active extravasation of contrast media from mesenteric vessels (Fig. 1.4), a mesenteric hematoma adjacent to a bowel wall thickening (devascularization), an abrupt termination (or

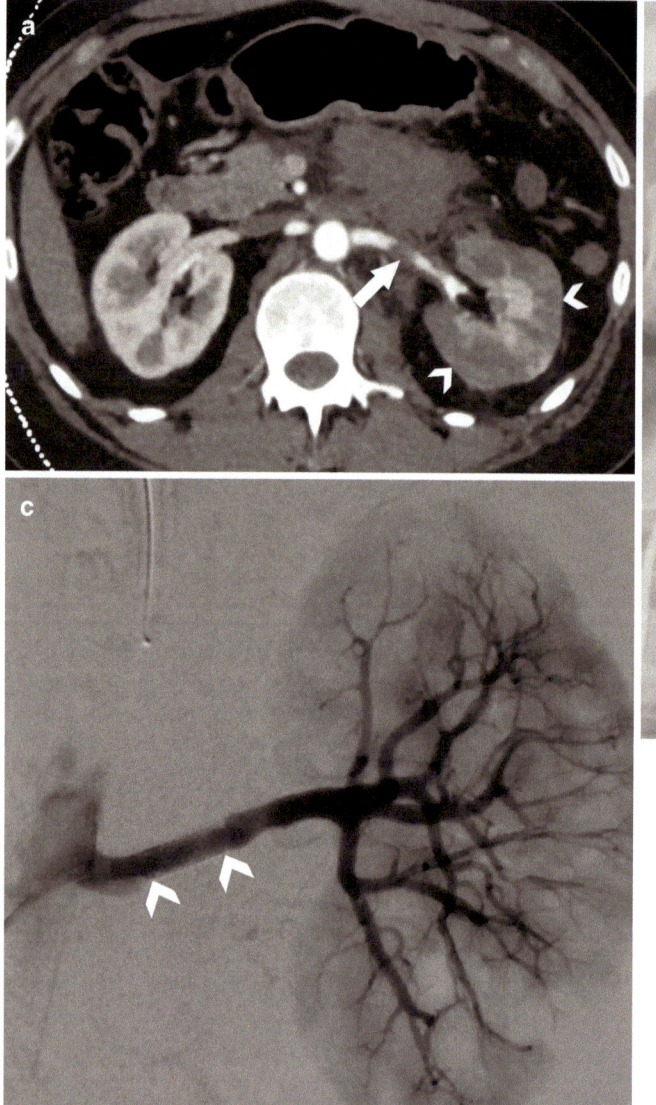

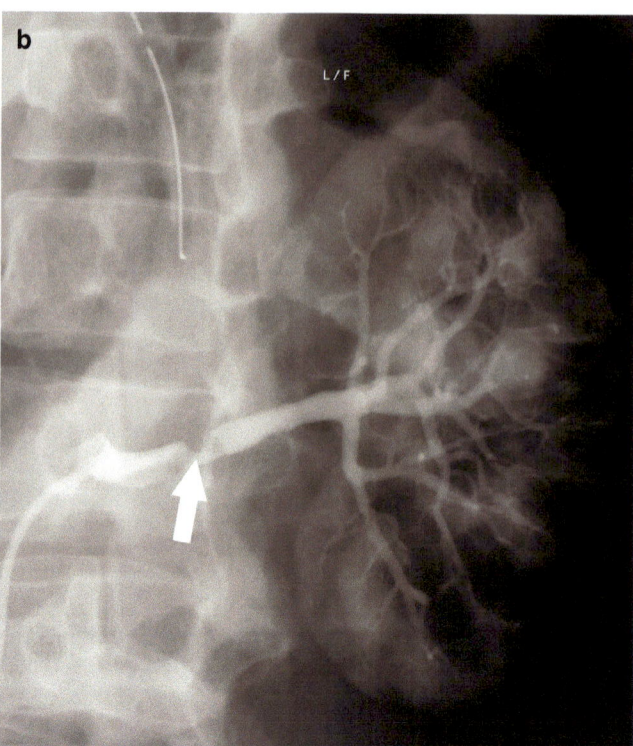

Fig. 1.2 Left renal artery injury (AAST Grade IV). 39 year-old man, admitted after a fall. Contrast enhanced CT, arterial phase (**a**), shows a thrombus occluding the renal artery (arrow) associated with an extended hypoperfusion of the renal cortex (arrowheads). Angiography coronal image (**b**) shows the site of the occlusion and the reperfusion (**c**) after stent placement (arrows)

a vascular beading) of mesenteric vessels, or in the presence of a high density fan-shaped interloop fluid. The two former signs are usually associated with the need for surgery [19].

Diaphragmatic Injuries

Diaphragmatic injuries are quite rare and can often be overlooked at admission CT, especially on the right side, where the sensitivity of CT has been reported as low as 50% (vs 78% on the left). Right-sided diaphragmatic injuries are associated with a worst outcome than the left-sided ones since they are usually encountered at higher trauma forces and associated with major liver laceration. CT signs of diaphragm rupture classically include a disruption of the diaphragm and the herniation of abdominal content into the chest, usually the liver on the right side and various intraperitoneal structures on the left (stomach, bowel, fat, spleen), associated with a cardiomediastinal shift on the contralateral side (Fig. 1.5). A direct contact of these structures on the posterior chest wall is referred to as "the dependent viscera sign." Since many non-traumatic situations may mimic a diaphragmatic injury, such

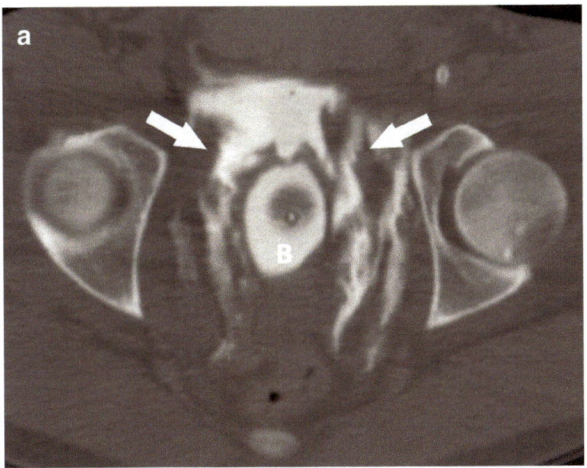
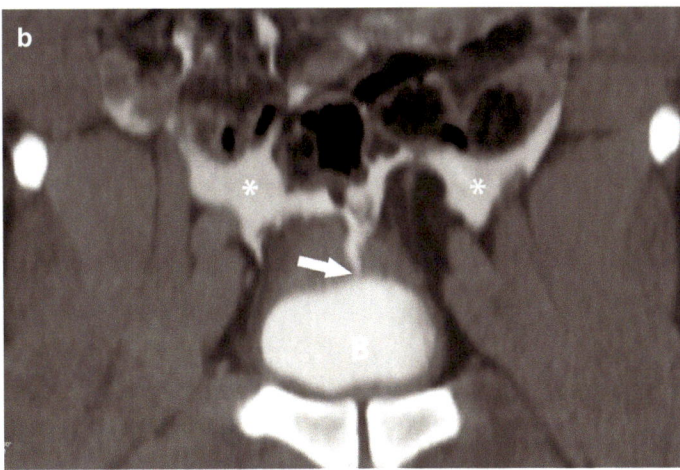

Fig. 1.3 Extraperitoneal and intraperitoneal bladder rupture. (**a**) Axial CT-cystographic image obtained after retrograde instillation of 250 mL of contrast media inside the bladder (**b**) through the urinary catheter, in a patient with pelvic fracture (not shown). Contrast media is spilling along the extraperitoneal lateral borders of the bladder (arrows). **b**)

Delayed coronal image reformation obtained 10 min after completion of a contrast-enhanced abdominal CT in another patient shows a leak of contrast media from the dome of the bladder (arrow) spreading into the intraperitoneal spaces (stars)

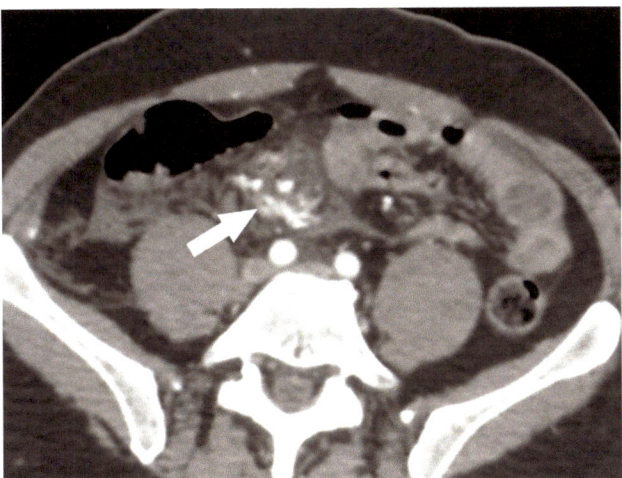

Fig. 1.4 AAST Grade V mesenteric injury. A 43-year-old man admitted after a motor vehicle collision. Contrast enhanced axial CT image (arterial phase) shows a hematoma in the mesenteric root with extravasation of contrast media from an actively bleeding mesenteric artery (arrow)

as a gastric distention, a phrenic nerve paresis, and a congenital hernia, identification of a constricted area of the ascended structure ("collar sign") will be helpful to assert the diagnosis of a diaphragmatic rupture [20].

Pancreatic Injuries

Due to its protected location in the retroperitoneal space, the pancreas is relatively rarely injured in blunt abdominal trauma. Abdominal CT is the standard diagnostic tool to assess pancreatic injury but is often falsely negative at admission. A progressive elevation of serum amylase and lipase should alert towards a potential pancreatic injury that could have been missed at initial CT and justify a repeat evaluation by CT, 24–48 h after trauma. The 5 grades AAST-pancreatic injury scale is based on the extent of the injury and on the presence and location of a duct injury (Grade III to IV). The involvement of the pancreatic duct is important to be assessed by imaging because of its implication on the patients' management (Fig. 1.6). A distal duct injury (Grade III, to the left of the superior mesenteric artery), when partial, may still be treated by drainage while a proximal duct injury usually requires surgery [21]. Unless CT shows a completely transected pancreas, the integrity of the main pancreatic duct can often not be well demonstrated by this method and must be further investigated by magnetic resonance cholangiopancreatography (MRCP), usually with secretin. Endoscopic retrograde cholangiopancreatography (ERCP) still remains the reference standard diagnostic tool to confirm a pancreatic duct injury; it has been recently recommended for stent placement therapy that might reduce the need for surgical resection [22].

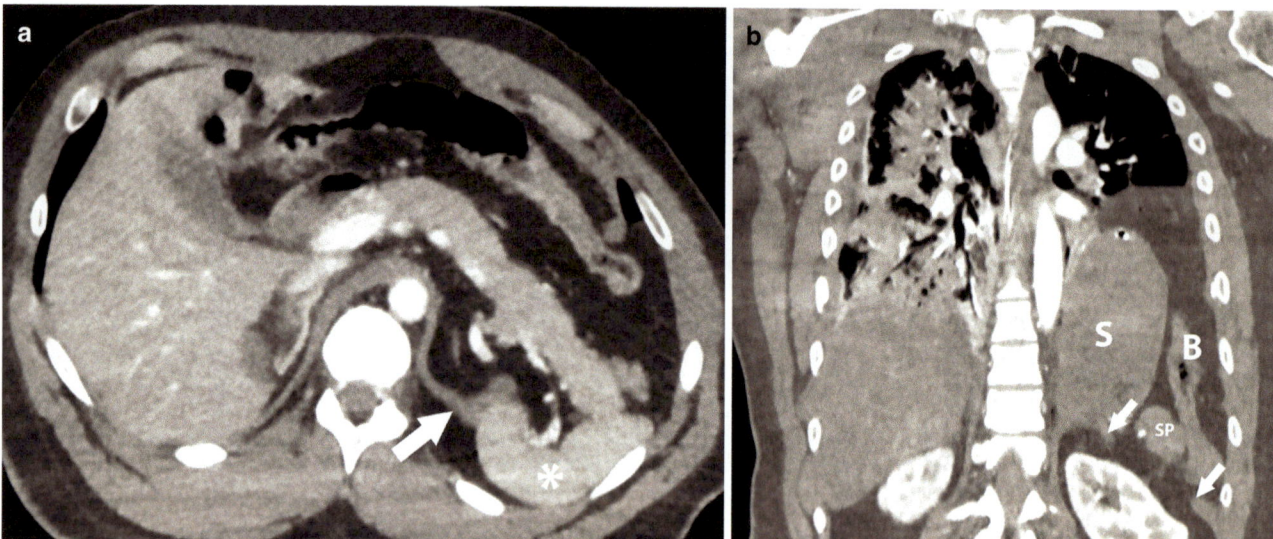

Fig. 1.5 Left hemidiaphragm rupture with organs herniation. A 29-year-old man admitted after a severe motor vehicle collision. Axial contrast-enhanced CT image (**a**) shows a discontinuity and thickening of the left hemidiaphragm (arrow) with a posterior displacement of the spleen (star), abutting the thoracic wall (dependent visceral sign). Coronal reformation image (**b**) shows the herniation of the stomach (S), the large bowel (B), and the spleen (SP), through a large diaphragmatic rent (arrows)

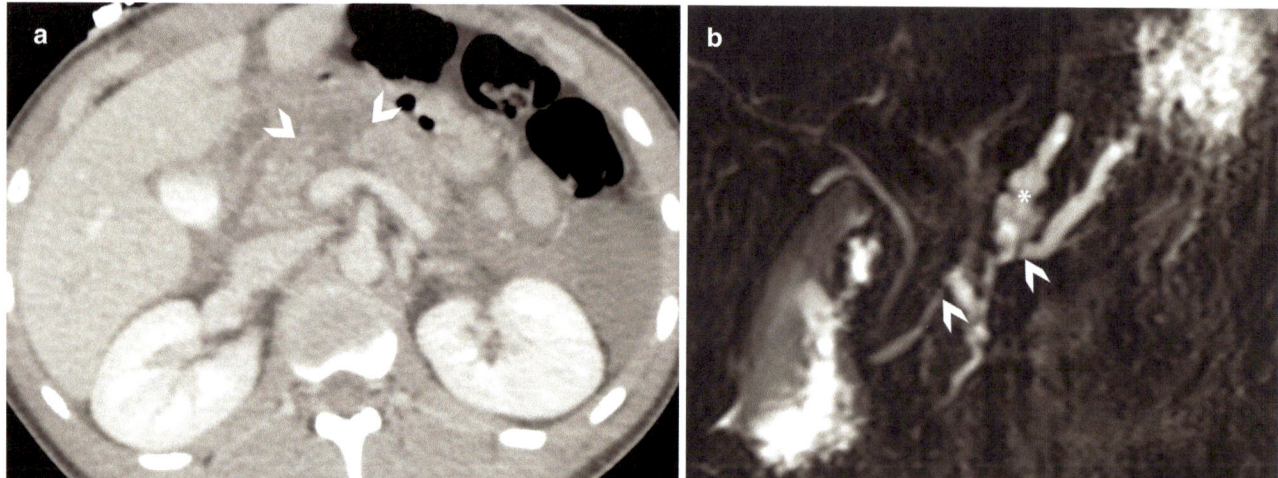

Fig. 1.6 AAST Grade IV pancreatic injury. A 22-year-old man admitted after a motor bike accident. Contrast-enhanced CT axial image (**a**) shows a non-enhancing area through the pancreatic neck (arrowheads). MRI-cholangiopancreatogram (MRCP) coronal oblique image (**b**), performed a couple of days later, shows a complete transection of the main pancreatic duct (arrows), with extravasation of the pancreatic juice (star)

CT is also useful for depiction of post-traumatic complications, especially those associated with undetected pancreatic duct injuries that may be suggested by pseudocysts, duct dilatations, or signs of chronic pancreatitis.

Take-Home Messages
- Knowledge of CT trauma grading systems plays a key role in the management of blunt abdominal trauma patients.
- Depiction of vascular injuries on CT is important for the therapeutic and clinical follow-up of abdominal trauma patients.
- While still limited in the current imaging armamentarium of the emergency radiologist, ultrasound with contrast agents and MRI have a looming role in the follow-up imaging and monitoring of blunt abdominal trauma patients.

1.2 Non-Traumatic Abdominal Pain

Vincent Mellnick

Learning Objectives
- Identify the most common conditions to cause abdominal pain and their imaging appearance, grouped by quadrant.
- Recognize acute conditions of the small and large bowel, including obstruction and ischemia.
- Diagnose gynecologic conditions that may present with acute abdominal or pelvic pain.

Key Points
- Chronic cholecystitis, xanthogranulomatous cholecystitis, and gangrenous cholecystitis may create a diagnostic challenge for interpreting radiologists, demanding knowledge of these entities.
- CT allows for localization of a transition point when the small or large bowel is obstructed. Adhesions and malignancy are the most common cause of obstruction of the small and large bowel, respectively.
- Small bowel ischemia and ischemic colitis are different diseases on the same spectrum and have often disparate causes, imaging appearance, and prognosis.

1.2.1 Modalities

Ultrasound is a useful first line test for right upper quadrant and flank pain as well as for evaluating potential gynecologic sources of abdominal pain. However, it is operator-dependent and may not be available at all centers at all hours of the day.

CT is truly the workhorse modality in the emergency department. Typically, intravenous contrast is indicated, unless clinical suspicion is high for renal colic or if there is a compelling contra-indication to contrast. While often a single, portal venous phase of contrast enhancement is obtained, arterial and venous phases may be acquired if gastrointestinal bleeding or bowel ischemia is suspected clinically. A pre-contrast scan or virtual non-enhanced series may be helpful in this setting as well.

MRI is often precluded in the evaluation of abdominal pain due to the acuity of emergency care, concerns regarding exam length, and potential for limited availability. However, it may play a role in stable patients, including pregnant patients and those with known inflammatory bowel disease.

1.2.2 Right Upper Quadrant

1.2.2.1 Acute Cholecystitis

When a patient presents with right upper quadrant pain, gallbladder pathology—specifically gallstones and/or cholecystitis—are often the first diagnosis considered by both clinicians and radiologists. This diagnosis can be made on multiple modalities, including CT and MRI, but frequently ultrasound is employed as a first line test. Findings of acute cholecystitis include a distended gallbladder, typically with associated sludge and/or stones, surrounding inflammation, and a sonographic Murphy's sign.

The diagnosis of acute cholecystitis may be more difficult in patients with superimposed chronic cholecystitis, in which case the gallbladder may be contracted rather than distended. Gangrenous cholecystitis may present with intramural gas and potentially a lack of Murphy's sign. As it may lead to perforation, an early diagnosis is important and is suggested by the presence of mucosal defects or frank wall discontinuity (Fig. 1.7). Xanthogranulomatous variant of cholecystitis can be difficult to differentiate from gallbladder cancer but is suggested by the presence of lipid-containing spaces in the thickened gallbladder wall [23].

1.2.2.2 Duodenal Ulcers

The most frequent site of peptic ulcer disease is the duodenal bulb, which may project into the hepatic hilum near the gallbladder. Given this proximity, inflammation of the duodenum may be mistaken for acute cholecystitis or cholangitis.

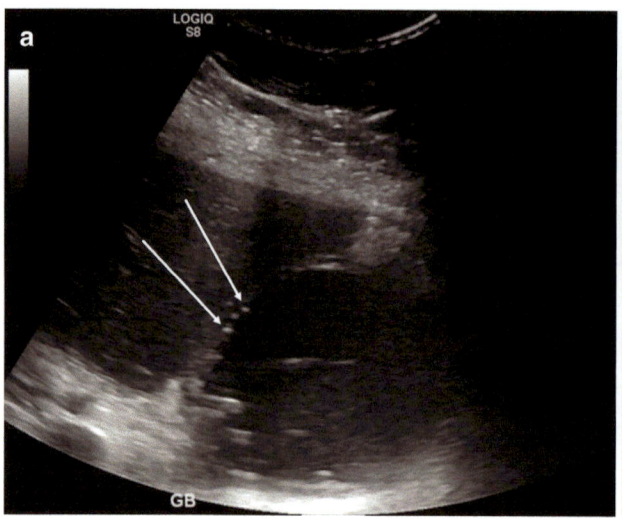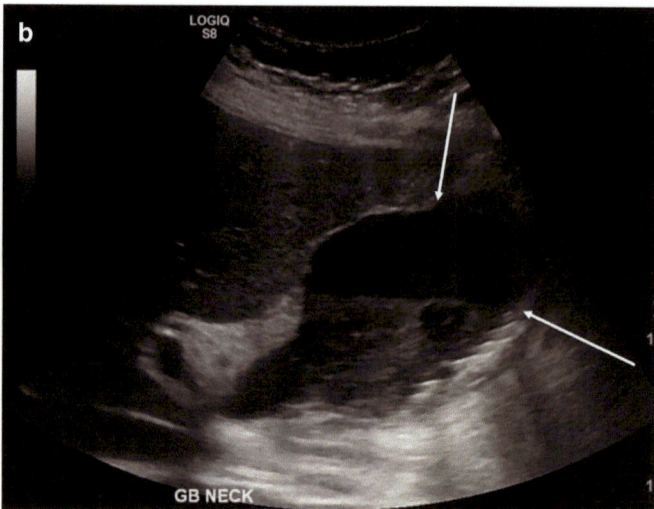

Fig. 1.7 Gangrenous cholecystitis. A 82-year-old man with 2-week history of right upper quadrant pain. Ultrasound images show layering sludge and stones with subtle echogenic reflectors (**a**, arrows) repre-senting intramural gas. There is also a contour abnormality of the gall-bladder fundus with mucosal discontinuity (**b**, arrows), consistent with a walled off perforation

The imaging findings of a peptic ulcer include duodenal wall thickening and adjacent fat stranding with a mucosal defect and outpouching [24]. When the duodenal bulb perforates, free retroperitoneal or intraperitoneal air and paraduodenal fluid may be seen. Chronically, duodenal ulcers may cause strictures and gastric outlet obstruction.

Notably, when peptic ulcers occur distal to the duodenal bulb (post-bulbar), consideration should be given to the possibility of Zollinger-Ellison syndrome, caused by a gastrin-secreting tumor [25]. Crohn disease involving the duodenum may also cause post-bulbar duodenal ulcers. Importantly, perforation of the post-bulbar duodenum typically presents with retroperitoneal gas and/or fluid collections in contrast to the intraperitoneal duodenal bulb.

One diagnosis that may mimic duodenal ulcers is that of groove pancreatitis ("cystic degeneration of the duodenum.") Thought to occur due to inflammation of intramural pancreatic rests, groove pancreatitis typically manifests with inflammation and cysts along the medial wall of the duodenum near its interface with the pancreas [26]. Chronic groove pancreatitis may result in strictures of the duodenum and/or distal common bile duct.

1.2.3 Left Upper Quadrant

1.2.3.1 Acute Pancreatitis

Acute pancreatitis is frequently considered in the patient presenting with left upper quadrant pain. CT is often the initial imaging modality to assess for complications of pancreatitis, including intrapancreatic and peripancreatic necrosis as well as fluid collections. Particularly when evaluating for parenchymal necrosis and vascular complications, intravenous

contrast is useful. MRI may aid in characterizing ductal anatomy and detecting obstructing masses. Potential pitfalls in the diagnosis of acute pancreatitis include atypical cases such as from autoimmune inflammation. These patients present with less severe inflammation, a smooth "sausage" appearance to the pancreas, elevated IgG4 levels, and potentially other autoimmune findings such as nephritis [27]. Ultimately in both typical and autoimmune pancreatitis, imaging follow-up may prove useful in evaluating for an underlying neoplasm.

1.2.3.2 Gastritis

The stomach can become inflamed due to a variety of insults. Common examples include nonsteroidal anti-inflammatory medications, *Helicobacter pylori* infection, and alcohol. Imaging findings include mucosal hyperemia, submucosal edema, and perigastric fat stranding. When determining abnormal thickening of the gastric wall, care must be taken to account for gastric distention. A collapsed stomach may appear to be abnormally thick, particularly the gastric antrum which has a more muscular wall and is more peristaltic than other portions of the stomach. Similar to the duodenum, inflammation may be accompanied by ulcers, manifesting a focal outpouching, potentially with signs of perforation and/or bleeding (Fig. 1.8).

1.2.4 Right Lower Quadrant Pain

1.2.4.1 Acute Appendicitis

Acute appendicitis is the most common cause of a surgical emergency in the right lower quadrant. Imaging has substantially decreased negative appendectomy rates and is performed with CT in many settings. However, ultrasound and/or MRI may be used in young or pregnant patients to avoid exposure to ionizing radiation. Findings on all three modalities include a dilated, fluid-filled appendix more than 6 mm in diameter with surrounding inflammation. In addition to providing a diagnosis of acute appendicitis, imaging can also stratify patients into non-operative management and identify complications. For instance, gangrenous appendicitis may present with decreased mucosal enhancement, intramural gas, and/or perforation. While most cases of appendicitis are caused by obstructing appendicoliths, appendicitis may occasionally be caused by tumors of the appendix or cecal base [28].

1.2.4.2 Cecal Inflammation

Right-sided diverticula are more common in young patients and, when inflamed, may clinically mimic acute appendicitis. Cecal diverticulitis may also be confused for appendicitis on imaging as well, manifesting with a blind-ending structure with inflammation arising from the base of the cecum [29]. However, careful localization of a normal, typically longer appendix separate from the more rounded diverticulum is key to making this diagnosis and guiding the patient to what is often non-operative treatment. Other causes of primary cecal inflammation includes epiploic appendagitis. Although more often seen in the left colon, an inflamed oval, fat-containing mass along the surface of the cecum should suggest this diagnosis. In neutropenic patients, focal colitis ("neutropenic colitis" or "typhlitis") can also present with localized inflammation in the right lower quadrant (Fig. 1.9). The clinical context and nondilated appendix may are important clues to this diagnosis.

1.2.4.3 Terminal Ileitis

The terminal ileum may become inflamed and clinically present similarly to acute appendicitis, often in the setting of Crohn disease. In this case, the inflammation usually manifests with asymmetric, nodular wall thickening with surrounding fat-stranding, potentially complicated by obstruction and/or penetrating disease. MRI may demonstrate increased T2 signal and diffusion restriction of the bowel wall in the acute phase. In addition to inflammatory bowel disease, the ileum may be inflamed due to infection, classically described with tuberculosis, Salmonella, and Yersinia species.

The terminal ileum may also become inflamed due to diverticulitis. This may occur due to acquired diverticula or Meckel diverticula, either of which may be a source of acute abdominal pain (Fig. 1.10). The key to this diagnosis is identifying a focal outpouching from the terminal ileum separate from the appendix surrounded by inflammation. Meckel diverticula may also present with intussusception, gastrointestinal bleeding, and volvulus of the small bowel [30].

1.2.5 Left Lower Quadrant Pain

1.2.5.1 Sigmoid Diverticulitis

Descending and/or sigmoid colon diverticulitis is one of most common causes of left lower quadrant abdominal pain. It manifests on imaging with an inflamed, rounded outpouching extending from the colon and may be complicated by bowel perforation and subsequent abscess formation. Chronically, fistulae may form from the colon to the adjacent bladder or other structures. Sometimes acute diverticulitis

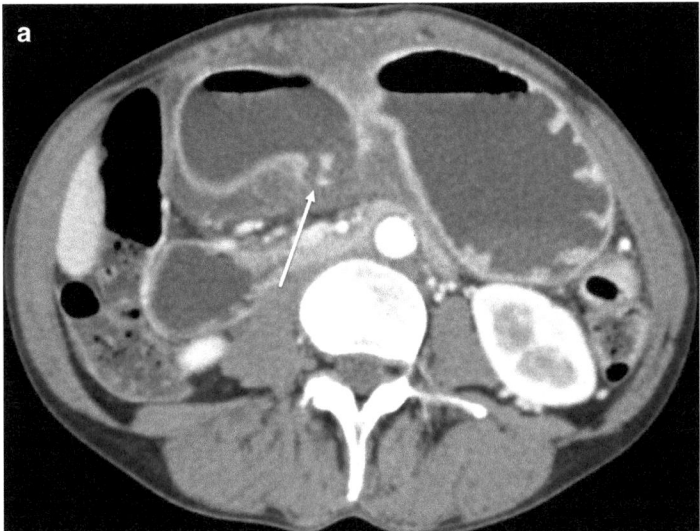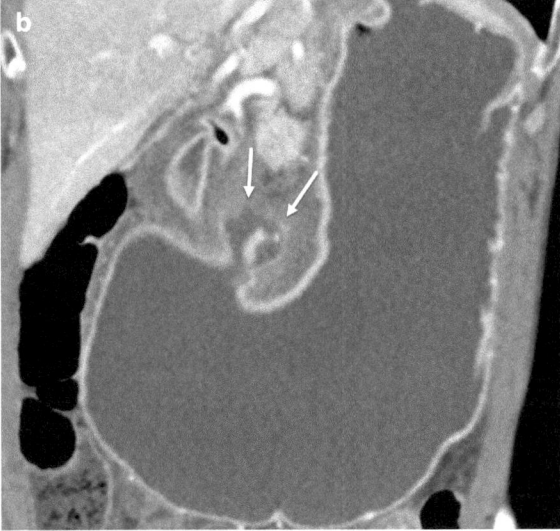

Fig. 1.8 Gastric ulcer. A 56-year-old man with epigastric pain and hematemesis. Axial (**a**) and coronal (**b**) CT images show a large outpouching from the posterior lesser curvature with surrounding wall thickening, consistent with a peptic ulcer. Note the high attenuation material in the ulcer crater (arrows). This active bleeding was confirmed endoscopically

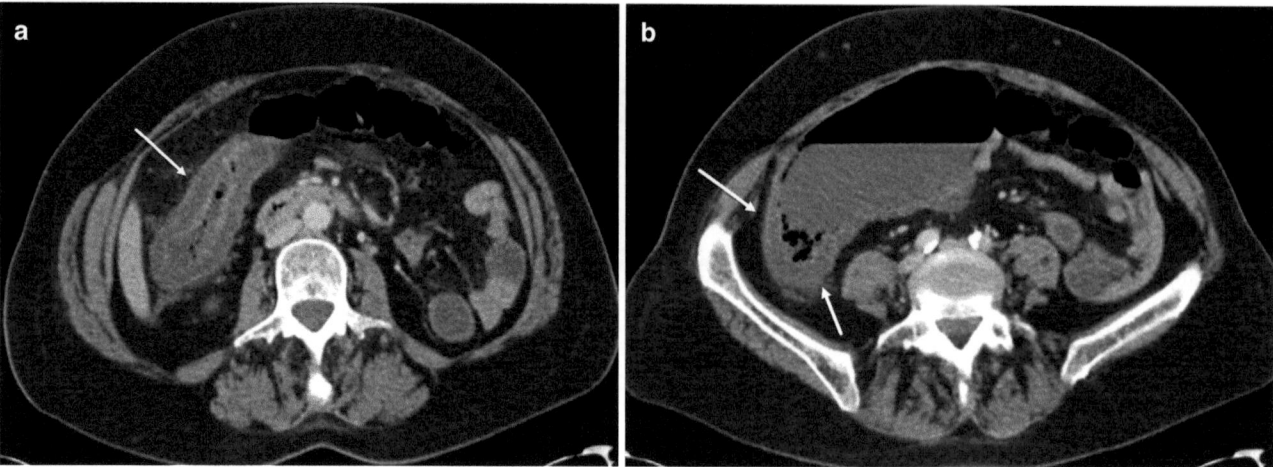

Fig. 1.9 Neutropenic colitis. A 32-year-old woman with leukemia and neutropenia after bone marrow transplant. Axial CT Images demonstrate wall thickening isolated to the proximal colon (**a**, **b**, arrows), a typical distribution for neutropenic colitis. The patient was managed conservatively with antibiotics

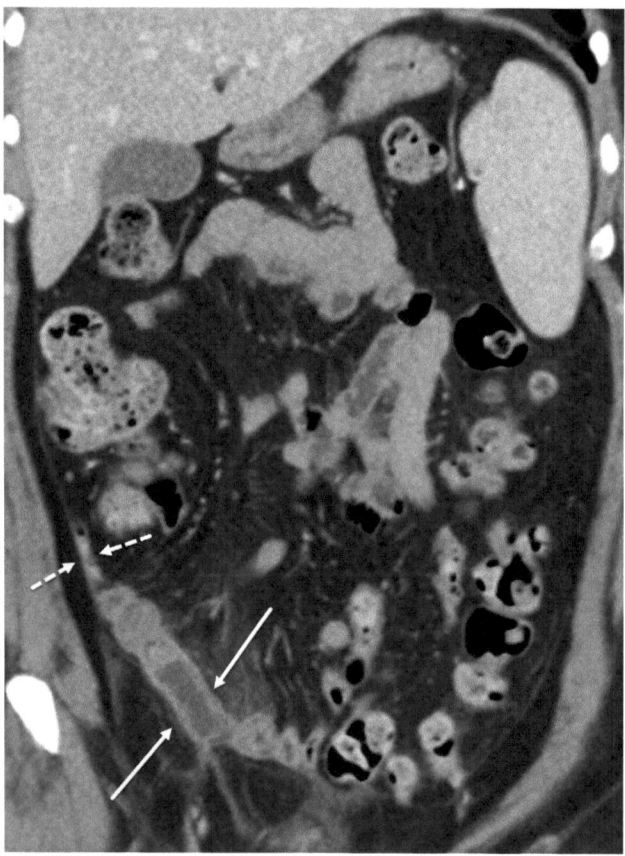

Fig. 1.10 Meckel diverticulitis. 28-year-old man with suspected appendicitis. Coronal CT image shows a thickened, inflamed terminal ileum, centered around a blind-ending structure in the right lower quadrant (arrows). This is separate from the normal appendix (dotted arrows) and was found to be a Meckel diverticulitis at surgery

can appear mass-like and may be difficult to differentiate from malignancy. In such cases, the presence of lymphadenopathy is a feature more commonly seen in adenocarcinoma, whereas the presence of diverticula in the affected segment more strongly suggests diverticulitis [31]. Chronically, sigmoid diverticulitis results in muscular hypertrophy and potentially stenosis of the lumen.

1.2.5.2 Epiploic Appendagitis

Epiploic appendages are small pouches of peritoneal fat arising from subserosa of the colon, largest in size in the sigmoid region. They can be seen on CT primarily when they are surrounded by fluid, or when they become inflamed and/or infarcted after getting torsed resulting in epiploic appendagitis. The most common CT finding is small round or oval fat attenuation lesion abutting the colonic wall with surrounding inflammation. A central area of high attenuation is commonly seen representing a centrally thrombosed vessel.

1.2.5.3 Pelvic Pain: Endometriosis

Endometriosis is an important cause of infertility and chronic pelvic pain. In addition to the ovaries, endometrial implants can involve the sigmoid colon, rectum, and cul-de-sac and therefore cause left lower quadrant and pelvic pain. These implants can be complicated by bleeding, inflammation, and eventually fibrosis and adhesions [32]. The classic sonographic appearance of an endometrioma is a homogenous, hypoechoic lesion with thin walls and posterior acoustic enhancement demonstrating low-level internal echoes and no internal blood flow. MRI is very useful in detecting small implants. Endometriomas appear T1 hyperintense with corresponding low signal on

T2-weighted imaging, referred to as "T2 shading." However, CT may simply demonstrate inflammation surrounding a mass or ill-defined area of bowel wall thickening.

1.2.5.4 Ovarian Torsion

Ovarian torsion typically occurs in younger patients, commonly—although not necessarily—in the setting of an underlying mass. Imaging signs of a torsed ovary include ovarian enlargement, peripheralized follicles, a twisted ovarian vascular pedicle, deviation of the uterus towards the side of the torsion and surrounding inflammation. Ultrasound may show reduced or absent Doppler signal within a torsed ovary [33]. However, incomplete or intermittent torsion may result in a false-negative Doppler exam.

1.2.6   Diffuse Abdominal Pain

1.2.6.1 Small Bowel Obstruction

Small bowel obstruction (SBO) is a common cause of hospital admissions for abdominal pain. There are numerous causes of SBO, with adhesions representing the majority of cases. Other causes include inflammatory bowel disease, internal and external hernias, tumors, intussusception, volvulus, and foreign bodies. The classic symptoms for SBO include diffuse abdominal pain, abdominal distention, and vomiting. However, such symptoms and laboratory findings have limited sensitivity and specificity for diagnosing SBO.

Although radiography and fluoroscopic exams may play a role in the diagnosis of SBO, CT has become the mainstay of imaging when this clinical situation is suspected. This allows for identification of dilated (>3 cm) small bowel leading to a transition point for the obstruction and potentially an underlying cause. Depending on the severity of the obstruction, there may be abrupt decompression after the transition point. In addition, CT allows for identification of patients with complications or who are at risk for them. One such example is patients with closed loop obstruction, in which both the inlet and outlet of an obstructed bowel segment are compressed, often by a single source, like an adhesion or hernia neck [34] (Fig. 1.11).

Ischemia complicating small bowel obstruction may manifest with nonspecific findings including bowel wall and mesenteric edema. Decreased bowel wall enhancement and intramural hemorrhage are more specific findings for ischemia in the setting of SBO. Extraluminal gas and/or well-defined fluid collections can be seen with perforation complicating SBO [35].

1.2.6.2 Colonic Obstruction

In contrast to SBO, colonic tumors are the most common cause of large bowel obstruction [36] (Fig. 1.12). Obstructing colon cancers are more common on the left than on the right, likely due to the progressively narrower lumen distally.

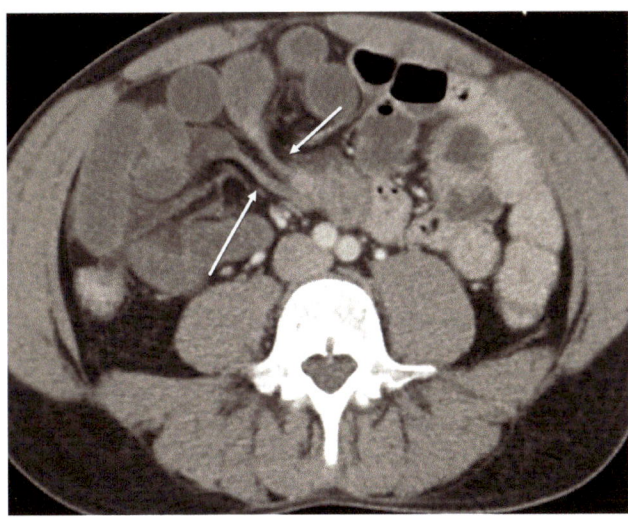

Fig. 1.11 Closed loop small bowel obstruction. A 43-year-old woman with abdominal pain and vomiting. Axial CT demonstrates clustered, dilated loops of small bowel in the right upper quadrant. The inlet and outlet of the obstruction occur at the same point (arrows), a configuration concerning for closed-loop obstruction. An adhesion was the underlying cause

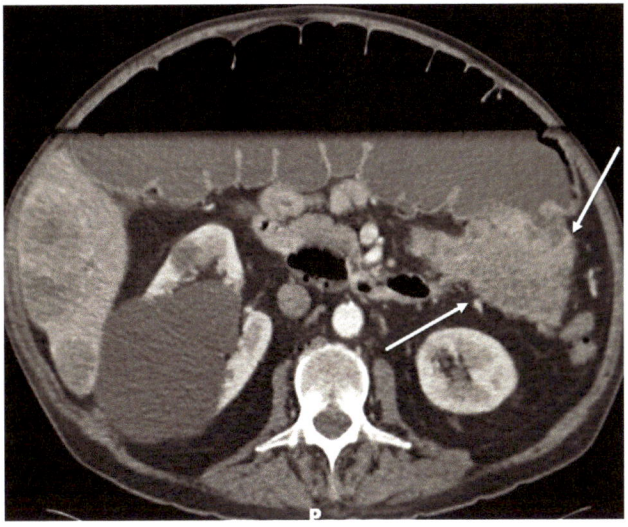

Fig. 1.12 Large bowel obstruction due to colon cancer. A 60-year-old man with abdominal distention. Axial CT shows a soft tissue mass at the splenic flexure (arrows) causing marked dilatation of the transverse colon. The patient underwent colonic stent placement, confirming an obstructing adenocarcinoma. Note metastases in the inferior right liver

Although most commonly seen with primary colonic adenocarcinoma, direct invasion from another primary tumor or extrinsic metastatic involvement of the colon may also result in intestinal obstruction. On CT, obstructing colon tumors result a mass with soft tissue attenuation in the submucosa as well as other evidence of malignancy, including lymphadenopathy and metastases.

After malignancy, colonic volvulus is the second most common cause of colonic obstruction. This most commonly occurs in the cecum and sigmoid colon. Cecal volvulus results from increased mobility and twisting of the proximal ascending colon. In addition to twisting of the proximal colon, cecal obstruction can also result from anterior folding of the cecum relative to the ascending colon, the so-called cecal bascule.

Closed loop obstruction of the sigmoid classically occurs in elderly patients, and often those who are chronically debilitated and constipated. The most common site of colonic volvulus, sigmoid volvulus may be a chronic process of twisting and untwisting, resulting in an indolent presentation. Similar to cecal volvulus, CT may demonstrate the colonic closed loop obstruction with a twist or "whirl" sign in the sigmoid mesentery. As in volvulus of any segment of the bowel, prompt decompression—either endoscopic or surgical—is the mainstay of treatment [37].

1.2.6.3 Acute Mesenteric Ischemia

Acute mesenteric ischemia (AMI) is a rare but deadly disease process. The surgical literature states that arterial thromboembolic causes are most common, followed by nonocclusive and venous causes. However, the incidence of nonocclusive ischemia is likely underestimated. Clinical symptoms of AMI are nonspecific. Classically, the patient presents with sudden onset of severe abdominal pain out of proportion to the clinical exam. Elevated lactate and d-dimer levels can be seen but are nonspecific for AMI.

CT angiography with IV contrast is the recommended test of choice in adults with suspected acute mesenteric ischemia. However, many patients will be imaged with routine portal venous phase imaging because the diagnosis was not suspected clinically. MR angiography has high sensitivity and specificity for diagnosing AMI but is typically not used in the emergency setting due to availability and length of exam. Therefore, it is best reserved for patients with iodinated contrast allergies.

Classic and specific imaging findings for occlusive AMI include a filling defect in the mesenteric arteries, with associated hypoenhancing or non-enhancing bowel wall (Fig. 1.13). Gas within the small bowel—pneumatosis intestinalis—may be seen with other conditions but may be an ominous sign of bowel infarction. Other, more nonspecific, findings include mesenteric congestion, ascites, and bowel wall thickening. These findings are more commonly seen with venous ischemia and/or reperfusion [38].

In contrast to small bowel ischemia, ischemic colitis is often caused by relatively mild episodes of hypotension. It is commonly self-limited but can manifest with full-thickness necrosis and peritonitis. While classically described in

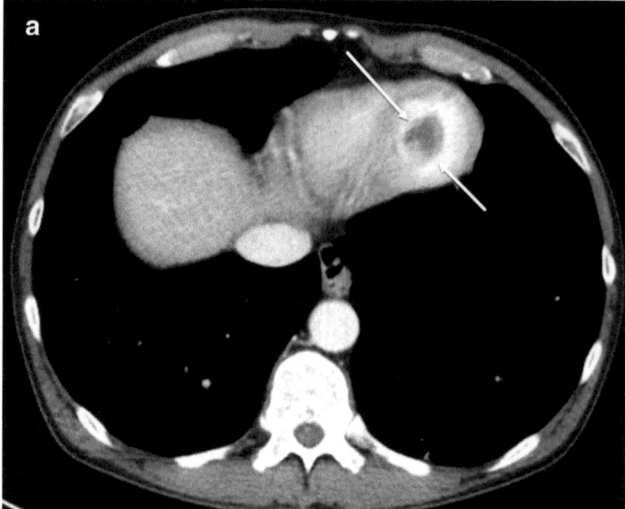

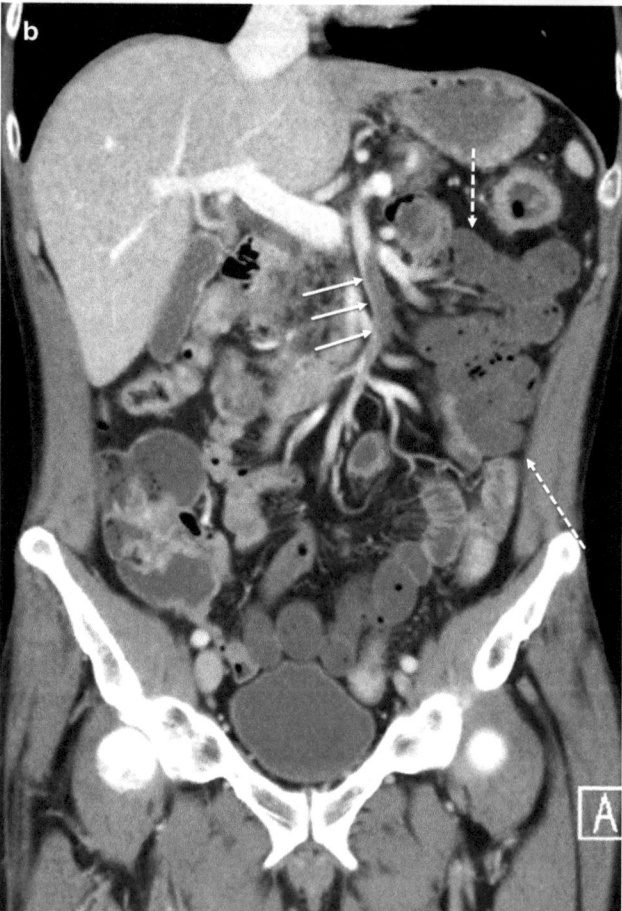

Fig. 1.13 Embolic small bowel ischemia. A 48 year-old woman with abdominal pain, elevated lactate. Axial CT shows a filling defect in the left ventricle (**a**, arrows). This has caused an embolism to the superior mesenteric artery (coronal CT **b**, arrows), resulting in small bowel ischemia. Note the hypoenhancing small bowel in the left upper quadrant (**b**, dotted arrows)

anatomic "water-shed" areas between major vascular beds, ischemic colitis can affect any portion of the colon. On imaging, ischemic colitis usually presents with wall thickening in more mild cases [39]. More severe cases can present with hypoenhancement, ileus, and pneumatosis.

> **Take-Home Messages**
> - While cholecystitis is a common reason for right upper quadrant pain, consider alternative causes of inflammation in this location, including peptic ulcers and cholangitis.
> - Cecal diverticulitis and inflammation of the terminal ileum may mimic acute appendicitis, both clinically and radiologically.
> - Bowel ischemia may have a variety of appearances, depending on the cause, severity, and chronicity.

1.2.7 Concluding Remarks

Imaging is a mainstay in the emergency department, both in trauma and non-trauma settings. CT is often the workhorse modality in both situations, but ultrasound and MRI are useful in select clinical presentations and patient populations. Emergency and general radiologists should have familiarity with CT signs of hollow viscous and solid organ injuries and grade them to help guide clinical management. Likewise, radiologists should know common conditions—and their mimics—that occur in each quadrant of the abdomen as well as conditions that can appear in multiple locations.

References

1. Holmes JF, Wisner DH, McGahan JP, Mower WR, Kuppermann N. Clinical prediction rules for identifying adults at very low risk for intra-abdominal injuries after blunt trauma. Ann Emerg Med. 2009;54(4):575–84.
2. Kortbeek JB, Al Turki SA, Ali J, Antoine JA, Bouillon B, Brasel K, et al. Advanced trauma life support, 8th edition, the evidence for change. J Trauma. 2008;64(6):1638–50.
3. Poletti PA, Mirvis SE, Shanmuganathan K, Takada T, Killeen KL, Perlmutter D, et al. Blunt abdominal trauma patients: can organ injury be excluded without performing computed tomography? J Trauma. 2004;57(5):1072–81.
4. Shanmuganathan K, Mirvis SE, Sherbourne CD, Chiu WC, Rodriguez A. Hemoperitoneum as the sole indicator of abdominal visceral injuries: a potential limitation of screening abdominal US for trauma. Radiology. 1999;212(2):423–30.
5. Boscak AR, Shanmuganathan K, Mirvis SE, Fleiter TR, Miller LA, Sliker CW, et al. Optimizing trauma multidetector CT protocol for blunt splenic injury: need for arterial and portal venous phase scans. Radiology. 2013;268(1):79–88.
6. Hamilton JD, Kumaravel M, Censullo ML, Cohen AM, Kievlan DS, West OC. Multidetector CT evaluation of active extravasation in blunt abdominal and pelvic trauma patients. Radiographics. 2008;28(6):1603–16.
7. Poletti PA, Kinkel K, Vermeulen B, Irmay F, Unger PF, Terrier F. Blunt abdominal trauma: should US be used to detect both free fluid and organ injuries? Radiology. 2003;227(1):95–103.
8. Shackford SR, Molin M. Management of splenic injuries. Surg Clin North Am. 1990;70(3):595–620.
9. Gavant ML, Schurr M, Flick PA, Croce MA, Fabian TC, Gold RE. Predicting clinical outcome of nonsurgical management of blunt splenic injury: using CT to reveal abnormalities of splenic vasculature. AJR Am J Roentgenol. 1997;168(1):207–12.
10. Lee JT, Slade E, Uyeda J, Steenburg SD, Chong ST, Tsai R, et al. American Society of Emergency Radiology Multicenter Blunt Splenic Trauma Study: CT and clinical findings. Radiology. 2021;299(1):122–30.
11. Mirvis SE, Whitley NO, Gens DR. Blunt splenic trauma in adults: CT-based classification and correlation with prognosis and treatment. Radiology. 1989;171(1):33–9.
12. Kozar RA, Crandall M, Shanmuganathan K, Zarzaur BL, Coburn M, Cribari C, et al. Organ injury scaling 2018 update: spleen, liver, and kidney. J Trauma Acute Care Surg. 2018;85(6):1119–22.
13. Davis KA, Fabian TC, Croce MA, Gavant ML, Flick PA, Minard G, et al. Improved success in nonoperative management of blunt splenic injuries: embolization of splenic artery pseudoaneurysms. J Trauma. 1998;44(6):1008–13; discussion 13-5.
14. Poletti PA, Becker CD, Arditi D, Terraz S, Buchs N, Shanmuganathan K, et al. Blunt splenic trauma: can contrast enhanced sonography be used for the screening of delayed pseudoaneurysms? Eur J Radiol. 2013;82(11):1846–52.
15. Fang JF, Wong YC, Lin BC, Hsu YP, Chen MF. The CT risk factors for the need of operative treatment in initially hemodynamically stable patients after blunt hepatic trauma. J Trauma 2006;61(3):547–53; discussion 53–4.
16. Poletti PA, Mirvis SE, Shanmuganathan K, Killeen KL, Coldwell D. CT criteria for management of blunt liver trauma: correlation with angiographic and surgical findings. Radiology. 2000;216(2):418–27.
17. Gross JA, Lehnert BE, Linnau KF, Voelzke BB, Sandstrom CK. Imaging of urinary system trauma. Radiol Clin N Am. 2015;53(4):773–88. ix
18. Tominaga GT, Crandall M, Cribari C, Zarzaur BL, Bernstein M, Kozar RA, et al. Organ injury scaling 2020 update: bowel and mesentery. J Trauma Acute Care Surg. 2021;91(3):e73-e7.
19. Alabousi M, Mellnick VM, Kashef Al-Ghetaa R, Patlas MN. Imaging of blunt bowel and mesenteric injuries: current status. Eur J Radiol. 2020;125:108894.
20. Killeen KL, Mirvis SE, Shanmuganathan K. Helical CT of diaphragmatic rupture caused by blunt trauma. AJR Am J Roentgenol. 1999;173(6):1611–6.
21. Lin BC, Hwang TL. Resection versus drainage in the management of patients with AAST-OIS grade IV blunt pancreatic injury: a single trauma Centre experience. Injury. 2022;53(1):129–36.
22. Biffl WL, Ball CG, Moore EE, Lees J, Todd SR, Wydo S, et al. Don't mess with the pancreas! A multicenter analysis of the management of low-grade pancreatic injuries. J Trauma Acute Care Surg. 2021;91(5):820–8.
23. O'Connor OJ, Maher MM. Imaging of cholecystitis. Am J Roentgenol. 2011;196(4):W367–W74.
24. Tonolini M, Ierardi AM, Bracchi E, Magistrelli P, Vella A, Carrafiello G. Non-perforated peptic ulcer disease: multidetector CT findings, complications, and differential diagnosis. Insights Imaging. 2017;8(5):455–69.
25. Davila A, Menias CO, Alhalabi K, Lall C, Pickhardt PJ, Lubner M, et al. Multiple endocrine neoplasia: spectrum of abdominal manifestations. AJR Am J Roentgenol. 2020;215(4):885–95.

26. Kim DU, Lubner MG, Mellnick VM, Joshi G, Pickhardt PJ. Heterotopic pancreatic rests: imaging features, complications, and unifying concepts. Abdom Radiol (NY). 2017;42(1):216–25.

27. Vlachou PA, Khalili K, Jang HJ, Fischer S, Hirschfield GM, Kim TK. IgG4-related sclerosing disease: autoimmune pancreatitis and extrapancreatic manifestations. Radiographics. 2011;31(5):1379–402.

28. Shademan A, Tappouni RF. Pitfalls in CT diagnosis of appendicitis: pictorial essay. J Med Imaging Radiat Oncol. 2013;57(3):329–36.

29. Pooler BD, Lawrence EM, Pickhardt PJ. Alternative diagnoses to suspected appendicitis at CT. Radiology. 2012;265(3):733–42.

30. Rossi P, Gourtsoyiannis N, Bezzi M, Raptopoulos V, Massa R, Capanna G, et al. Meckel's diverticulum: imaging diagnosis. AJR Am J Roentgenol. 1996;166(3):567–73.

31. Gryspeerdt S, Lefere P. Chronic diverticulitis vs. colorectal cancer: findings on CT colonography. Abdom Imaging. 2012;37(6):1101–9.

32. Mason BR, Chatterjee D, Menias CO, Thaker PH, Siegel CL, Yano M. Encyclopedia of endometriosis: a pictorial rad-path review. Abdom Radiol (NY). 2020;45(6):1587–607.

33. Dawood MT, Naik M, Bharwani N, Sudderuddin SA, Rockall AG, Stewart VR. Adnexal torsion: review of radiologic appearances. Radiographics. 2021;41(2):609–24.

34. Elsayes KM, Menias CO, Smullen TL, Platt JF. Closed-loop small-bowel obstruction: diagnostic patterns by multidetector computed tomography. J Comput Assist Tomogr. 2007;31(5):697–701.

35. Scaglione M, Galluzzo M, Santucci D, Trinci M, Messina L, Laccetti E, et al. Small bowel obstruction and intestinal ischemia: emphasizing the role of MDCT in the management decision process. Abdom Radiol (NY). 2022;47(5):1541–55.

36. Verheyden C, Orliac C, Millet I, Taourel P. Large-bowel obstruction: CT findings, pitfalls, tips and tricks. Eur J Radiol. 2020;130:109155.

37. Wortman JR, Dhyani M, Ali SM, Scholz FJ. Pearls and pitfalls in multimodality imaging of colonic volvulus. Radiographics. 2020;40(4):1039–40.

38. Srisajjakul S, Prapaisilp P, Bangchokdee S. Comprehensive review of acute small bowel ischemia: CT imaging findings, pearls, and pitfalls. Emerg Radiol. 2022;29(3):531–44.

39. Taourel P, Aufort S, Merigeaud S, Doyon FC, Hoquet MD, Delabrousse E. Imaging of ischemic colitis. Radiol Clin N Am. 2008;46(5):909–24. vi

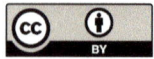

Imaging Infectious Disease of the Abdomen (Including COVID-19)

2

Rubal Rai, Ramandeep Singh, Peter F. Hahn, Avinash Kambadakone, and Richard M. Gore

Learning Objectives
- To understand the imaging spectrum of different types of infections and their potential mimics in the abdomen and pelvis.
- To understand differentiating features of abdominal infections with imaging in various organs in the abdomen and pelvis taking into consideration relevant clinical background information and the main risk factors.

2.1 Introduction

Intra-abdominal infections are the second leading cause of death in critical care settings with the incidence in the USA estimated to be 3.5 million cases per year [1]. In both developing and developed countries with a myriad of etiologies, abdominal infections pose a high risk of morbidity and mortality. Impairments to the immune system, potentially lead to higher rates and impact long-term outcomes in predisposing conditions such as malignancy or immunocompromise [2–4]. Predisposing host factors include barrier disruption, such as skin or mucosa, anatomic obstruction, pre-existing malignancies, immunosuppression including chemotherapy, surgical procedures, interventions, and medical device site infections. The common infectious agents can be categorized into viral including COVID-19, bacterial including gram-negative and positive, acid-fast bacilli, and nosocomial such as clostridium difficile, fungal such as candida, aspergillus, mucor and parasitic such as echinococcus. The organ systems and sites involved with infections include gastrointestinal and genitourinary tracts, hepatobiliary, pancreas, peritoneum, retroperitoneum, and abdominal wall. Based on the organ system involvement diverse imaging modalities can be utilized including plain radiographs, fluoroscopy, ultrasound (US), computed tomography (CT) including dual energy, magnetic resonance imaging (MRI), and molecular imaging techniques such as positron emission tomography (PET). Distinct imaging features about the site and etiology of infection can help clinch early diagnosis and improve patient outcomes. The purpose of this chapter is to discuss the underlying risk factors and mechanisms of infections and to present the variety of imaging manifestations of abdominal and pelvic infections.

2.2 Risk Factors for Infections

Abdominal infections can occur de novo or in a setting of numerous risk factors such as barrier disruption, such as skin or mucosa, anatomic obstruction, pre-existing malignancies, tumor burden, immunosuppression including chemotherapy, surgical procedures, interventions, and medical device site infections [5].

2.2.1 Barrier Disruption

The cornerstone defense mechanism for the body against infections includes the skin and mucosal surfaces. The destruction of these barriers by predisposing conditions such as trauma, catheter placement, vascular compromise, malignancy, radiation therapy, and chemotherapy [6]. The mucosal barrier injury occurs in four phases: inflammation, apoptosis, ulceration, and healing [7].

R. Rai · R. Singh · P. F. Hahn · A. Kambadakone
Department of Radiology, Massachusetts General Hospital, Boston, MA, USA
e-mail: Rsingh17@mgh.harvard.edu; phahn@partners.org; akambadakone@mgh.harvard.edu

R. M. Gore (✉)
Department of Radiology, Northwestern University Feinberg School of Medicine, Evanston, IL, USA

© The Author(s) 2023
J. Hodler et al. (eds.), *Diseases of the Abdomen and Pelvis 2023-2026*, IDKD Springer Series,
https://doi.org/10.1007/978-3-031-27355-1_2

2.2.2 Anatomic Obstruction

The presence of anatomic obstructions such as gastrointestinal, hepatobiliary, and urinary tracts can be a predisposing factor for post-obstructive infections. Small or large bowel obstruction which can be due to adhesions, strictures, or tumors can be challenging to clinically manage as it can contribute to bowel ischemia, perforation, fistulas, peritonitis, and abdominopelvic abscesses, typically polymicrobial. Hepatobiliary obstruction can result in recurrent cholangitis and hepatic abscesses. Urinary tract obstruction may cause hydronephrosis which can progress to complicated pyelonephritis, and renal and prostatic abscesses [5].

2.2.3 Vascular Compromise

Vascular occlusion can lead to poor circulation and thereby ischemia and infarction which facilitates infection in an organ. Decrease in arterial flow from iatrogenic, thrombus, or malignant causes while venous compromise can from direct tumor extension or mass effect result in complications such as bowel perforation and abscess formation [8].

2.2.4 Pre-existing Malignancy

While solid organ malignancies such as carcinoma and sarcoma commonly lead to disruption of natural barriers and obstruction, hematological malignancies, such as lymphoma, acute myeloid leukemia, and chronic lymphocytic leukemia can cause severe prolonged immunosuppression and neutropenia in addition to barrier disruption, thereby predisposing to infections.

2.2.5 Immunosuppression

Chemotherapy and marrow infiltration-induced immunosuppression causes febrile neutropenia with an absolute neutrophil count <of 1500 cells per mm^3 (severe neutropenia <500 cells per mm^3)[9]. This clinical condition can lead to polymicrobial bacterial infections commonly enteric Gram-negative bacteria, *Staphylococcus aureus*, and clostridium [3, 10, 11]. Additionally, viral infections and invasive fungal infections, such as candida and aspergillus, can occur[12, 13]. Imaging features of these infections can help detect and manage any potential complications.

2.2.6 Prior Radiation

Acute radiation leads to inflammation and mucosal barrier injury depending upon the dose and the field of radiation, thereby causing the entry of infectious pathogens into the body and bloodstream [14]. The most common manifestations of acute radiation injury include mucositis, esophagitis, and esophageal dysmotility, colitis, and anorectal complications. Chronic radiation can lead to fibrosis with stricture or fistula formation causing obstruction, stasis, and viscus perforation, superinfection, and abscess formation [14, 15]. Another potential mechanism of chronic radiation-induced injury that may predispose to infection is vascular sclerosis leading to tissue hypoperfusion. Some of the radiation-induced changes such as small bowel wall thickening and mucosal hyperenhancement, and luminal narrowing [15].

2.2.7 Medical Devices

Medical devices including drainage and peritoneal dialysis catheters, vascular access catheters, stents, and shunts can not only be the vehicle for introducing infectious pathogens such as skin-colonizing staphylococci but can also complicate the management [16]. Superficial infections can spread along the skin or abdominal wall muscles and cause peritonitis and abdominopelvic abscesses. While biliary stents can lead to cholangitis and recurrent obstruction, ureteric stents and percutaneous nephrostomy tubes can cause acute and chronic pyelonephritis and bacteremia [17, 18]. Timely diagnosis with multimodality imaging can help in surveillance of these infections and prevention of complications.

2.2.8 Surgery

The global incidence of surgical site infections is 11 % [19]. These can be minor such as surgical wound infections or major such as anastomotic bowel and biliary leaks which may need additional surgical interventions. Presence of adhesions, obstruction, leaks, and fistula can predispose to surgical site infection. Imaging can help identify, characterize, and manage these complications.

2.3 Imaging in Abdominal Infections

Imaging plays an essential role in evaluating infections within the abdomen and pelvis and can facilitate early detection and management, thus truly adding value to patient care with potential to improve outcomes. Although abdominal radiographs have been largely replaced by cross-sectional imaging, they play an important role for the surveillance of bowel obstruction and pneumoperitoneum and to evaluate implanted devices and catheters [20]. Ultrasound is additional imaging modality which can be used as bed side technique to assess hepatobiliary, genitourinary, and gynecologic infections and related pathologies. For assessment of gastrointestinal infectious etiologies, ultrasound is however limited due to the inability of sound to travel through the bowel gas. Other factors limiting usage of this technique include operator dependence, patient compliance, and body habitus. Thereby, for the workup of patients with abdominal infections and for nonspecific complaints such as abdominal pain, fever, or unknown sepsis, contrast-enhanced CT (CECT) has become the diagnostic modality of choice. Recently, dual energy CT (DECT) with material density images and iodine quantification can help detect and evaluate infectious disease processes. MRI is a useful problem-solving tool for better characterization for hepatobiliary or pancreatic infections and to differentiate from infection mimics such as inflammatory or autoimmune etiologies and malignancies [21]. While CT remains the preferred imaging modality, MRI can not only help with the diagnosis of microbial infection but also in the longitudinal tracking of the bacterial infection [22]. For the bacterial and viral infections, MRI can help in detection of local inflammation, edema formation, and tissue characterization such as assessment of water content and diffusivity as manifestation of immune response. While radiation dose accompanying the CT scan, could favor use of MRI in certain clinical circumstances, longer acquisition time and compromised image quality due to motion artifacts, need of longer breath hold and following commands can limit the diagnostic utility of MRI. Radionuclide studies, such as using indium-111 white blood cell scan, are most useful for vascular graft infection, and their larger use have been superseded by cross-sectional imaging[23]. Combination of radionuclide uptake with SPECT/CT can improve localization while FDG PET/CT can both localize and quantitate the degree of infection [24]. White light imaging and linked color imaging endoscopy have been used, for example, in diagnosis of *Helicobacter pylori* infection with high sensitivity and specificity. Functional imaging largely remains a research tool with clinical potential uncertain for diverse infectious conditions.

2.3.1 Gastrointestinal Tract Infections

Gastrointestinal tract immune system is dependent upon a number of components which include gastric acid, bowel flora, and motility apart from the humoral and cell-mediated immune defenses [25]. Disruption of any of these protective mechanisms can ensue an infectious disease process. Compared to immunocompetent individuals, gastrointestinal infections in immunosuppression leads to a high rate of morbidity and mortality. Common pathogens infecting the gastrointestinal tract causing colitis include Gram-negative bacilli such as shigella (*S. dysenteriae, S. flexneri, S. boydii, and S. sonnei*), *Escherichia coli*, *Clostridium difficile*, and Salmonella and viruses such as cytomegalovirus (CMV) [26]. In developing countries, mycobacterial tuberculosis infections are common involving most frequently causing terminal ileitis and cecal colitis, lymphadenopathy, and peritonitis. Imaging manifestations of bacterial infections on CECT and MRI include bowel wall thickening, with enhancement and edema, fat stranding, perforation, abscess, neutropenic enterocolitis, and secondary peritonitis. Accurate diagnosis is based on a combination of clinical history, symptoms, imaging findings, and serological and laboratory tests. The management is most often conservative, and interventions and surgery are reserved for complications such as perforation or bleeding.

Apart from the bowel wall, perirectal and perianal infections can also occur with pre-existing conditions such as cancer and radiation presenting as diarrhea, tenesmus, and hematochezia [27]. Acute proctitis (<6 months) occurs due to mucosal inflammation, and chronic proctitis occurs due to

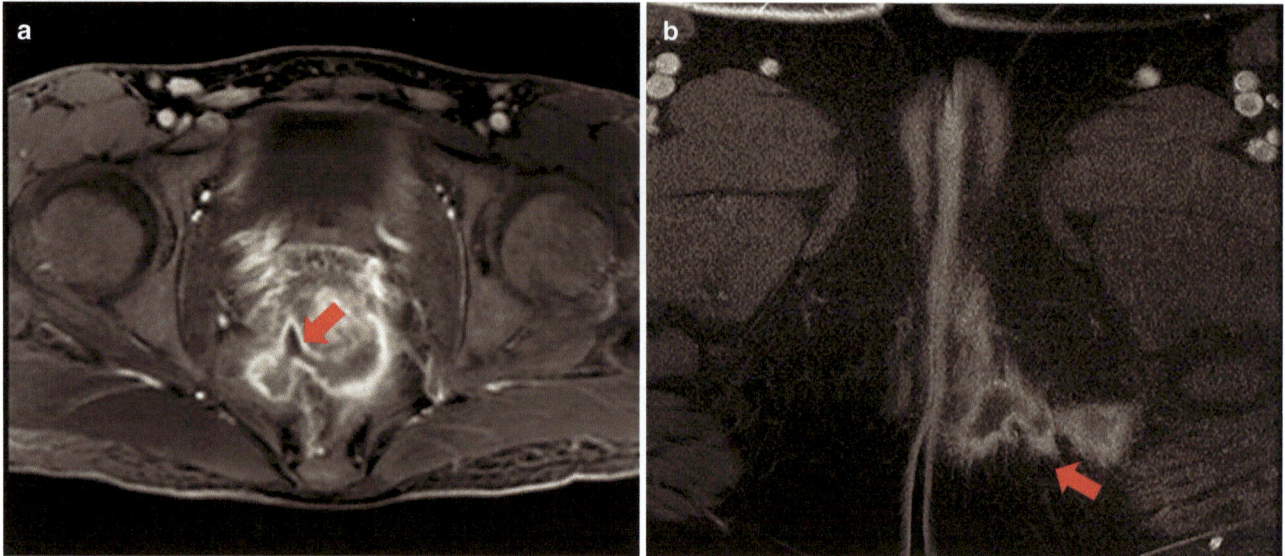

Fig. 2.1 Axial post-gadolinium T1-weighted fat-suppressed image (**a**, **b**) showing perianal abscess (red arrow) in the left ischiorectal fossa extending superiority into the perirectal region in a patient of Crohn's disease. The perianal fistula track is located at 5 o'clock position on the left side

microvascular insufficiency from obliterative endarteritis [28]. The resulting vascular compromise leads to intestinal ischemia, transmural fibrosis and possibly strictures, ulcerations, fistulas, and perforation [28]. CECT demonstrates mural stratification and wall thickening at the radiation site. Fistulas can be better evaluated with fluoroscopy. MRI with high soft-tissue resolution can delineate the extent and degree of sphincter involvement of fistulous tracts and perirectal and perianal abscesses (Fig. 2.1) [29].

2.3.1.1 Clostridioides Difficile Colitis

C. difficile, a Gram-positive anaerobic infection commonly occurs after a few weeks of use of antibiotics that disrupt the normal bowel flora and is most common cause of nosocomial bowel infections (Fig. 2.2) [30]. While often the infection can be mild, it is not infrequent that it can be fulminant leading to hypotension, or ileus to necessitate hospitalization [31]. The severe manifestations of infection include megacolon, perforation, and septicemia, with mortality rates of up to 25% [31] Usually, the infection involves the entire colon and less commonly segmental [30, 31]. CECT features include mucosal ulcers, pseudomembrane, wall thickening, submucosal edema, mucosal hyperenhancement, and pericolic fat stranding, which later evolve to lack of enhancement and sloughing. The transmural edema with wall thickening along with mucosal hyperemia produce the "accordion sign" where the orally administered contrast is trapped between edematous haustral folds [32]. Presence of irregular mucosal with polypoid protrusions can result in wall nodularity and "thumbprinting" on contrast enema and radiographs [32]. Radiologically, if the colonic diameter is more than 6 cm,

toxic megacolon is suspected. The management is usually medical, except for complicated cases where surgery may be required.

2.3.1.2 Neutropenic Enterocolitis

Neutropenic enterocolitis is also called as neutropenic colitis or typhlitis and is a potentially life-threatening complication of chemotherapy, more commonly seen in hematological malignancies such as acute myeloid leukemia and following cytotoxic chemotherapy. The condition occurs in severely neutropenic patients (cell count <500 cells per mm^3) typically in the third week of chemotherapy [33]. The most common site of involvement is cecum and patients often present with right lower quadrant pain [34]. The risk of this condition is increased in the presence of prior inflammation such as diverticulitis, malignancy, and postoperative state [33]. The infection is most commonly polymicrobial although bacterial organisms such as Gram-negative bacilli, Gram-positive cocci, and anaerobes, and fungal pathogens such as candida can also cause the condition [33]. Multipronged approach of clinical, laboratory, and imaging features is critical for diagnosis. CECT is the imaging modality of choice with findings including wall thickening, submucosal edema, mucosal hyperenhancement, fat stranding in the region of cecum and ascending colon with possible terminal ileum involvement (Fig. 2.3). The complications can include perforation, pneumatosis, extraluminal gas, and pericolic fluid [32, 35]. For pediatric population, thickened bowel wall of more than 10 mm on US with clinical and laboratory findings can provide diagnosis [36]. Imaging differentials include cecal diverticulitis and pseudomembranous colitis.

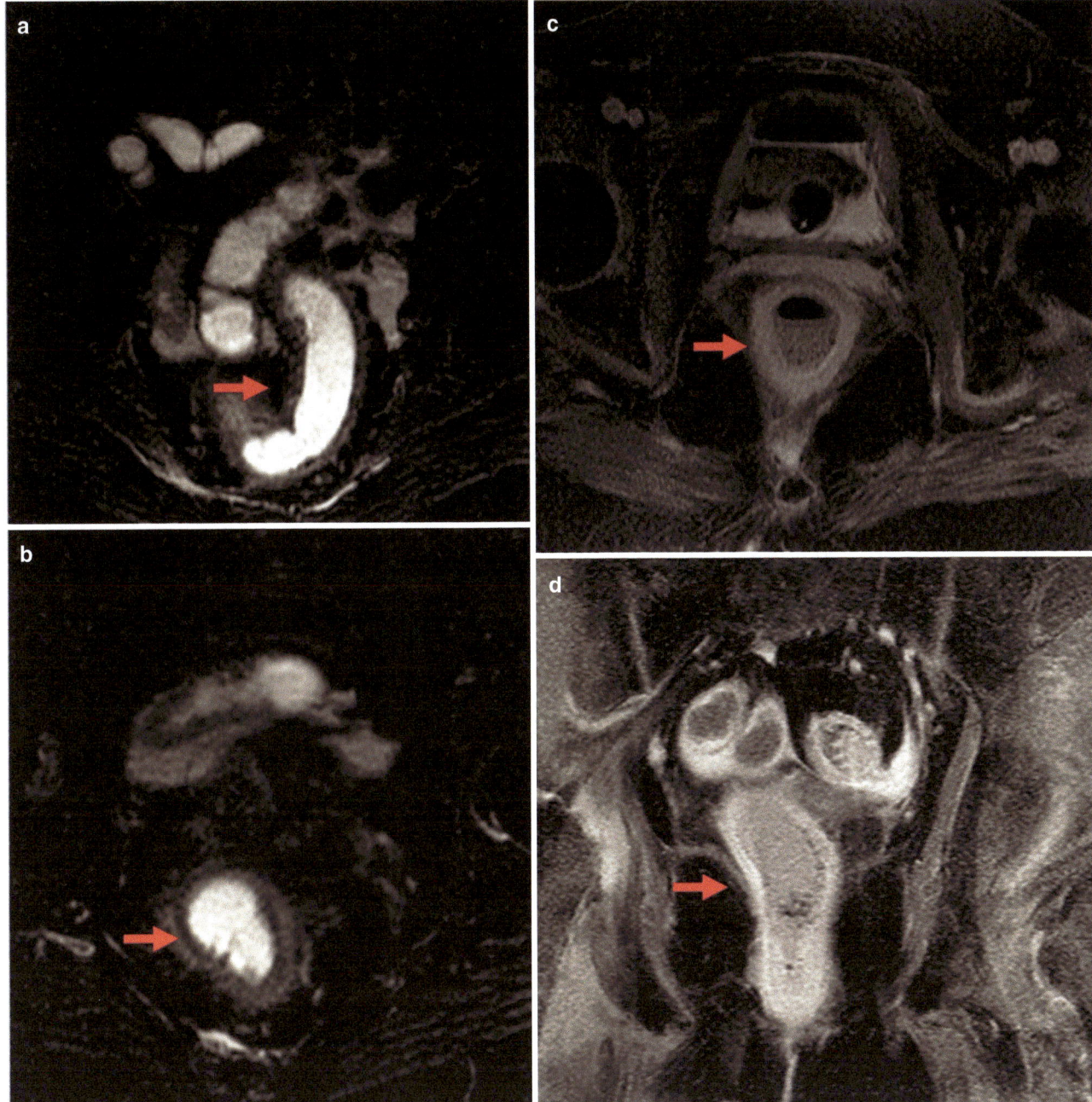

Fig. 2.2 Axial T2-weighted fat-suppressed images (**a**, **b**) of an elderly female with clostridium difficile colitis following prolonged use of antibiotics show diffuse wall thickening of the rectosigmoid colon with evidence of enhancement on axial (**c**) and coronal (**d**) fat-suppressed post-contrast T1-weighted image

2.3.1.3 Gastrointestinal Tuberculosis

Due to factors such as stasis, presence of lymphoid tissue, and closer contact of bacilli with the enteric mucosa, the most common site of tubercular involvement in gastrointestinal tract is ileocecal region in about 64% of cases [37]. The lesions can be ulcerative and ulcero-hypertrophic in bowel and show confluent granulomas and caseation necrosis in the bowel and adjacent lymph nodes[38]. Rarely, duodenum and esophagus can be involved. Plain X-ray abdomen may show enteroliths, features of obstruction like dilated bowel loops with multiple air fluid levels or presence of air under diaphragm in case of perforation. There may be evidence of calcification as calcified lymph nodes, calcified granulomas, and hepatosplenomegaly. On barium studies, accelerated intestinal transit; hyper-segmentation of the barium column, precipitation, flocculation and dilution of the barium, stiffened and thickened folds, narrowing of bowel lumen and strictures can be seen. CECT and CT enterography can show

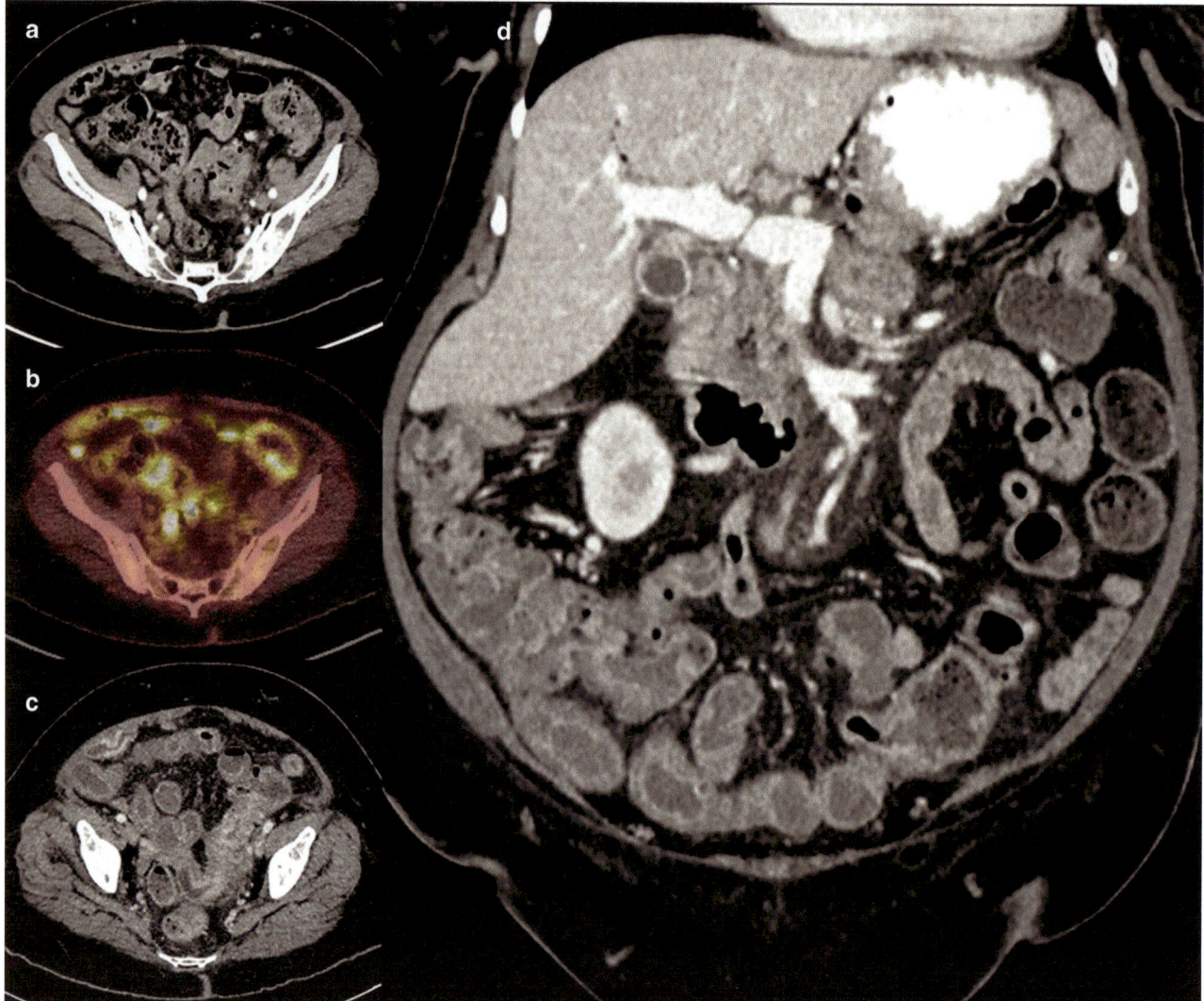

Fig. 2.3 Axial post-contrast CT (**a**) and PET (**b**) image showing colonic wall thickening and uptake within the small bowel and colon which worsens on follow-up post-contrast CT axial (**c**) and coronal (**d**) image obtained 2 weeks later in a patient of necrotizing enterocolitis

wall thickening in the cecum and terminal ileum with asymmetric thickening of the IC valve and associated lymphadenopathy with areas of low attenuation suggestive of caseous necrosis (Fig. 2.4) [39, 40]. Strictures can be seen in ileum and sometimes jejunum.

2.3.1.4 Viral Enterocolitis

Viral infections such as CMV have a high morbidity and mortality (42%), commonly affecting the colon, stomach, and esophagus [41]. CECT and MRI imaging features are non-specific including wall thickening, ascites, and lymphadenopathy. In complicated cases, mucosal ulcers and ischemia or perforation-related changes can occur. Differential diagnosis apart from other infectious etiologies include graft versus host disease in a setting of stem cell transplant.

Another common viral agent which affects the gastrointestinal tract is Norovirus, causing gastroenteritis[42]. Non-specific CT findings include low attenuation small bowel wall thickening and distension with fluid [43]. Differential diagnosis includes neoplastic bowel infiltration and mural hemorrhage where the bowel wall is hyperdense [44].

Recently, COVID-19 commonly affects the gastrointestinal tract and could at times precede pulmonary involvement. While CECT is the modality of choice for the detection of bowel involvement, US and MRI can help management and follow-up. CECT findings include involvement of ascending colon, transverse colon, and descending colon with features of bowel wall thickening, mucosal hyperenhancement, low attenuation submucosal edema, bowel dilation, pericolic fat stranding and lymphadenopathy [45, 46]. Complications

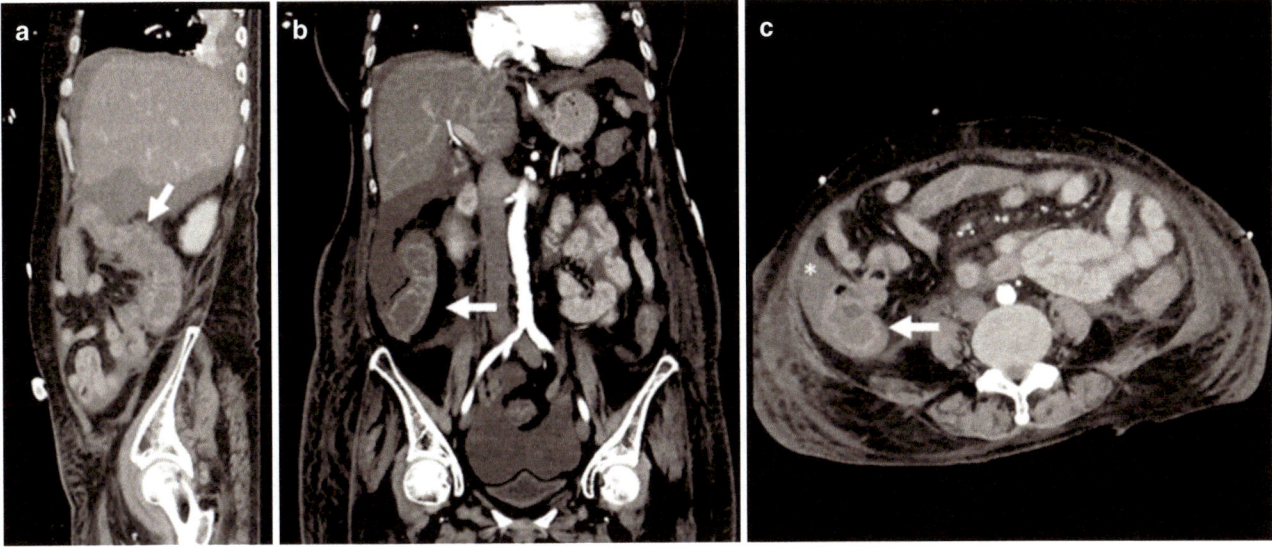

Fig. 2.4 An adult male patient with tuberculous colitis demonstrating diffuse colonic wall thickening (white arrow) and ascites (*) on sagittal (**a**), coronal (**b**), and axial post-contrast (**c**) images

such as pneumatosis intestinalis are rare and can secondarily be contributed by chronic bowel ischemia, obstruction, and autoimmune etiologies. Portal and mesenteric vein thrombosis are typically seen in COVID-19 infection [47]. Isolated case reports of appendicitis have also been reported [48].

2.3.1.5 Fungal Infections

In patients with acute leukemia, diabetes, cancer and immunocompromised states, fungal infections in the gastrointestinal tract are increasingly common with pathogens including Aspergillus, Candida, and Mucor [49, 50]. CECT shows gastrointestinal tract wall thickening and stranding, lymphadenopathy, peritoneal and retroperitoneal thickening, hepatic and splenic microabscesses, vascular compromise, and infarcts [51]. Both aspergillus and mucor are angio-invasive with highest mortality in about half the cases with mucor. Additionally, large ulcers with irregular edges can be seen within the stomach and the colon. Candida infections can cause ulcers, peritonitis, and infarcts in solid organs [52].

2.3.2   Hepatobiliary Infections

Hepatobiliary infections comprise of infectious cholangitis, hepatitis (acute and chronic viral), bacterial, mycobacterial, parasitic (such as echinococcal and amoebiasis), fungal, and gastrointestinal or systemic infections involving the liver secondarily due to portal circulation and the organ [53].

2.3.2.1 Liver Abscesses

The routes of spread of liver abscess include biliary, hematogenous, or contiguous with infections resulting from bacterial or fungal colonization [21]. Predisposing factors

include the presence of malignancy, biliary tract disease, post-interventions, and surgery. While CECT is the imaging modality of choice, MRI can provide information on possible communication of abscesses with the biliary tract and to differentiate hepatic abscesses from necrotic metastases. Compared to the latter, abscesses demonstrate a rather thin and homogeneous wall, and greater restricted diffusion with lower ADC values [54]. Area of diffusion restriction on MRI correlate with high T2 signal while in necrotic tumors these correlates to intermediate T2 signal intensity. For abscesses larger than 6 cm, or risk of impending perforation, percutaneous drainage is often required [55]. Fungal infections such as hepatosplenic candidiasis, the most common form of chronic disseminated candidiasis usually sets in a predisposing hematologic malignancy after chemotherapy [56]. The typical manifestation includes multifocal peripheral hepatic, splenic, and renal cortical microabscesses demonstrable on US, CT, and MRI [57]. US shows microabscesses as hypoechoic or as a "bull's eye" lesion with peripheral hypoechoic fibrosis and central hyperechoic inflammation [58]. CECT and MRI can demonstrate innumerable tiny microabscesses, hypoattenuating on CT and variable on MRI: T1 hypointense ad T2 hyperintense when acute and hypointense peripheral rim on T1 and T2 with central hyperintensity on T1-weighted images when subacute and hypointense on all sequences when in chronic phase. These can calcify in chronic phase with differentials including metastases, lymphoma, and sarcoidosis.

2.3.2.2 Cholangitis

Obstructing stones, malignant or non-malignant stricture, biliary stents, and choledochojejunostomy can lead to acute or ascending cholangitis presenting with Charcot's triad including abdominal pain, fever, and jaundice [59]. Acute suppurative cholangitis refers to cholangitis with the presence of pus in the biliary tract occurring in elderly patients >70 years of age, smokers, and in patients with impacted biliary stones or procedure related [51, 60]. Common bacterial agents include *E. coli* (31%), *Klebsiella pneumoniae, Enterococcus faecalis*, and Streptococcus species. Indwelling plastic biliary stents predispose to enterococcus and polymicrobial infections [60]. CECT and MRI images show central, diffuse, or segmental biliary ductal dilation with smooth symmetric and diffuse bile duct wall thickening most pronounced in

the central ducts. While the ductal dilation can be assessed on US, early, and intense enhancement of the thickened bile duct walls and the liver parenchyma may demonstrate wedge-shaped peripheral patchy peribiliary enhancement, most marked in the arterial phase. US and MR cholangiopancreatography (MRCP) can determine the presence of tumors or stones in the central bile ducts (Fig. 2.5). Pus may be seen on CT as hyperdense material within the distended ducts. Inspissated bile or sludge may also be hyperdense on CT; MRI, especially DWI, can be more specific for identifying purulent material, as it demonstrates restricted diffusion

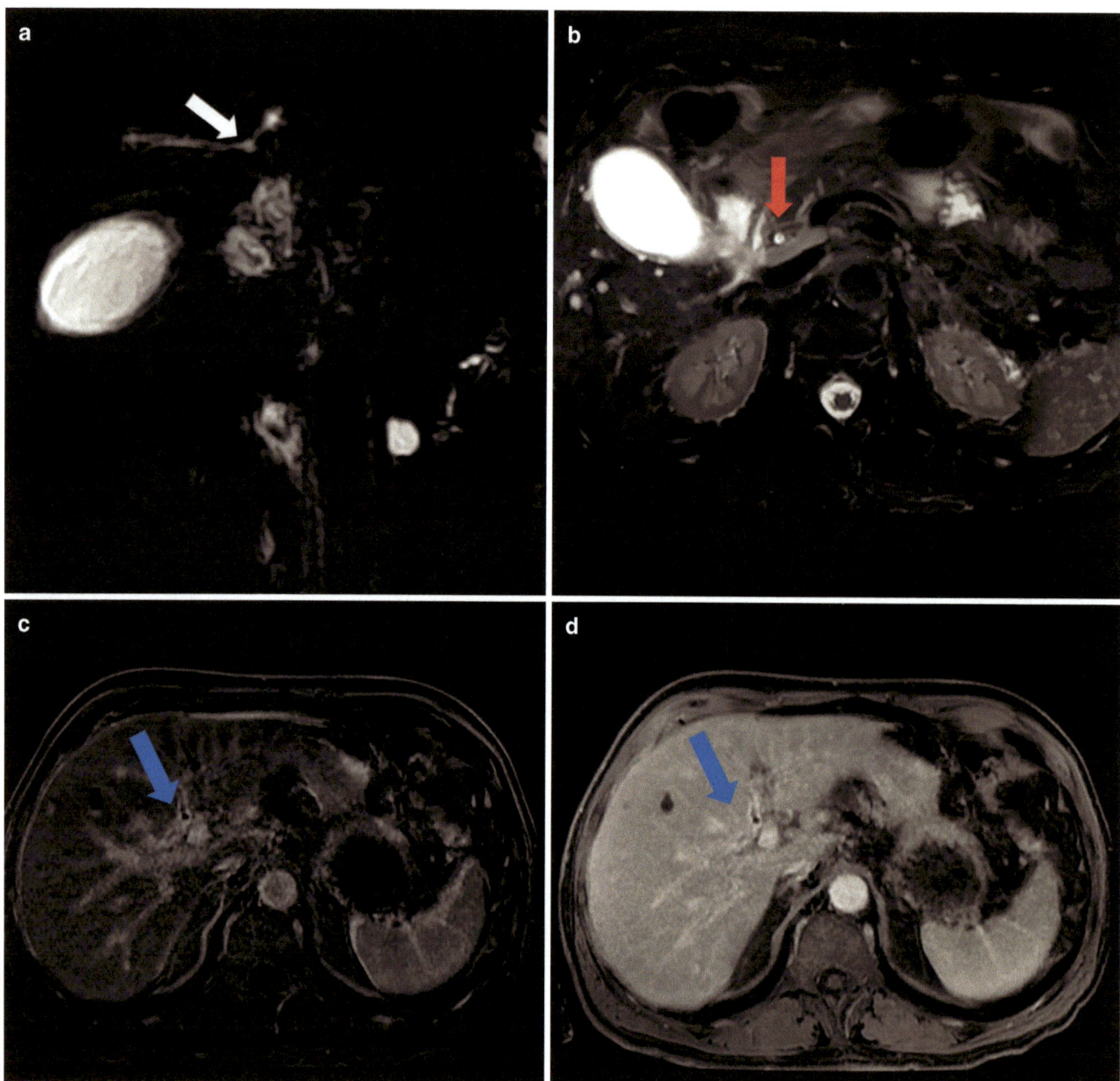

Fig. 2.5 An adult female with cholangitis. Coronal MRCP (**a**) image showing left-sided mild ductal dilatation. The plastic stent can be visualized in the common bile duct on axial T2-weighted image (**b**). Axial subtracted (**c**) and non-subtracted (**d**) fat-suppressed post-contrast delayed images show the biliary thickening and enhancement

with very low signal intensity on ADC map but no internal enhancement. Cholangitis can be complicated by bacteremia and sepsis, hepatic abscesses, portal vein thrombosis, and bile peritonitis [60].

2.3.2.3 Viral Infections

Viral hepatitis can result from hepatitis A virus infection commonly in developing countries and reactivation of hepatitis B and hepatitis C in patients with known chronic hepatitis after receiving chemotherapy [59, 60]. The resultant periportal edema and parenchymal injury can be seen on US as "starry sky" appearance due to increased echogenicity of the portal triads, and on MRI as diffusely heterogeneous signal intensity of the liver with hyperintense T2 signal. CECT and post-contrast MRI images show early and heterogenous hepatic enhancement. Recently, COVID-19 has been shown to cause liver injury due to its cytopathic effect with elevation of liver enzymes such as ALT, AST, and GGT. There have been reports of moderate micro-vesicular steatosis and lobular and portal activity in liver biopsy specimens of COVID-19 patients [61, 62].

2.3.2.4 Parasitic Infections

There are a number of parasitic infections that can affect the liver and biliary tree with the most common being amebic infection, hydatid disease, schistosomiasis, fascioliasis, and clonorchiasis [63, 64]. Amoebiasis, an infection of the large intestine can spread to the liver leading to abscess formation appearing on US as solitary, unilocular, and hypoechoic round or oval mass commonly in right hepatic lobe. There may be evidence of internal echoes and posterior acoustic enhancement. Associated diaphragmatic disruption with rupture into the pleural space or pericardium is highly suggestive of an amebic liver abscess [64]. CT appearance is of a circumscribed lesion with central fluid attenuation and peripheral rim enhancement (target" or "double-rim" appearance) with or without septations, fluid-debris levels, and rarely gas or hemorrhage [58]. MRI shows central low T1- and high T2-signal, peripheral rim enhancements and perilesional edema. The amoebic abscess usually responds to medical management with drainage needed for larger ones. In a setting of a suspected liver abscess with associated thickening/inflammation of the right colon, an amebic abscess should be considered.

Echinococcal liver disease is caused by echinococcosis granulosus and multilocularis infections. On US, the appearance can range from a pure cyst to a lesion that mimics a solid mass [65]. Echinococcal cysts can be easily differentiated from simple hepatic cysts by the presence of a wall of varying thickness and additional signs such as the presence of daughter cysts demonstrating a "spoke-wheel" pattern [64]. Another is the "water-Lily" sign, in which wavy float-

ing membranes are seen within the hydatid cavity resulting from detachment of the endocyst. When the patient is repositioned, multiple echogenic foci can be seen to move within the hydatid cavity giving the "snowstorm" sign. These echogenic foci result from rupture of daughter cysts that leads to scolices passing into the hydatid cyst fluid forming a white sediment that is then referred to as "hydatid sand." When the hydatid cyst degenerates and becomes nonviable, it can appear heterogeneous with hypoechoic and hyperechoic content, mimicking a solid mass. This is the "ball of wool" sign. Finally, a hydatid cyst can partially or completely calcify over time [66]. If the calcifications are more central in location, that usually indicates a nonviable cyst. CT shows high attenuation of the echinococcal cyst walls and the internal floating membranes with peripheral enhancement and non-enhancing central content. Daughter cysts and calcifications similar to that on US can be seen. MRI shows a T1 and T2 hypointense peripheral rim of pericyst with internal floating membranes and daughter cysts. The *E. multilocularis* can infiltrate along the biliary tracts towards the hepatic hilum and cause peritoneal seeding of infection, transdiaphragmatic intrathoracic spread of disease, and superinfection (Fig. 2.6) [67].

2.3.3 Genitourinary Tract Infections

2.3.3.1 Obstructive Uropathy

Obstructive uropathy due to the presence of tumor, ureteral reflux from loss of the ureterovesical junction competency, indwelling catheters and stents, and pelvic radiation can predispose to urinary tract infections. The level of urinary tract obstruction can be the ureter, bladder, or urethra, leading to urinary stasis, a major risk for bacterial colonization and infection [68]. Additionally, urinary tract obstruction also impairs the renal function. The obstruction at the level of ureters can occur due to retroperitoneal adenopathy, pelvic or ureteric malignancies or radiation-induced stricture [69]. The major diagnostic imaging modalities include US and CECT which can demonstrate hydroureteronephrosis and asymmetric nephrogram for detection of ureteral obstruction. In lower urinary tract obstruction, such as due to prostatomegaly or strictures, US can also help evaluate the presence of post-void residual urine. The filling defects in the collecting system or ureters including mass lesion or stones can be better assessed on CT urography using a split bolus technique or a 3-phase study. The level of obstruction and etiologies pertaining to soft-tissue mass can be better evaluated with MRI. Accuracy in diagnosis helps in clinical management typically requiring decompression using retrograde ureteral stents or percutaneous nephrostomy tubes.

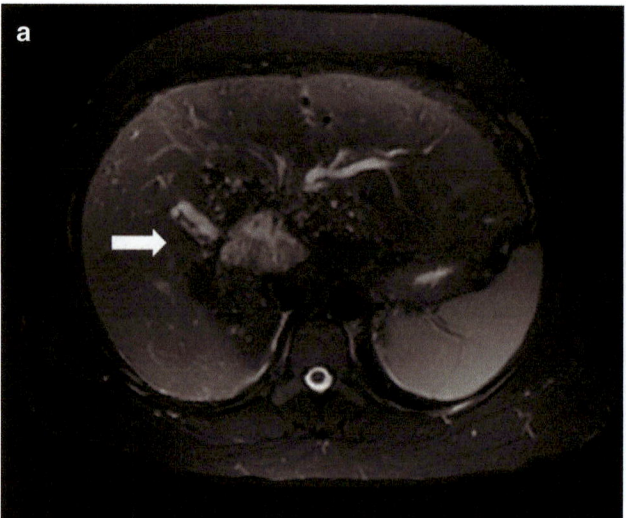
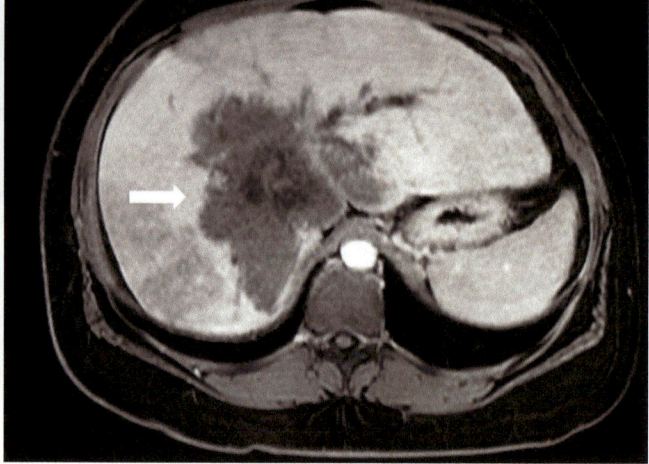

Fig. 2.6 Axial T2-weighted image (**a**) of an adult male shows hyperintense complex solid and cystic lesion infiltrating along the bile ducts (white arrow) with mild ductal dilatation in a patient with *Echinococcus*

multilocularis infection. Axial delayed post-contrast image (**b**) shows heterogenous enhancement

2.3.3.2 Renal and Urinary Bladder Infections

Urinary bladder infections can occur with *E. coli* and other Gram-positive cocci, Gram-negative enterobacteriaceae and candida [70]. The predisposing factors for urinary bladder infection include indwelling Foley's catheter or suprapubic catheter, obstructive uropathy, and prior surgical interventions such as bladder tumor resection with or without intestinal urinary pouches. While the bacterial infections frequently can be diagnosed early and effectively managed, fungal organisms such as *C. albicans* can lead to renal microabscesses or larger abscesses, fungal balls or chronic disseminated candidiasis [54]. [71]. Renal infections can occur due to ascending urinary tract infection or hematogenous dissemination. The initial presentation of renal infection is pyelonephritis which can evolve and complicate into renal abscess in the setting of bacteremia or fungemia. Prompt and early diagnosis can ensure medical management with favorable outcome prior to the development of complications that may need percutaneous or surgical aspiration [72]. On US, the presence of pyelonephritis demonstrates a heterogenous appearance of renal cortex with reduced flow on Doppler. On CECT and MRI, the appearance is of a wedge-shaped or rounded area of streaky cortical enhancement (Fig. 2.7). The presence of renal abscess can demonstrate central hypodensity on CT and T2 hyperintensity on MRI with evidence of diffusion restriction.

2.3.3.3 Prostatic Infections

Infections in the prostate gland can occur contiguously such as from urethra or bladder infections or secondary to procedures such as cystoscopy, prostate biopsy, urethral/suprapubic catheter placement, brachytherapy, cryotherapy, or

radiation [73]. Chemotherapy and bacteremia are additional systemic factors in cancer patients that increase the risk of developing prostatic abscess. Clinically, patients present with dysuria, urgency, frequency, sensation of incomplete voiding, and suprapubic or perineal pain. On CT and MRI, the inflamed gland can demonstrate enlarged and edematous appearance. The presence of central hypoechoic areas on US, low attenuation on CT and T2 hyperintensity on MRI correlate with possibility of a prostatic abscess. MRI provides better imaging characterization for prostatic abscess assessment, and both CT and MRI can demonstrate a unilocular or multilocular rim enhancing collection commonly in the transition zone or central zone of the prostate (Fig. 2.8) [73].

2.3.4 Peritoneal and Abdominal Wall Infections

Intra-abdominal and abdominal wall infections can occur due to secondary involvement from adjacent site or in a setting of immunosuppression, cancer, radiation, and interventions such as paracentesis, surgery, and medical devices. The inflammation of the peritoneum (peritonitis) can be infectious or non-infectious such as due to irritation by blood or bile. The gastrointestinal etiologies for peritonitis include bowel obstruction and perforation and anastomotic dehiscence. Additional causes include cancer, ischemia, infectious enterocolitis, ulcers, and radiation can lead to bowel perforation. Surgery, indwelling peritoneal dialysis catheters, non-tunneled catheters and shunts also predispose to infection. The complicated peritonitis can lead to a systemic

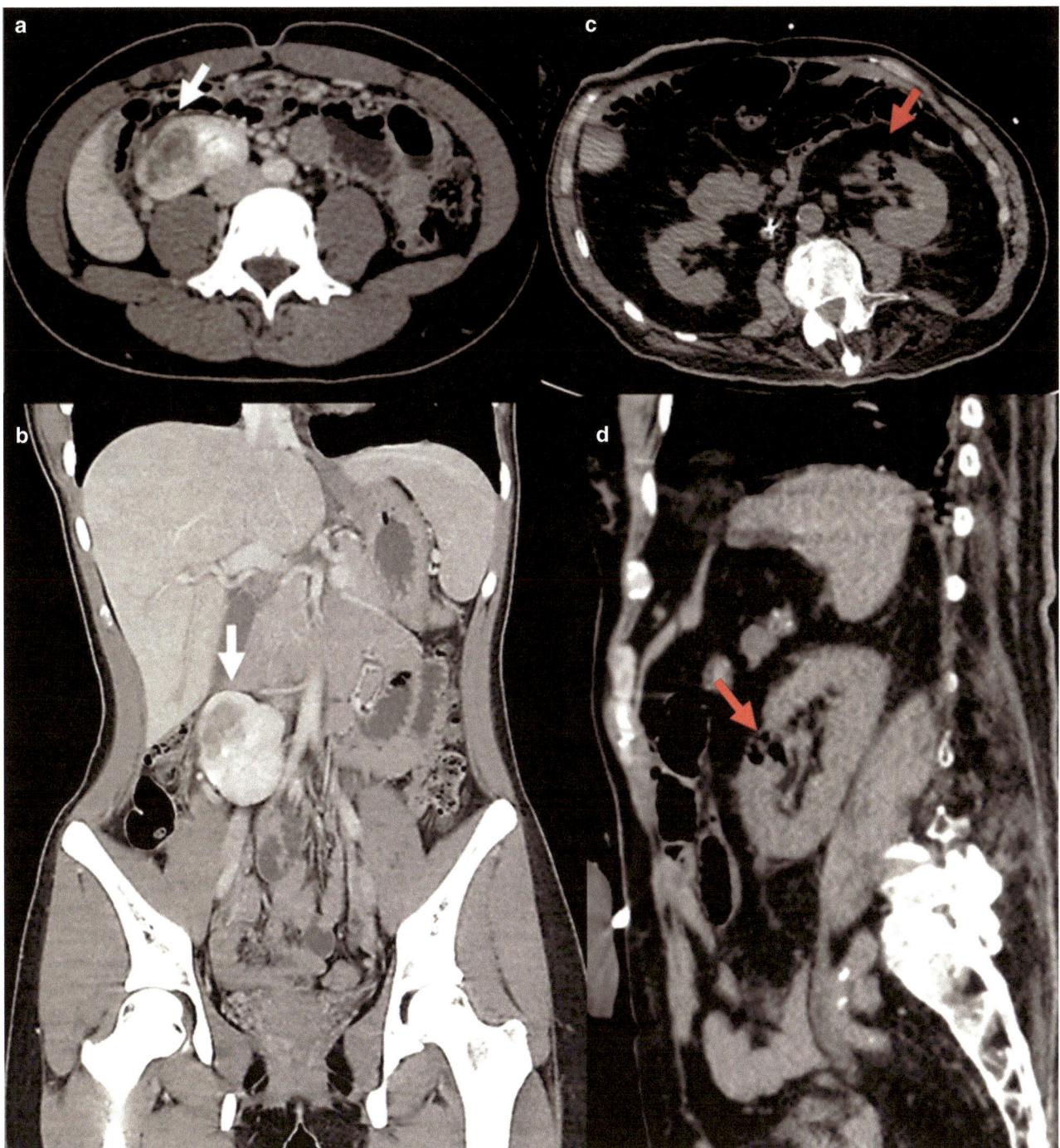

Fig. 2.7 Axial (**a**) and coronal (**b**) post-contrast CT images of an adult male shows heterogenous focus of evolving renal abscess at the upper pole of the ectopic single kidney. Axial (**c**) and coronal (**d**) non-contrast CT images of an adult male with diabetes shows air within the anterior interpolar cortex of the left kidney suggesting emphysematous pyelonephritis and evolving abscess

inflammatory response that with a mortality rate of up to 30% [73, 74]. Patients present with generalized abdominal pain, tenderness, guarding, and fever. Pathogens in peritonitis depend upon the cause, as pathogens in the upper gastrointestinal tract differ than those of the lower. US can be used to evaluate for ascites and collections, and to guide aspiration, but CECT is the modality of choice in imaging peritonitis to identify a source and look for intra-abdominal abscesses. Typical imaging features are ascites, peritoneal enhancement, and thickening, which is typically smooth with infectious etiology, but could less commonly be nodular or irregular, a feature favoring carcinomatosis.

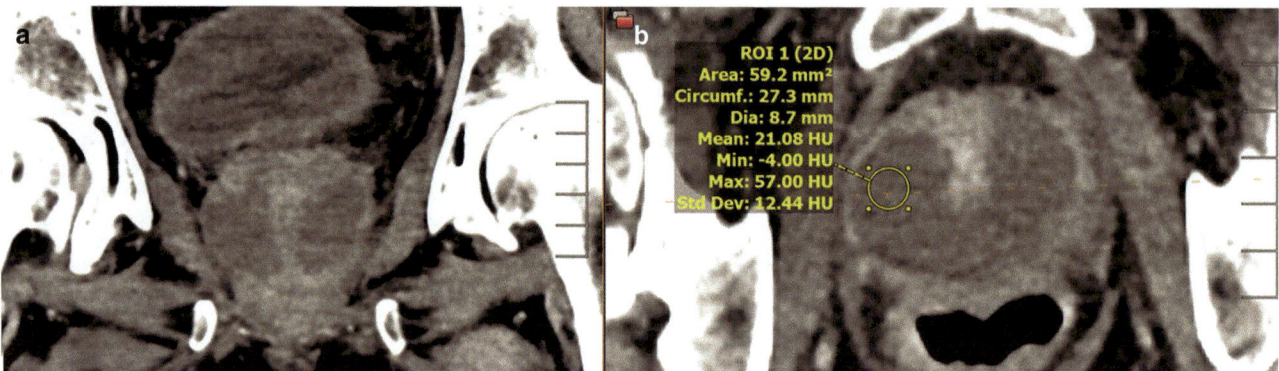

Fig. 2.8 Coronal (**a**) and axial (**b**) post-contrast CT images of an adult male showing low attenuation within the prostate gland consistent with prostatic abscess

2.3.4.1 Peritoneal Devices

Patients with advanced abdominal malignancies often develop refractory ascites requiring indwelling peritoneal catheters associated with a significantly increased infection risk. Simple fluid collections or ill-defined fluid around devices can be due to seromas and post-surgical changes; however, the development of an enhancing wall or new gas pockets without recent intervention is concerning for abscess formation. Additional peritoneal devices include peritoneal infusion catheters, dialysis catheters, ventriculo-peritoneal shunts, and surgical drains; any of those can be complicated by peritonitis from translocation of skin flora or from bowel perforation, albeit the latter is rare. Peritonitis is also an uncommon risk following percutaneous gastrostomy tube placement. Management consists of antibiotics and removal of the causative device, with surgery in cases of frank perforation.

2.3.4.2 Intra-abdominal Abscesses

Non-visceral abscesses are polymicrobial and either peritoneal or retroperitoneal with the former due to a complication of peritonitis and/or perforation. Retroperitoneal abscesses can be caused by hollow viscous perforation or by hematogenous, lymphatic, or local spread of infection. Clinical symptoms include fever and abdominal discomfort. For example, a perirectal abscess may cause diarrhea, and an abscess in contiguity with the bladder may cause urinary symptoms. CECT and MR imaging demonstrate a rim enhancing fluid collection with surrounding inflammatory changes. For

>3 cm abscess, drainage is required. If untreated, abscesses may extend to adjacent structures, erode into vessels (causing pseudoaneurysms, hemorrhage, and thrombosis), rupture, or less commonly fistulize, eventually leading to bacteremia and septic shock with high mortality rates [74].

2.3.4.3 Abdominal Wall Infections

Skin and soft-tissue infections (SSTI) in the abdominal wall can be very serious in immunocompromised patients, particularly those with vascular pathologies such as endarteritis obliterans (seen with radiation therapy). SSTIs include cutaneous infections in addition to deeper subcutaneous, muscular, and fascial infections such as cellulitis, necrotizing fasciitis, and pyomyositis. Deep SSTI infections can be caused by skin injury or skin disruption from surgery, catheter and line insertions, radiation treatment, and primary or metastatic tumors. Cellulitis is a clinical diagnosis, but imaging features include skin thickening with subcutaneous fat stranding, edema, and inflammation. The presence of subcutaneous gas on non-contrast CT that spreads along fascial planes is usually worrisome for necrotizing fasciitis, requiring early and aggressive management with drainage and surgical debridement (Fig. 2.9). Vesicocutaneous and enterocutaneous fistulas due to tumors, radiation therapy, or surgical complications can lead to SSTIs. Imaging with US, CT, or MRI can be helpful in delineating the predisposing factor, differentiating acute versus fibrotic fistula track as well as the number and relationships of tracts, and evaluating for any associated drainable abscesses.

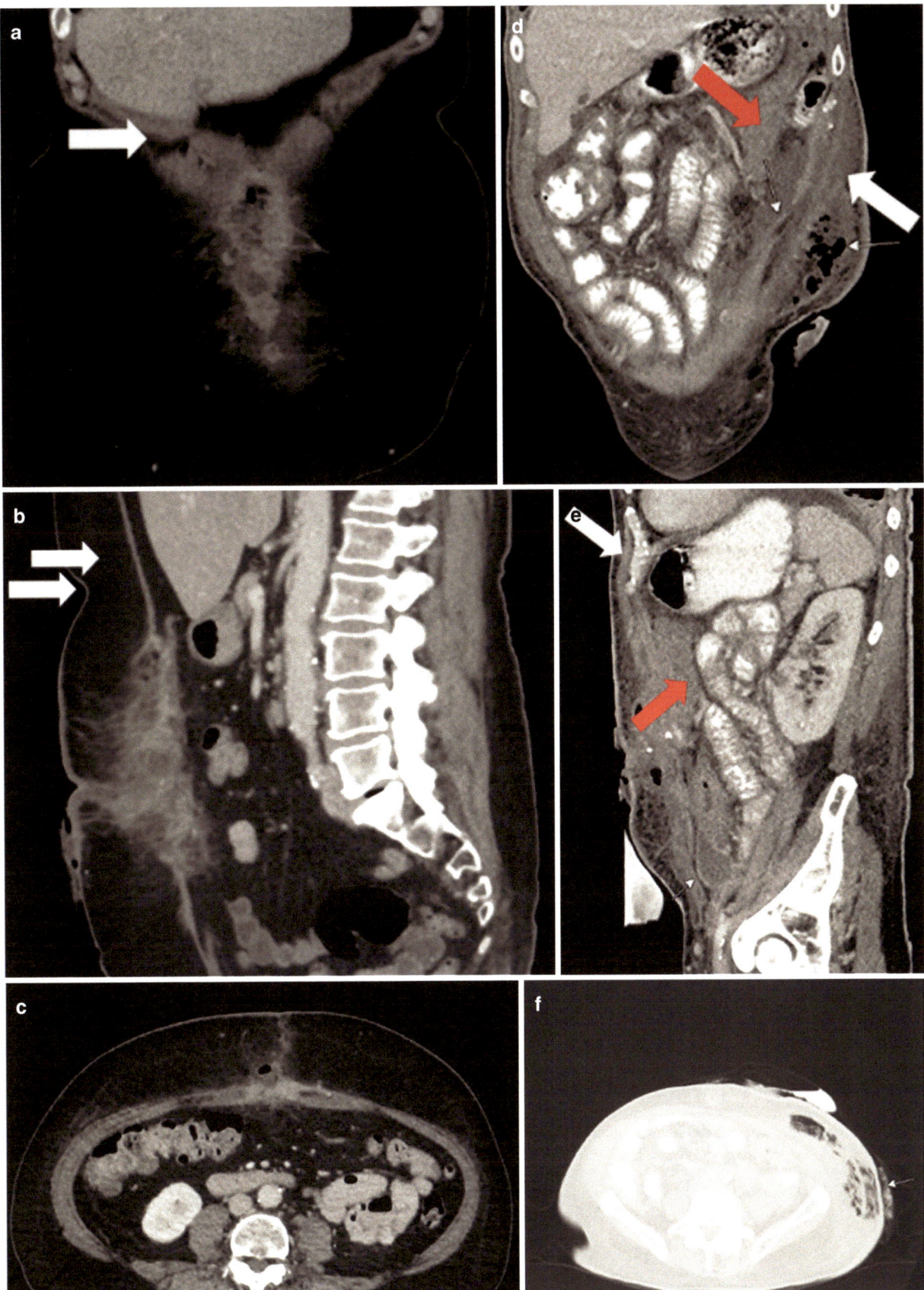

Fig. 2.9 Coronal (**a**, **d**), sagittal (**b**, **e**) and axial (**c**, **f**) post-contrast CT images of two adult female patients showing anterior abdominal wall air and fluid containing collections (white Arrows). Note the peritoneal enhancement and thickening (red arrows)

2.4 Conclusion

Radiologists should be familiar with the risks of infection and identify the most common imaging manifestations of infections. Imaging plays an important role in diagnosis, management, and prognosis of infectious processes in the abdomen and pelvis in patients with oncologic conditions, including those affecting the gastrointestinal, hepatobiliary, and genitourinary systems, in addition to non-visceral and abdominal wall infections, and those associated with medical devices, radiation, and surgical procedures.

> **Take-Home Messages**
> - Infections of the abdomen and pelvis have significant impact on patient morbidity and mortality.
> - Imaging plays an important role in the diagnosis and management of patients with intra-abdominal infections.
> - Imaging manifestation of abdominal infections can be varied depending on the type of microbial, pathogenesis, and organ system involved.
> - Early recognition of imaging signs of infection along with identification of mimics is essential for prompt diagnosis and management.

References

1. Intra-abdominal infections market—global industry analysis S, share, growth, trends, and forecast 2017–2025: intra-abdominal infections market; 2022. https://www.transparencymarketresearch.com/intraabdominal-infections-market.html. Accessed.
2. Siegel RL, Miller KD, Jemal A. Cancer statistics, 2020. Cancer J Clin. 2020;70(1):7–30. https://doi.org/10.3322/caac.21590.
3. Rolston KVI. Infections in cancer patients with solid tumors: a review. Infect Dis Ther. 2017;6(1):69–83. https://doi.org/10.1007/s40121-017-0146-1.
4. Safdar A, Armstrong D. Infectious morbidity in critically ill patients with cancer. Crit Care Clin. 2001;17(3):531–70. https://doi.org/10.1016/s0749-0704(05)70198-6.
5. Itani M, Menias CO, Mellnick VM, El Zakhem A, Elsayes K, Katabathina V, et al. Imaging of abdominal and pelvic infections in the cancer patient. Abdominal Radiol. 2021;46(6):2920–41. https://doi.org/10.1007/s00261-020-02896-7.
6. Reed D, Sen J, Lassiter K, Thomas T, Harr E, Daniels E, et al. Prospective initiative to reduce mucosal barrier injuries and bloodstream infections in patients with hematologic malignancy receiving inpatient chemotherapy. JCO Oncol Pract. 2020;16(3):e306–e12. https://doi.org/10.1200/jop.19.00344.
7. Blijlevens NMA, Donnelly JP, De Pauw BE. Mucosal barrier injury: biology, pathology, clinical counterparts and consequences of intensive treatment for haematological malignancy: an overview. Bone Marrow Transpl. 2000;25(12):1269–78. https://doi.org/10.1038/sj.bmt.1702447.
8. Abdol Razak N, Jones G, Bhandari M, Berndt M, Metharom P. Cancer-associated thrombosis: an overview of mechanisms, risk factors, and treatment. Cancers. 2018;10(10):380. https://doi.org/10.3390/cancers10100380.
9. Lustberg MB. Management of neutropenia in cancer patients. Clin Adv Hematol Oncol. 2012;10(12):825–6.
10. Baker TM, Satlin MJ. The growing threat of multidrug-resistant Gram-negative infections in patients with hematologic malignancies. Leukemia Lymphoma. 2016;57(10):2245–58. https://doi.org/10.1080/10428194.2016.1193859.
11. Sutton SH. Infections associated with solid malignancies. Infectious complications in cancer patients. Springer International Publishing; 2014. p. 371–411.
12. Cumbo TA, Segal BH. Prevention, diagnosis, and treatment of invasive fungal infections in patients with cancer and neutropenia. J Natl Compreh Cancer Network. 2004;2(5):455–69. https://doi.org/10.6004/jnccn.2004.0036.
13. Reusser P. Current concepts and challenges in the prevention and treatment of viral infections in immunocompromised cancer patients. Support Care Cancer. 1997;6(1):39–45. https://doi.org/10.1007/s005200050130.
14. Shadad AK. Gastrointestinal radiation injury: prevention and treatment. World J Gastroenterol. 2013;19(2):199. https://doi.org/10.3748/wjg.v19.i2.199.
15. Iyer R. Radiation injury: imaging findings in the chest, abdomen and pelvis after therapeutic radiation. Cancer Imaging. 2006;6(Special Issue A):S131–S9. https://doi.org/10.1102/1470-7330.2006.9095.
16. Stewart PS, Bjarnsholt T. Risk factors for chronic biofilm-related infection associated with implanted medical devices. Clin Microbiol Infect. 2020;26(8):1034–8. https://doi.org/10.1016/j.cmi.2020.02.027.
17. Lamarca A, Rigby C, McNamara MG, Hubner RA, Valle JW. Impact of biliary stent-related events in patients diagnosed with advanced pancreatobiliary tumours receiving palliative chemotherapy. World J Gastroenterol. 2016;22(26):6065. https://doi.org/10.3748/wjg.v22.i26.6065.
18. Bahu R, Chaftari A-M, Hachem RY, Ahrar K, Shomali W, El Zakhem A, et al. Nephrostomy tube related pyelonephritis in patients with cancer: epidemiology, infection rate and risk factors. J Urol. 2013;189(1):130–5. https://doi.org/10.1016/j.juro.2012.08.094.
19. Gillespie BM, Harbeck E, Rattray M, Liang R, Walker R, Latimer S, et al. Worldwide incidence of surgical site infections in general surgical patients: a systematic review and meta-analysis of 488,594 patients. Int J Surg. 2021;95:106136. https://doi.org/10.1016/j.ijsu.2021.106136.
20. Boermeester MA, Gans SL, Stoker J, Boermeester MA. Plain abdominal radiography in acute abdominal pain; past, present, and future. Int J Gen Med. 2012;525 https://doi.org/10.2147/ijgm.s17410.
21. Lardière-Deguelte S, Ragot E, Amroun K, Piardi T, Dokmak S, Bruno O, et al. Hepatic abscess: diagnosis and management. J Visc Surg. 2015;152(4):231–43. https://doi.org/10.1016/j.jviscsurg.2015.01.013.
22. Frickenstein AN, Jones MA, Behkam B, McNally LR. Imaging inflammation and infection in the gastrointestinal tract. Int J Mol Sci. 2019;21(1) https://doi.org/10.3390/ijms21010243.
23. Puges M, Bérard X, Ruiz J-B, Debordeaux F, Desclaux A, Stecken L, et al. Retrospective study comparing WBC scan and 18F-FDG PET/CT in patients with suspected prosthetic vascular graft infection. Eur J Vasc Endovasc Surg. 2019;57(6):876–84. https://doi.org/10.1016/j.ejvs.2018.12.032.
24. Kouijzer IJE, Mulders-Manders CM, Bleeker-Rovers CP, Oyen WJG. Fever of unknown origin: the Value of FDG-PET/CT. Semin Nucl Med. 2018;48(2):100–7. https://doi.org/10.1053/j.semnuclmed.2017.11.004.
25. Bodey GP, Fainstein V, Guerrant R. Infections of the gastrointestinal tract in the immunocompromised patient. Annu Rev Med. 1986;37(1):271–81. https://doi.org/10.1146/annurev.me.37.020186.001415.

26. Schmidt-Hieber M, Bierwirth J, Buchheidt D, Cornely OA, Hentrich M, Maschmeyer G, et al. Diagnosis and management of gastrointestinal complications in adult cancer patients: 2017 updated evidence-based guidelines of the Infectious Diseases Working Party (AGIHO) of the German Society of Hematology and Medical Oncology (DGHO). Ann Hematol. 2017;97(1):31–49. https://doi.org/10.1007/s00277-017-3183-7.

27. Loureiro RV, Borges VP, Tomé AL, Bernardes CF, Silva MJ, Bettencourt MJ. Anorectal complications in patients with haematological malignancies. Eur J Gastroenterol Hepatol. 2018;30(7):722–6. https://doi.org/10.1097/meg.0000000000001133.

28. Dayani M, Porouhan P, Farshchian N. Management of radiation-induced proctitis. J Family Med Primary Care. 2019;8(7):2173. https://doi.org/10.4103/jfmpc.jfmpc_333_19.

29. Tonolini M, Bianco R. MRI and CT of anal carcinoma: a pictorial review. Insights Imaging. 2012;4(1):53–62. https://doi.org/10.1007/s13244-012-0199-3.

30. Delgado A, Reveles IA, Cabello FT, Reveles KR. Poorer outcomes among cancer patients diagnosed with Clostridium difficile infections in United States community hospitals. BMC Infect Dis. 2017;17(1) https://doi.org/10.1186/s12879-017-2553-z.

31. Czepiel J, Dróżdż M, Pituch H, Kuijper EJ, Perucki W, Mielimonka A, et al. Clostridium difficile infection: review. Eur J Clin Microbiol Infect Dis. 2019;38(7):1211–21. https://doi.org/10.1007/s10096-019-03539-6.

32. Thoeni RF, Cello JP. CT imaging of colitis. Radiology. 2006;240(3):623–38. https://doi.org/10.1148/radiol.2403050818.

33. Nesher L, Rolston KVI. Neutropenic enterocolitis, a growing concern in the era of widespread use of aggressive chemotherapy. Clin Infect Dis. 2012;56(5):711–7. https://doi.org/10.1093/cid/cis998.

34. Davila ML. Neutropenic enterocolitis. Curr Treatment Options Gastroenterol. 2006;9(3):249–55. https://doi.org/10.1007/s11938-006-0043-2.

35. Horton KM, Corl FM, Fishman EK. CT evaluation of the colon: inflammatory disease. RadioGraphics. 2000;20(2):399–418. https://doi.org/10.1148/radiographics.20.2.g00mc15399.

36. McCarville MB, Spunt SL, Pappo AS. Rhabdomyosarcoma in Pediatric Patients. Am J Roentgenol. 2001;176(6):1563–9. https://doi.org/10.2214/ajr.176.6.1761563.

37. Horvath KD, Whelan RL. Intestinal tuberculosis: return of an old disease. Am J Gastroenterol. 1998;93(5):692–6. https://doi.org/10.1111/j.1572-0241.1998.207_a.x.

38. Sharma K, Sinha S, Sharma A, Prasad K, Rana S, Sharma M, et al. Multiplex PCR for rapid diagnosis of gastrointestinal tuberculosis. J Global Infect Dis. 2013;5(2):49. https://doi.org/10.4103/0974-777x.112272.

39. Leder RA, Low VHS. Tuberculosis of the abdomen. Radiol Clin North Am. 1995;33(4):691–705. https://doi.org/10.1016/s0033-8389(22)00613-3.

40. Nagi B, Kochhar R, Bhasin DK, Singh K. Colorectal tuberculosis. Eur Radiol. 2003;13(8):1907–12. https://doi.org/10.1007/s00330-002-1409-z.

41. Torres HA, Kontoyiannis DP, Bodey GP, Adachi JA, Luna MA, Tarrand JJ, et al. Gastrointestinal cytomegalovirus disease in patients with cancer: A two decade experience in a tertiary care cancer center. Eur J Cancer. 2005;41(15):2268–79. https://doi.org/10.1016/j.ejca.2005.07.011.

42. Haessler S, Granowitz EV. Norovirus gastroenteritis in immunocompromised patients. New Engl J Med. 2013;368(10):971. https://doi.org/10.1056/nejmc1301022.

43. Tajiri H, Kiyohara Y, Tanaka T, Etani Y, Mushiake S. Abnormal computed tomography findings among children with viral gastroenteritis and symptoms mimicking acute appendicitis. Pediatr Emergency Care. 2008;24(9):601–4. https://doi.org/10.1097/pec.0b013e3181850cc8.

44. Finkelstone L, Wolf E, Stein MW. Etiology of small bowel thickening on computed tomography. Can J Gastroenterol. 2012;26(12):897–901. https://doi.org/10.1155/2012/282603.

45. Caruso D, Zerunian M, Pucciarelli F, Lucertini E, Bracci B, Polidori T, et al. Imaging of abdominal complications of COVID-19 infection. BJR Open. 2021;2(1):20200052. https://doi.org/10.1259/bjro.20200052.

46. Rha SE, Ha HK, Lee S-H, Kim J-H, Kim J-K, Kim JH, et al. CT and MR imaging findings of bowel ischemia from various primary causes. RadioGraphics. 2000;20(1):29–42. https://doi.org/10.1148/radiographics.20.1.g00ja0629.

47. Ignat M, Philouze G, Aussenac-Belle L, Faucher V, Collange O, Mutter D, et al. Small bowel ischemia and SARS-CoV-2 infection: an underdiagnosed distinct clinical entity. Surgery. 2020;168(1):14–6. https://doi.org/10.1016/j.surg.2020.04.035.

48. Pautrat K, Chergui N. SARS-CoV-2 infection may result in appendicular syndrome: chest CT scan before appendectomy. J Visceral Surg. 2020;157(3):S63–S4. https://doi.org/10.1016/j.jviscsurg.2020.04.007.

49. Lamps LW, Lai KKT, Milner DA. Fungal infections of the gastrointestinal tract in the immunocompromised host. Adv Anatomic Pathol. 2014;21(4):217–27. https://doi.org/10.1097/pap.0000000000000016.

50. Friedman S. Emerging fungal infections: new patients, new patterns, and new pathogens. J Fungi. 2019;5(3):67. https://doi.org/10.3390/jof5030067.

51. Yeom DH, Oh HJ, Son YW, Kim TH. What are the risk factors for acute suppurative cholangitis caused by common bile duct stones? Gut Liver. 2010;4(3):363–7. https://doi.org/10.5009/gnl.2010.4.3.363.

52. Prescott RJ, Harris M, Banerjee SS. Fungal infections of the small and large intestine. J Clin Pathol. 1992;45(9):806–11. https://doi.org/10.1136/jcp.45.9.806.

53. Talwani R, Gilliam BL, Howell C. Infectious diseases and the liver. Clin Liver Dis. 2011;15(1):111–30. https://doi.org/10.1016/j.cld.2010.09.002.

54. Park HJ, Kim SH, Jang KM, Lee SJ, Park MJ, Choi D. Differentiating hepatic abscess from malignant mimickers: value of diffusion-weighted imaging with an emphasis on the periphery of the lesion. J Magn Reson Imaging. 2013;38(6):1333–41. https://doi.org/10.1002/jmri.24112.

55. Lübbert C, Wiegand J, Karlas T. Therapy of liver abscesses. Visceral Med. 2014;30(5):334–41. https://doi.org/10.1159/000366579.

56. Cornely OA, Bangard C, Jaspers NI. Hepatosplenic candidiasis. Clin Liver Dis. 2015;6(2):47–50. https://doi.org/10.1002/cld.491.

57. Moore NJE, Leef JL, Pang Y. Systemic candidiasis. RadioGraphics. 2003;23(5):1287–90. https://doi.org/10.1148/rg.235025162.

58. Bächler P, Baladron MJ, Menias C, Beddings I, Loch R, Zalaquett E, et al. Multimodality imaging of liver infections: differential diagnosis and potential pitfalls. RadioGraphics. 2016;36(4):1001–23. https://doi.org/10.1148/rg.2016150196.

59. Ely R, Long B, Koyfman A. The emergency medicine–focused review of cholangitis. J Emergency Med. 2018;54(1):64–72. https://doi.org/10.1016/j.jemermed.2017.06.039.

60. Patel NB, Oto A, Thomas S. Multidetector CT of emergent biliary pathologic conditions. RadioGraphics. 2013;33(7):1867–88. https://doi.org/10.1148/rg.337125038.

61. Xu Z, Shi L, Wang Y, Zhang J, Huang L, Zhang C, et al. Pathological findings of COVID-19 associated with acute respiratory distress syndrome. Lancet Respir Med. 2020;8(4):420–2. https://doi.org/10.1016/s2213-2600(20)30076-x.

62. Behzad S, Aghaghazvini L, Radmard AR, Gholamrezanezhad A. Extrapulmonary manifestations of COVID-19: radiologic and clinical overview. Clin Imaging. 2020;66:35–41. https://doi.org/10.1016/j.clinimag.2020.05.013.

63. Mortelé KJ, Segatto E, Ros PR. The infected liver: radiologic-pathologic correlation. RadioGraphics. 2004;24(4):937–55. https://doi.org/10.1148/rg.244035719.

64. Doyle DJ, Hanbidge AE, O'Malley ME. Imaging of hepatic infections. Clin Radiol. 2006;61(9):737–48. https://doi.org/10.1016/j.crad.2006.03.010.

65. Brunetti E, Kern P, Vuitton DA. Expert consensus for the diagnosis and treatment of cystic and alveolar echinococcosis in humans. Acta Tropica. 2010;114(1):1–16. https://doi.org/10.1016/j.actatropica.2009.11.001.

66. Pedrosa I, Saíz A, Arrazola J, Ferreirós J, Pedrosa CS. Hydatid disease: radiologic and pathologic features and complications. RadioGraphics. 2000;20(3):795–817. https://doi.org/10.1148/radiographics.20.3.g00ma06795.

67. Mehta P, Prakash M, Khandelwal N. Radiological manifestations of hydatid disease and its complications. Trop Parasitol. 2016;6(2):103. https://doi.org/10.4103/2229-5070.190812.

68. Heyns CF. Urinary tract infection associated with conditions causing urinary tract obstruction and stasis, excluding urolithiasis and neuropathic bladder. World J Urol. 2011;30(1):77–83. https://doi.org/10.1007/s00345-011-0725-9.

69. Chitale SV, Scott-Barrett S, Ho ETS, Burgess NA. The management of ureteric obstruction secondary to malignant pelvic disease. Clin Radiol. 2002;57(12):1118–21. https://doi.org/10.1053/crad.2002.1114.

70. Falagas ME, Vergidis PI. Urinary tract infections in patients with urinary diversion. Am J Kidney Dis. 2005;46(6):1030–7. https://doi.org/10.1053/j.ajkd.2005.09.008.

71. Orlowski HLP, McWilliams S, Mellnick VM, Bhalla S, Lubner MG, Pickhardt PJ, et al. Imaging spectrum of invasive fungal and fungal-like infections. RadioGraphics. 2017;37(4):1119–34. https://doi.org/10.1148/rg.2017160110.

72. Lee SH, Jung HJ, Mah SY, Chung BH. Renal abscesses measuring 5 cm or less: outcome of medical treatment without therapeutic drainage. Yonsei Med J. 2010;51(4):569. https://doi.org/10.3349/ymj.2010.51.4.569.

73. Ackerman AL, Parameshwar PS, Anger JT. Diagnosis and treatment of patients with prostatic abscess in the post-antibiotic era. Int J Urol. 2017;25(2):103–10. https://doi.org/10.1111/iju.13451.

74. Sartelli M. A focus on intra-abdominal infections. World J Emergency Surg. 2010;5(1):9. https://doi.org/10.1186/1749-7922-5-9.

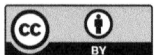

Advances in Molecular Imaging and Therapy and Its Impact in Oncologic Imaging

3

Irene A. Burger and Thomas A. Hope

Learning Objectives
- To understand the theranostic concept and the potential differences between alpha and beta therapy.
- To know about the advantages and limitations of receptor PET-based patient selection.
- Review the developing role of PET-based response assessment.
- To learn about the evidence, pearls and pitfalls of morphology-based response assessment.
- To introduce the role of combining DWI with receptor targeted PET in patient evaluation.

3.1 Introduction

With the introduction of the combination of anatomical imaging with CT and molecular imaging based on positron emission tomography (PET) in the early 2000, there was a steady increase in clinical applications in oncology. The most commonly used tracer is fluorodeoxyglucose [^{18}F]-FDG, taken up by cells with high expression of insulin-independent glucose transporter (GLUT1, 2, or 3), if the patient was fasting for at least 4 h. GLUT expression, however, is also increased in a variety of inflammatory lesions, reducing the specificity. Despite intensive research for a more specific tracer for malignant tissue compared to FDG [1, 2] the high sensitivity was still not reached by any other approach for lymphomas and most solid tumors. Only for tumors with a usually low metabolic activity (neuroendocrine tumors (NET) and prostate cancer (PCa)), alternative approaches based on receptor-based imaging have been established: targeting the prostate-specific membrane antigen (PSMA) for PCa and somatostatin receptor 2 (SSTR-2) imaging for NET. These targets are currently also in the focus of a theranostic approach; we would like to focus in the first part of this chapter. The second part will be focused on response assessment with both morphologic and molecular imaging in general and for specific therapeutic approaches.

3.2 Introduction to Theranostics

Theranostics refers to the use of molecules for both imaging and therapy. Although this was originally developed over 75 years ago with the introduction of iodine therapy (I-123 for imaging and I-131 for treatment), it was the development of SSTR-2 targeted imaging agents and subsequent therapy, which led to the renewed focus on radioligand therapies (RLTs). In general, most theranostic agents have a ligand that targets a protein overexpressed on the surface of a tumor. These ligands are then labeled with either a radionuclide used for imaging or a radionuclide used for therapy. The most common imaging radionuclides used clinically for theranostics are positron emitting (β^+) used in PET and include fluorine-18, gallium-68, and copper-64. Although gamma emitters (γ) can also be used, including technetium-99m and indium-111, the field has focused on PET radiopharmaceuticals. Radionuclides for therapy are broken down into alpha (α) and beta (β^-) emitters. Beta emitters, which emit an electron, include yttrium-90, lutetium-177, and iodine-131. Alpha emitters, which emit a helium atom, include actinium-225, lead-212, and radium-223.

Theranostics is considered a personalized therapy, as patients are selected using the imaging study to demonstrate the presence of the target, before the treatment is administered.

I. A. Burger (✉)
Department of Nuclear Medicine, Kantonsspital Baden, Baden, Aarau, Switzerland
e-mail: Irene.burger@ksb.ch

T. A. Hope
Department of Radiology and Biomedical Imaging, University of California, San Francisco, San Francisco, CA, USA
e-mail: Thomas.Hope@ucsf.edu

© The Author(s) 2023
J. Hodler et al. (eds.), *Diseases of the Abdomen and Pelvis 2023-2026*, IDKD Springer Series,
https://doi.org/10.1007/978-3-031-27355-1_3

This allows one to have some understanding of how patients will respond to treatment. For example, in patients with prostate cancer, higher uptake on the pre-treatment PSMA PET have a better response to PSMA-targeted RLT [3].

3.2.1 Therapeutic Radionuclides

There are many factors that influence which radionuclide groups use for RLT, including half-life, chemistry, and the distance the emitted particle travels. Having a half-life that enables central synthesis and distribution is critical for commercialization and is why radionuclides such as astatine-211, with its 7 h half-life, is not frequently utilized. Lutetium-177 has a 6.6-day half-life, allowing for central synthesis. The distance the emitted particle is also important and impacts treatment efficacy. Yttrium-90 emits a beta particle that travels over 1 cm, while the lutetium-177 beta particle travels between 1 and 2 mm. This means that yttrium-90 would be better at treating larger lesions than lutetium-177 and may explain the higher rate of renal toxicity with yttrium-90 that has been reported [4]. Alpha particles have a very high energy but deposit their doses over a much shorter distance, typically 50–70 micrometers. This shorter range has led some to believe that alpha particles might be able to kill single cells, but it must be remembered that the majority of the energy is deposited at the Bragg peak, at the end of the path, so the deposited energy is mostly 1 to 2 cells away from the cell of origin. Nonetheless, there is considerable interest in alpha particles given their potential for higher efficacy due to the high energy deposition [5–7]. There is currently one Phase III study evaluating [^{225}Ac]-DOTATATE in patients with gastroenteropancreatic (GEP) neuroendocrine tumors (NETs) (NCT05477576).

Key Points

The currently most commonly used radionuclide for RLT is Lutetium-177—a beta emitting nuclide with a half-life of 6.6 days. Yttrium-90, also a beta emitter, has a higher energy and could be used for larger lesions, or targets with more distance (spheres). And Actinium-225 is an alpha emitting nuclide, with the potential of higher efficacy but also more potential side effects.

3.2.2 Unique Role of Dosimetry

One unique aspect of many RLTs is that they can be directly imaged after treatment in order to measure the actual dose deposited in the tumors. Although this is also true for I-131 in

thyroid cancer, it was performed infrequently with thyroid patients. Of particular interest is lutetium-177, which has a 12% gamma emission, allowing for high quality post-treatment images. As software is developed that makes quantifying dosimetry more streamlined, it is hoped that this approach will be incorporated into clinical practice. Currently, post-treatment imaging is used mostly qualitatively to determine if there has been evidence of progression or response, rather than to modulate administered activity based on measured dosimetry from the previously administered cycle. It should be noted that alpha emitters such as actinium-225 are difficult to image using SPECT/CT due to their low gamma emissions and much lower administered activities. There is significant work underway to try to improve our ability to image alpha emitters.

3.2.3 Current Theranostic Agents and Agents in Development

There are two major applications for theranostics in clinic today: [^{177}Lu]-DOTATATE (Lutathera, Novartis) and [^{177}Lu]-PSMA-617 (Pluvicto, Novartis) RLT. [^{177}Lu]-DOTATATE targets the SSTR in patients with NETs and is used in patients who progress after somatostatin analog therapy. [^{177}Lu]-DOTATOC is a nearly identical agent, which is currently being evaluated in two Phase III trials (NCT03049189 and NCT04919226). Yttrium-90 labeled compounds have been evaluated but have been largely replaced with lutetium-177 labeled compounds. [^{177}Lu]-PSMA-617 targets PSMA in patients with metastatic castration-resistant prostate cancer (mCRPC) and was shown to prolong life in patients after chemotherapy and androgen receptor targeted therapies in the VISION trial [8]. [^{177}Lu]-PSMA-I&T is a similar compound currently being evaluated in two Phase III studies in the pre-chemotherapy mCRPC setting (NCT05204927 and NCT04647526). [^{177}Lu]-PSMA-617 is also being evaluated in the metastatic castration-sensitive setting (NCT04720157).

There are a number of exciting targets outside of PSMA which are currently being evaluated. Radioligands targeting the fibroblast activation protein (FAP) are of interest, as the target is expressed across multiple cancer types rather than being specific to a cancer like SSTR and PSMA. There is limited evidence of efficacy to date with small retrospective series published to date [9, 10]. [^{177}Lu]-FAP-2286 is being evaluated in a dose expansion Phase I trial (NCT04939610). Other targets in evaluation includes the gastrin-releasing peptide receptor [11], C-X-C motif chemokine receptor 4 (CXCR4) [12, 13] and urokinase-type plasminogen activator receptor (uPAR) [14]. It is unclear if any of these compounds will have the clinical impact of SSTR and PSMA-targeted RLTs, but there is considerable investment being made in the field.

3.2.4 Patient Selection for Internal Radiotherapy

The use of the targeted imaging to select patients for RLT has been adopted very early on. The NETTER trial that lead to the approval for [177Lu]-DOTATATE for midgut NET selected patients with well-differentiated tumors Grade 1-2 and high uptake based on SSTR-scintigraphy [15]. The concensus statement by the North American Neuroendocrine Tumor Society (NANETS) and the Society of Nuclear Medicine and Molecular Imaging (SNMMI) agreed that positivity on SSTR imaging is defined as an intensity in uptake in sites of disease that exceeds the normal liver for both imaging modalities [111In]-pentetreotide single-photon emission computer tomography (SPECT) or [68Ga]-DOTATATE PET [16]. However, already for neuro-endocrine disease several authors suggested that imaging the target is fundamental, but not enough [17]. Tumor heterogeneity and dedifferentiation in the course of a malignant disease lead to tumor parts that lost the expression of the target, and therefore cannot be detected by the receptor PET. Therefore, a combination with FDG PET/CT is suggested, in patients with only faint uptake or negative lesions on [68Ga]-DOTATATE [18].

Also the VISION trial leading to the approval for [177Lu]-PSMA-617 used the corresponding [68Ga]-PSMA-11 PET scan for patient selection [8]. Eligible patients had PSMA-positive metastatic lesions and no PSMA-negative lesions; PSMA-positive status was defined as uptake greater than that of liver parenchyma in one or more metastatic lesions of any size in any organ system. Given that based on these criteria only 12% of the patients were excluded due to PET criteria, the discussion was opened, if the costs of [68Ga]-PSMA-11 PET are justified and needed, if the patient exclusion is so low. On the contrary, given that bone metastasis are often not well seen on CT, the additional value of FDG PET/CT might even be higher for PCa than NET patients. Preliminary results for studies selecting patients based on [68Ga]-PSMA-11 and FDG PET showed indeed a slightly higher PSA response rate compared to the VISION trial (TheraP: 65%, compared to VISION: 46%) [19]. Follow-up data on the TheraP trial now published further support that patients with an SUVmean ≥10 on PSMA PET had an excellent response to [177Lu]-PSMA-617, while patients with FDG active disease larger than ≥200 mL did worse in both arms (Cabazitaxel and [177Lu]-PSMA-617), indicating that the combination of metabolic and receptor PET information might be a good way to tailor therapy intensity in the future [3].

3.3 Monitoring Disease

The World Health Organization (WHO) recognized the need for standardized criteria across clinical trials very early, publishing the initial "WHO handbook for reporting results of cancer treatment" in 1979 [20]. Since then, a number of guidelines and updates have been published.

3.3.1 Response Based on Morphology

The most commonly applied response criteria for systemic disease are Response Evaluation Criteria In Solid Tumors (RECIST) that have been updated to RECIST 1.1 [21]. Based on the changes of target and non-target lesions patients are categorized in four groups: complete response (CR), partial response (PR), stable disease (SD), and progressive disease (PD) (Table 3.1). To simplify readouts only five target lesions (TL), maximum two in the same organ, are assessed by the maximum diameter. Lymph nodes are measured by the short axis and need to be larger than 1.5 cm to be considered as target lesions. Sclerotic bone lesions are considered non-target lesions (NTL), as well as cystic lesions, if they do not have large solid components. The sum of all diameters from TLs need to decrease more than 30% to be considered as a partial response or increase by 20% (more than 5 mm) to indicate progressive disease.

3.3.2 Response Based on Morphology for Immunotherapy

Chemotherapies directly kill tumor cells leading to shrinkage of tumor volume depending on the efficacy of the therapy. Immunotherapies activate the immune system of the patient with different response patterns depending on the mechanism of drug action [22]. Morphologic response after immunotherapy will often need more time compared to conventional therapies due to an initial increase in volume due to infiltration of inflammatory cells into the tumor (Fig. 3.1).

Table 3.1 Response according to RECIST1.1

Response	RECIST 1.1
PD	Increase of TL diameters by ≥20% (with at least an increase of 5 mm), progressive NTL, new lesions.
SD	No PR or PD
PR	Decrease of TL diameters by ≥30%, no new lesions.
CR	Disappearance of all extranodal TLs, all LN <1 cm, no progressive NTL, normalization of tumor marker

For accurate interpretation of the response pattern, understanding of the drug mechanism is crucial. Therapeutics leading to an increasing migration of T-cells into the tumor (CTLA-4 blocking, e.g., Ipilimumab) will be more likely to have an initial increase in tumor size [23]. iRECIST is based on RECIST 1.1 to select TL and NTL, if however PD is seen on first follow-up, this is inter-preted as iUPD (Unconfirmed Progressive Disease), only if tumor increase of more than 30% is confirmed on the second follow-up (4–8 weeks later) a confirmed progression iCPD will be noted (Fig. 3.2). If the tumor remains stable, iUPD will remain the interpretation and only if criteria for partial or complete response are met, iPR or iCR will be given [22].

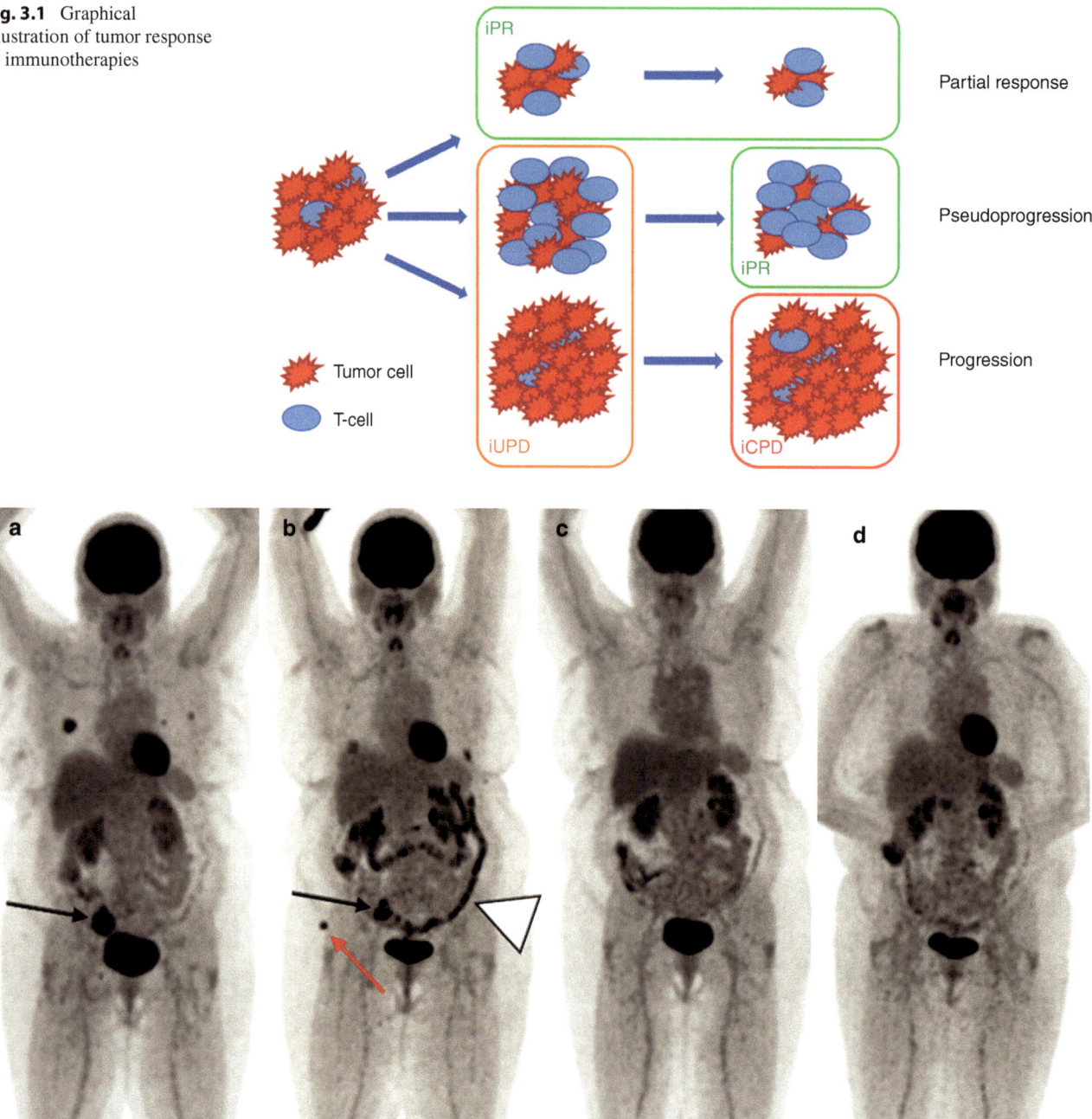

Fig. 3.1 Graphical illustration of tumor response to immunotherapies

Fig. 3.2 Maximum intensity projection (MIP) images in a patient with melanoma treated with nivolumab. Baseline imaging demonstrates a peritoneal nodal that resolves at the first time point (black arrow, **a** and **b**). A new lesion is seen at the 3-month PET (**b**, red arrow) which is consistent with unconfirmed progressive disease (iUPD). All diseases resolve on subsequent imaging (**c**, **d**). Note that the patient developed immune-related colitis (**b**, white arrowhead)

Key Points
Initial progression after start of immunotherapy has to be confirmed after 4–8 weeks to distinguish pseudo-progression from confirmed progression.

Besides accurate interpretation of early pseudoprogression, the recognition of immune-related response (irR) is crucial as well. Inflammatory changes can result in activation of sarcoidosis with enlarged lymph nodes (Fig. 3.3) or adrenalitis with enlarged suprarenal glands. This is not only challenging for morphologic imaging but also for PET/CT since irR can show intensive ^{18}F-fluorodeoxyglucose (FDG) uptake [23]. Immunotherapies are already a clinically established option for patients with melanoma or lung cancer. However, more indications also for abdominal diseases will follow soon, such as prostate cancer (Sipuleucel-T), kidney cancer (nivolumab), or bladder cancer (pembrolizumab).

3.3.3 Response Based on FDG PET

Numerous publications showed a good correlation between the decrease in ^{18}F-FDG accumulation in tumor lesions and therapy response [24]. Therefore, PET response evaluation was postulated, including EORTC PET response recommendations (1999) and the PET response criteria in solid tumors (PERCIST) pioneered by Wahl et al. in 2009 [25]. Both methods follow the model of RECIST with four adapted response categories: complete metabolic response (CMR), partial metabolic response (PMR), stable metabolic disease (SMD), and progressive metabolic disease (PMD). Numerous studies compared the original EORTC PET criteria with PERCIST showing similar results (Table 3.2). However, the use of PERCIST seems preferable for clinical trials due to a better standardization [26]. Both methods recommend the use of standardized uptake values (SUV) normalized to the lean body mass (SUL). However, if possible PERCIST favors the use of an SUL_{peak} (average value in the hottest 1cm^3 sphere within the tumor), instead of SUL_{max} (only one maximum voxel) to reduce the intrinsic variability.

Despite all these efforts, one has to recognize that PERCIST assessment has not been used to evaluate response in clinical trials yet. As a primary or secondary endpoint for prospective studies, we still rely on morphologic imaging.

It is important to note that all these recommendations are focusing on ^{18}F-FDG PET for the evaluation of metabolic response of solid tumors. Tumor dedifferentiation does not correlate with receptor expression in the same way like ^{18}F-FDG. Therefore, PERCIST per se is not necessarily applicable for the increasing use of receptor imaging in oncologic diseases, for example, SSTR PET for NETs or PSMA for prostate cancer.

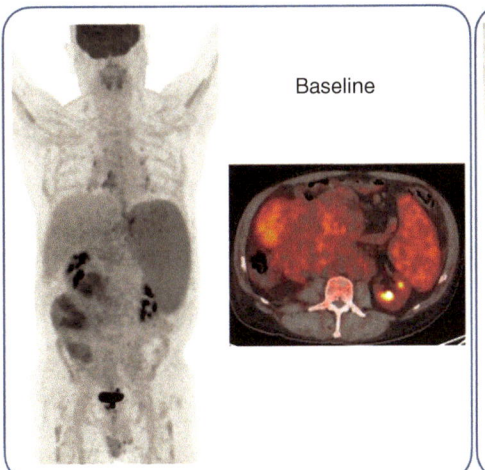 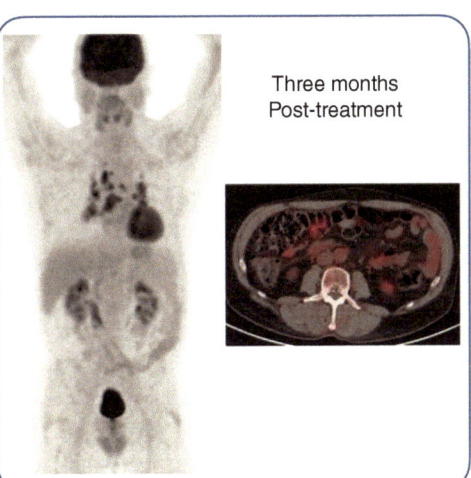

Fig. 3.3 Maximum intensity projection (MIP) images and axial fused images through the mid abdomen in a patient with Mantle Cell Lymphoma treated with pembrolizumab. Baseline imaging demonstrates splenomegaly and a large abdominal mass. Three months after treatment initiation, the has been resolution of the abdominal mass and the splenomegaly, and development of numerous mediastinal hypermetabolic nodes consistent with a sarcoid-like reaction

Baseline

Three months
Post-treatment

Table 3.2 Response according to PERCIST

Response	PERCIST - Based on SUL$_{peak}$ (SUL$_{max}$)
PMD	SUL increase by at least 30% and increase by at least 0.8 SUL units of the target lesion/or increase in target lesion size by 30%/or development of at least one new lesion/or unequivocal progression of non-target lesions.
SMD	Increase or decrease of SUL by less than 30%.
PMR	Decrease of SUL by ≥30% and at least 0.8 SUL units difference/and no new FDG-avid lesions/and no increase in size >30% of the target lesion/and no increase in SUL or size of non-target lesion.
CMR	FDG uptake indistinguishable from surrounding background and SUL less than liver.

3.4   Monitoring Liver Disease After SIRT

Selective internal radiotherapy (SIRT) using yttrium-90 resins or glass microspheres is an increasingly used palliative therapy option for patients with non-resectable primary liver tumors or metastatic hepatic disease. Clinical evaluation of patients prior to SIRT includes contrast-enhanced CT of the chest and the abdomen to rule out extensive extrahepatic disease, liver MRI to assess tumor burden and selective angiography to evaluate vascular anatomy and hepatic shunt with technetium-99m labeled aggregated macroalbumin [^{99m}Tc]-MAA) [27, 28].

3.4.1   Monitoring SIRT with CT/MRI

Early response assessment after SIRT using anatomical imaging can be limited due to delayed reduction in tumor size and initial pseudoprogression due to edema and sharper demarcation of tumor boundaries on conventional imaging (Fig. 3.4). Early investigations with serial ceCT images showed a maximum decrease in tumor size at 3–21 months (median 12 months), concluding that blood tumor markers (e.g., CEA for colorectal metastasis) were superior in therapy response assessment compared to ceCT [28].

The calculation of arterial perfusion (AP) using dynamic contrast-enhanced CT prior to SIRT was the best predictor for good treatment response and overall survival in patients [29]. Furthermore, follow-up perfusion CT showed a significant decrease of AP in hepatic metastasis 4 weeks after SIRT in patients with long-term response, compared to non-

responders [30]. Dual-energy CT is a new technology, allowing the creation of iodine maps as promising tools to evaluate and quantify tumor viability, utilizing iodine maps measuring the amount of iodine per lesion. Although this approach requires validation and standardization, it showed promising first results for hepatic radiofrequency ablation [31] and could also be a promising tool for SIRT therapy response assessment.

Functional MRI was suggested to be used to assess response to SIRT, as well. A post-therapeutic increase in ADC$_{min}$ of more than 22%, 4 weeks after SIRT was significantly associated with a superior overall survival (18 vs. 5 months, $p < 0.001$), while tumor size did not show any significant decrease after 4 weeks [32].

3.4.2   Monitoring SIRT with PET

Early on FDG PET was used to assess the reduction of hepatic metastatic load after SIRT [33]. Such studies displayed superior early response assessment with FDG PET/CT compared to ceCT [34, 35]. Other groups investigated the PET-based volume-metrics such as the metabolic tumor volume (MTV) or the total lesion glycolysis rate (TLG) and came to the conclusion that those parameters correlate better with outcome compared to plain tumor size or SUV$_{max}$[36]. For accurate response assessment with FDG PET potential pitfalls have to be considered. To name the two most prominent limitations: False-negative results caused by partial volume effects in small lesions (<1 cm) or diabetes and false-positive results caused by abscess formation or inflammatory changes [37]. However, a combination of FDG PET/CT with ceCT can solve most of these limitations.

Despite the fact that earlier prediction of response to SIRT with FDG PET is possible, there is no established clinical role for FDG PET in assessing tumor response after SIRT. This might be attributable to a lack of additional treatment options. Therefore, early knowledge of a limited response to this palliative therapy will change treatment only in very few cases. Nevertheless, it is crucial to know the potential limitations and possibilities of the various imaging modalities to prevent false interpretation of early morphologic changes in the accurate judgment of therapeutic response.

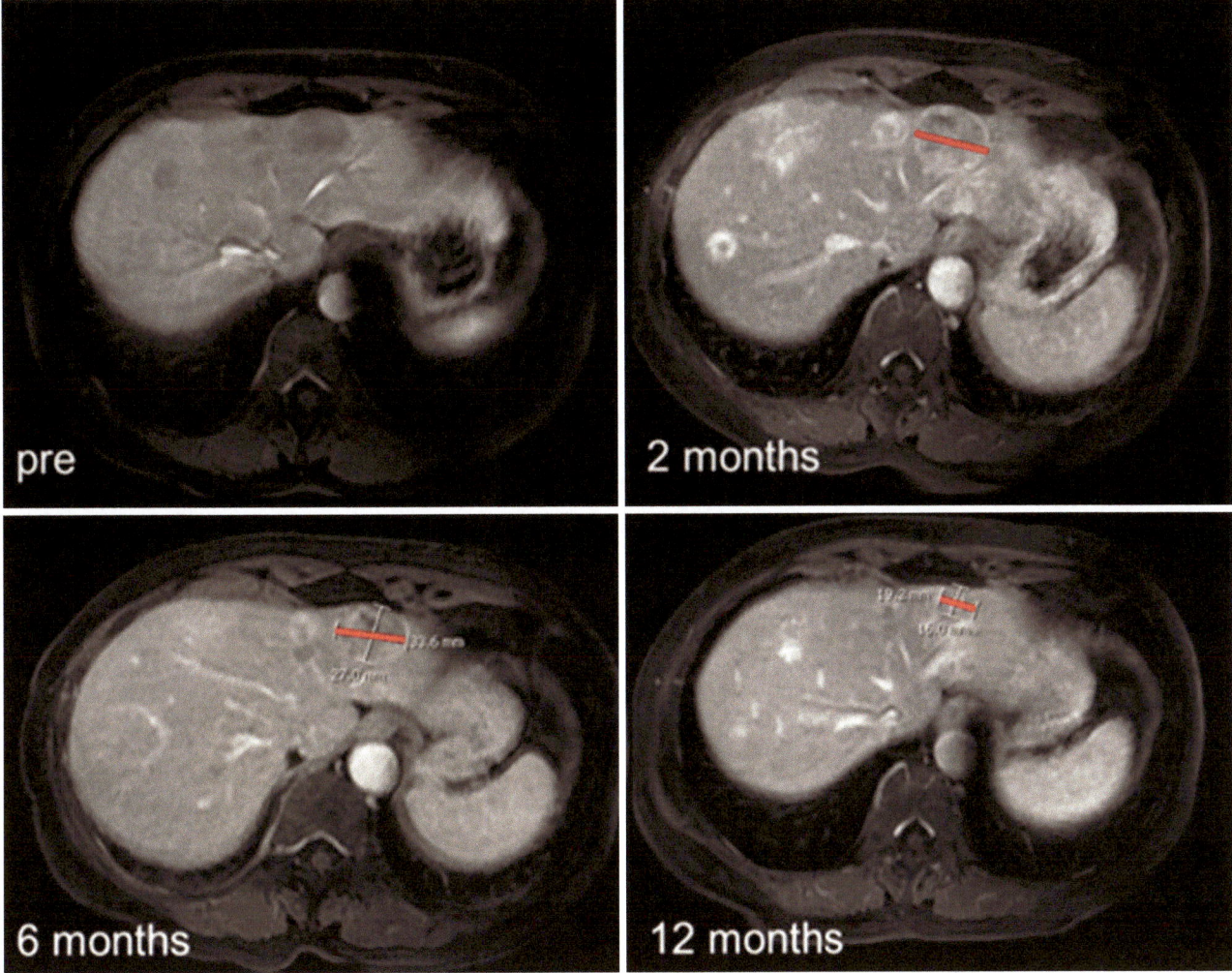

Fig. 3.4 Axial post-contrast MRI before, and 2, 6, and 12 months after SIRT therapy, showing the long standing pseudoprogression over 6 months, with improved delineation of metastases on the first scan after SIRT and final partial morphologic response after 12 months

3.5 Monitoring Neuroendocrine Tumors

NETs are a heterogeneous tumor type classified based on their grade and their site of origin. Grade is broken into three categories: Grade 1 referring to well-differentiated tumors with a Ki-67 less than 2, Grade 2 for well-differentiated tumors with a Ki-67 between 3 and 20, and Grade 3 for poorly differentiated tumors with a Ki-67 greater than 20. Recently, Grade 3 has been broken down into well differentiated and poorly differentiated tumors. The most common site of origin for NETs are the small bowel and the pancreas. Prior to the approval of [177Lu]-DOTATATE, somatostatin analogs (SSAs), and everolimus were used for small bowel NETs, and SSAs, everolimus, sunitinib, and capecitabine/temozolomide for pancreatic NETs. Everolimus is also indicated for the treatment of bronchial NETs. It should be noted that in all clinical trials for NETs, the primary endpoint has been progression-free survival using RECIST-based evaluation.

The NETTER-1 trial investigated the efficacy of peptide receptor radionuclide therapy (PRRT) with [177Lu]-DOTATATE compared to 60 mg of sandostatin. The primary endpoint was progression-free survival where was defined as primary endpoint documented with either CT or MRI. An

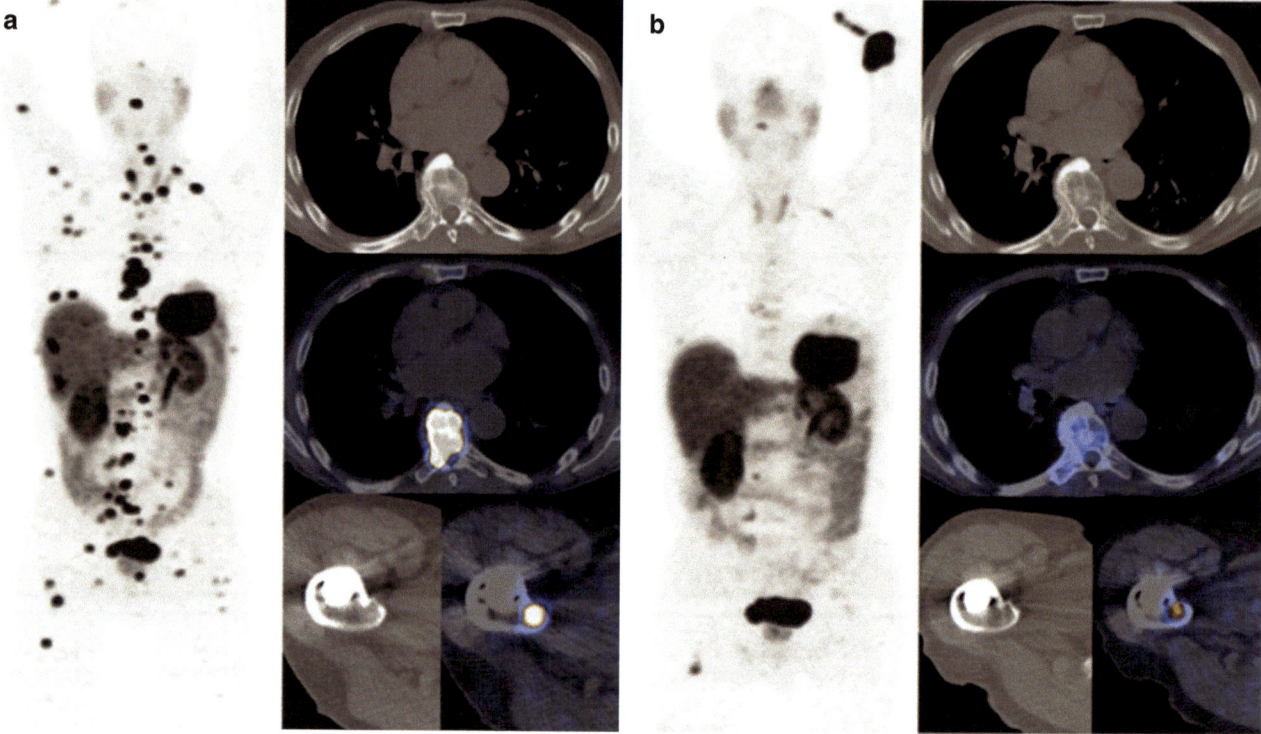

Fig. 3.5 ^{68}Ga-DOTATATE MIP images of a patient before (**a**) and 12 months after (**b**) PRRT with ^{177}Lu-Dotatate. Not the excellent response of most of the bone metastasis to therapy, without significant changes on CT

increase of progression-free survival fraction from 10.8% in the sandostatin arm to 65.2% with [^{177}Lu]-DOTATATE was observed at 20 months. One important issue with NETs is that the disease can be slow growing, particularly in Grade 1 and 2 patients, and therefore the detection of small changes in tumor volume can be clinically significant although hard to tell. Because of the slow growth in disease, some groups have started to suggest replacing RECIST with tumor growth rate as an endpoint [38]. Due to the slow rate of growth, using the most reproducible imaging modality available is important, and for patients with liver dominant disease hepatobiliary phase MRI is the optimal imaging modality [39].

Similar to SIRT and immunotherapies, the morphologic response can lag significantly behind physiologic changes. Additionally, pseudoprogression can confound interpretation due to edema and improved tumor delineation of liver lesions. This is crucial since progression under therapy is a potential reason to stop current treatment according to the European Neuroendocrine Tumor Society (ENETS) consensus guidelines. Therefore, a harmonization and combination of anatomical and molecular imaging as well as biomarkers was suggested for monitoring PRRT [40]. No standardized procedures have been established yet on how to interpret molecular imaging (e.g., ^{68}Ga-DOTATATE PET/CT) results after PRRT. Only one publication summarizing results of 33 patients undergoing early therapy response assessment with ^{68}Ga-DOTATATE after 1 cycle of PRRT has been published so far. They came to the conclusion that a decrease of the tumor to spleen ratio ($SUV_{T/S}$) correlated well with progression-free survival ($p = 0.002$), while a decrease in SUV_{max} did not reach significance [41] (Fig. 3.5). Therefore at this time, evaluation of response is still base on cross-sectional imaging, and SSTR PET can be acquired 9–12 months after the completion of treatment as a new baseline [16, 42].

3.6 Monitoring Metastasized Prostate Cancer

3.6.1 Conventional Monitoring of Metastasized Prostate Cancer with CT and Bone Scans

Imaging response assessment for prostate cancer is notoriously difficult on anatomical imaging and therefore plays only secondary role for treatment evaluation in new drug trials that commonly focus on overall survival (OS) as primary endpoint instead and for early stages now metastasis-free survival (MFS) as a primary endpoint [43, 44]. For standardized response assessment, the Prostate Cancer Clinical Trials Working Group 3 (PCWG-3) published an updated version in 2016 [45]. The recommendations for extraskeletal disease are still in line with the RECIST 1.1 criteria, with the exception that up to 5 lesions per site (e.g., lung, lymph node, liver) should be measured to address the disease heterogeneity. Lymph nodes are considered measurable with a short axis of ≥1.5 cm and visceral lesions have to be ≥1.0 cm to be considered target lesions. Lymph nodes between 1 and 1.5 cm can be considered malignant but only as non-target lesions. Given that sclerotic lesions can increase under therapy and persist for a long time on CT only lytic lesions ≥1.0 cm can be considered target lesions based on CT. To assess response, bone scans are incorporated into the PCWG-3 assessment. Given that healing bone metastases will initially react with increasing mineralization (Fig. 3.6). This will therefore also increase the activity on ^{99m}Tc-bone scans or ^{18}F-NaF PET/CT, the so called tumor flare, typically lasting for 3 months after therapy but can be seen as late as 6 months after treatment [46]. An initial increase in lesions after 8 weeks on a new therapy is therefore interpreted as a bone flare and progression on bone scans defined only after confirmation of at least 2 new lesions twice (2+2 rule).

Key Points
Sclerotic bone lesions on CT should not be considered as target lesions for response assessment. New sclerotic lesions after therapy change are not considered progressive disease. A confirmation is needed due to the flair phenomenon.

Based on analysis of the data from the PREVAIL trial investigating the effect of enzalutamide in chemotherapy naïve man, Rathkopf et al. not only demonstrate the robustness of the PCWG criteria but also a high positive correlation between rPFS and OS 0.89 by Spearman ρ [47]. Based on this data, several trials now use rPFS based on the PCWG-3 criteria as their primary endpoints including studies for Lu-PSMA-617 [8].

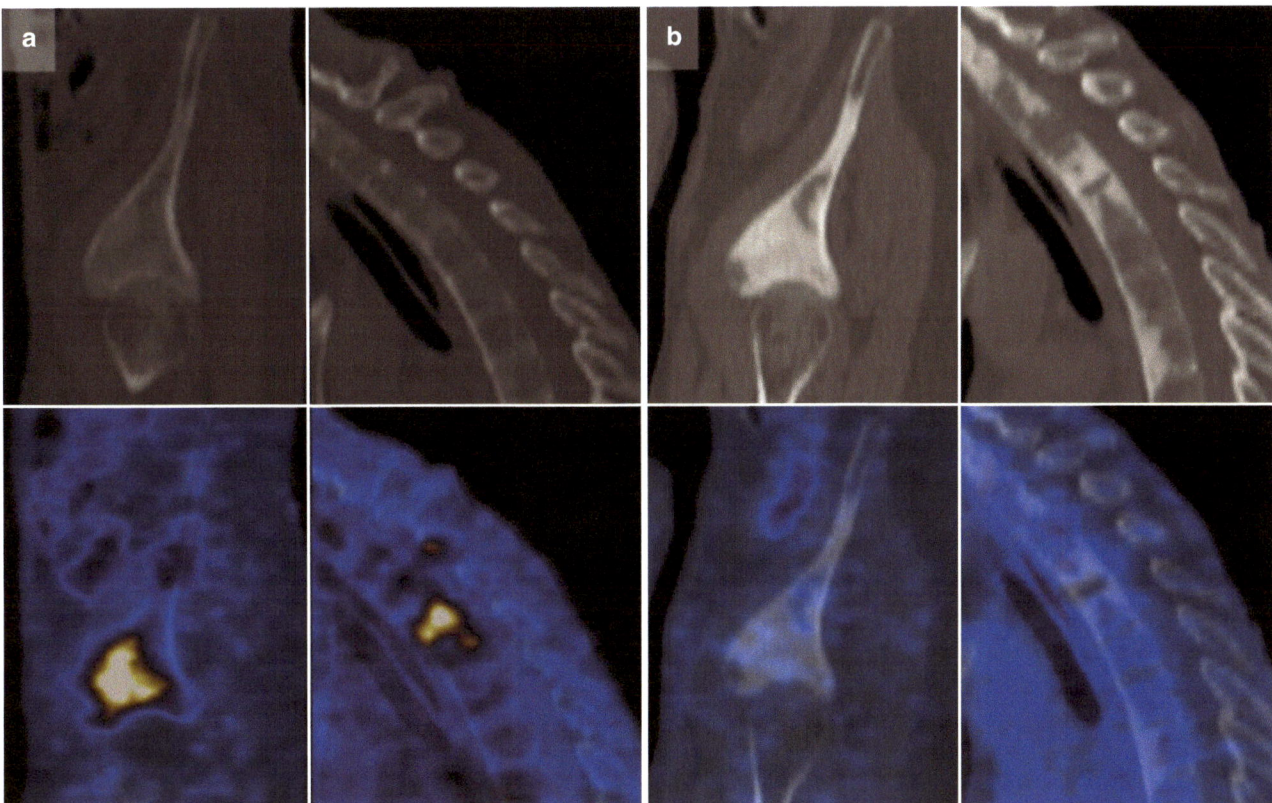

Fig. 3.6 Sagittal CT and PET/CTs of bone metastasis before (**a**) and after (**b**) chemotherapy showing increasing and new sclerotic lesions with a complete decrease on FDG PET consistent with good metabolic response

3.6.2 Monitoring Metastasized Prostate Cancer with PET/CT

The use of FDG PET/CT is very limited in prostate cancer patients since only a small subgroup of highly dedifferentiated tumors will have increased glucose uptake. Assessment of nodal, visceral, and osseous metastasis with one exam is possible with ^{18}F or ^{11}C-Choline or ^{68}Ga-prostate-specific membrane antigen (PSMA) PET/CT. A good correlation between apoptosis and decrease in SUV on ^{11}C-Choline PET/CT scans was shown after neoadjuvant docetaxel chemotherapy and complete androgen blockade in locally advanced prostate cancer patients [48]. The prospective use of Choline PET/CT for response assessment of standardized docetaxel first-line chemotherapy on the other hand showed no correlation between changes in Choline uptake and clinical assessments of progression based on RECIST 1.1 and PSA values [49].

The clinical utility of ^{68}Ga-PSMA PET for treatment response is not established, yet (Fig. 3.7). First investigations showed promising results using ^{68}Ga-PSMA PET to evaluate [223]Ra therapy response [50]. The use of ^{68}Ga-PSMA PET for response assessment to androgen-deprivation therapy (ADT) will need careful prospective evaluation since preliminary invitro results showed that ADT is increasing the cellular expression of PSMA; therefore, a novel "tumor flare" might be observed in these patients [51]. With RECIP 1.0 based on the appearance of new lesions and the change in PSMA-positive tumor volume (+20% for DP and -30% for PR), a simple algorithm was proposed incorporating PSA and PSMA PET information to improve response assessment [52].

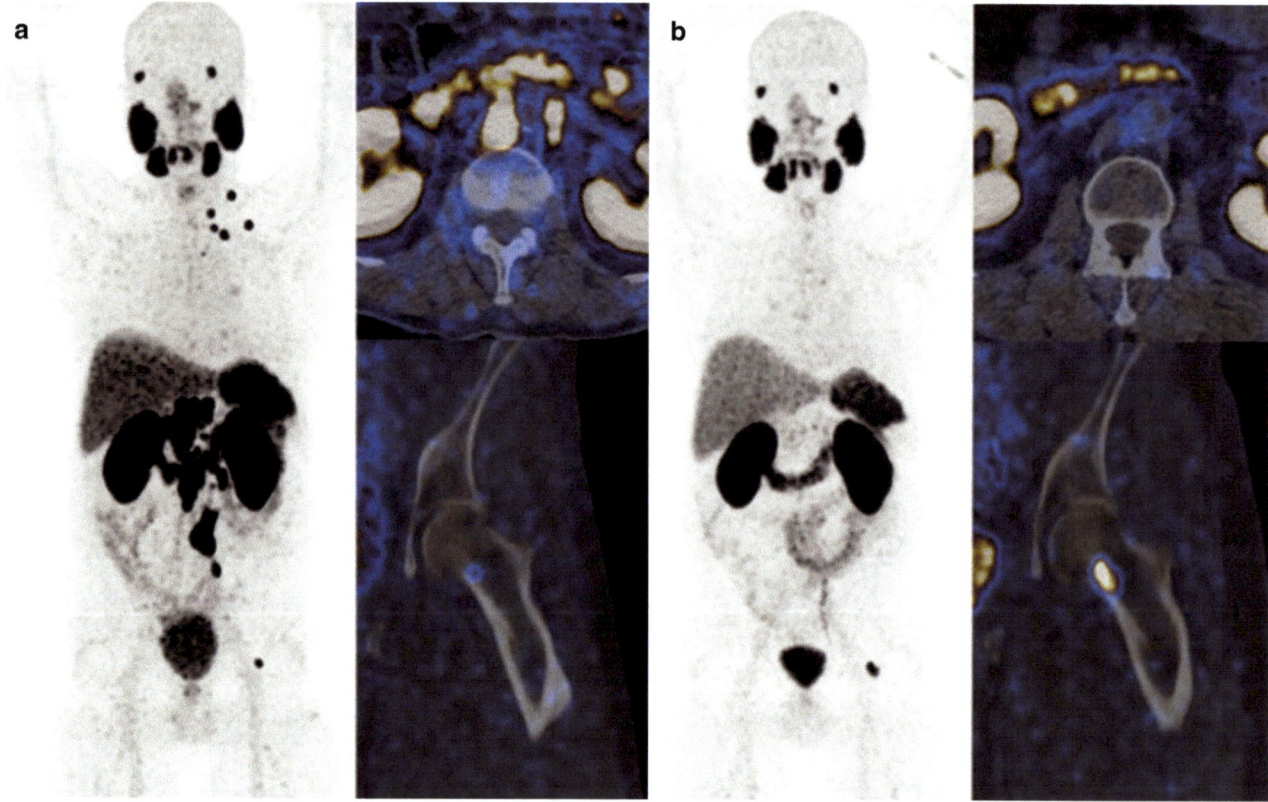

Fig. 3.7 ^{68}Ga-PSMA PET before (**a**) and after (**b**) two cycles of ^{177}Lu-PSMA therapy with heterogeneous response: significant reduction in PSMA expression and size in all lymph node metastasis, however increase in PSMA expression and size of the bone metastasis

3.7   The Role of MRI and PET/MRI for Response Evaluation

There has been historically limited interest in the combination of diffusion-weighted imaging (DWI) and FDG PET in the setting of PET/MRI as restricted diffusion often mirrors elevated metabolism as measured on PET. Therefore when performing an FDG PET/MRI, there is little value in performing DWI. In the setting of theranostics, patients are imaged with targeted radiopharmaceuticals as described above, for example, PSMA- and SSTR-targeted agents. In this setting, there can be additional information from DWI that is not captured with the PET imaging. Additionally, NETs and mCRPC is heterogeneous in its hypermetabolism and diffusion restriction; therefore, MRI can detect disease that is not visualized on PET. For example, in Fig. 3.8, this patient with well-differentiated Grade 3 NET has extensive liver disease that is not FDG positive.

The same is true in prostate cancer. Figure 3.9 shows a patient with innumerable liver metastases imaged using PET/MRI. The lesions have uptake less than the background liver, but are clearly seen on DWI, and so the patient is not a good candidate for PSMA RLT. This is an important approach for patient selection, as patients with PSMA-negative disease can be missed if only PSMA PET is used for screening. The TheraP trial used the combination of FDG and PSMA PET and excluded patients who had FDG-positive/PSMA-negative disease [19]: TheraP a randomized, open-label, Phase II trial. However, it is not always possible to image patients with both PSMA and FDG PET in order to select patients, and therefore an alternative that allows one to visualize PSMA-negative disease is needed. DWI imaging may be able to help replace FDG PET in order to find PSMA-negative disease.

Although this case demonstrates that DWI can detect PSMA-negative disease, the liver is not the main issue, as

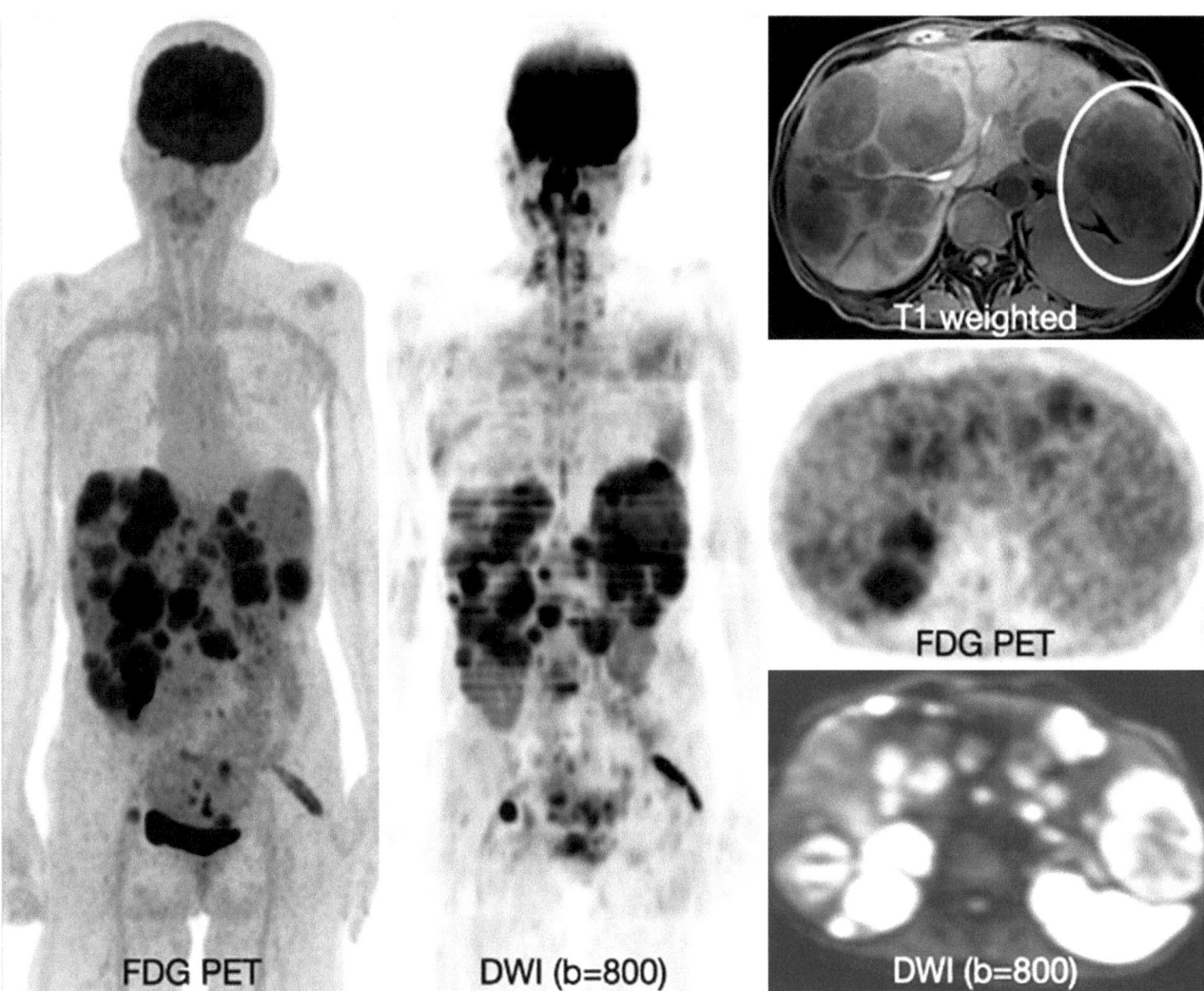

Fig. 3.8   FDG PET/MRI performed in a patient with a well-differentiated G3 NET. FDG PET demonstrates extensive FDG avid liver disease, but DWI demonstrates multiple additional masses in the liver, which do not demonstrate hypermetabolism

cross-sectional imaging can easily evaluate for liver metasta-ses. Much more clinically relevant is bone disease. In PSMA PET, it is difficult to determine if a bone lesion is expressing low levels of PSMA (i.e., PSMA negative) or if the bone lesion has been treated and has a low cellularity. The prior would por-tend a poor outcome, while the latter would not. In Fig. 3.10, you can see how DWI can detect PSMA-negative disease in the bones that would otherwise not be able to be detected.

> **Key Points**
> DWI can be a very helpful tool to determine PSMA-negative disease. Especially for bone lesions, this could be of significant added value since the vitality of these lesions can't be evaluated on CT.

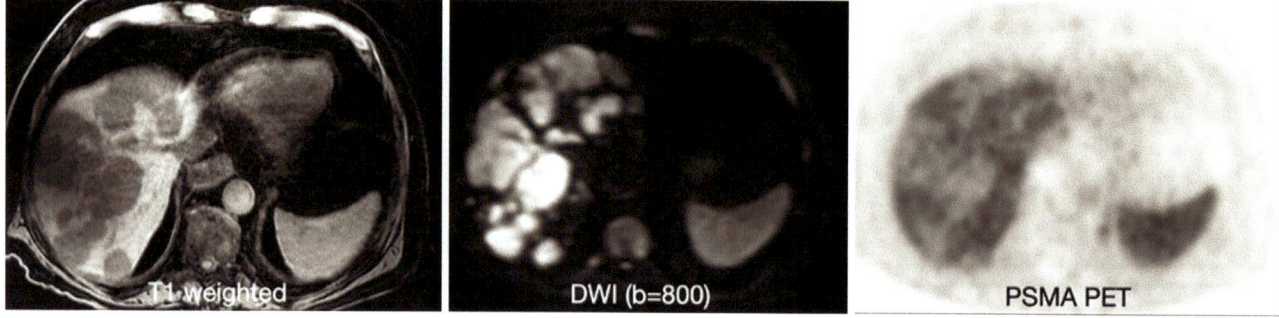

Fig. 3.9 PSMA PET/MRI with whole-body DWI, demonstrate multiple restricting liver lesions on the $b = 800$ image. These lesions do not dem-onstrate uptake on PSMA PET. This patient would not be a good candidate for PSMA RLT

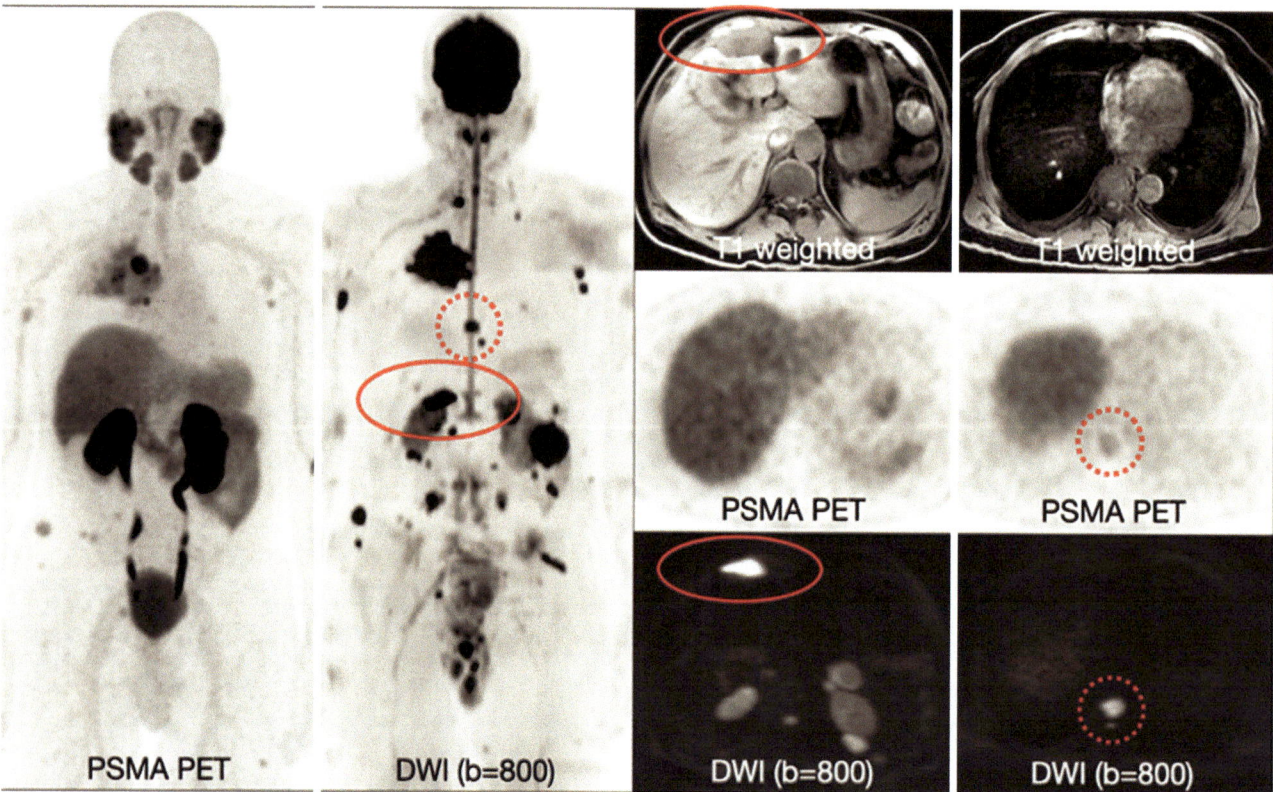

Fig. 3.10 PSMA PET/MRI in a 59-year-old man being evaluated for PSMA RLT. The PSMA PET demonstrates PSMA avid lung disease, but the whole-body DWI demonstrates numerous additional sites of metastatic disease that are not PSMA avid. There is PSMA-negative disease immediate anterior to the liver that markedly restricts diffusion (solid red circle). In particular, note how DWI can detect osseous metastases that is only minimally positive on PSMA PET (dotted red circle)

What may end up being most valuable in terms of using diffusion-weighted imaging for imaging of patients with theranostics is the ability to follow patients over time. In many centers, it is not feasible to image patients using PSMA- or SSTR-PET at multiple timepoints, and moreover, this approach would miss PSMA-negative disease that might develop. In this setting, following patients using whole-body MRI may be preferred. The METastasis Reporting and Data System for Prostate Cancer (MET-RADS-P) has already been developed to use whole-body DWI as response criteria [53]. In addition to assessing anatomic changes for nodal and visceral lesions similar to RECIST, MET-RADS-P incorporates WB DWI as a key imaging technique for evaluating bone response, which has been limited using conventional imaging (e.g., CT and bone scan) [54]. The combined use of targeted PET and whole-body DWI holds significant promise for both patient selection and response assessment in patients undergoing RLT.

3.8 Concluding Remarks

With the introduction of hybrid imaging, the use of different PET tracers to assess metabolism or receptor expression has expanded a lot. The potential to use the same molecules in a second step not only for diagnosis but also therapy is currently generating a novel momentum. The optimal combination of morphologic and molecular information for patient selection for therapy as well as monitoring disease has still to be determined. A profound understanding of the tumor biology as well as imaging possibilities is key for optimal patient care.

> **Take-Home Messages**
> - Systemic therapy response assessment with imaging is generally based on morphology. With the introduction of non-cytotoxic therapies, response patterns became very heterogeneous.
> - Especially immunotherapy or local therapy of liver metastasis such as SIRT can lead to an initial pseudoprogression as a part of the response pattern with delayed morphologic response.
> - In analogy to RECIST, response criteria have been proposed for FDG PET/CT (PERCIST) and shown to correlate with outcome. PERCIST might be a good surrogate marker for response, however until now no clinical prospective trials are based on FDG PET/CT for solid tumors.
> - Morphologic assessment of bone metastasis is only possible for lytic lesions with a soft-tissue component. New sclerotic lesions on CT are not necessarily a sign of tumor progression but might be a sign of response of previously occult lesions.

References

1. Hicks RJ. Beyond FDG: novel PET tracers for cancer imaging. Cancer Imaging. 2003;4:22–4. https://doi.org/10.1102/1470-7330.2003.0032.
2. Burger IA, Zitzmann-Kolbe S, Pruim J, Friebe M, Graham K, Stephens A, et al. First clinical results of (D)-18F-Fluoromethyltyrosine (BAY 86-9596) PET/CT in patients with non-small cell lung cancer and head and neck squamous cell carcinoma. J Nucl Med. 2014;55:1778–85. https://doi.org/10.2967/jnumed.114.140699.
3. Buteau JP, Martin AJ, Emmett L, Iravani A, Sandhu S, Joshua AM, et al. PSMA and FDG-PET as predictive and prognostic biomarkers in patients given [(177)Lu]Lu-PSMA-617 versus cabazitaxel for metastatic castration-resistant prostate cancer (TheraP): a biomarker analysis from a randomised, open-label, phase 2 trial. Lancet Oncol. 2022; https://doi.org/10.1016/S1470-2045(22)00605-2.
4. Bodei L, Kidd M, Paganelli G, Grana CM, Drozdov I, Cremonesi M, et al. Long-term tolerability of PRRT in 807 patients with neuroendocrine tumours: the value and limitations of clinical factors. Eur J Nucl Med Mol Imaging. 2015;42:5–19. https://doi.org/10.1007/s00259-014-2893-5.
5. Ballal S, Yadav MP, Bal C, Sahoo RK, Tripathi M. Broadening horizons with (225)Ac-DOTATATE targeted alpha therapy for gastroenteropancreatic neuroendocrine tumour patients stable or refractory to (177)Lu-DOTATATE PRRT: first clinical experience on the efficacy and safety. Eur J Nucl Med Mol Imaging. 2020;47:934–46. https://doi.org/10.1007/s00259-019-04567-2.
6. Kratochwil C, Bruchertseifer F, Rathke H, Hohenfellner M, Giesel FL, Haberkorn U, et al. Targeted alpha-therapy of metastatic castration-resistant prostate cancer with (225)Ac-PSMA-617: swimmer-plot analysis suggests efficacy regarding duration of tumor control. J Nucl Med. 2018;59:795–802. https://doi.org/10.2967/jnumed.117.203539.
7. Sathekge M, Bruchertseifer F, Vorster M, Lawal IO, Knoesen O, Mahapane J, et al. Predictors of overall and disease-free survival in metastatic castration-resistant prostate cancer patients receiving (225)Ac-PSMA-617 radioligand therapy. J Nucl Med. 2020;61:62–9. https://doi.org/10.2967/jnumed.119.229229.
8. Sartor O, de Bono J, Chi KN, Fizazi K, Herrmann K, Rahbar K, et al. Lutetium-177-PSMA-617 for metastatic castration-resistant prostate cancer. N Engl J Med. 2021;385:1091–103. https://doi.org/10.1056/NEJMoa2107322.
9. Baum RP, Schuchardt C, Singh A, Chantadisai M, Robiller FC, Zhang J, et al. Feasibility, biodistribution, and preliminary dosimetry in peptide-targeted radionuclide therapy of diverse adenocarcinomas using (177)Lu-FAP-2286: first-in-humans results. J Nucl Med. 2022;63:415–23. https://doi.org/10.2967/jnumed.120.259192.
10. Fendler WP, Pabst KM, Kessler L, Fragoso Costa P, Ferdinandus J, Weber M, et al. Safety and efficacy of 90Y-FAPI-46 radioligand therapy in patients with advanced sarcoma and other cancer entities. Clin Cancer Res. 2022;28:4346–53. https://doi.org/10.1158/1078-0432.CCR-22-1432.
11. Dalm SU, Bakker IL, de Blois E, Doeswijk GN, Konijnenberg MW, Orlandi F, et al. 68Ga/177Lu-NeoBOMB1, a novel radiolabeled GRPR antagonist for theranostic use in oncology. J Nucl Med. 2017;58:293–9. https://doi.org/10.2967/jnumed.116.176636.
12. Buck AK, Grigoleit GU, Kraus SK, Schirbel A, Heinsch M, Dreher N, et al. C-X-C motif chemokine receptor 4-targeted radioligand therapy in patients with advanced T-cell lymphoma. J Nucl Med. 2022; https://doi.org/10.2967/jnumed.122.264207.
13. Merkx RIJ, Rijpkema M, Franssen GM, Kip A, Smeets B, Morgenstern A, et al. Carbonic anhydrase IX-targeted alpha-radionuclide therapy with 225Ac inhibits tumor growth in a renal cell carcinoma model. Pharmaceuticals (Basel). 2022;15. https://doi.org/10.3390/ph15050570.

14. Persson M, Juhl K, Rasmussen P, Brandt-Larsen M, Madsen J, Ploug M, et al. uPAR targeted radionuclide therapy with (177) Lu-DOTA-AE105 inhibits dissemination of metastatic prostate cancer. Mol Pharm. 2014;11:2796–806. https://doi.org/10.1021/mp500177c.

15. Strosberg J, El-Haddad G, Wolin E, Hendifar A, Yao J, Chasen B, et al. Phase 3 Trial of (177)Lu-Dotatate for midgut neuroendocrine tumors. N Engl J Med. 2017;376:125–35. https://doi.org/10.1056/NEJMoa1607427.

16. Hope TA, Bodei L, Chan JA, El-Haddad G, Fidelman N, Kunz PL, et al. NANETS/SNMMI consensus statement on patient selection and appropriate use of (177)Lu-DOTATATE peptide receptor radionuclide therapy. J Nucl Med. 2020;61:222–7. https://doi.org/10.2967/jnumed.119.240911.

17. Zhang J, Liu Q, Singh A, Schuchardt C, Kulkarni HR, Baum RP. Prognostic value of (18)F-FDG PET/CT in a large cohort of patients with advanced metastatic neuroendocrine neoplasms treated with peptide receptor radionuclide therapy. J Nucl Med. 2020;61:1560–9. https://doi.org/10.2967/jnumed.119.241414.

18. Kaewput C, Vinjamuri S. Role of combined (68)Ga DOTA-peptides and (18)F FDG PET/CT in the evaluation of gastroenteropancreatic neuroendocrine neoplasms. Diagnostics (Basel). 2022;12. https://doi.org/10.3390/diagnostics12020280.

19. Hofman MS, Emmett L, Sandhu S, Iravani A, Joshua AM, Goh JC, et al. [(177)Lu]Lu-PSMA-617 versus cabazitaxel in patients with metastatic castration-resistant prostate cancer (TheraP): a randomised, open-label, phase 2 trial. Lancet. 2021;397:797–804. https://doi.org/10.1016/S0140-6736(21)00237-3.

20. WHO handbook for reporting results of cancer treatment; 1979.

21. Eisenhauer EA, Therasse P, Bogaerts J, Schwartz LH, Sargent D, Ford R, et al. New response evaluation criteria in solid tumours: revised RECIST guideline (version 1.1). Eur J Cancer. 2009;45:228–47. https://doi.org/10.1016/j.ejca.2008.10.026.

22. Seymour L, Bogaerts J, Perrone A, Ford R, Schwartz LH, Mandrekar S, et al. iRECIST: guidelines for response criteria for use in trials testing immunotherapeutics. Lancet Oncol. 2017;18:e143–e52. https://doi.org/10.1016/S1470-2045(17)30074-8.

23. Wong ANM, McArthur GA, Hofman MS, Hicks RJ. The advantages and challenges of using FDG PET/CT for response assessment in melanoma in the era of targeted agents and immunotherapy. Eur J Nucl Med Mol Imaging. 2017;44:67–77. https://doi.org/10.1007/s00259-017-3691-7.

24. Rymer B, Curtis NJ, Siddiqui MR, Chand M. FDG PET/CT can assess the response of locally advanced rectal cancer to neoadjuvant chemoradiotherapy: evidence from meta-analysis and systematic review. Clin Nucl Med. 2016;41:371–5. https://doi.org/10.1097/RLU.0000000000001166.

25. Wahl RL, Jacene H, Kasamon Y, Lodge MA. From RECIST to PERCIST: evolving considerations for PET response criteria in solid tumors. J Nucl Med. 2009;50(Suppl 1):122S–50S. https://doi.org/10.2967/jnumed.108.057307.

26. Pinker K, Riedl C, Weber WA. Evaluating tumor response with FDG PET: updates on PERCIST, comparison with EORTC criteria and clues to future developments. Eur J Nucl Med Mol Imaging. 2017;44:55–66. https://doi.org/10.1007/s00259-017-3687-3.

27. Stubbs RS, Cannan RJ, Mitchell AW. Selective internal radiation therapy with 90yttrium microspheres for extensive colorectal liver metastases. J Gastrointest Surg. 2001;5:294–302.

28. Boppudi S, Wickremesekera SK, Nowitz M, Stubbs R. Evaluation of the role of CT in the assessment of response to selective internal radiation therapy in patients with colorectal liver metastases. Australas Radiol. 2006;50:570–7. https://doi.org/10.1111/j.1440-1673.2006.01630.x.

29. Morsbach F, Pfammatter T, Reiner CS, Fischer MA, Sah BR, Winklhofer S, et al. Computed tomographic perfusion imaging for the prediction of response and survival to transarterial radioembo-lization of liver metastases. Invest Radiol. 2013;48:787–94. https://doi.org/10.1097/RLI.0b013e31829810f7.

30. Reiner CS, Morsbach F, Sah BR, Puippe G, Schaefer N, Pfammatter T, et al. Early treatment response evaluation after yttrium-90 radioembolization of liver malignancy with CT perfusion. J Vasc Interv Radiol. 2014;25:747–59. https://doi.org/10.1016/j.jvir.2014.01.025.

31. Lee SH, Lee JM, Kim KW, Klotz E, Kim SH, Lee JY, et al. Dual-energy computed tomography to assess tumor response to hepatic radiofrequency ablation: potential diagnostic value of virtual non-contrast images and iodine maps. Invest Radiol. 2011;46:77–84. https://doi.org/10.1097/RLI.0b013e3181f23fcd.

32. Schmeel FC, Simon B, Sabet A, Luetkens JA, Traber F, Schmeel LC, et al. Diffusion-weighted magnetic resonance imaging predicts survival in patients with liver-predominant metastatic colorectal cancer shortly after selective internal radiation therapy. Eur Radiol. 2017;27:966–75. https://doi.org/10.1007/s00330-016-4430-3.

33. Wong CY, Qing F, Savin M, Campbell J, Gates VL, Sherpa KM, et al. Reduction of metastatic load to liver after intraarte-rial hepatic yttrium-90 radioembolization as evaluated by [18F] fluorodeoxyglucose positron emission tomographic imaging. J Vasc Interv Radiol. 2005;16:1101–6. https://doi.org/10.1097/01.RVI.0000168104.32849.07.

34. Annunziata S, Treglia G, Caldarella C, Galiandro F. The role of 18F-FDG-PET and PET/CT in patients with colorectal liver metastases undergoing selective internal radiation therapy with yttrium-90: a first evidence-based review. ScientificWorldJournal. 2014;2014:879469. https://doi.org/10.1155/2014/879469.

35. Szyszko T, Al-Nahhas A, Canelo R, Habib N, Jiao L, Wasan H, et al. Assessment of response to treatment of unresectable liver tumours with 90Y microspheres: value of FDG PET versus computed tomography. Nucl Med Commun. 2007;28:15–20. https://doi.org/10.1097/MNM.0b013e328011453b.

36. Fendler WP, Philippe Tiega DB, Ilhan H, Paprottka PM, Heinemann V, Jakobs TF, et al. Validation of several SUV-based parameters derived from 18F-FDG PET for prediction of survival after SIRT of hepatic metastases from colorectal cancer. J Nucl Med. 2013;54:1202–8. https://doi.org/10.2967/jnumed.112.116426.

37. Dierckx R, Maes A, Peeters M, Van De Wiele C. FDG PET for monitoring response to local and locoregional therapy in HCC and liver metastases. Q J Nucl Med Mol Imaging. 2009;53:336–42.

38. Dromain C, Pavel ME, Ruszniewski P, Langley A, Massien C, Baudin E, et al. Tumor growth rate as a metric of progression, response, and prognosis in pancreatic and intestinal neuroendo-crine tumors. BMC Cancer. 2019;19:66. https://doi.org/10.1186/s12885-018-5257-x.

39. Morse B, Jeong D, Thomas K, Diallo D, Strosberg JR. Magnetic resonance imaging of neuroendocrine tumor hepatic metastases: does hepatobiliary phase imaging improve lesion conspicuity and interob-server agreement of lesion measurements? Pancreas. 2017;46:1219–24. https://doi.org/10.1097/MPA.0000000000000920.

40. Hicks RJ, Kwekkeboom DJ, Krenning E, Bodei L, Grozinsky-Glasberg S, Arnold R, et al. ENETS consensus guidelines for the standards of care in neuroendocrine neoplasia: peptide receptor radionuclide therapy with radiolabeled somatostatin analogues. Neuroendocrinology. 2017; https://doi.org/10.1159/000475526.

41. Haug AR, Auernhammer CJ, Wangler B, Schmidt GP, Uebleis C, Goke B, et al. 68Ga-DOTATATE PET/CT for the early pre-diction of response to somatostatin receptor-mediated radionu-clide therapy in patients with well-differentiated neuroendocrine tumors. J Nucl Med. 2010;51:1349–56. https://doi.org/10.2967/jnumed.110.075002.

42. Hope TA, Bergsland EK, Bozkurt MF, Graham M, Heaney AP, Herrmann K, et al. Appropriate use criteria for somatostatin receptor PET imaging in neuroendocrine tumors. J Nucl Med. 2018;59:66–74. https://doi.org/10.2967/jnumed.117.202275.

43. de Bono JS, Logothetis CJ, Molina A, Fizazi K, North S, Chu L, et al. Abiraterone and increased survival in metastatic prostate cancer. N Engl J Med. 2011;364:1995–2005. https://doi.org/10.1056/NEJMoa1014618.

44. Parker C, Nilsson S, Heinrich D, Helle SI, O'Sullivan JM, Fossa SD, et al. Alpha emitter radium-223 and survival in metastatic prostate cancer. N Engl J Med. 2013;369:213–23. https://doi.org/10.1056/NEJMoa1213755.

45. Scher HI, Morris MJ, Stadler WM, Higano C, Basch E, Fizazi K, et al. Trial design and objectives for castration-resistant prostate cancer: updated recommendations from the Prostate Cancer Clinical Trials Working Group 3. J Clin Oncol. 2016;34:1402–18. https://doi.org/10.1200/JCO.2015.64.2702.

46. Costelloe CM, Chuang HH, Madewell JE, Ueno NT. Cancer response criteria and bone metastases: RECIST 1.1, MDA and PERCIST. J Cancer. 2010;1:80–92.

47. Rathkopf DE, Beer TM, Loriot Y, Higano CS, Armstrong AJ, Sternberg CN, et al. Radiographic progression-free survival as a clinically meaningful end point in metastatic castration-resistant prostate cancer: the PREVAIL randomized clinical trial. JAMA Oncol. 2018;4:694–701. https://doi.org/10.1001/jamaoncol.2017.5808.

48. Schwarzenbock SM, Knieling A, Souvatzoglou M, Kurth J, Steiger K, Eiber M, et al. [11C]Choline PET/CT in therapy response assessment of a neoadjuvant therapy in locally advanced and high risk prostate cancer before radical prostatectomy. Oncotarget. 2016;7:63747–57. https://doi.org/10.18632/oncotarget.11653.

49. Schwarzenbock SM, Eiber M, Kundt G, Retz M, Sakretz M, Kurth J, et al. Prospective evaluation of [11C]Choline PET/CT in therapy response assessment of standardized docetaxel first-line chemotherapy in patients with advanced castration refractory prostate cancer. Eur J Nucl Med Mol Imaging. 2016;43:2105–13. https://doi.org/10.1007/s00259-016-3439-9.

50. Bieth M, Kronke M, Tauber R, Dahlbender M, Retz M, Nekolla SG, et al. Exploring new multimodal quantitative imaging indices for the assessment of osseous tumour burden in prostate cancer using 68Ga-PSMA-PET/CT. J Nucl Med. 2017; https://doi.org/10.2967/jnumed.116.189050.

51. Meller B, Bremmer F, Sahlmann CO, Hijazi S, Bouter C, Trojan L, et al. Alterations in androgen deprivation enhanced prostate-specific membrane antigen (PSMA) expression in prostate cancer cells as a target for diagnostics and therapy. EJNMMI Res. 2015;5:66. https://doi.org/10.1186/s13550-015-0145-8.

52. Gafita A, Rauscher I, Weber M, Hadaschik B, Wang H, Armstrong WR, et al. Novel framework for treatment response evaluation using PSMA-PET/CT in patients with metastatic castration-resistant prostate cancer (RECIP 1.0): an international multicenter study. J Nucl Med. 2022; https://doi.org/10.2967/jnumed.121.263072.

53. Padhani AR, Lecouvet FE, Tunariu N, Koh DM, De Keyzer F, Collins DJ, et al. METastasis reporting and data system for prostate cancer: practical guidelines for acquisition, interpretation, and reporting of whole-body magnetic resonance imaging-based evaluations of multiorgan involvement in advanced prostate cancer. Eur Urol. 2017;71:81–92. https://doi.org/10.1016/j.eururo.2016.05.033.

54. Yoshida S, Takahara T, Ishii C, Arita Y, Waseda Y, Kijima T, et al. METastasis reporting and data system for prostate cancer as a prognostic imaging marker in castration-resistant prostate cancer. Clin Genitourin Cancer. 2020;18:e391–e6. https://doi.org/10.1016/j.clgc.2019.12.010.

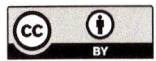

Benign and Malignant Diseases of the Colon and Rectum

4

Ulrike Attenberger and Inês Santiago

Learning Objectives
- To provide an overview of the most common benign and malignant conditions of the colon and rectum on cross-sectional imaging (CT and MRI).
- To understand the current role of cross-sectional imaging in the detection, characterization, and differentiation of colorectal diseases.

4.1 Benign Diseases of the Colon and Rectum

4.1.1 Inflammatory Diseases of the Colon and Rectum

CT is a valuable diagnostic tool for the detection and characterization of different inflammatory conditions of the colon, including appendicitis, diverticulitis, epiploic appendagitis, chronic inflammatory bowel diseases (IBDs), as well as infectious and non-infectious colitis. CT plays an important role in detection of acute conditions including extraluminal complications and extraintestinal manifestations of inflammatory bowel disease. Despite the significant overlap in imaging findings of inflammatory bowel diseases, their findings may differ in their primary localization within the gastrointestinal tract, length of segmental involvement, degree of wall thickening, mural enhancement pattern, and extraintestinal involvement. Therefore, understanding of leading disease patterns and specific imaging features can allow accurate diagnosis.

4.1.1.1 Chronic Inflammatory Bowel Diseases

Inflammatory bowel diseases (IBD) are a group of chronic disorders that cause relapsing inflammation in the gastrointestinal tract and comprise three major subgroups of Crohn's disease, ulcerative colitis, and unclassified. Environmental changes, genetic factors, intestinal microbiota alterations, and immune system deregulation contribute to the initiation and progression of inflammation and subsequent fibrosis [1]. Despite of the considerable overlap between the imaging findings in Crohn's disease and ulcerative colitis, there are often certain features that can help differentiate them (Table 4.1, see also Fig. 4.1) [2].

4.1.1.2 Infectious Colitis

Infectious colitis, as its name suggests, is caused by an infection due to bacterial, viral, fungal, or parasitic agents, leading to inflammation of the colon. Although cross-sectional imaging is not the primary diagnostic tool, and imaging findings are often non-specific, standard abdominal CT may be required to assess disease extent and severity, extraluminal complications, and especially to rule out other causes of acute abdomen [3]. Typical imaging findings regardless of the infective cause are: diffuse wall thickening with homogeneous enhancement, pericolonic fat stranding, gas-fluid levels, and ascites [3].

Pseudomembranous Colitis

Pseudomembranous colitis is an acute, potentially life-threatening nosocomial infectious colitis caused by toxins produced by an unopposed proliferation of *Clostridium difficile* bacteria. In recent years, it has become a significant clinical problem, mostly due to the increased use of prophylactic and broad-spectrum antibiotics. Imaging features include marked wall thickening (which is usually more extensive compared to other infectious and non-infectious

U. Attenberger (✉)
Department of Diagnostic and Interventional Radiology, University Hospital Bonn, Bonn, Germany
e-mail: ulrike.attenberger@ukbonn.de

I. Santiago
Radiology Department, Champalimaud Foundation, Lisbon, Portugal
e-mail: ines.santiago@neuro.fchampalimaud.org

© The Author(s) 2023
J. Hodler et al. (eds.), *Diseases of the Abdomen and Pelvis 2023-2026*, IDKD Springer Series,
https://doi.org/10.1007/978-3-031-27355-1_4

Table 4.1 Characteristics of Crohn's disease and ulcerative colitis

	Crohn's disease	Ulcerative colitis
Site of origin	Terminal ileum	Rectum
Bowel involvement	The entire gastrointestinal tract with small bowel (terminal ileum) in 70–80%	Rectum in 95%, terminal ileum involvement in pancolitis ("backwash ileitis")
Upper part of GIT	Rarely	Never
Distal ileum	Very common	"Backwash ileitis"
Colon	Common	Always
Rectum	Rarely	Always
Distribution	Discontinuous "skip lesions"	Continuous distribution from rectum up
Bowel wall involvement (inflammation)	Transmural	Mucosal and submucosal
Mural thickening	1–2 cm	7–8 mm
Intestinal complications	Strictures (fibrotic, stenotic), fissures and fistulas, deep ulcers, cobblestone appearance, abscesses, perianal disease	Toxic megacolon, hemorrhage
Perianal involvement	Perirectal stranding, fistulas	Perianal complications are rare

colitis), low-attenuation mural thickening corresponding to mucosal and submucosal edema, the "accordion sign" (oral contrast media trapped between the thickened colon wall folds), and the "target sign" (or "double halo sign") (Fig. 4.2). Extracolonic features include ascites and pericolonic stranding, which may be relatively mild compared to the degree of colon wall thickening. Most commonly, the entire colon is affected. In severe cases, complications like intramural gas formation (pneumatosis coli), toxic megacolon, and perforation (pneumoperitoneum) may occur [4].

4.1.1.3 Non-infectious Colitis

Non-infectious colitis refers to the heterogeneous group of colonic inflammation caused by various causes other than infections (pathogenic organisms), for example, ischemic, drug-induced or immune-mediated.

Ischemic Colitis

Ischemic colitis is a condition in which inflammatory injury of the colon results from interruption and/or insufficient blood supply. It is more likely to occur in the elderly with atherosclerotic disease and/or low-flow state (e.g., due to heart disease). Low-flow state and non-occlusive vessel disease may lead to ischemic colitis in watershed areas while complete vessel occlusion produces an involvement of the dependent vascular territory (e.g., in the territory of the supe-

rior mesenteric artery). Imaging findings are mostly non-specific: uniform bowel wall thickening, "target sign" (low-density ring of submucosal edema between enhancing mucosa and serosa), bowel dilatation, pneumatosis coli (in severe cases), pericolic fluid or fat stranding, mesenteric edema, and/or asities (Fig. 4.2). Multiphase CT angiography has to be performed to identify the level of vessel occlusion and procedural planning.

Drug-Induced Colitis

The dramatic increase in pharmaceutical medical therapies (e.g., immune-modulating therapies with biologics, chemotherapeutics, nonsteroidal anti-inflammatory drugs) has led to an increased frequency of gastrointestinal adverse effects. Medical history and clinical presentation supported by imaging findings are the key to the diagnosis. Cross-sectional imaging may be required for the assessment of (peri-)colonic involvement, associated complications and to exclude other causes of acute abdomen (e.g., ischemic causes) [5]. Imaging findings are generally based on those seen in other infectious and non-infectious colitis (Fig. 4.2).

Neutropenic Colitis

Neutropenic colitis (also known as typhlitis) is a severe necrotizing inflammation occurring primarily in neutropenic patients. It mostly originates in the cecum and extends to the ascending colon, appendix, or terminal ileum [6]. As morphologic imaging findings are similar to that of other infectious and non-infectious colitis, medical history (e.g., immunodeficiency) is necessary to establish the diagnosis.

Radiation Colitis and Proctitis

Radiation colitis is the inflammatory injury of the colon and rectum caused by radiation therapy, which may occur between 6 months to 5 years after treatment. Depending on the onset, radiation colitis may be classified as acute or chronic. Cross-sectional imaging may be indicated for the assessment of extracolonic involvement and other complications. Imaging findings in the acute phase include nonspecific wall thickening and pericolonic stranding; in the chronic phase, short or long strictures, colonic lumen narrowing, ulcerations, and/or fistulas may be present [7].

Graft-Versus-Host Disease

Intestinal graft-versus-host disease (GvHD) is a common, potentially life-threatening complication after hematopoietic stem cell transplantation, which may affect the entire gastrointestinal tract (large bowel involvement is present in ~25% of cases). Imaging findings are non-specific and include: moderate bowel wall thickening with mucosal enhancement, mesenteric edema, vascular engorgement, and/or pneumatosis intestinalis in severe cases (Fig. 4.2) [8].

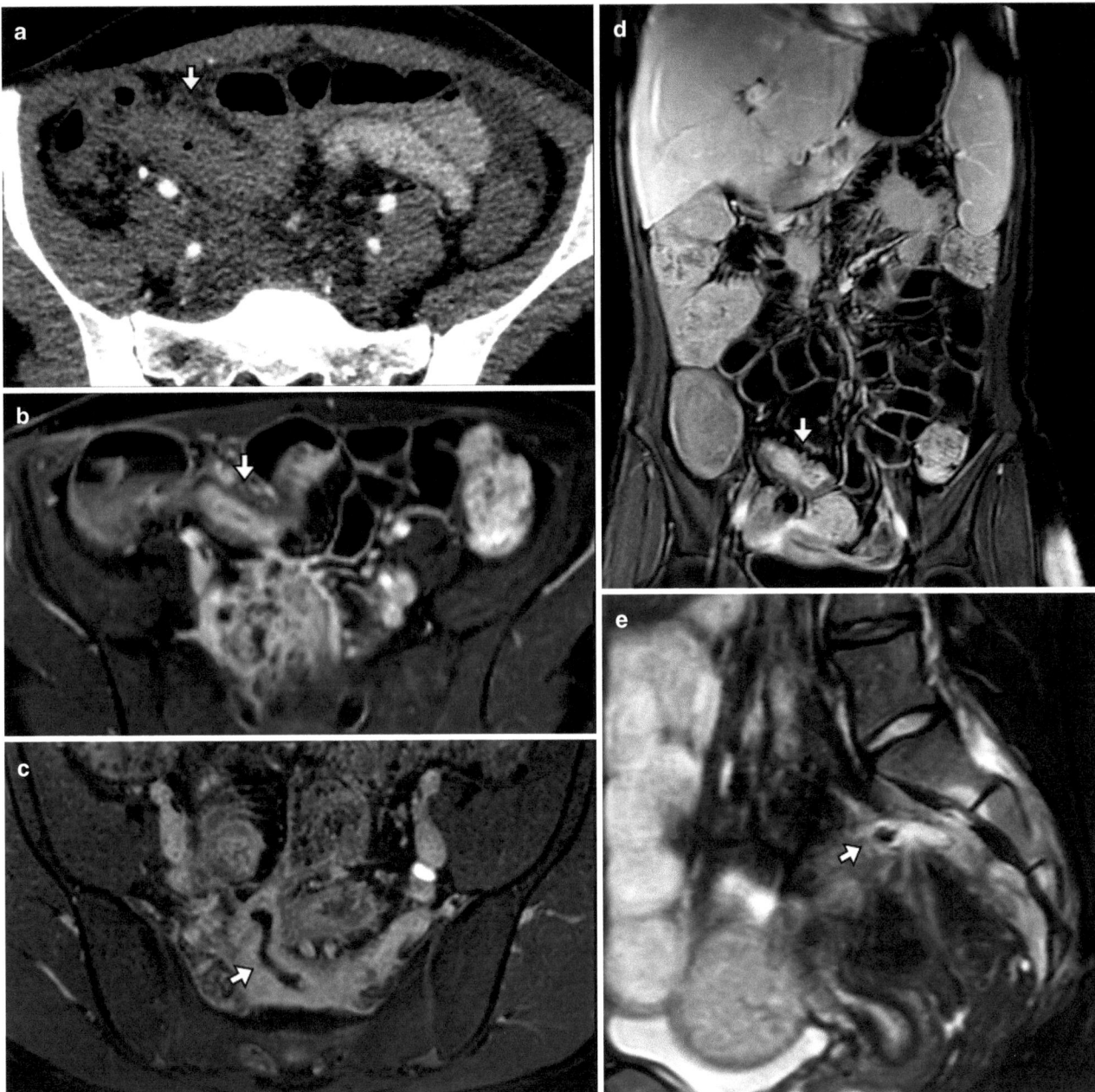

Fig. 4.1 A 24-year-old female patient with known history of Crohn's disease. Axial contrast-enhanced CT with positive oral contrast (**a**), axial (**b**), and coronal (**d**) contrast-enhanced MR-enterography images with neutral oral contrast show stratified mural thickening with hyper-enhancement of the terminal ileum (arrows) and presacral abscess formation (**c**, **e**) (arrows). Findings are consistent with active inflammatory Crohn's disease

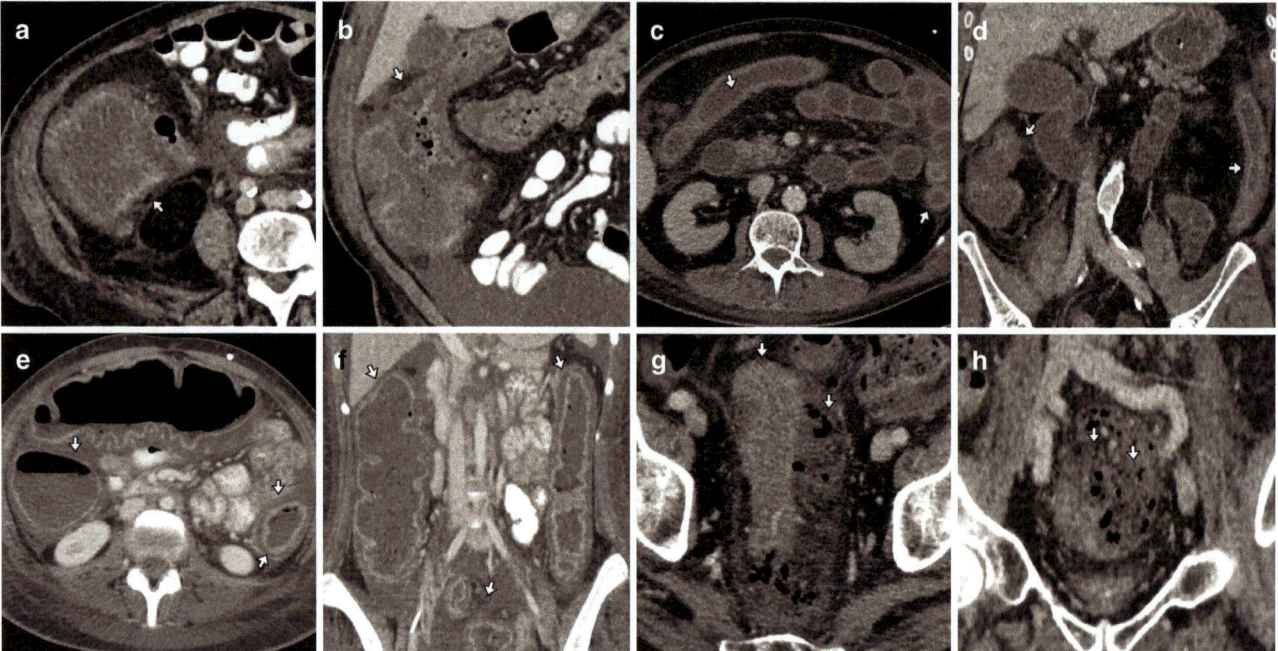

Fig. 4.2 Composed figure shows different types of inflammatory colitis (**a, c, e, g**: axial images, **b, d, f, h**: coronal images). (**a, b**) A 77-years-old female patient with abdominal pain. Images show distension, wall thickening, and submucosal edema with surrounding stranding involving the colon ascendens (arrows) without occlusion of the mesenterial arteries (not shown). Colonoscopy confirmed ischemic colitis. (**c, d**) A 59-year-old male patient with history of allogeneic stem cell transplantation presents with sepsis and intestinal bleeding. Images show diffuse bowl wall thickening with submucosal edema affecting the entire nondilated small and large bowl (arrows). Given the medical history and other clinical findings including biopsy, bowel graft versus host disease was the final diagnosis. (**e, f**) A 22-year-old female patient with sepsis and long-term treatment at the intensive care unit presents with abdominal distension and diarrhea. Images show thick-walled, mildly dilated, fluid-filled colon with mucosal enhancement and minor pericolic stranding. The entire colon is involved (pancolitis, arrows). As the stool test for *Clostridium difficile* toxin was positive, pseudomembranous colitis was the final diagnosis. (**g, H**) A 71-year-old male with metastatic melanoma and known drug-induced pneumonitis under immune-checkpoint-inhibitor therapy (ICI; Nivolumab) presents with new-onset of gastrointestinal bleeding. Images show extensive wall thickening and enhancement of the sigmoid colon (arrows) with surrounding fat stranding and diffuse inflammatory pericolic formation including pneumoperitoneum due to perforation. Perforated ICI-induced colitis was the final clinical diagnosis

---

Key Point
CT plays an essential role in the detection and characterization of inflammatory conditions, including extraluminal complications and extraintestinal manifestations.

Key Point
CT is the method of choice to evaluate diverticulitis and allows accurate classification and guide treatment.

4.1.2   Diverticular Disease and Diverticulitis

Diverticular disease is one of the most common gastroenterological disorders in the Western world. In case of acute abdomen and suspicious diverticular disease, ultrasound is routinely followed by CT, further clinical decision-making, and risk stratification. Based on the classification of diverticular disease (CDD), a differentiation can be made between uncomplicated (type 1), complicated (type 2), and chronic (type 3) diverticular disease (Fig. 4.3) [9]. In this context, CT allows the detection of associated microabscesses, macroabscesses, and free perforation as they determine the further therapeutic approach.

4.1.3   Benign Mucosal Colonic Polyp

Since the majority of colorectal cancer are believed to arise within benign adenomatous polyps that develop slowly over many years following the "adenoma to carcinoma" sequence, they are the primary target lesions for colorectal screening. Cross-sectional imaging with introduction of virtual colonoscopy (CT and MRI colonography) are promising techniques and play an increasingly important role in both symptomatic and screening patients for the selection of the appropriate therapeutic procedure (see the Abstract Book IDKD 2018).

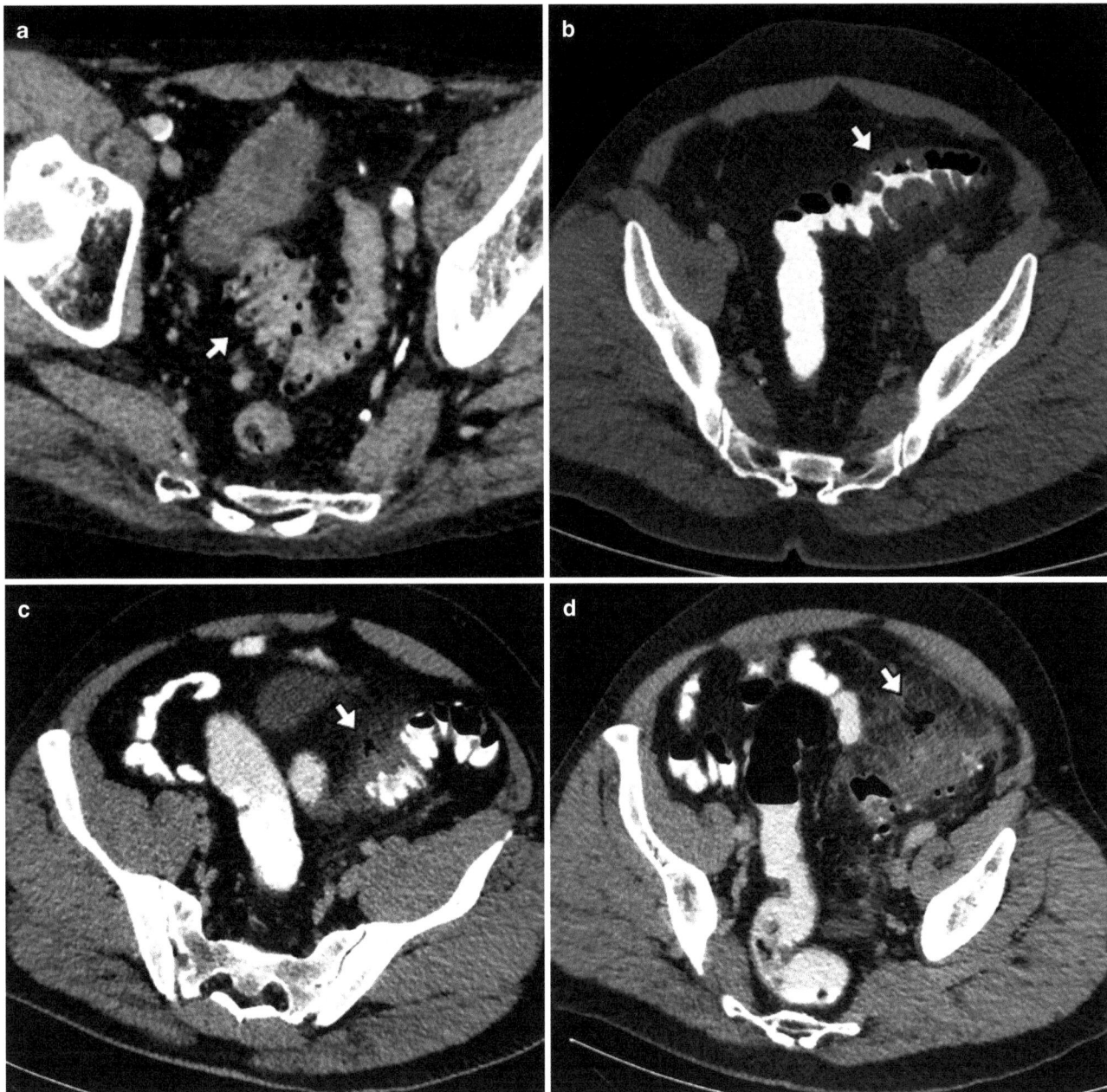

Fig. 4.3 (**a**) A 56-year-old asymptomatic patient with uncomplicated diverticular disease. The axial contrast-enhanced CT image shows multiple diverticula (arrow) of the sigmoid without associated inflammation. (**b**) A 63-year-old with intermittent pain localized in the left lower abdomen and elevated blood inflammatory markers. The contrast-enhanced axial CT image after the administration of positive rectal contrast shows bowel wall thickening and fat stranding (arrow). Findings are consistent with acute complicated diverticulitis with phlegmonous peridiverticulitis Type 1b. (**c**) A 60-year-old patient with severe abdominal pain, located in the left lower abdomen, fever, nausea, and elevated blood inflammatory markers. The contrast-enhanced axial CT image after the administration of positive rectal contrast material shows diverticulitis with bowel wall thickening, fat stranding, and covered perforation with small abscess (≤1 cm) and minimal paracolic air (arrow). Findings are consistent with acute complicated diverticulitis Type 2a. (**d**) A 57-year-old patient with severe abdominal pain, fever, nausea, and elevated blood inflammatory markers. Axial CT image shows acute complicated diverticulitis with phlegmonous peridiverticulitis and paracolic abscess (>1 cm, arrow). Findings are consistent with acute complicated diverticulitis Type 2b

Key Point

Cross-sectional imaging techniques with the introduction of virtual colonoscopy are promising techniques and are playing an increasing role.

4.2   Malignant Diseases of the Colon and Rectum

4.2.1   Rectal Cancer

Colorectal cancer is the third most common cancer in men and the second most common in women [10]. Nowadays, rectal MRI plays a leading role in the evaluation of rectal cancer, especially in primary local staging and assessment of response to chemotherapeutic treatment.

4.2.1.1   Elective Rectal Cancer Staging

In primary staging (pre-operative setting), MRI is important for the evaluation of tumor location and morphology, T and N category, involvement of the mesorectal fascia (MRF), extramural vascular invasion (EMVI), mucin content, and involvement of the pelvic sidewall and anal sphincter complex (Fig. 4.4). Therefore, rectal MRI is particularly performed for (1) selecting patients with locally advanced rectal cancer who are suitable for treatment with neoadjuvant chemotherapy; (2) guiding surgical planning; and (3) identifying poor prognostic factors, including EMVI, mucin content, and CRM status [10]. The prognosis of rectal cancer is directly related to mesorectal tumor infiltration and circumferential resection margins (CRMs).

Key Point

Rectal MRI plays a key role in local staging of rectal cancer and allows selection of an appropriate treatment strategy. Moreover, it allows to identify poor prognostic factors including MRF and EMVI.

4.2.2   Colon Cancer

Colon cancer is the fourth most commonly diagnosed cancer worldwide and the fifth deadliest, representing 5.8% of all cancer deaths [11]. Its incidence is 3 to 4 times higher in developed countries, making it a marker of socioeconomic development [11].

The diagnosis of colon cancer is either driven by symptoms or screening. Optical colonoscopy is the diagnostic gold standard, with detection rates of (pre)cancerous lesions >95% [12]. CT colonography may be a good alternative, particularly in patients with structural problems or comorbidities, and a good adjunct to incomplete examinations, with comparable sensitivity for lesions >10 mm [13].

Clinical staging of colorectal cancer is the most important predictor of survival and relies on the TNM system proposed by the AJCC/UICC, which is based on the pathologic analysis of the resected specimen [14]. Imaging plays an essential role, not only for surgery planning in eligible patients, but also for distant staging, detection of pre- and postoperative complications, and oncologic follow-up.

4.2.2.1   Elective Colon Cancer Staging

CT is the mainstay for colon cancer staging, but accurate T and N staging has always been a challenge and MRI has not demonstrated better results [15, 16]. Given surgery remains primary curative treatment for all TN stages, more than getting the T and N stages right, the radiologist should provide the multidisciplinary team with all the relevant information for a successful curative surgery or, alternatively, with the detailed baseline information to monitor systemic treatment. In the absence of IV contrast contraindications, a weight and concentration-adjusted acquisition in the portal venous phase of enhancement should be sufficient, oral contrast being considered unnecessary by the great majority of experts [17].

Most colon cancers present as a polyp (Fig. 4.5) or as an asymmetrical or concentrical wall thickening, the latter with lumen caliber reduction and loss of the normal layered appearance of the bowel wall (Fig. 4.6). Relative enhancement varies, most non-mucinous tumors being hyper to isoenhancing (78%) (Figs. 4.5 and 4.6) and most mucinous tumors being iso to hypoenhancing (84%) compared to adjacent bowel wall (Fig. 4.7) [18]. Enhancement pattern is usually heterogeneous, particularly in mucinous tumors (Fig. 4.7). Intratumoral calcification is unusual but relatively more frequent in mucinous tumors [18].

No reliable radiologic lymph node involvement criteria have been established so far although several have been investigated [16, 19].

The success of curative R0 resection relies on detailed imaging delineation of tumor boundaries, including any involved surrounding organs or structures (Fig. 4.8). Attention should be paid to other colon segments, particularly proximal to tumor

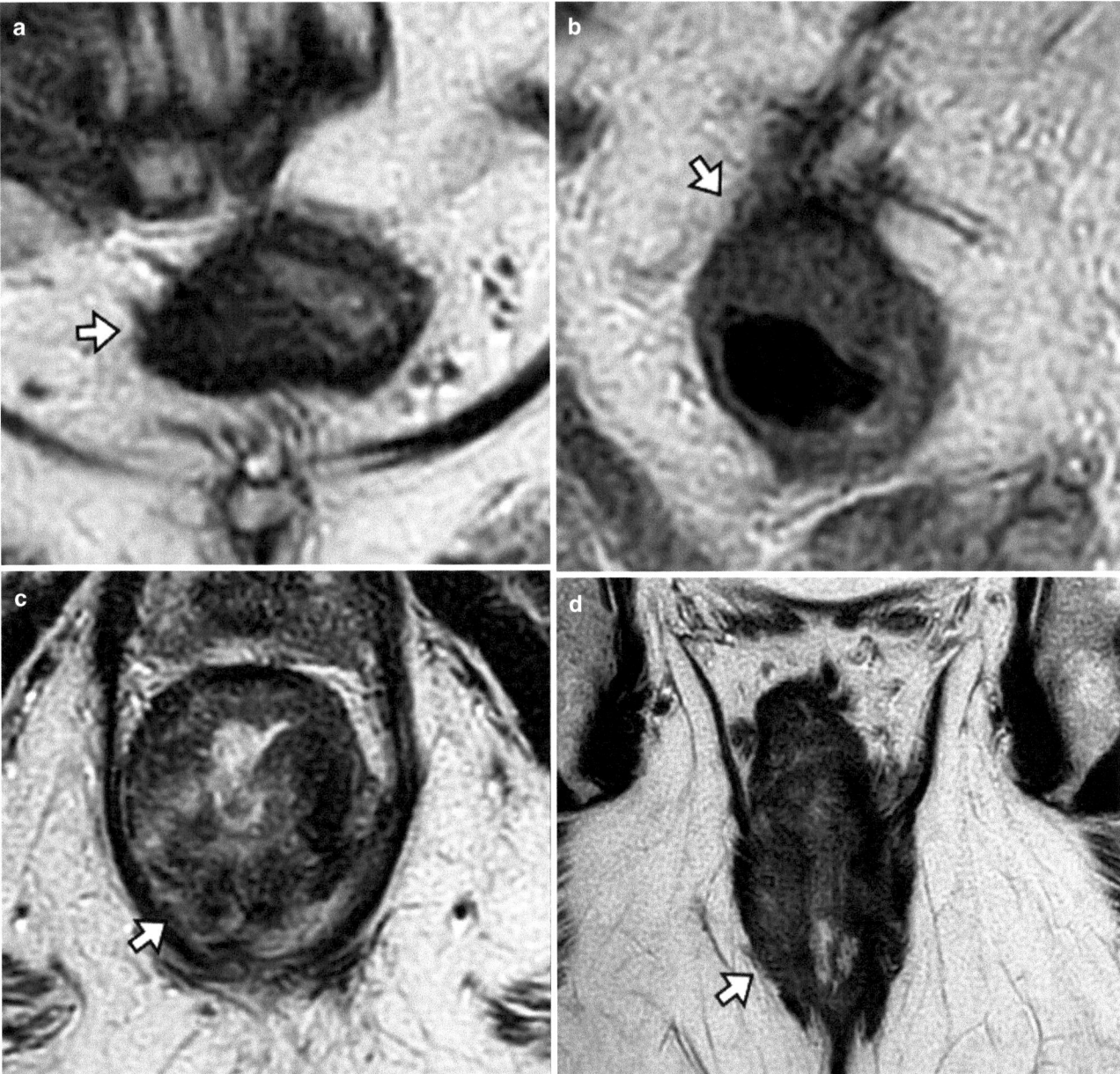

Fig. 4.4 Rectal MR images (axial T2-weighted images) show different tumor stages from four different patients. (**a**) The axial T2-weighed image shows a tumor within the middle rectum infiltrating the muscularis propria (T2). (**b**) The axial T2-weighted image shows a tumor within the middle rectum with infiltration beyond the muscularis propria (T3c), with negative MRF infiltration and positive EMVI. (**c, d**) The axial and coronal T2-weighted images show a tumor within the low rectum infiltrating beyond the muscularis propria and invading the external sphincter, internal sphincter complex, and the levator ani muscle (T4b)

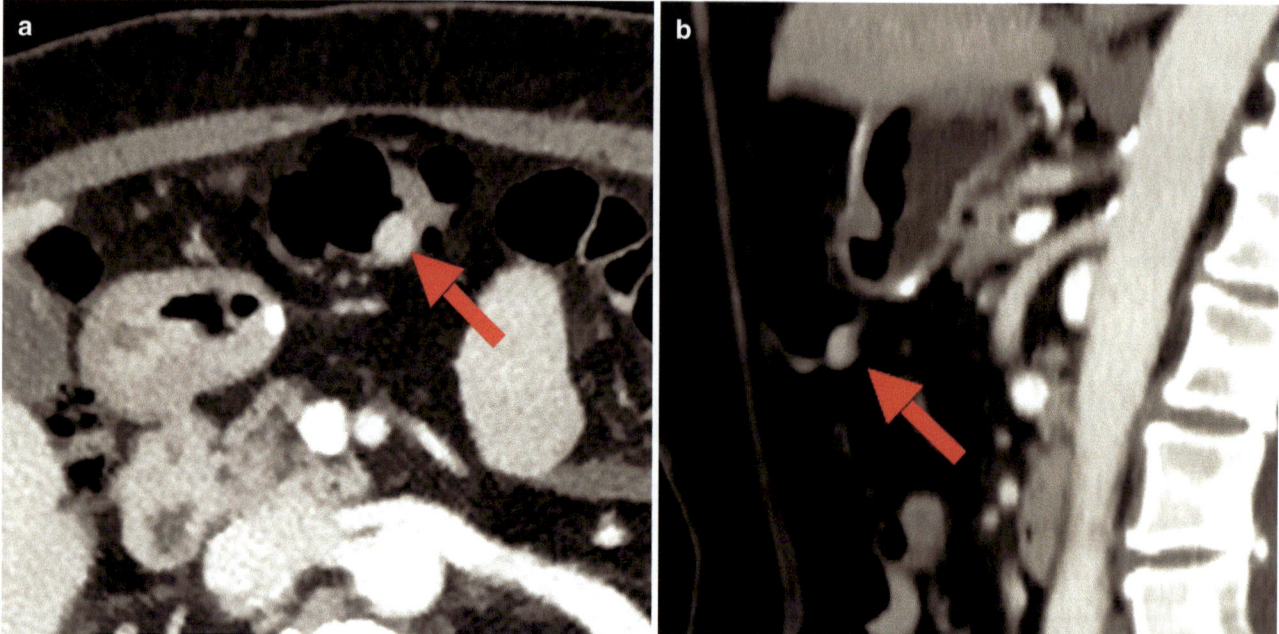

Fig. 4.5 A 66-year-old female patient referred for colon cancer staging after screening colonoscopy detected a small, biopsy conformed, adenocarcinoma. (**a**) Axial and (**b**) sagittal cropped CT images acquired on the portal venous phase of enhancement depict a 10 mm polypoid, homogeneously hyperenhancing, lesion of the transverse colon (red arrow). Patient underwent laparoscopic right hemicolectomy and pathology revealed a G1 pT2N0 tumor

in incomplete colonoscopies, not to miss additional lesions. Other details that matter for the selection of the best surgical approach include: specific tumor location, lesion size, and the particularities of mesenteric vascular anatomy, for which multiplanar reformations and maximum intensity projections, especially in coronal plane, may be quite illustrative [20].

4.2.2.2 Colon Cancer Presenting as Acute Abdomen

Colon cancer may present as a surgical emergency in up to 40% of cases, which occurs more frequently in the elderly population [21]. Obstruction and perforation, the most common presentations, are considered high-risk features and are linked to poorer recurrence-free survival, higher surgical morbidity and mortality, and stoma formation [21]. Other complications include acute appendicitis, ischemic colitis, and intussusception [22].

CT can localize an obstructing lesion with high sensitivity (96%) and specificity (93%) [22]. Left-sided malignancies are more likely to be obstructive. Obstructive lesions manifest with an intestinal caliber transition point at tumor level and upstream dilatation. A cecal lumen exceeding 12–15 cm, more likely to occur in patients with a competent ileo-cecal valve, should be an alert for imminent rupture, as should be the presence of any area of wall hypoenhancement [23].

Although perforation may occur proximal to an obstructing tumor, it more commonly occurs at the tumor site itself, due to necrosis and tissue friability [24]. It is the most lethal complication of colon cancer, with mortality rates as high as 50% due to secondary fecal peritonitis [21]. On CT, a focal defect in the bowel wall may be observed, accompanied by adjacent fat stranding, extraluminal air, and a variable amount of fluid. Perforation may be free or localized, the latter with eventual abscess formation and/or fistulation [21]. Oral contrast or contrast per rectum may help document a perforation but lack of extravasation of contrast does not rule it out, making its clinical utility questionable.

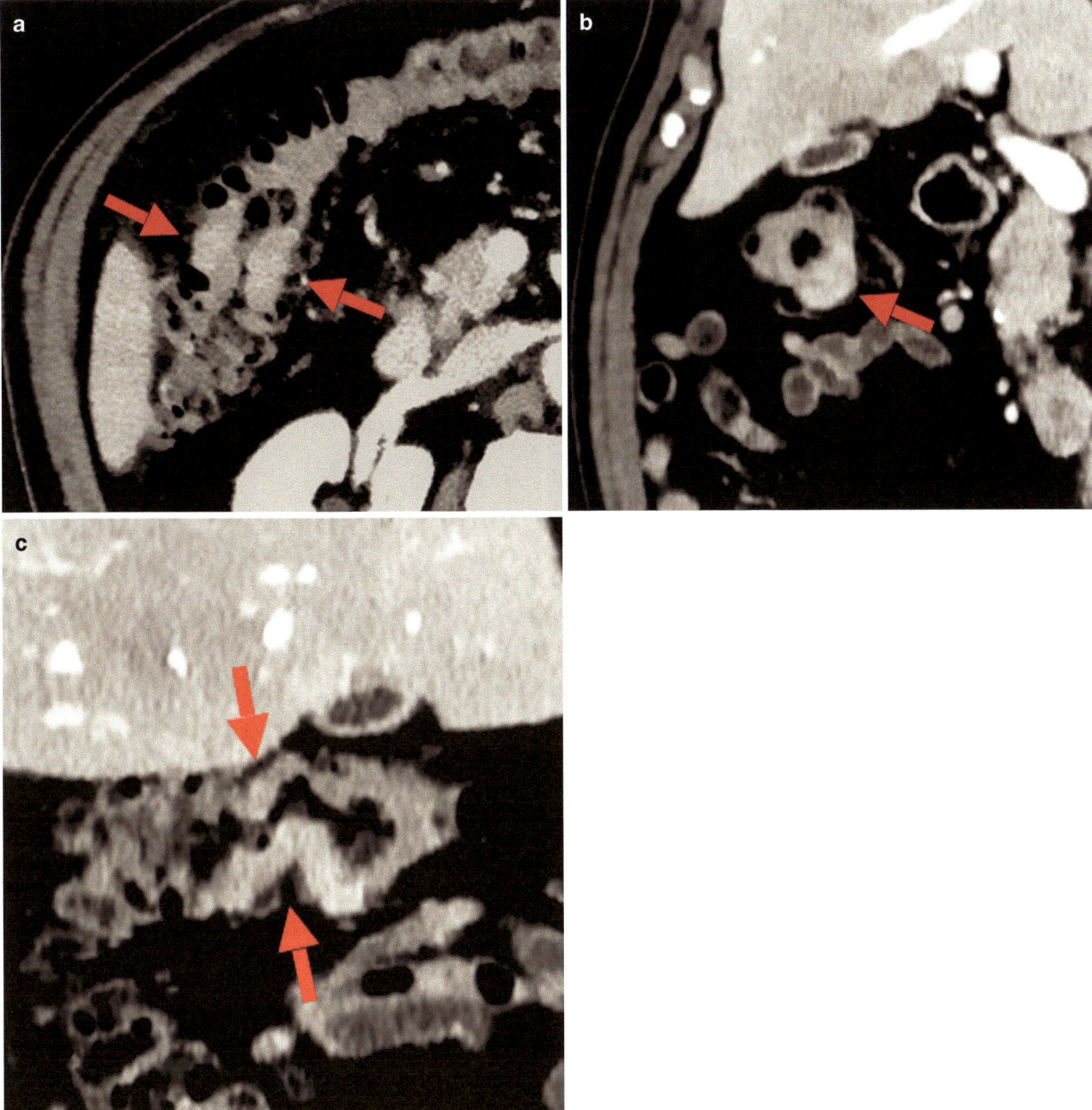

Fig. 4.6 An 81-year-old male patient referred for colon cancer staging after screening colonoscopy revealed an ulcerated tumor of the transverse colon. (**a**) Axial, (**b**) oblique sagittal, and (**c**) oblique coronal cropped CT images acquired on the portal venous phase of enhancement. An asymmetrical hyperenhancing, mildly heterogeneous, wall thickening at the hepatic flexure of the colon is observed, associated with focal lumen caliber reduction. Although clinically staged as T2, right hemicolectomy revealed a pT3 N0 specimen

Key Point

Precise T and N staging with CT for colon cancer is challenging. However, it is highly valuable for M staging, planning curative surgery, diagnosing pre- and postoperative complications, assessing response to systemic treatment, and for long-term follow-up.

4.2.3 Evaluation of Response to Neoadjuvant Therapy in Rectal Cancer

Given the established advantage regarding local recurrence rates, standard treatment for locally advanced rectal cancer involves a combination of neoadjuvant radiation and chemotherapy, prior to total mesorectal excision (TME). It

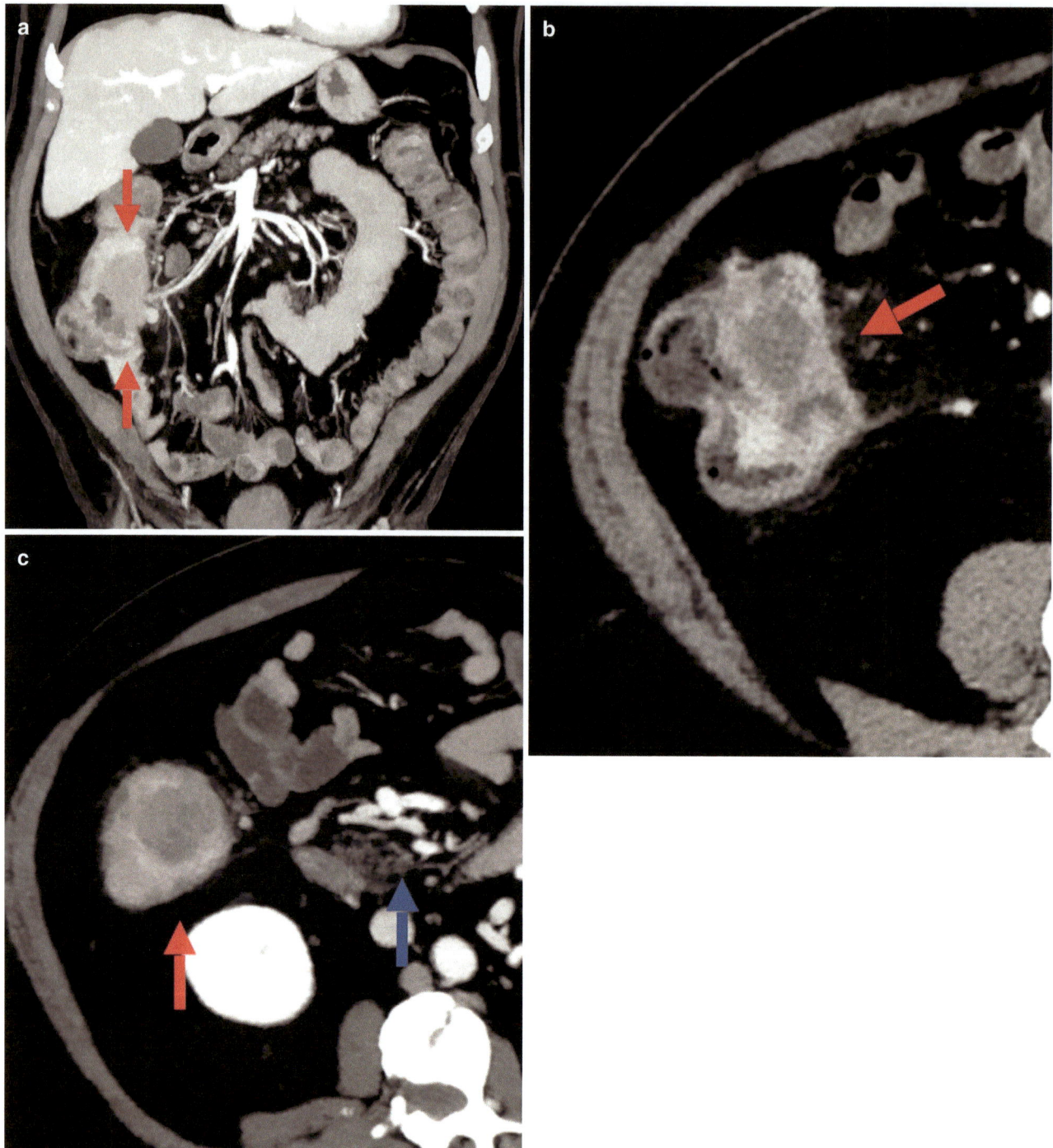

Fig. 4.7 Male patient, 50 years of age, presenting with vomiting and epigastric pain with 2-month duration. Endoscopy found no abnormalities. Colonoscopy revealed a bulky, ulcerated, and stenosing lesion of the ascending colon, which could not be passed with the colonoscope. (**a**) Coronal maximum intensity projection, (**b**) axial, and (**c**) axial maximum intensity projection portal venous phase CT images depicting an 8 cm bulky, irregular, heterogeneous lesion (red arrows) involving the cecum and ascending colon, with areas of hyper-, iso-, and hypoenhancement. In (**c**), the colic arteries cross the superior mesenteric vein posteriorly (blue arrow), an important information for laparoscopic surgery planning. Laparoscopic right hemicolectomy revealed a mucinous pT3N0 specimen

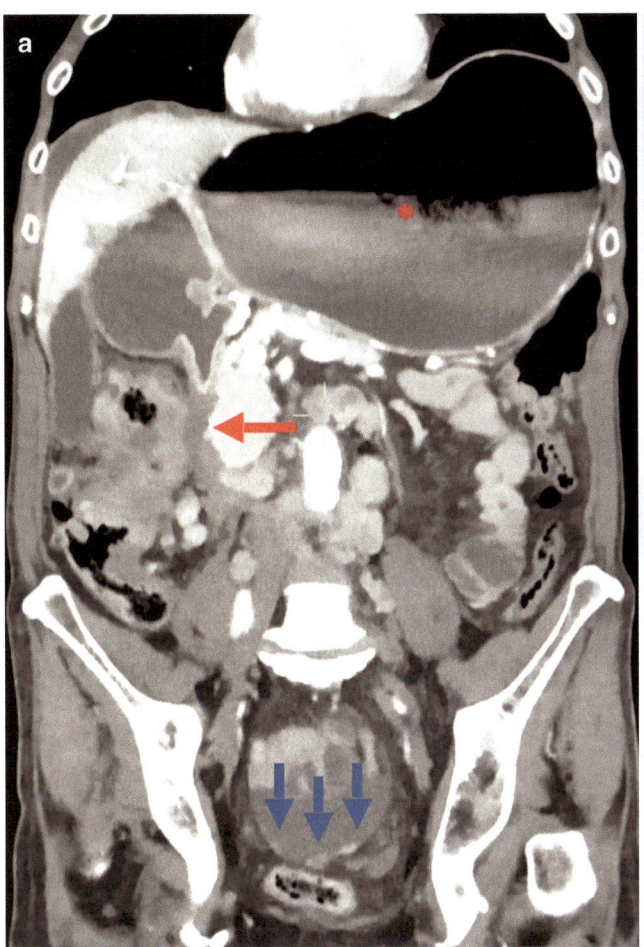

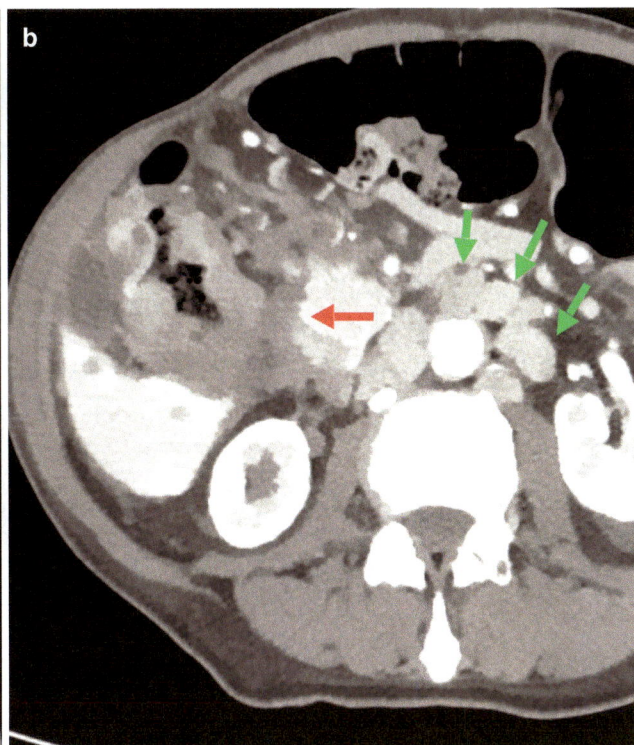

Fig. 4.8 A 84-year-old patient presenting with nausea and vomiting. (**a**) Coronal and (**b**) axial CT images acquired on the portal venous phase of enhancement. Bulky, circumferential, heterogeneously iso- to hyperenhancing lesion of the ascending colon (red arrows) invading the root of the mesentery, the head of the pancreas, and the 1st, 2nd, and 3rd portions of the duodenum (red arrows), causing severe stenosis with pronounced upstream dilatation—notice the distended stomach (*). The lesion was stenotic itself and could not be passed with the colonoscope, but no upstream small bowel distention was observed because of the stenosing effect on the duodenum. Peritoneal carcinomatosis is visible in the pelvis (blue arrows in **a**), as are bulky, retroperitoneal lymphadenopathies (green arrows in **b**)

induces downsizing and downstaging of the disease in most patients, and in a variable proportion of them, 10–25% in most series, it leads to a complete response [11]. There are two main drives to re-stage rectal cancer after neoadjuvant therapy (NAT): to detect changes in the relation between the tumor and adjacent structures that may permit a less mutilating, yet still curative surgery; and to offer, in dedicated centers, the option of non-operative management to clinical complete responders [11].

4.2.3.1 Technique
Assessment of response to NAT prior to surgery relies on clinical evaluation, MR imaging and, in "Watch-and-Wait" dedicated centers, also on rectoscopy. The post-NAT MR imaging evaluation, just as in the staging setting, relies on high resolution T2-weighted images acquired in sagittal, parallel, and perpendicular planes relative to the tumor bed. For the identification of clinical complete responses, the use of

diffusion-weighted imaging (DWI) may be of additional value, and given it is very sensitive to motion and air-induced susceptibility, patient preparation is determinant [25]. We recommend fasting for 6 h, a small enema 20 min before acquisition, and the administration of a spasmolytic agent in the absence of contraindications [25].

4.2.3.2 Re-staging to Plan Surgery
After NAT, the tumor may move away from anatomical landmarks or structures in a favorable manner. For instance, its inferior border may shift cranially making TME with a colo-anal anastomosis a possibility. Also, whenever a fat cushion becomes visible between the tumor bed and the mesorectal fascia at re-staging, or whenever the mesorectal fascia is reached only by very thin hypointense fibrotic spiculae, the specificity for a non-involved margin at pathology after TME may be 100% (Fig. 4.9a, b) [25]. On the other hand, whenever dense hypointense "fibrosis" reaches the mesorectal fascia, a

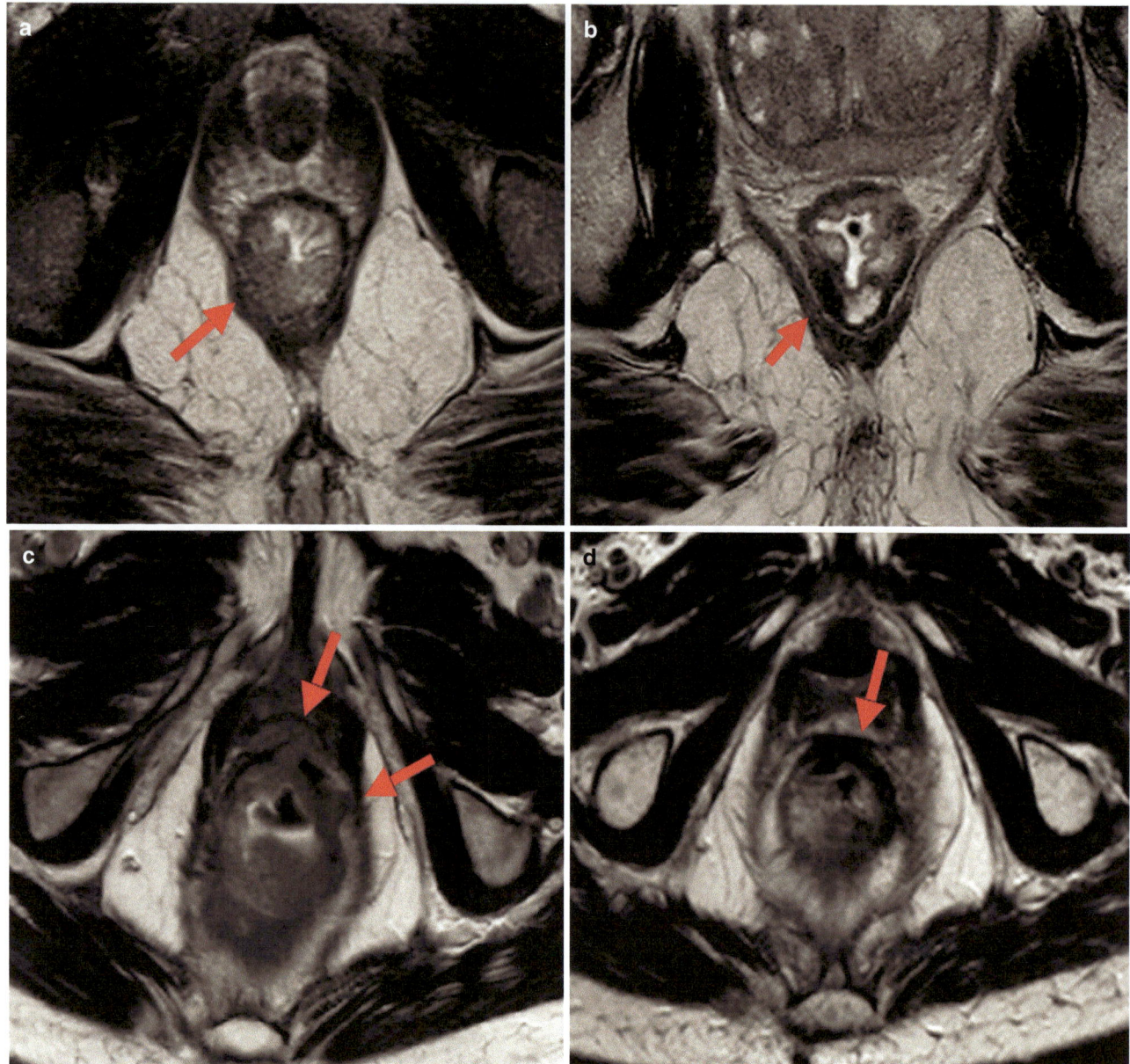

Fig. 4.9 Staging (**a**) and 11 weeks post-NAT re-staging (**b**) MR oblique axial T2-weighted images depicting a low rectal cancer. The tumor reached and pushed the right levator laterally at staging examination (arrow in **a**). After NAT, it regressed, and a thin fat plane became visible between it and the *levator* (arrow in **b**). Patient underwent abdominoperineal excision and an ypT2N0R0 specimen was obtained; another case of a very low rectal tumor invading the posterior wall of the vagina and the left *levator* at staging examination (arrows in **c**). Twelve weeks post-NAT, it regressed but a relatively large surface of contact between the hypointense fibrotic tumor bed and the posterior wall of the vagina was still apparent (arrow in **d**). Anteriorly extended abdominoperineal excision specimen showed a ypT3 tumor <1 mm from the anterior mesorectal fascia

resection beyond TME plane should be planned to achieve negative margins (Fig. 4.9c, d) [25].

It is also very important to evaluate the pelvic lymph nodes in the obturator and internal iliac compartments. Data from the Lateral Node Study Consortium found that internal iliac lymph nodes with a short axis >4 mm post-NAT were associated with a 52% likelihood of lateral local recurrence and that obturator lymph nodes with a short axis >6 mm post-NAT were associated with a higher 5-year rate of distant metastases, re-igniting the discussion on the need to remove lateral nodes surgically during TME in selected patients, which is not standard practice in western countries (Fig. 4.10) [26].

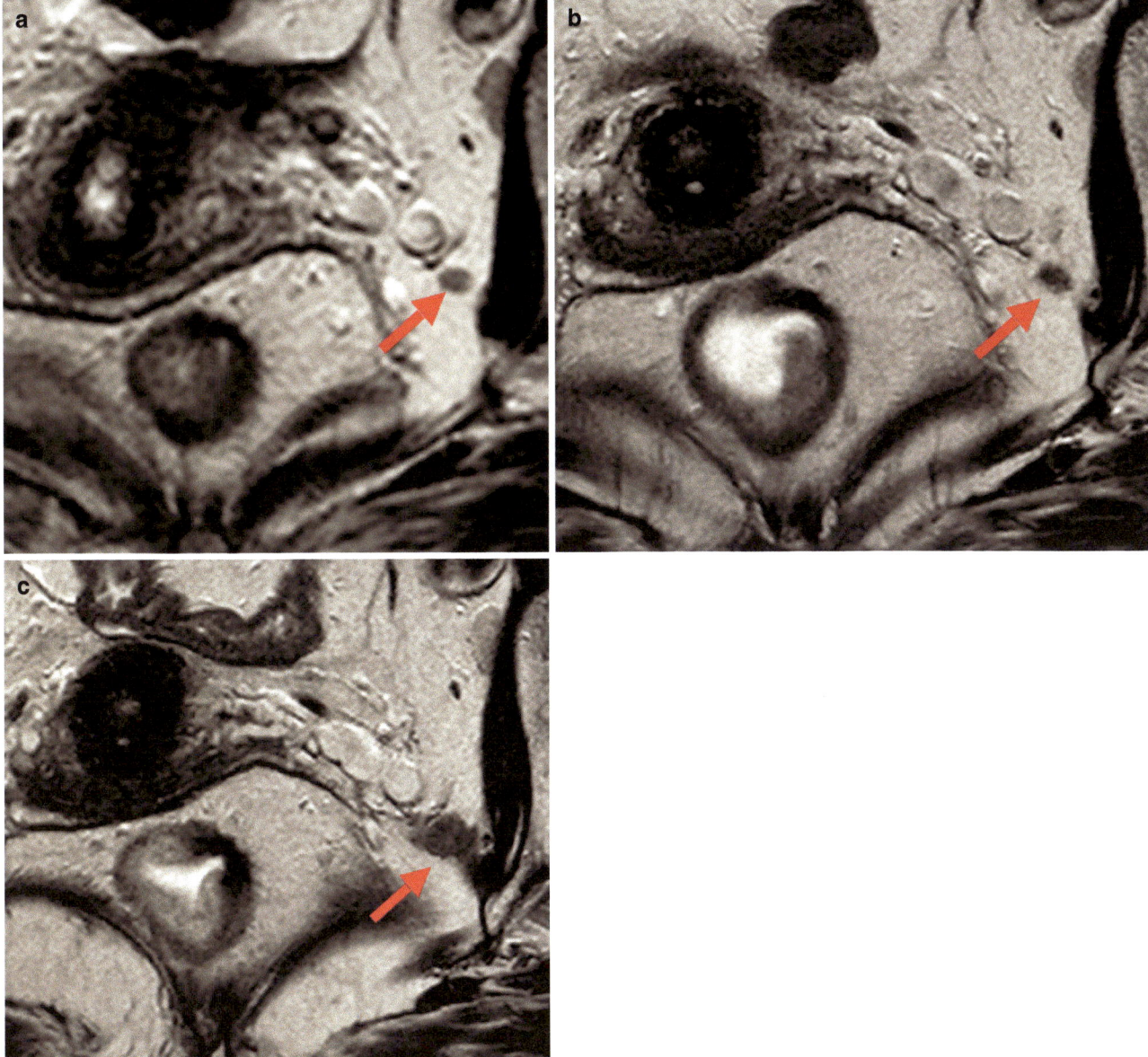

Fig. 4.10 Patient with a mid-rectal cancer and an uncharacteristic 5 mm lymph node in the left iliac compartment on staging oblique axial T2-weighted MR imaging (arrow in **a**). Lymph node became heterogeneously hypointense after irradiation but remained 5 mm in short axis (arrow in **b**). At 1-year follow-up imaging, a clear lateral nodal recurrence became apparent (arrow in **c**). Retroperitoneal and lung metastasis were detected concomitantly

4.2.3.3 The Prognostic Value of Re-staging MR Imaging

Different assessment methods may be utilized to evaluate response of the primary tumor but the most important is the T2-weighted imaging-based magnetic resonance tumor regression grade (mrTRG) (Fig. 4.11), mrTRGs 4 and 5 being associated with worse patient survival [26].

Regarding low rectal cancer in particular, an mrTRG1-2 plus a tumor regression from an "unsafe" to a "safe" plane on post-NAT MR imaging is very specific for a non-involved margin at pathology (Fig. 4.12) [27].

4.2.3.4 Re-staging to Select Patients for Non-operative Management

In a variable proportion of locally advanced rectal cancer patients, there are no signs of viable tumor after NAT. In the observational studies available, the clinical criteria with the highest specificity for a pathologic complete response or a sustained clinical complete response over time are a flat white scar with or without telangiectasia at rectoscopy; and a smooth "normalized" tumor bed at digital rectal examination [28]. Regarding MR imaging, the most specific criteria depend on the analysis of T2-weighted images. They are the following:

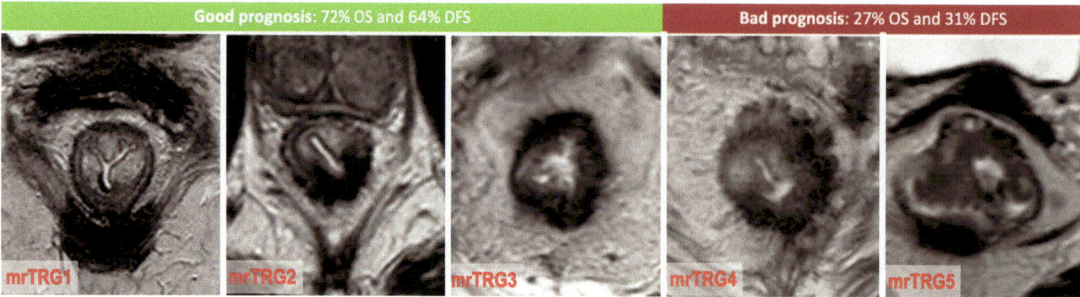

Fig. 4.11 MrTRG scale examples on oblique axial T2-weighted cropped images. MrTRG1—linear crescentic 1–2 mm endoluminal scar; mrTRG2—dense hypointense fibrosis with no obvious intermediate tumor signal intensity; mrTRG3—>50% fibrosis and visible intermediate tumor signal intensity; mrTRG4—slight response (mostly intermediate tumor signal intensity); mrTRG5—no response or tumor growth [5, 7]

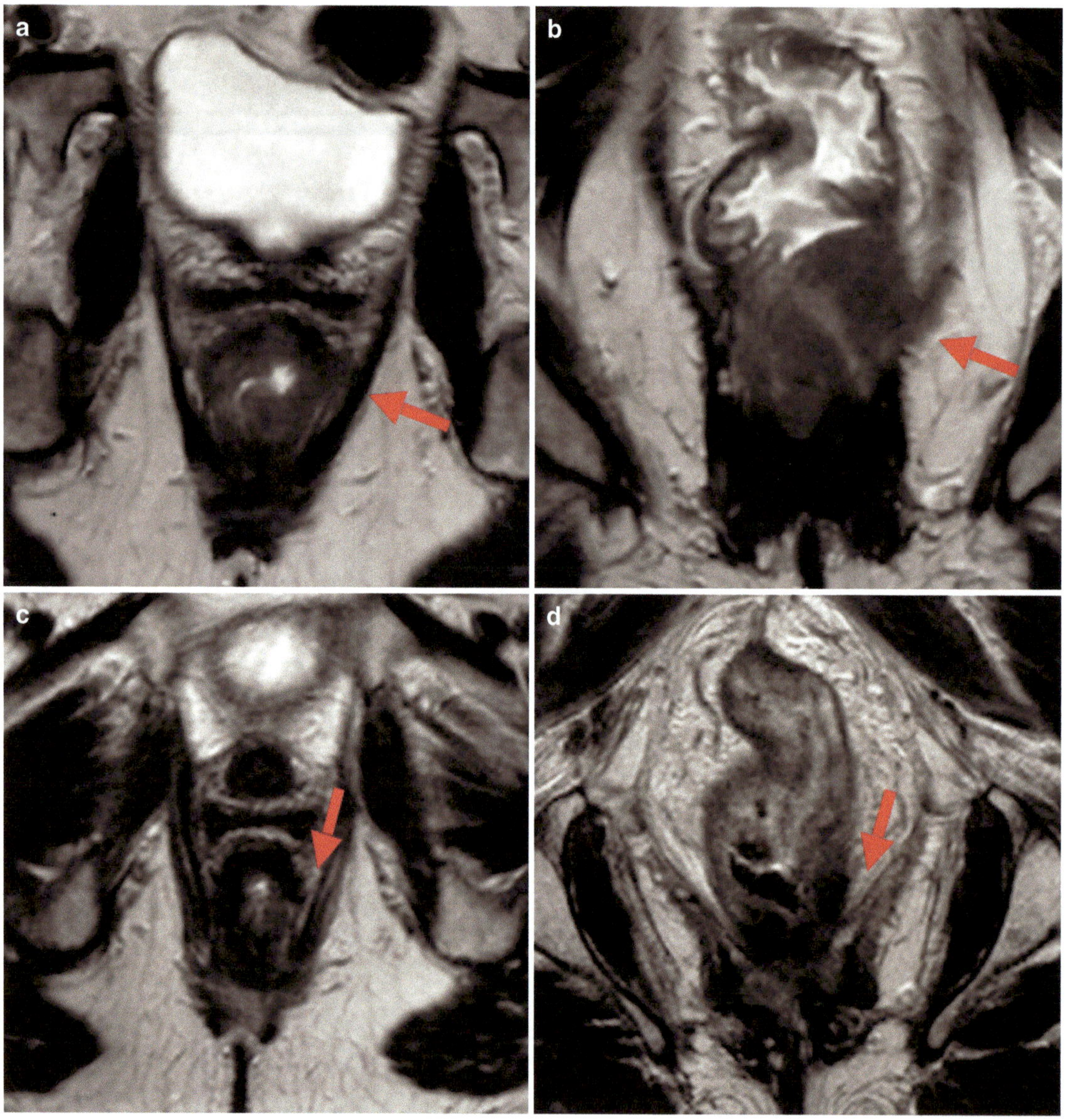

Fig. 4.12 A 55-year-old female with low rectal cancer invading the internal sphincter and the left *levator* [red arrows in **a** (oblique axial) and **b** (coronal T2-weighted images)] who underwent NAT and was restaged at 10 weeks. Tumor regressed from an "unsafe" to a "safe" resection plane, given a thin fat cushion became visible between the tumor bed and the levator (red arrows in **c** and **d**). An abdominoperineal excision was performed and a ypT3N0R0 resection specimen was obtained. Tumor was 3 mm away from the radial resection margin

– an mrTRG1, corresponding either to a linear/crescentic 1–2 mm hypointense scar on the endoluminal aspect of the rectal wall or to its normalization (rarely observed in our experience) [29].
– a positive split scar sign, corresponding to a specific layered reorganization of the rectal wall at tumor bed [30].

The lack or residual high signal intensity at high b value DWI images supports a complete response, but it is not specific.

An example of a patient with strict criteria for a complete response is provided in Fig. 4.13.

> **Key Point**
> Re-staging MRI after neoadjuvant therapy in rectal cancer may document sufficient tumoral regression to support less mutilating curative surgery and help identify clinical complete responders for non-operative management in dedicated centers.

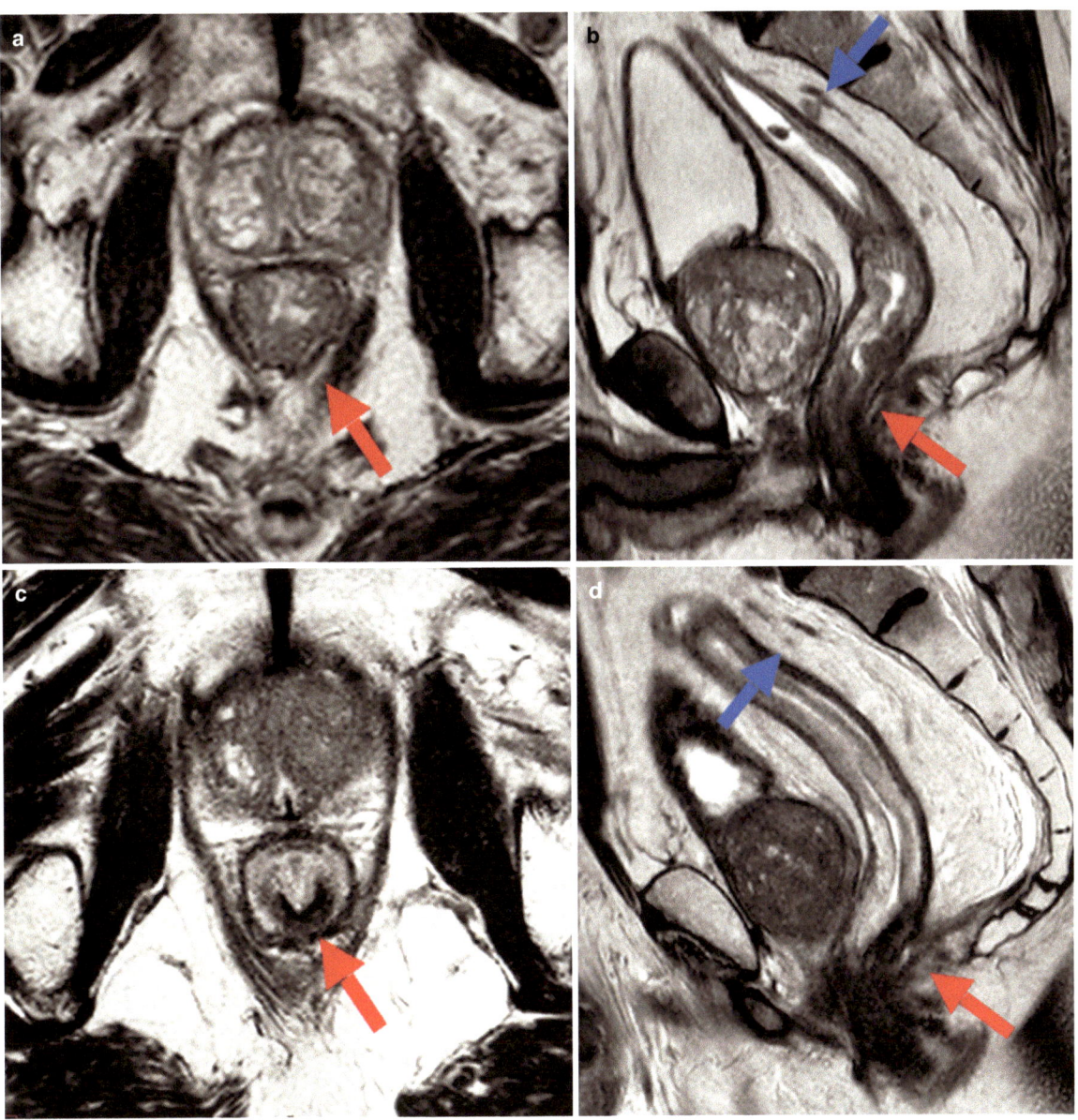

Fig. 4.13 Oblique axial (**a**) and sagittal (**b**) T2-weighted images from a 68-year-old male patient with an mrT2 tumor (red arrows) involving the postero-bilateral wall at 4 cm from the anal verge. Patient was N1a (blue arrow in **b**) and EMVI negative. After NAT, at 11 weeks, digital rectal examination was normal, and response on MR imaging was considered mrTRG1 and split scar sign positive on axial and sagittal T2-weighted imaging (**c** and **d**). The positive high rectal lymph node regressed to 2 mm in size (blue arrow in **d**). No high signal intensity at tumor bed was found on DWI (**e**) (red arrow points to "star-shaped" normal luminal hyperintensity). At rectoscopy (**f**), a flat white scar with overhanging telangiectasia is observed (between arrows). These are the typical MR imaging and rectoscopy findings of a clinical complete response

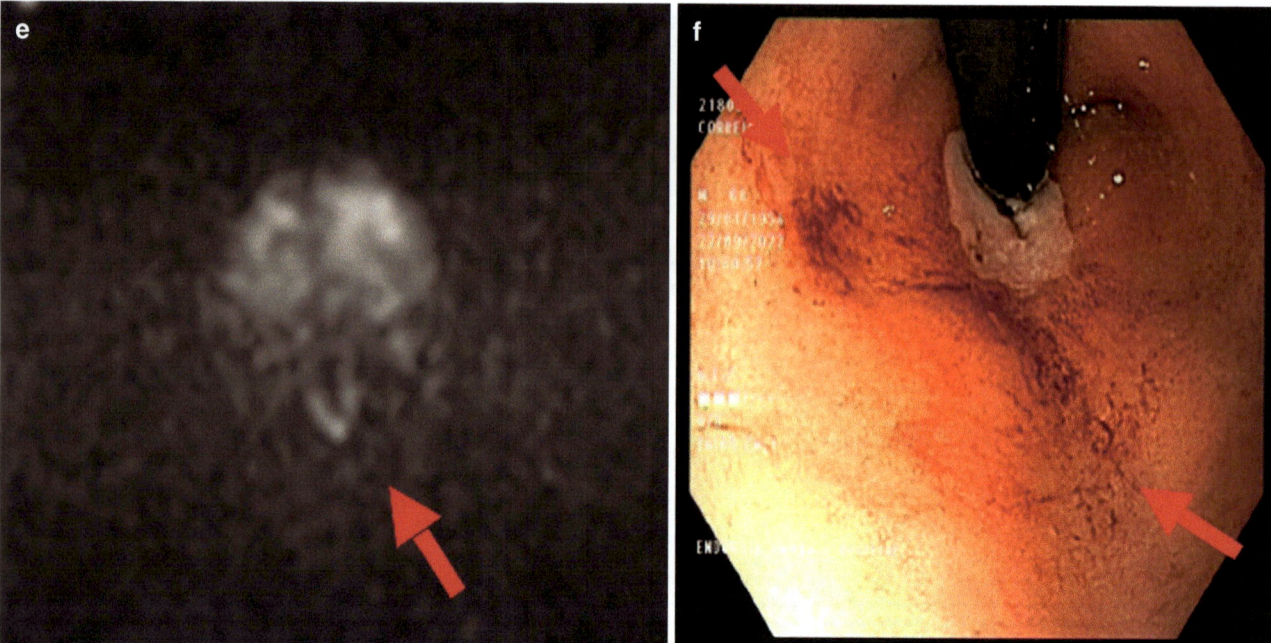

Fig. 4.13 (continued)

4.3   Concluding Remarks

Benign and malignant diseases of the colon and rectum include a wide spectrum of neoplastic and inflammatory disorders. Cross-sectional imaging techniques (including CT and MRI) play a crucial role in imaging of benign and malignant diseases of the colon and rectum for the primary diagnosis, risk stratification, procedural planning, treatment response evaluation, and the assessment of related extraluminal and extraintestinal pathologies and complications. Despite the significant overlap in imaging findings of different bowel conditions, understanding of leading disease patterns and specific imaging features can allow accurate diagnosis and, therefore, patients' management.

complications, distant staging, response assessment in those selected for systemic therapy and follow-up.
- Rectal MRI plays a key role in the pre-treatment local staging of rectal cancer and enables assessment of poor prognostic factors including MRF and EMVI.
- Re-staging of rectal cancer after neoadjuvant therapy may help select patients for less mutilating surgery or for non-operative management when an mrTRG 1/split scar positive tumor bed is observed without diffusion restriction.

Take-Home Messages
- Abdominal CT and MRI are standard care for patients with colon and rectum diseases for primary diagnosis and assessment of complications. They allow accurate and reliable diagnosis of different colorectal diseases, including their localization, extension, in-depth mural involvement, enhancement pattern, and also associated pericolonic and extraintestinal findings.
- CT is the imaging workhorse in colon cancer. It allows adequate planning of curative resection in eligible patients, pre- and postoperative diagnose of

References

1. Loftus EV. Clinical epidemiology of inflammatory bowel disease: incidence, prevalence, and environmental influences. Gastroenterology. 2004;126(6):1504–17.
2. Panizza PSB, Viana PCC, Horvat N, et al. Inflammatory bowel disease: current role of imaging in diagnosis and detection of complications: gastrointestinal imaging. Radiographics. 2017;37(2):701–2.
3. Maddu KK, Mittal P, Shuaib W, Tewari A, Ibraheem O, Khosa F (2014) Colorectal emergencies and related complications: a comprehensive imaging review—imaging of colitis and complications. AJR Am J Roentgenol 203(6):1205–1216.
4. Kawamoto S, Horton KM, Fishman EK. Pseudomembranous colitis: spectrum of imaging findings with clinical and pathologic correlation. Radiographics. 1999;19(4):887–97.
5. McGettigan MJ, Menias CO, Gao ZJ, Mellnick VM, Hara AK. Imaging of drug-induced complications in the gastrointestinal system. Radiographics. 2016;36(1):71–87.

6. Vogel MN, Goeppert B, Maksimovic O, et al. CT features of neutropenic enterocolitis in adult patients with hematological diseases undergoing chemotherapy. Rofo. 2010;182(12):1076–81.

7. Capps GW, Fulcher AS, Szucs RA, Turner MA. Imaging features of radiation-induced changes in the abdomen. Radiographics. 1997;17(6):1455–73.

8. Brodoefel H, Bethge W, Vogel M, et al. Early and late-onset acute GvHD following hematopoietic cell transplantation: CT features of gastrointestinal involvement with clinical and pathological correlation. Eur J Radiol. 2010;73(3):594–600.

9. Lembcke B. Diagnosis, differential diagnoses, and classification of diverticular disease. Viszeralmedizin. 2015;31(2):95–102.

10. Horvat N, Carlos Tavares Rocha C, Clemente Oliveira B, Petkovska I, Gollub MJ. MRI of rectal cancer: tumor staging, imaging techniques, and management. Radiographics. 2019;39(2):367–87.

11. Morgan E, Arnold M, Gini A, et al. Global burden of colorectal cancer in 2020 and 2040: incidence and mortality estimates from GLOBOCAN. Gut. 2022; https://doi.org/10.1136/gutjnl-2022-327736.

12. Simon K. Colorectal cancer development and advances in screening. Clin Interv Aging. 2016;11:967–76.

13. Haan MC de, Pickhardt PJ, Stoker J (2015) CT colonography: accuracy, acceptance, safety and position in organised population screening. Gut 64(2):342–350.

14. Tong G-J, Zhang G-Y, Liu J, et al. Comparison of the eighth version of the American Joint Committee on Cancer manual to the seventh version for colorectal cancer: A retrospective review of our data. World J Clin Oncol. 2018;9(7):148–61.

15. Hunter C, Siddiqui M, Georgiou Delisle T, et al. CT and 3-T MRI accurately identify T3c disease in colon cancer, which strongly predicts disease-free survival. Clin Radiol. 2017;72(4):307–15.

16. Santiago IA, Rodrigues ER, Germano AS, et al. High-risk features in potentially resectable colon cancer: a prospective MDCT-pathology agreement study. Abdom Radiol (NY). 2016;41(10):1877–90.

17. Unterrainer M, Deroose CM, Herrmann K, et al. Imaging standardisation in metastatic colorectal cancer: a joint EORTC-ESOI-ESGAR expert consensus recommendation. Eur J Cancer. 2022;176:193–206.

18. Ko EY, Ha HK, Kim AY, et al. CT differentiation of mucinous and nonmucinous colorectal carcinoma. AJR Am J Roentgenol. 2007;188(3):785–91.

19. Hong EK, Landolfi F, Castagnoli F, et al. CT for lymph node staging of colon cancer: not only size but also location and number of lymph node count. Abdom Radiol (NY). 2021;46(9):4096–105.

20. Fernandez LM, Ibrahim RNM, Mizrahi I, DaSilva G, Wexner SD. How accurate is preoperative colonoscopic localization of colonic neoplasia? Surg Endosc. 2019;33(4):1174–9.

21. Yang KM, Jeong M-J, Yoon KH, Jung YT, Kwak JY. Oncologic outcome of colon cancer with perforation and obstruction. BMC Gastroenterol. 2022;22(1):247.

22. Kim SW, Shin HC, Kim IY, Kim YT, Kim C-J. CT findings of colonic complications associated with colon cancer. Korean J Radiol. 2010;11(2):211–21.

23. Herring W. Learning radiology: recognizing the basics/ William Herring, MD, FACR, Vice Chairman and Residency Program Director, Albert Einstein Medical Center, Philadelphia, Pennsylvania. 3rd ed. Philadelphia, PA: Elsevier; 2016.

24. Taydas O, Unal E, Onur MR, Akpinar E. Role of computed tomography in intestinal obstruction. Istanbul Med J. 2018;19(2):105–12.

25. Santiago I, Rodrigues B, Barata M, et al. Re-staging and follow-up of rectal cancer patients with MR imaging when "Watch-and-Wait" is an option: a practical guide. Insights Imaging. 2021;12(1):114.

26. Schaap DP, Boogerd LSF, Konishi T, et al. Rectal cancer lateral lymph nodes: multicentre study of the impact of obturator and internal iliac nodes on oncological outcomes. Br J Surg. 2021;108(2):205–13.

27. Battersby NJ, How P, Moran B, et al. Prospective validation of a low rectal cancer magnetic resonance imaging staging system and development of a local recurrence risk stratification model: the MERCURY II study. Ann Surg. 2016;263(4):751–60.

28. van der Sande ME, Maas M, Melenhorst J, Breukink SO, van Leerdam ME, Beets GL. Predictive value of endoscopic features for a complete response after chemoradiotherapy for rectal cancer. Ann Surg. 2021;274(6):e541–7.

29. Jang JK, Choi SH, Park SH, et al. MR tumor regression grade for pathological complete response in rectal cancer post neoadjuvant chemoradiotherapy: a systematic review and meta-analysis for accuracy. Eur Radiol. 2020;30(4):2312–23.

30. Santiago I, Barata M, Figueiredo N, et al. The split scar sign as an indicator of sustained complete response after neoadjuvant therapy in rectal cancer. Eur Radiol. 2020;30(1):224–38.

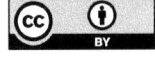

Indeterminate Retroperitoneal Masses

5

Christina Messiou and Wolfgang G. Kunz

Learning Objectives
- To describe the most common indeterminate retroperitoneal mass lesions and to highlight features which should raise suspicion for retroperitoneal sarcoma
- To outline safe practice for tissue diagnosis
- To understand the diagnostic value of imaging modalities in the differential diagnosis
- To comprehend the diagnostic limits of imaging in differentiating retroperitoneal pathologies

5.1 Introduction

The retroperitoneum can host a broad spectrum of pathologies and masses can grow to a substantial size before presenting symptoms and signs such as abdominal swelling, early satiety, hernias, testicular swelling, nerve irritation, or lower limb swelling. Due to increased use of cross-sectional imaging, retroperitoneal (RP) masses may also be incidental findings. Although soft-tissue sarcomas (STS) are rare, in the RP they can account for up to a third of tumors and must therefore be considered as a differential diagnosis [1]. In 291 patients with indeterminate RP mass lesions, 79.4% were mesenchymal (55.8% were adipocytic (liposarcoma, angiomyolipoma, myelolipoma), and 36.8% non-adipocytic (schwannoma, leiomyosarcoma, desmoid, other sarcomas)); 53.3% were non-mesenchymal (metastatic carcinoma, lymphoma, germ cell, other) [2]. STS patients treated at high volume centers have significantly better survival and functional outcomes and therefore any suspicion for STS should trigger early referral [3].

Contrast-enhanced CT is the modality of choice, yet MRI can clarify involvement of muscle, bone, or neural foramina. [18]F FDG PET/CT is not routinely indicated, however, for lesions which are inaccessible to percutaneous biopsy it can differentiate between intermediate/high-grade lesions and low grade/benign lesions, but critically it is unable to differentiate between low grade and benign lesions [4].

This chapter aims to describe the most common indeterminate RP mass lesions and to highlight features which should raise suspicion for RP sarcoma.

5.2 Retroperitoneal Space

The RP space is divided into four anatomically separate compartments [5]: the posterior pararenal space is encompassed by the posterior parietal peritoneum. The anterior pararenal space extends to the transversalis fascia [5]. The perirenal space is encapsulated by the perirenal fascia. The anterior pararenal space contains visceral organs that mainly originate from the dorsal mesentery, i.e., the pancreas and the descending and ascending parts of the colon. The perinephric space is bounded anteriorly by Gerota's fascia and posteriorly by Zuckerkandl's fascia [5]. It contains the kidneys and adrenal glands. The perinephric space is home to bridging septa and a network of lymphatic vessels, which may facilitate the spread of disease processes to or from adjacent spaces. The perinephric space is limited caudally by the merging of Gerota's and Zuckerkandl's fascias and therefore does not continue into the pelvic region [5]. The posterior pararenal space is bound by the transversalis fascia on its posterior face. Anatomic communication between the posterior pararenal space and the structures of the flank wall may be established. A fourth space surrounds the large vessels,

C. Messiou
Department of Radiology, The Royal Marsden Hospital, London, UK
e-mail: Christina.Messiou@rmh.nhs.uk

W. G. Kunz (✉)
Department of Radiology, University Hospital, LMU Munich, Munich, Bavaria, Germany
e-mail: wolfgang.kunz@med.lmu.de

© The Author(s) 2023
J. Hodler et al. (eds.), *Diseases of the Abdomen and Pelvis 2023-2026*, IDKD Springer Series,
https://doi.org/10.1007/978-3-031-27355-1_5

the aorta, and the inferior vena cava. This space has a lateral boundary with the perirenal spaces and ureters and extends cranially into the posterior mediastinum [5]. Some diseases, for example, RP fibrosis, are largely limited to this space. Depending on the definition, some sources refer to a fifth space, which includes the muscular structures with psoas and quadratus lumborum muscles.

> **Key Point**
> *Recognizing the retroperitoneal origin of masses is crucial to narrow down the list of differential diagnoses.*

5.3   Tissue Diagnosis

Apart from RP liposarcoma and renal angiomyolipoma, accurate characterization of indeterminate RP masses on imaging alone is challenging [2]. Therefore, a tissue diagnosis is imperative, and image-guided percutaneous coaxial core needle biopsy is safe and preferred. If a diagnosis of STS is suspected radiologically, the biopsy should preferentially be performed at a specialist sarcoma center to expedite final diagnosis through expert pathology review. Multiple needle cores (ideally 4–5 at 16G) should be obtained to allow for histologic and molecular subtyping. Although percutaneous core biopsy is accurate for diagnosis, under-grading of pathologies such as sarcoma is recognized due to sampling error [6, 7]. Use of functional imaging techniques such as ^{18}F-Fluorodeoxyglucose PET/CT and contemporary robotic-assisted CT-guided biopsy techniques have immense potential to improve sampling of the most deterministic tumor elements [8]. The RP route is preferred and the transperitoneal approach only utilized following discussion at multidisciplinary tumor boards when the tumor is inaccessible via the retroperitoneum. Risk of needle track seeding when the RP route is respected is minimal and core needle biopsy does not negatively influence outcome [9].

Fine-needle aspiration (FNA) cytology rarely yields sufficient diagnostic information and is not recommended. An open or laparoscopic surgical incision/excision biopsy of an RP mass is discouraged as it exposes the peritoneal cavity to contamination and distorts planes of dissection if subsequent completion surgery is necessary [10]. Incision or excision biopsy of an indeterminate RP mass should only be performed after specialist sarcoma multidisciplinary review.

> **Key Point**
> *Percutaneous core needle biopsy of indeterminate retroperitoneal masses is safe and does not adversely affect outcomes.*

5.4   Adipocytic Tumors

As a substantial proportion of mesenchymal RP masses are adipocytic (55.8%), it is useful to establish early whether there is abnormal macroscopic fat associated with an indeterminate RP mass [2, 11]. This should include careful interrogation of whether the fat containing mass originates from the kidney or adrenal leading to a more reassuring diagnosis of benign renal angiomyolipoma (AML) or adrenal myelolipoma (ML), respectively. The presence of renal cortical defects and prominent vessels strengthens the diagnosis of the AML [12] and adrenal ML tend to be more well defined than RP liposarcoma. If the adipocytic mass is not arising from the solid viscera, a diagnosis of RP liposarcoma should be considered and referral to a soft-tissue sarcoma unit made.

Expansile macroscopic fat external to the solid abdominal viscera is highly suspicious for well-differentiated liposarcoma and the presence of solid enhancing elements suggests dedifferentiation (Fig. 5.1). In adults over 55, liposarcoma is the commonest RP sarcoma, accounting for up to 70% of RP sarcomas [13]. Well-differentiated liposarcoma does not metastasize but can dedifferentiate and develop high-grade non-adipocytic elements with potential to metastasize. Well and dedifferentiated liposarcoma characteristically harbor supernumerary ring and/or giant chromosomes in relation to amplification of several genes in the 12q13–15 region. These include MDM2, CDK4, and HMGA2, which can be of diagnostic use [14]. Calcifications may be present and can indicate dedifferentiation or may reflect sclerosing or inflammatory variants of WDL [15]. The presence of fat is not always immediately apparent, and careful evaluation is crucial. Failure to recognize the presence of abnormal fat is the commonest reason for misdiagnosis and mismanagement. If the well-differentiated component is not recognized, incomplete resection may follow which deprives the patient of potentially curative surgery. Furthermore, several foci of dedifferentiation can be misinterpreted as multifocal disease contraindicating surgery or leading to piecemeal resection; however, this usually represents separate foci of dedifferentiation within a single contiguous liposarcoma with well-differentiated elements between the solid masses. This is treated as unifocal disease [10].

Absence of macroscopic fat in an RP mass does not exclude a diagnosis of RP liposarcoma. This may represent disease that has dedifferentiated throughout or a sclerosing subtype. Anatomic constraints within the retroperitoneum limit the ability to achieve wide resection margins. As a consequence, local recurrence of RPS is more frequent than for extremity sarcoma and represents the leading cause of death [16]. Tumor grade and macroscopic complete resection are the two most important and consistent independent factors that predict oncological outcome. Other factors include patient age, tumor subtype, microscopic resection margins, tumor size, primary or recurrent disease, multifocality, mul-

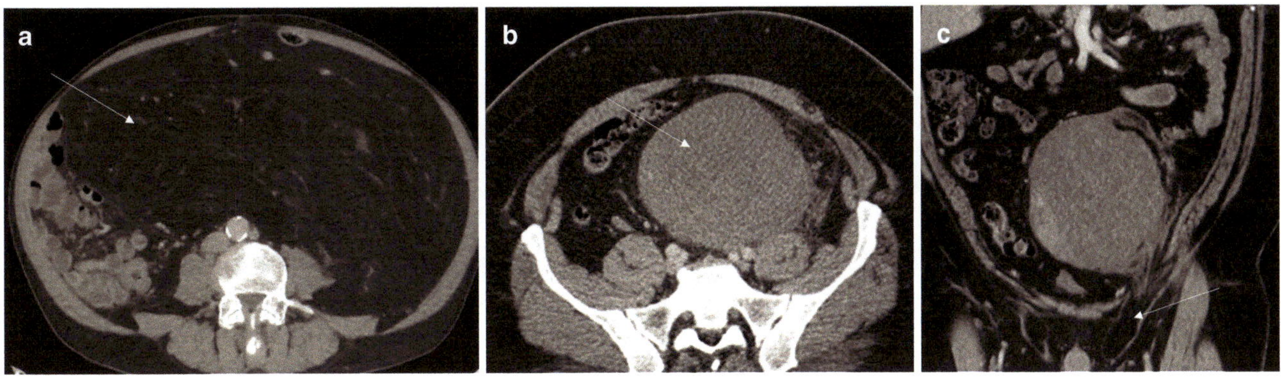

Fig. 5.1 Liposarcoma. Well-differentiated liposarcoma typically appears as a relatively bland fat density mass with minimal internal complexity, displacing adjacent structures (**a**). In contrast, dedifferentiated liposarcoma in another patient appears as a solid mass (**b**). The diagnosis of the solid mass seen in image **b** is challenging until the well-differentiated component extending into the left inguinal canal is identified (**c**)

timodality treatment and centralized multidisciplinary management in a specialist sarcoma center [14]. In liposarcomas, local recurrence dictates outcome as the main mode of disease recurrence (70% 5-year local recurrence), while systemic metastases are rare (10–15% 5-year distant disease recurrence) [17]. Although rare in the retroperitoneum, benign fat-containing extragonadal dermoids, hibernomas, extramedullary hematopoiesis, and lipomas can also mimic RP liposarcomas. Therefore, biopsy must always be performed.

> **Key Point**
>
> *Absence of macroscopic fat in a retroperitoneal mass does not exclude a diagnosis of liposarcoma. This may represent disease that has dedifferentiated throughout.*

5.5 Other Soft-Tissue Sarcomas

Leiomyosarcoma (LMS) is the second most common RP sarcoma accounting for up to 15% of all RPS. The exception is in younger adults where LMS can supersede liposarcoma. LMS usually arise from the IVC below the level of the hepatic veins (Fig. 5.2), but they do also arise from smaller vessels such as the renal veins or less commonly the gonadal veins [18]. LMS commonly have an exophytic component, which can make differentiation from extrinsic compression challenging. Unlike liposarcomas where local recurrence dictates outcome, LMS are much less likely to recur locally but systemic metastases, usually to the lungs, are much more common [14]. After LMS, the remaining 5% of RPS are composed of much rarer sarcoma subtypes. The commonest of these are described below.

Synovial sarcoma is the fifth commonest sarcoma overall, typically affecting young adults (15–40 years). Despite the name, the tissue of origin is not synovium but undifferentiated mesenchyme; it simply most resembles adult synovium microscopically. Synovial sarcoma is a high-grade tumor with 5-year survival rates of less than 50% [19, 20]. Imaging findings are generally those of a non-specific heterogeneous mass; however, many display smooth well-defined margins with cystic contents, leading to an erroneous diagnosis of a benign ganglion or myxoma [21] (Fig. 5.3). 30% contain calcification [21]. Changes compatible with hemorrhage are seen in 40% of cases and fluid-fluid levels are seen in around 20% of lesions [22]. As with other STSs the lung is the main site of metastasis, which occurs in over 50% of patients and 25% of patients present with metastatic disease. Synovial sarcoma is one of the few sarcomas which commonly spread to regional lymph nodes, occurring in up to 20% of cases [20, 21].

Undifferentiated Pleomorphic Sarcomas (UPS) (formerly known as malignant fibrous histiocytomas) are high-grade sarcomas which are thought to represent a heterogeneous group of poorly differentiated tumors which may be the poorly differentiated endpoints of many mesenchymal lineages. As the morphological pattern is shared by many poorly differentiated neoplasms, it is important to exclude pleomorphic variants of more common tumor types (i.e., sarcomatoid renal cell carcinoma). Most UPSs in the retroperitoneum are now considered to represent dedifferentiated liposarcoma [23, 24]. In view of this, a histological diagnosis of RP poorly differentiated sarcoma warrants close correlation with clinical history to see if there is a history of well-differentiated liposarcoma. Immunohistochemistry for MDM2 and CDK4 gene products, and cytogenetic analysis to assess MDM2 gene amplification status may also be beneficial. This has prognostic implications as dedifferentiated liposarcoma tends to be less aggressive than other pleomorphic sarcomas [25].

The finding of a large, well-circumscribed solid, vascular tumor, particularly with prominent feeding vessels should introduce the possibility of solitary fibrous tumor (Fig. 5.4). The presence of fat may suggest lipomatous hemangiopericytoma, a subtype of SFT [26].

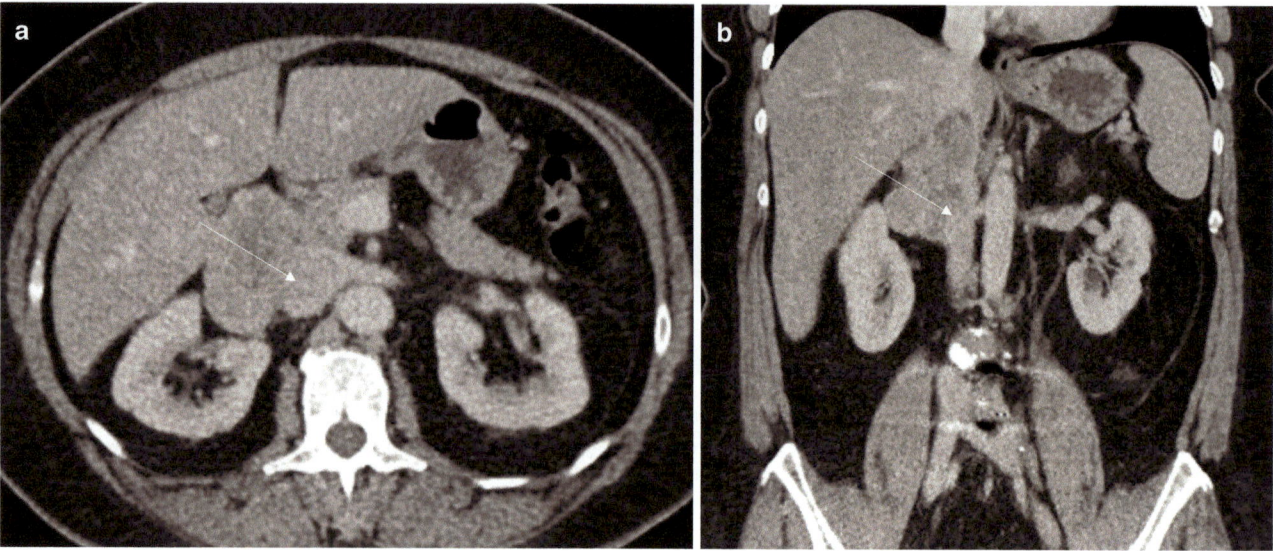

Fig. 5.2 Leiomyosarcoma of the inferior vena cava. Retroperitoneal leiomyosarcomas usually arise from the inferior vena cava. In this case the mass relating to the right lateral wall of the inferior vena cava has an exophytic (**a**) and endoluminal (**b**) component

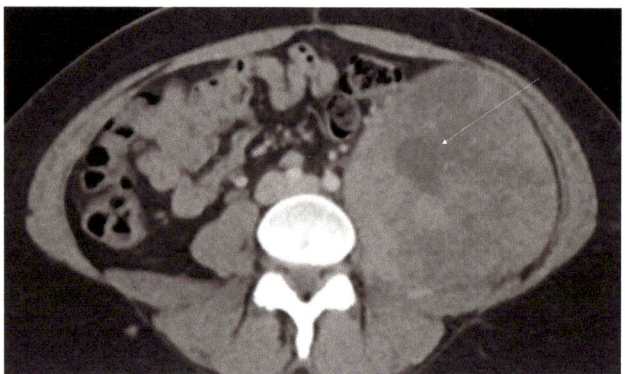

Fig. 5.3 Synovial sarcoma. Large left-sided retroperitoneal mass in a 30-year-old lady was biopsy-proven synovial sarcoma. Cystic looking change is common (A) which together with well-defined margins can lead to a misdiagnosis of benign neurogenic tumor. Therefore, biopsy of indeterminate retroperitoneal masses is mandatory for accurate diagnosis

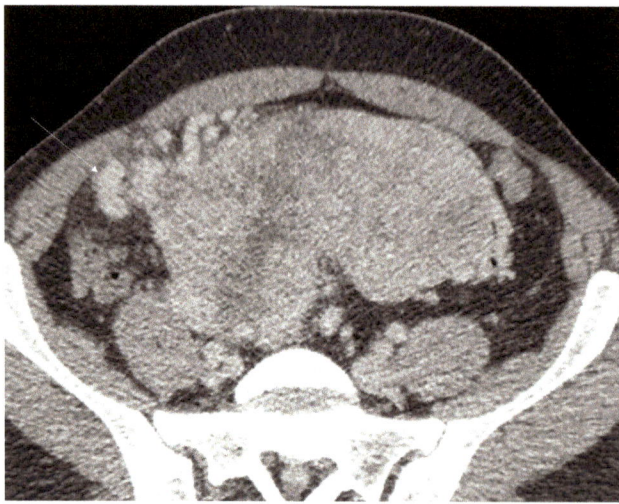

Fig. 5.4 Solitary fibrous tumor. Characteristically, solitary fibrous tumours are greater than 10 cm at presentation and avidly enhancing with prominent surrounding tumor vasculature

> **Key Point**
> *Liposarcoma and leiomyosarcoma are the commonest soft-tissue sarcomas occurring in the retroperitoneum.*

5.6 Neurogenic Tumors

Neurogenic tumors make up 10%–20% of primary RP masses [27] and manifest at a younger age and are more frequently benign. They develop from the nerve sheath, ganglionic or paraganglionic cells, and are commonly observed along the sympathetic nerve system, in the adrenal medulla, or in the organs of Zuckerkandl [28].

Schwannomas represent benign masses that arises from the perineural sheath and account for 6% of RP neoplasms [27]. They usually present without symptoms and occur around the second to fifth decade. It is an encapsulated tumor along the nerve. Degenerative changes can be present (i.e., ancient schwannomas), as well as hemorrhage, cystic changes, or calcification. Schwannomas are often found in the paravertebral region. They demonstrate variable homogeneous or heterogeneous contrast enhancement [27]. Cystic areas appear hyperintense on T2-weighted sequences whereas cellular areas appear hypointense on T1- and T2-weighted images [29].

Malignant nerve sheath tumors include malignant schwannoma, neurogenic sarcoma, and neurofibrosarcoma. Half develop spontaneously and half originate from neurofibroma, ganglioneuroma, or prior radiation [28]. Ongoing enlargement, irregular boundaries, pain, heterogeneous appearance, and infiltration in surrounding structures raise suspicion for malignancy, in particular for neurofibromatosis type 1 (NF1) patients [27].

Neurofibromas are a benign nerve sheath tumors that are either unifocal (90%) or part of NF1. About a third of single and all multifocal tumors are associated with NF1 [27]. They are unencapsulated solid tumors consisting of nerve sheath and collagen bundles on pathology. Variable myxoid degeneration exists and cystic degeneration is infrequent. On imaging, it presents as a well-circum-scribed, homogeneous, low attenuating lesion (about 25 HU), resulting from lipid-rich components. On T2-weighted sequences, the periphery has higher signal owing to myxoid degeneration [27]. Malignant transformation is more frequent with neurofibroma than schwannoma, particularly in NF1 patients [27]. An example of an RP neurofibroma is shown (Fig. 5.5).

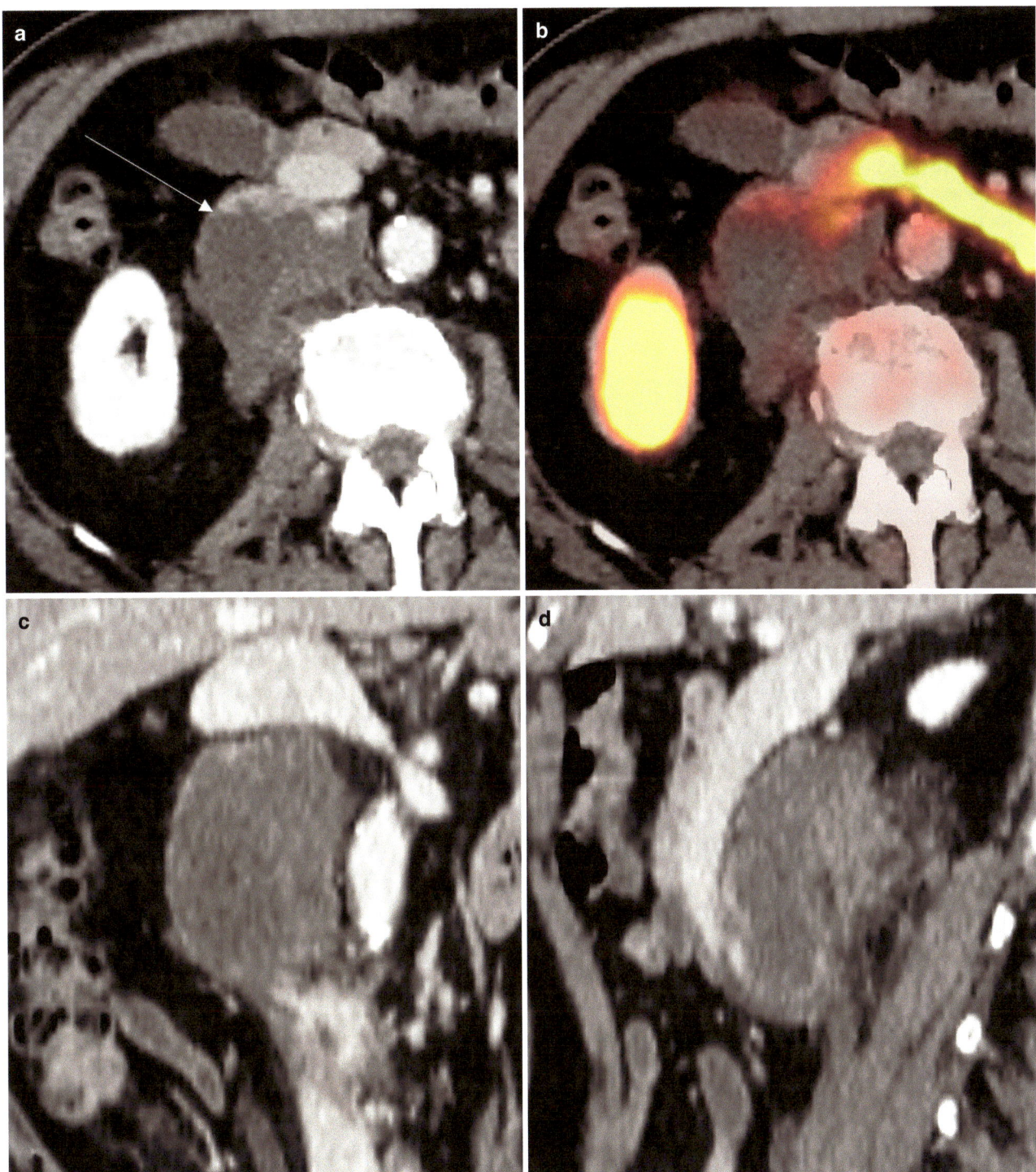

Fig. 5.5 Neurofibroma. Neurofibromas typically present as hypodense masses with no or minimal contrast enhancement (**a, c, d**). The patient had originally been examined for metastatic prostate cancer; there was no PSMA expression of the mass (**b**). Neurofibromas are not encapsu-lated and tend to be less well defined, in contrast to other neurogenic tumors like schwannomas. Local infiltration of adjacent structures makes resections difficult

Ganglioneuroma is a rare benign tumor that arises from the sympathetic ganglia [27]. Most commonly asymptomatic, it can sometimes produce hormones such as catecholamines, vasoactive peptides, or androgenic hormones. The most common sites are retroperitoneum and mediastinum. In the retroperitoneum, the tumor is frequently located along the paravertebral sympathetic ganglia. At imaging, it presents as a well-circumscribed, sometimes lobulated, low attenuating mass [27]. Necrosis and hemorrhage are rare, and there is variable contrast enhancement. On T2-weighted sequences, ganglioneuromas demonstrate variable signal, which depends on the myxoid, cellular, and collagen composition.

Paragangliomas are tumors in an extra-adrenal location that arise from chromaffin cells, where tumors that arise from cells of the adrenal medulla are referred to as pheochromocytomas [27]. About 40% of paragangliomas secrete high levels of catecholamines, leading to symptoms such as headache, palpitations, excessive sweating, and elevated urinary metabolites. Paragangliomas can be associated with NF1, multiple endocrine neoplasia syndrome, and von Hippel–Lindau syndrome [27]. The most frequent retroperitoneal location is the organs of Zuckerkandl. On imaging, they typically present as large well-defined lobular tumors and may contain areas of hemorrhage and necrosis; hence, variable signal is observed on T2-weighted sequences. Its hypervascular nature frequently results in intense contrast enhancement [27]. The tumor frequently has a heterogeneous appearance due to hemorrhages. Radionuclide imaging performed with m-iodobenzylguanidine (MIBG) or 18F-DOPA shows high uptake in paragangliomas [30]. Paragangliomas are more aggressive and metastasize in up to 50% of cases. An example of an RP extra-adrenal paraganglioma with strong DOPA decarboxylase activity is shown (Fig. 5.6).

> **Key Point**
> *Retroperitoneal neurogenic tumors are commonly observed along the sympathetic nerve system, in the adrenal medulla, or in the organs of Zuckerkandl.*

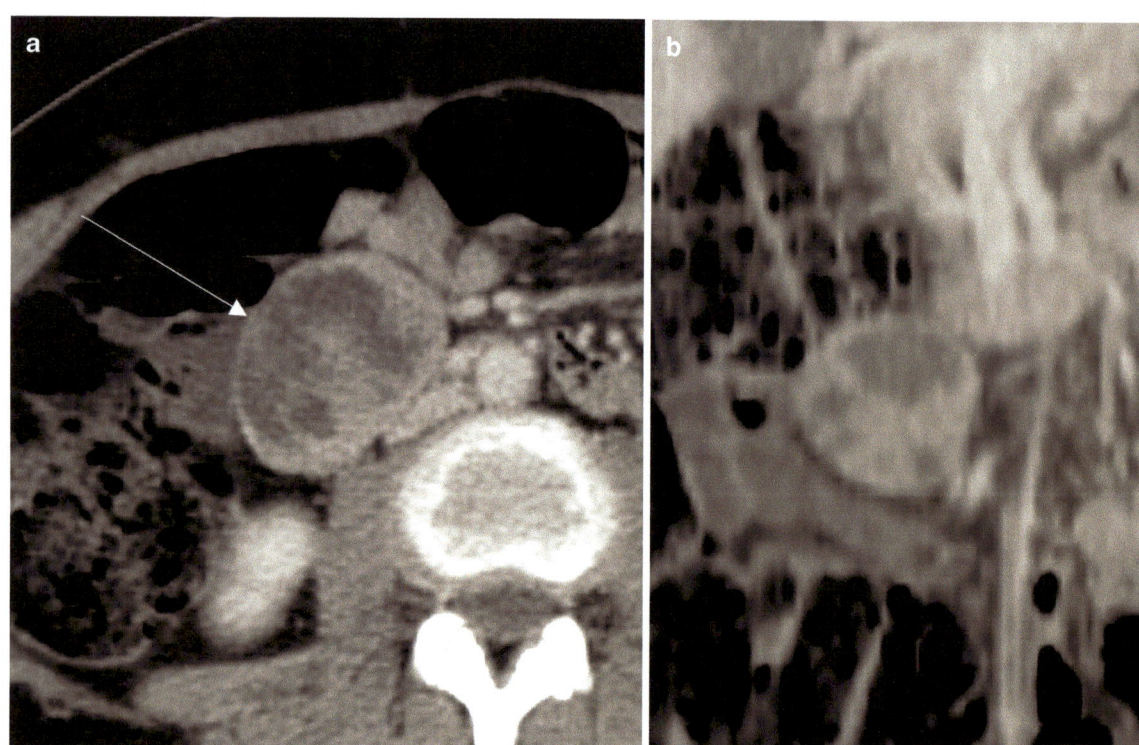

Fig. 5.6 Paraganglioma. Retroperitoneal paragangliomas can manifest in extraadrenal locations. It typically presents as well-circumscribed mass with variable extent of cystic components, enhancing septa or solid components (**a**, **b**). 18F-DOPA imaging typically detects strong DOPA decarboxylase activity (**c**, **d**)

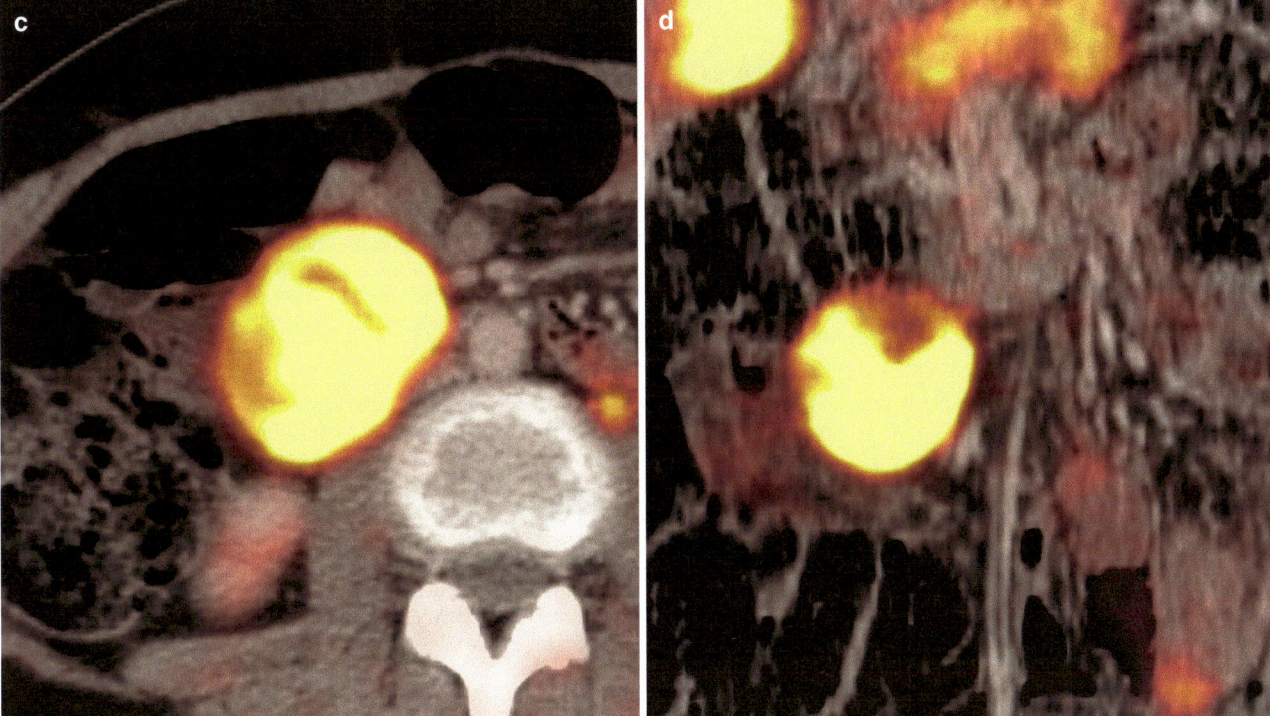

Fig. 5.6 (continued)

5.7 Miscellaneous

Among the most common RP masses are lymphomas. These are highly prevalent and less frequently indeterminate, yet tissue diagnosis remains a cornerstone of management. The hematological malignancies may also present with RP manifestations of posttransplant lymphoproliferative disease, extraosseous myelomas or extramedullary leukemias (i.e., extramedullary disease manifestations) [27]. This disease group typically manifests as solid masses in the form of lymphadenopathy yet may also contain liquid intralesional components as a result of necrosis in highly aggressive hematological malignancies. Benign tumors include lymphangiomas, benign germ cell tumors, or sex cord tumors [27]. For the latter two, serological tumor markers may aid in narrowing the list of differentials. Other rare nonneoplastic masses may include pseudotumoral lipomatosis, RP fibrosis, extramedullary hematopoiesis, IgG4-related disease, or Erdheim-Chester disease [27]. The latter two can have a characteristic imaging appearance with soft-tissue bands surrounding the kidneys in the perinephric space. Finally, the RP space may also represent a location for metastatic spread of disease. Most notably, these include lymph node metastasis from a large group of abdominal and pelvic malignancies. The most common primary, non-lymphoid malignancies to metastasize to the RP space outside of lymph nodes are melanomas and urogenital malignancies.

5.8 Concluding Remarks

The retroperitoneum can host a broad spectrum of pathologies, and the radiologist plays a pivotal role in providing a differential diagnosis and guiding management. Although STS are rare, in the retroperitoneum they can account for up to a third of cases in some series. The commonest RPS, liposarcoma and LMS, have characteristic imaging appearances; however, there are many other STS that can occur in the RP. It is unreasonable and unnecessary to expect that all radiologists should recognize these rarer subtypes. Instead, referral to specialist sarcoma units is recommended where the diagnosis of an RP mass remains indeterminate.

Take Home Messages

- Recognizing the retroperitoneal origin of masses is crucial to narrow down the list of differential diagnoses.
- Percutaneous core needle biopsy of indeterminate RP masses is safe and does not adversely affect outcomes.
- Liposarcoma and leiomyosarcoma are the commonest soft-tissue sarcomas occurring in the retroperitoneum. Absence of macroscopic fat in a retroperitoneal mass does not exclude a diagnosis of liposarcoma. This may represent disease that has dedifferentiated throughout.
- Retroperitoneal neurogenic tumors are commonly observed along the sympathetic nerve system, in the adrenal medulla, or in the organs of Zuckerkandl.
- The large variety of rare RP masses and overlap of imaging appearance highlights the limitations of non-invasive diagnostic tests and underlines the need for minimally invasive tissue diagnosis.

Key Point

The large variety of rare retroperitoneal masses and overlap of imaging appearance highlights the limitations of non-invasive diagnostic tests and underlines the need for minimally invasive tissue diagnosis.

References

1. Van Roggen JF, Hogendoorn PC. Soft tissue tumours of the retroperitoneum. Sarcoma. 2000;4(1-2):17–26. https://doi.org/10.1155/S1357714X00000049.
2. Morosi C, Stacchiotti S, Marchiano A, Bianchi A, Radaelli S, Sanfilippo R, et al. Correlation between radiological assessment and histopathological diagnosis in retroperitoneal tumors: analysis of 291 consecutive patients at a tertiary reference sarcoma center. Eur J Surg Oncol. 2014;40(12):1662–70. https://doi.org/10.1016/j.ejso.2014.10.005.
3. Gutierrez JC, Perez EA, Moffat FL, Livingstone AS, Franceschi D, Koniaris LG. Should soft tissue sarcomas be treated at high-volume centers? An analysis of 4205 patients. Ann Surg. 2007;245(6):952–8. https://doi.org/10.1097/01.sla.0000250438.04393.a8.
4. Ioannidis JP, Lau J. 18F-FDG PET for the diagnosis and grading of soft-tissue sarcoma: a meta-analysis. J Nucl Med. 2003;44(5):717–24.
5. Tirkes T, Sandrasegaran K, Patel AA, Hollar MA, Tejada JG, Tann M, et al. Peritoneal and retroperitoneal anatomy and its relevance for cross-sectional imaging. Radiographics. 2012;32(2):437–51. https://doi.org/10.1148/rg.322115032.
6. Strauss DC, Qureshi YA, Hayes AJ, Thway K, Fisher C, Thomas JM. The role of core needle biopsy in the diagnosis of suspected soft tissue tumours. J Surg Oncol. 2010;102(5):523–9. https://doi.org/10.1002/jso.21600.
7. Schneider N, Strauss DC, Smith MJ, Miah AB, Zaidi S, Benson C, et al. The adequacy of core biopsy in the assessment of smooth muscle neoplasms of soft tissues: implications for treatment and prognosis. Am J Surg Pathol. 2017;41(7):923–31. https://doi.org/10.1097/PAS.0000000000000867.
8. Johnston EW, Basso J, Winfield J, McCall J, Khan N, Messiou C, et al. Starting CT-guided robotic interventional oncology at a UK centre. Br J Radiol. 2022;95(1134):20220217. https://doi.org/10.1259/bjr.20220217.
9. Wilkinson MJ, Martin JL, Khan AA, Hayes AJ, Thomas JM, Strauss DC. Percutaneous core needle biopsy in retroperitoneal sarcomas does not influence local recurrence or overall survival. Ann Surg Oncol. 2015;22(3):853–8. https://doi.org/10.1245/s10434-014-4059-x.
10. Bonvalot S, Raut CP, Pollock RE, Rutkowski P, Strauss DC, Hayes AJ, et al. Technical considerations in surgery for retroperitoneal sarcomas: position paper from E-Surge, a master class in sarcoma surgery, and EORTC-STBSG. Ann Surg Oncol. 2012;19(9):2981–91. https://doi.org/10.1245/s10434-012-2342-2.
11. Messiou C, Moskovic E, Vanel D, Morosi C, Benchimol R, Strauss D, et al. Primary retroperitoneal soft tissue sarcoma: Imaging appearances, pitfalls and diagnostic algorithm. Eur J Surg Oncol. 2017;43(7):1191–8. https://doi.org/10.1016/j.ejso.2016.10.032.
12. Katabathina VS, Vikram R, Nagar AM, Tamboli P, Menias CO, Prasad SR. Mesenchymal neoplasms of the kidney in adults: imaging spectrum with radiologic-pathologic correlation. Radiographics. 2010;30(6):1525–40. https://doi.org/10.1148/rg.306105517.
13. Strauss DC, Hayes AJ, Thway K, Moskovic EC, Fisher C, Thomas JM. Surgical management of primary retroperitoneal sarcoma. Br J Surg. 2010;97(5):698–706. https://doi.org/10.1002/bjs.6994.
14. Miah AB, Hannay J, Benson C, Thway K, Messiou C, Hayes AJ, et al. Optimal management of primary retroperitoneal sarcoma: an update. Expert Rev Anticancer Ther. 2014;14(5):565–79. https://doi.org/10.1586/14737140.2014.883279.
15. Craig WD, Fanburg-Smith JC, Henry LR, Guerrero R, Barton JH. Fat-containing lesions of the retroperitoneum: radiologic-pathologic correlation. Radiographics. 2009;29(1):261–90. https://doi.org/10.1148/rg.291085203.
16. Swallow CJ, Strauss DC, Bonvalot S, Rutkowski P, Desai A, Gladdy RA, et al. Management of Primary Retroperitoneal Sarcoma (RPS) in the Adult: An Updated Consensus Approach from the Transatlantic Australasian RPS Working Group. Ann Surg Oncol. 2021; https://doi.org/10.1245/s10434-021-09654-z.
17. Singer S, Antonescu CR, Riedel E, Brennan MF. Histologic subtype and margin of resection predict pattern of recurrence and survival for retroperitoneal liposarcoma. Ann Surg. 2003;238(3):358–70; discussion 70-1. https://doi.org/10.1097/01.sla.0000086542.11899.38.
18. Ganeshalingam S, Rajeswaran G, Jones RL, Thway K, Moskovic E. Leiomyosarcomas of the inferior vena cava: diagnostic features on cross-sectional imaging. Clin Radiol. 2011;66(1):50–6. https://doi.org/10.1016/j.crad.2010.08.004.
19. Van Slyke MA, Moser RP Jr, Madewell JE. MR imaging of periarticular soft-tissue lesions. Magn Reson Imaging Clin N Am. 1995;3(4):651–67.
20. Weiss SW, Goldblum JR. Malignant tumors of uncertain type. Soft Tissue Tumors. 4th ed. Mosby; 2001.
21. Kransdorf MJ, Murphey MD, Synovial tumors. Imaging of soft tissue tumors. Lippincott Williams & Wilkins; 2005.
22. Jones BC, Sundaram M, Kransdorf MJ. Synovial sarcoma: MR imaging findings in 34 patients. AJR Am J Roentgenol. 1993;161(4):827–30. https://doi.org/10.2214/ajr.161.4.8396848.
23. Coindre JM, Mariani O, Chibon F, Mairal A, De Saint Aubain Somerhausen N, Favre-Guillevin E, et al. Most malignant fibrous histiocytomas developed in the retroperitoneum are dedifferentiated liposarcomas: a review of 25 cases initially diagnosed as

malignant fibrous histiocytoma. Mod Pathol. 2003;16(3):256–62. https://doi.org/10.1097/01.MP.0000056983.78547.77.

24. Binh MB, Guillou L, Hostein I, Chateau MC, Collin F, Aurias A, et al. Dedifferentiated liposarcomas with divergent myosarcomatous differentiation developed in the internal trunk: a study of 27 cases and comparison to conventional dedifferentiated liposarcomas and leiomyosarcomas. Am J Surg Pathol. 2007;31(10):1557–66. https://doi.org/10.1097/PAS.0b013e31804b4109.

25. McCormick D, Mentzel T, Beham A, Fletcher CD, Dedifferentiated liposarcoma. Clinicopathologic analysis of 32 cases suggesting a better prognostic subgroup among pleomorphic sarcomas. Am J Surg Pathol. 1994;18(12):1213–23. https://doi.org/10.1097/00000478-199412000-00004.

26. Wignall OJ, Moskovic EC, Thway K, Thomas JM. Solitary fibrous tumors of the soft tissues: review of the imaging and clinical features with histopathologic correlation. AJR Am J Roentgenol. 2010;195(1):W55–62. https://doi.org/10.2214/AJR.09.3379.

27. Rajiah P, Sinha R, Cuevas C, Dubinsky TJ, Bush WH Jr, Kolokythas O. Imaging of uncommon retroperitoneal masses. Radiographics. 2011;31(4):949–76. https://doi.org/10.1148/rg.314095132.

28. Improta L, Tzanis D, Bouhadiba T, Abdelhafidh K, Bonvalot S. Overview of primary adult retroperitoneal tumours. Eur J Surg Oncol. 2020;46(9):1573–9. https://doi.org/10.1016/j.ejso.2020.04.054.

29. Czeyda-Pommersheim F, Menias C, Boustani A, Revzin M. Diagnostic approach to primary retroperitoneal pathologies: what the radiologist needs to know. Abdom Radiol (NY). 2021;46(3):1062–81. https://doi.org/10.1007/s00261-020-02752-8.

30. Kunz WG, Auernhammer CJ, Nölting S, Pfluger T, Ricke J, Cyran CC. Phäochromozytom und Paragangliom. Der Radiologe. 2019; https://doi.org/10.1007/s00117-019-0569-7.

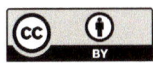

Diffuse Liver Disease

6

David Bowden and Cäcilia S. Reiner

Learning Objectives
- To know MR techniques useful to quantify liver steatosis, iron overload, and fibrosis.
- To learn about less common liver storage diseases.
- Discuss the MR imaging appearance of focal lesions in the cirrhotic liver and the use of the standardized reporting system LI-RADS.
- Learn about diffuse vascular liver disease causing liver parenchyma alteration.

6.1 Metabolic and Storage Diseases

6.1.1 Steatosis

Non-alcoholic fatty liver disease (NAFLD) represents a global epidemic which is now estimated to affect up to 25% of the world's adult population. Approximately 1 in 5 patients with NAFLD will develop non-alcoholic steatohepatitis (NASH), soon expected to overtake viral hepatitis as the leading cause of cirrhosis worldwide [1]. Non-invasive assessment of NAFLD is therefore of increasing importance given the limitations and risks associated with liver biopsy, in order to enable the diagnosis and monitoring of affected individuals. Although unenhanced computed tomography (CT) may allow the identification of individuals with moderate to severe steatosis, a threshold of 48 Hounsfield Units (HU) being highly specific for its

detection, given the associated radiation burden it is an impractical modality for large-scale monitoring and may be confounded by the co-existence of other materials such as iron [2] (Fig. 6.1). However, advances in magnetic resonance imaging (MRI) have enabled a more comprehensive assessment of steatosis. The most widely utilized technique is that of dual gradient-echo imaging, in which images are acquired with fat and water proton signals being either "in-phase" or "out-of-phase," the latter usually being acquired first. Voxels containing both fat and water appear relatively hypointense in the "out-of-phase" images due to signal cancellation, a result of the differing precession frequencies of fat and water protons, thereby enabling the identification of either diffuse or geographic steatosis within the parenchyma (Fig. 6.2).

However, while this may be a useful technique for the subjective assessment of steatosis, multiple confounding factors—including $T2^*$ decay, of particular importance if iron overload is present—limit its use for the reliable quanti-

D. Bowden
Department of Radiology, Cambridge University Hospitals, Cambridge, UK

C. S. Reiner (✉)
Institute of Diagnostic and Interventional Radiology, University Hospital Zurich, Zurich, Switzerland
e-mail: caecilia.reiner@usz.ch

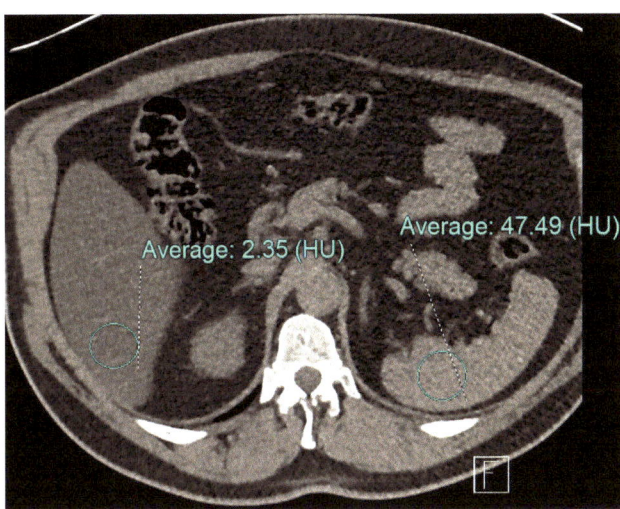

Fig. 6.1 Unenhanced CT image of severe steatosis demonstrating hepatic attenuation more than 10HU less than the spleen, and far below the proposed threshold of 48HU for moderate-severe steatosis

J. Hodler et al. (eds.), *Diseases of the Abdomen and Pelvis 2023-2026*, IDKD Springer Series,
https://doi.org/10.1007/978-3-031-27355-1_6

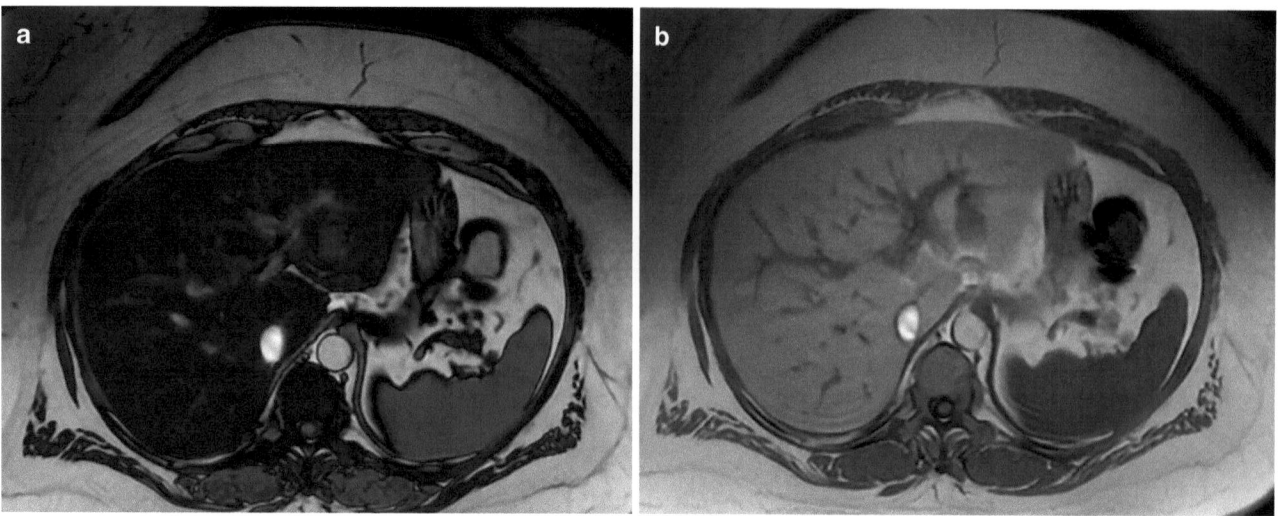

Fig. 6.2 Dual gradient-echo T1-weighted images of severe steatosis. (**a**) Out-of-phase image demonstrating marked liver parenchymal signal drop when compared with the in-phase image (**b**)

fication of fat and have led to the development of more complex sequences which account for these factors. Each major MR vendor has developed variations of a rapid breath-hold multi-echo technique which enables the measurement of the proton density fat fraction (PDFF)—defined as the fraction of mobile triglyceride protons relative to those of water (IDEAL IQ/GE, mDixon-Quant/Philips, and Multiecho VIBE Dixon/Siemens). Using a derived map, measurement of PDFF values is as simple as drawing an ROI within the parenchyma, allowing for variations in fat distribution, with proposed intervals for histological steatosis grading being grade 0 (normal, 0–6.4%), grade 1 (mild, 6.5–17.4%), grade 2 (moderate, 17.5–22.1%), and grade 3 (severe, 22.2% or greater)—Fig. 6.3. PDFF values using this technique have been well validated as a biomarker of steatosis, including when compared with histopathological and MR spectroscopy results [3].

6.1.2 Iron Overload

Due to the formation of free radicals, excess iron accumulation within body tissues is toxic and may result in organ damage—in particular to the liver, heart, and pancreas. It arises most commonly from either excessive intestinal absorption (e.g., hereditary hemochromatosis, iron supplementation) or chronic blood transfusions (e.g., patients with hemoglobinopathies or other red cell disorders). In the case of the latter, a form of hemosiderosis, iron accumulates predominantly within the reticuloendothelial system of the liver and other organs and while its measurement is required as part of the monitoring of therapy, is less damaging to the liver than to other organs such as the heart. As a result of abnormal metabolism, the presence of chronic liver disease

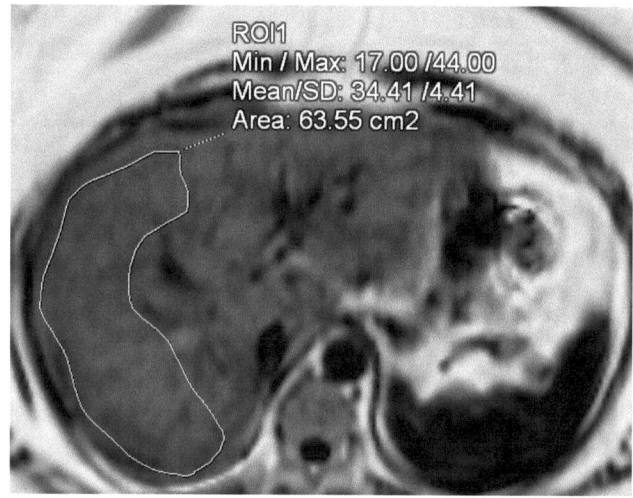

Fig. 6.3 Severe steatosis. Proton density fat fraction (PDFF) map derived using the multi-echo IDEAL IQ (GE) technique. ROI placement avoiding major vessels provides a simple percentage of fat within the parenchyma, in this case 34%

in itself, arising from NAFLD, alcohol-related liver disease or other causes, may also lead to iron accumulation which can further accelerate disease progression [4]. Evaluation of hepatic iron is therefore of importance in both the diagnosis and monitoring of patients at risk of iron overload.

While liver biopsy has historically represented the gold standard for its assessment, non-invasive methods such as MRI which are also less prone to sampling error are desirable. In addition, iron may not be distributed evenly throughout the liver parenchyma and pathological methods used in its precise quantification result in the destruction of specimens, precluding histological analysis. The presence of iron particles within tissues results in tiny inhomogeneities within the magnetic field, leading to rapid dephasing of protons, shortening of T1, T2, and T2* relaxation times and therefore an increase in R2*, the rate of T2* relaxation. During the acquisition of dual gradient-echo images as previously described, signal loss is therefore visible in the second, in-phase acquisition and a qualitative assessment of iron overload is possible (Fig. 6.4). The presence of concomitant steatosis, which results in signal loss in the first (out-of-phase) image, will however confound the appearance and more sophisticated techniques are required for formal quantification. While a full review is beyond the scope of this chapter, techniques such as those already described for steatosis quantification also allow the calculation of iron content. Multipoint Dixon techniques such as IDEAL-IQ (GE) not only provide a PDFF map in a single breath hold,

but also a simultaneous R2* map upon which ROIs can be placed to calculate mean R2* values for the liver parenchyma (Fig. 6.4). These values are then converted to a Liver Iron Concentration (LIC) value using a simple calibration formula. While it is unconfirmed which of several calibration formulae is most appropriate, evidence suggests differences between the results are small and for practical purposes any may be used [5]. Alternatively, spin echo techniques such as R2 relaxometry (e.g., Ferriscan®, Resonance Health) are also available and show excellent correlation with LIC values, but have the disadvantages of additional cost, long (up to 20 min) acquisition times that limit its use in difficult patients, off-site centralized analysis, and the lack of radiologist input to scrutinize images for significant findings such as HCC.

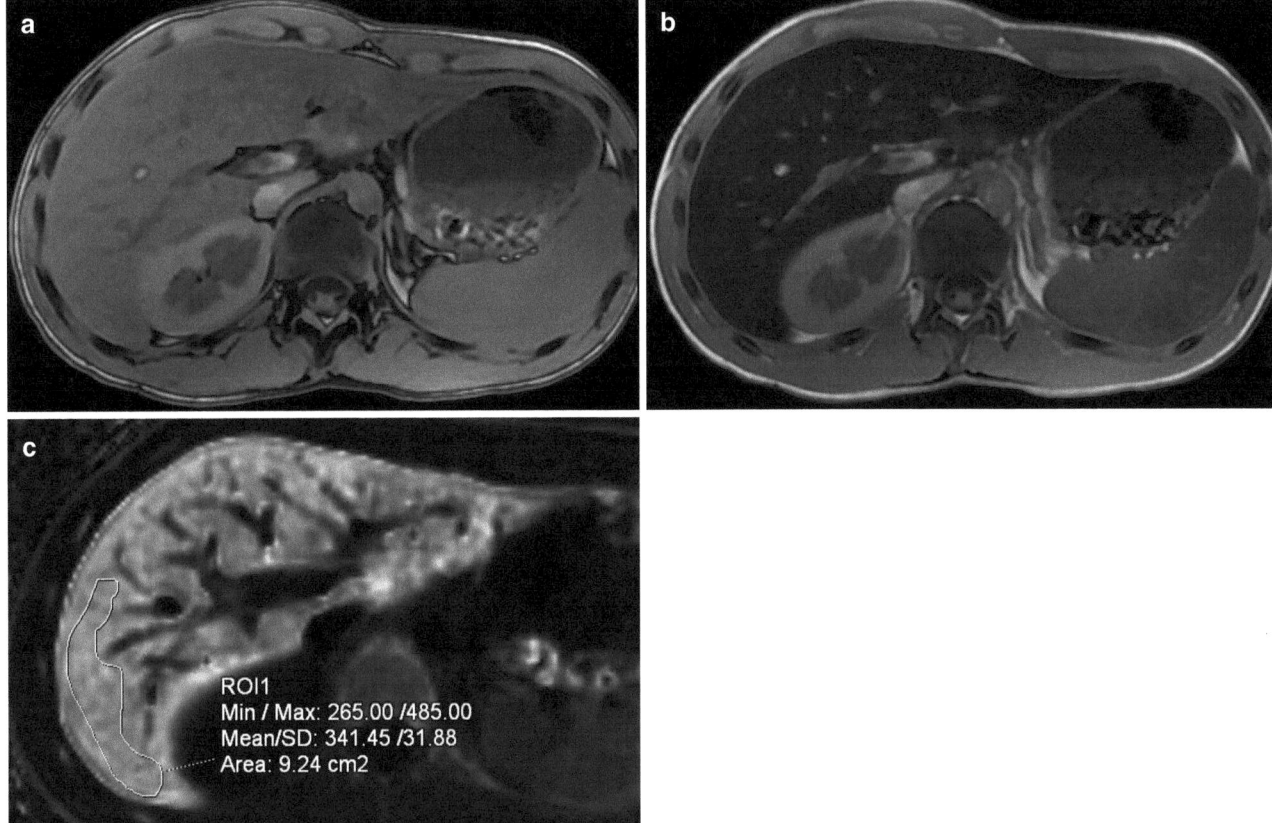

Fig. 6.4 Hepatic and splenic iron overload. Dual gradient-echo images of iron deposition in a patient who has received multiple blood transfusions. (a) Out-of-phase, (b) in-phase images. Due to dephasing of protons as a result of magnetic field inhomogeneity in the presence of iron, signal drop occurs within the liver parenchyma between the first (out-of-phase) and second (in-phase) echoes. Similar change is seen within the spleen as a result of iron deposition within the reticuloendothelial system following chronic transfusions. (c) Formal measurement of liver iron concentration. ROI placement on the R2* map derived using the multi-echo IDEAL IQ (GE) technique allows for liver iron concentration measurement, following conversion using a calibration formula. In this case, the R2* value = 341 s^{-1} (Normal <67 s^{-1} at 1.5 T), equivalent to 8.9 mg Fe/g dry liver (normal <1.8 mg Fe/g)—equivalent to severe overload

Key Points

For both iron and fat quantification, MR techniques have proven the most robust and include multi-echo single breath-hold acquisitions, available via each MR vendor, which unlike CT and MR are able to account for confounding variables. Given the rising epidemic of NAFLD, their inclusion as standard in liver imaging protocols is to be encouraged.

6.1.3 Wilson's Disease

Wilson's disease, or progressive hepatolenticular degeneration, is a rare autosomal recessive disorder of metabolism in which copper accumulates in multiple organs, in particular within the liver but also within the brain, kidney, and cornea. As a result, a spectrum of pathophysiologic changes occurs including steatosis, chronic active hepatitis and ultimately, cirrhosis. Imaging findings are somewhat non-specific and overlap significantly with chronic liver disease of other etiologies. These include an irregular capsular contour, T2 hypo/T1 hyperintense nodules and parenchymal heterogeneity with increased echogenicity at ultrasound. It has however been suggested that a relative lack of caudate lobe hypertrophy may be a more specific feature [6].

6.1.4 Amyloidosis

Amyloidosis refers to a spectrum of diseases in which extracellular accumulation of the fibrillar protein amyloid occurs, which may be either focal or diffuse and may involve several organs or be limited to one. Its most common forms are the AL type (amyloid light chain, formerly known as primary amyloidosis), associated with plasma cell dyscrasias, or AA type (amyloid A, formerly secondary amyloidosis) arising from systemic inflammation. Infiltration within the liver occurs predominantly along the sinusoids and results in the non-specific signs of hepatomegaly, increased echogenicity

at US with hypoattenuation at CT mimicking steatosis and heterogeneous enhancement following contrast medium administration. Elastography demonstrates increased hepatic stiffness which may be heterogeneous, diffuse or more focal and may therefore have a role in assessment of affected patients for liver involvement [7].

Key Points

Wilson's disease and amyloidosis have non-specific imaging findings which overlap significantly with other etiologies of liver disease although in the correct clinical context MR Elastography may show promise in the identification of liver involvement with amyloidosis.

6.1.5 Gaucher Disease

Gaucher disease is a rare lysosomal storage disorder in which a cell membrane glycosphingolipid accumulates within reticuloendothelial macrophages ("Gaucher cells") due to a hereditary deficiency in the GBA1 enzyme. Of the three types, type 1 is the most common in which Gaucher cells accumulate within the liver, spleen, and bone marrow and result in several clinical manifestations such as anemia, hepatosplenomegaly, and avascular necrosis of bone. Since the advent of enzyme replacement therapy, MRI has played a key role in the monitoring of response to treatment, both via the volumetric analysis of the liver and spleen as well as evaluation for malignancy. Gaucher disease may result in cirrhosis and is associated with an increased risk of solid organ malignancy, including HCC, in the context of both cirrhotic and non-cirrhotic livers [8]. Differentiation of HCC from benign entities such as focal nodular hyperplasia may be very challenging given the overlap in imaging features. In addition, focal accumulation of Gaucher cells within the liver and spleen may result in the so-called Gaucheromas, nodules which have highly variable imaging appearances, and which are a diagnosis of exclusion (Fig. 6.5).

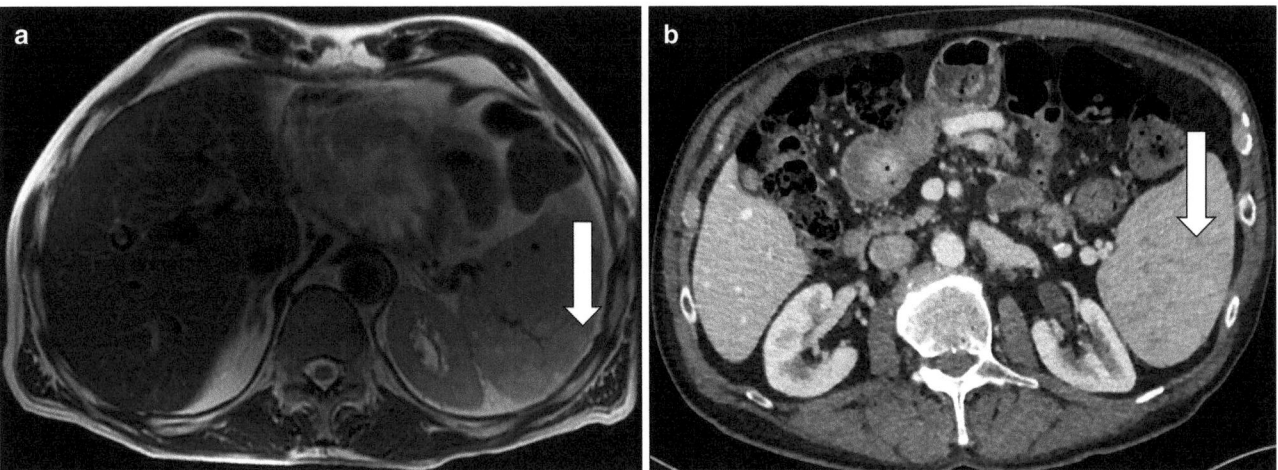

Fig. 6.5 (**a, b**) Gaucheromas within the spleen. (**a**) Axial T2-weighted image demonstrates multiple well-defined T2 hyperintense lesions (arrow), which appear relatively hypoenhancing in portal venous phase CT (**b**)

6.2 Cirrhosis

6.2.1 Imaging of Pre-stages of Cirrhosis

Regardless of etiology, chronic liver injury leads to inflammation and hepatocellular damage with resultant fibrosis and regeneration of hepatocytes. Stage 4 fibrosis, or cirrhosis, represents the end stage of this process and as described previously, Hepatitis B, C and alcohol-related liver disease are likely to be soon overtaken by NAFLD as its leading cause. Early detection and monitoring of fibrosis is therefore of critical importance. Although previously liver biopsy has been regarded as the gold standard for its evaluation, non-invasive techniques are desirable given the risks associated with biopsy and sampling error, fibrosis frequently having a heterogeneous distribution. While ultrasound techniques such as transient elastography (Fibroscan®) or 2D shear wave elastography are readily available, performance is poor in the presence of ascites or obesity and such techniques are also limited by small sample size and operator factors.

MR elastography has emerged as the most accurate technique for the non-invasive detection and staging of fibrosis, enables sampling of the entire liver, including in the presence of obesity and ascites, and is able to provide additional information on the geographic distribution of fibrosis [9]. Low frequency acoustic waves are transmitted through the abdominal wall overlying the liver using an acoustic driver, resulting in shear wave propagation through the parenchyma. Using a 2D gradient-echo sequence, 60 Hz motion-encoding gradients are synchronized to the driver motion in order to acquire images of propagating waves; magnitude and phase images are then used to derive a stiffness map at four adjacent slice locations, each in a single breath hold (Fig. 6.6). During post-processing, a confidence map is overlaid on the map to exclude unreliable data. The reader then draws an ROI on the confidence map, excluding large vessels, the liver edge, perihepatic tissues/fissures, and artifacts. A weighted mean of values derived from the four slices is then calculated to provide overall liver stiffness. While stiffness values have a relatively narrow range for each stage of fibrosis, its accuracy for both "ruling in" the presence of significant fibrosis and "ruling out" cirrhosis is excellent [10]. Drawbacks include the need for meticulous technique—in particular driver placement and slice location—and the presence of iron, which results in signal loss. While spin echo techniques may mitigate the latter if mild, commercial availability is limited and more severe cases of iron overload will still result in failure (Fig. 6.7). Further pitfalls include the presence of biliary obstruction, inflammation, or congestion due to right-sided heart failure, all of which may increase hepatic stiffness. Results therefore always require interpretation in the overall clinical context.

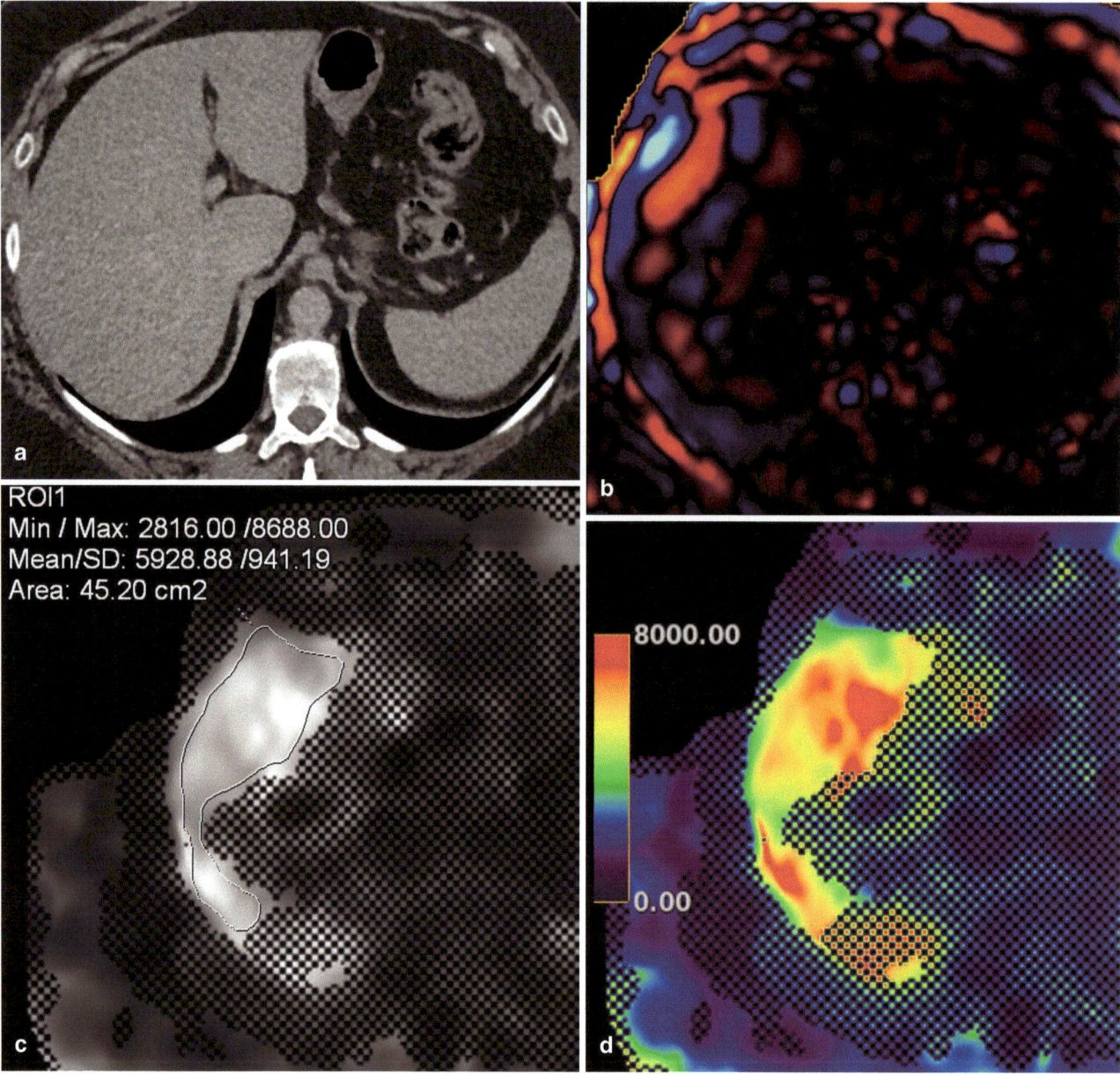

Fig. 6.6 MR Elastography of cirrhosis in a patient with normal liver morphology. (**a**) Portal venous phase CT image demonstrates a relatively normal morphology, with a lack of capsular irregularity, lobar atrophy/hypertrophy, or splenomegaly. (**b**) MRE wave image, required to inspect data quality. (**c**) Grey-scale elastogram: ROI placement avoiding the liver edge and major vessels allows measurement of hepatic stiffness in pascals, in this case 5.9 kPa (>5.0 kPa = stage 4 fibrosis/cirrhosis). (**d**) Color elastogram, used to analyze the distribution of hepatic stiffness which in some cases may provide additional information regarding etiology. Scale is in Pascals

6.2.2   Imaging of Cirrhosis

Cirrhosis is the result of chronic damage to the liver, characterized by progressive fibrosis of the liver parenchyma with ongoing regeneration. Beside the etiologies of cirrhosis described above other causes are hemochromatosis or biliary and cryptogenic diseases. On imaging, the liver may appear normal at an early stage of cirrhosis. With disease progression, heterogeneity and surface nodularity are observed. Because of the unique ability of the liver to regenerate in cirrhosis, the liver harbors a spectrum of hepatocellular nodules, most of which are regenerative. Due to the ongoing distortion of the liver parenchyma, the liver surface appears nodular, or lobular in most of the cases. Caudate lobe hypertrophy is the most characteristic morphologic feature of liver cirrhosis [11]. Alteration of blood flow results in typical morphologic abnormalities: segmental hypertrophy involving the lateral segments of the left lobe (segment 2, 3), and segmental atrophy affecting the right lobe (segment 6, 7) and medial segment of the left lobe (segment 4). Other typical

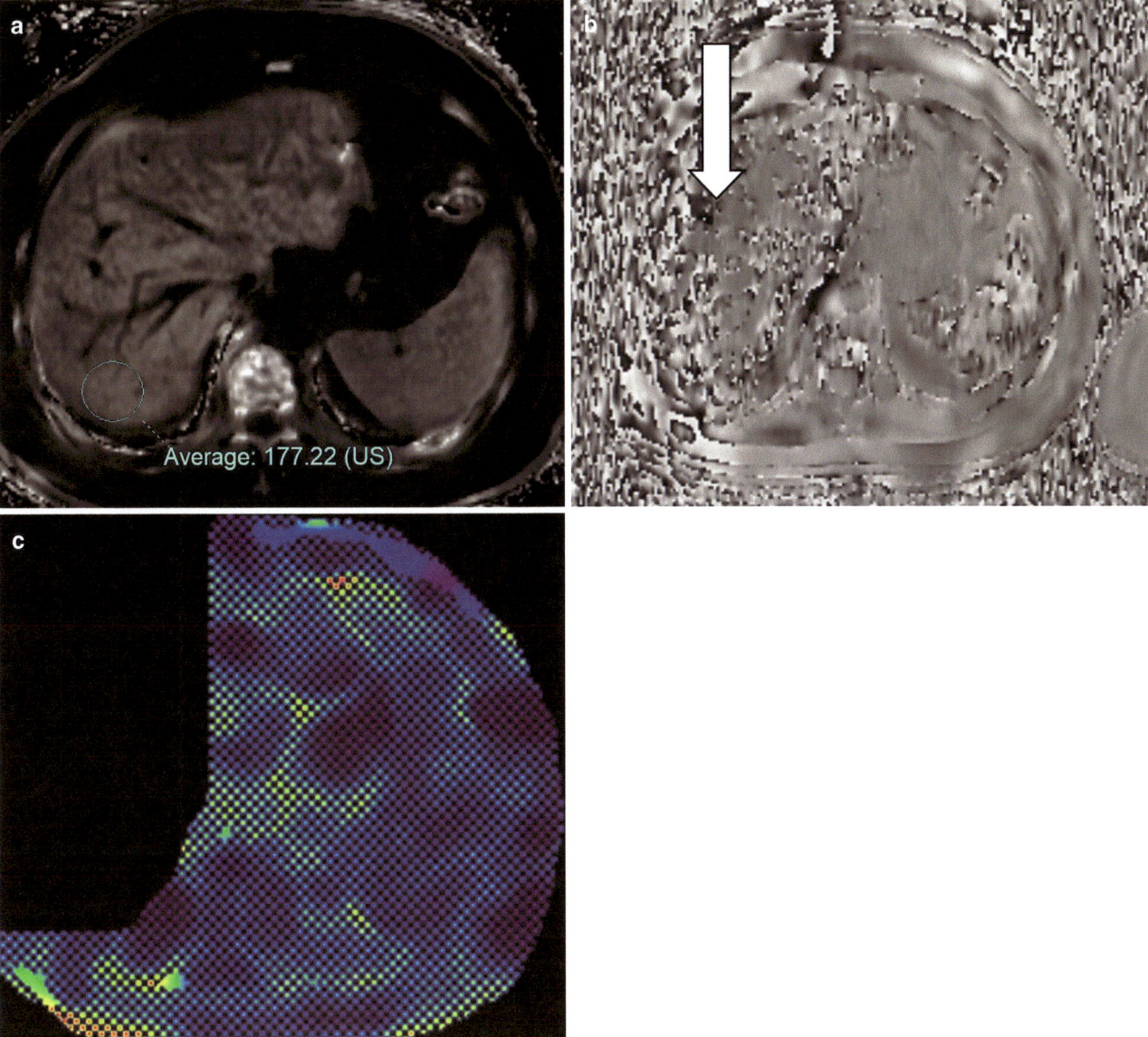

Fig. 6.7 Failure of MRE in a patient with iron overload. (**a**) R2* map derived from IDEAL IQ (GE) acquisition demonstrates an R2* value of 177 s⁻¹, equating to a liver iron concentration of = 4.7 mg Fe/g dry weight (DW), moderate iron overload (normal <1.8 mg/g DW). (**b**) Phase image shows diffuse signal loss within the liver parenchyma, visible in the color elastogram (**c**) as a signal void

findings include enlargement of hilar periportal space, the right posterior notch-sign and generalized widening of the interlobar fissures. Less typical distribution of segmental atrophy and hypertrophy is seen in primary sclerosing cholangitis, where the distribution follows in part the distribution of the bile duct involvement, for example, atrophy of segments 2 and 3 or 5 and 7 may be seen. The segmental compensatory hypertrophy associated with atrophy of other liver parts may appear as pseudotumoral enlargement. In 25% of cirrhosis, the liver shape and contour appear normal on CT or MRI.

Lymphadenopathy can appear in the liver hilum and peripancreatic region, which may mimic neoplastic lymph nodes, if the lymph nodes are large. Portal hypertension due to increased vascular resistance at the level of the hepatic sinusoids causes complications such as ascites, development of portosystemic shunts at the distal esophagus and the gastric fundus, via periumbilical veins and left gastric vein. Other shunts include splenorenal collaterals, hemorrhoidal veins, abdominal wall, and retroperitoneal collaterals [11]. These collateral veins are seen as enhancing tortuous vessels. The typical nodular liver contour and liver shape of cirrhosis as well as its vascular complications can be seen on ultrasound, CT, or MRI. MRI very well depicts fibrotic bands between regenerative nodules as T2 hyperintense and progressively or delayed enhancing structures.

6.3 Focal Lesions in Cirrhotic Liver

6.3.1 Regenerative Nodules

Regenerative nodules in a cirrhotic liver play a role in the stepwise carcinogenesis of HCC, most frequently through dedifferentiation from regenerative nodule, low-grade dysplastic nodule, high-grade dysplastic nodule to HCC. Most regenerative nodules do not progress in the dedifferentiation process. They are macronodular (≥9 mm) or micronodular (3–9 mm). Most regenerative nodules are not seen as distinct nodules on CT or MRI, but rather as nodular appearance of the liver parenchyma. MRI detects regenerative nodules with a higher sensitivity than US or CT. Regenerative nodules are usually iso- to hypointense on T2-weighted images and isointense on T1-weighted images. Variable signal intensity on T1-weighted images is due to lipid, protein, or copper content leading to a T1-weighted hyperintense appearance or iron deposition in the so-called siderotic nodules with a hypointense appearance on T1-weighted and T2-weighted images. Using extracellular gadolinium-containing contrast agent, regenerative nodules show the same contrast behavior as the background liver. After administration of hepatocyte-specific contrast material regenerative nodules usually enhance to the same degree as adjacent liver [12]. Some regenerative nodules—the so-called focal nodular hyperplasia like nodules—may also show arterial enhancement and increased uptake of hepatocyte-specific contrast agent compared to the surrounding liver, which may make them difficult to differentiate from hepatocellular carcinoma [13].

6.3.2 Dysplastic Nodules

Dysplastic nodules are regenerative nodules that contain atypical hepatocytes, measuring at least 1 mm, not meeting histologic criteria for malignancy. They are classified as low- or high-grade dysplastic nodules. High-grade dysplastic nodules are considered premalignant. The differentiation between a regenerative nodule and a low-grade dysplastic nodule is difficult due to similar appearance on MRI. Dysplastic nodules are rarely detected on CT. Dysplastic nodules usually are hypovascular. In high-grade dysplastic nodules, arterial vascularization can increase leading to arterial hyperenhancement on imaging. Using hepatocyte-specific MR contrast agents, dysplastic nodules show variable signal intensity in the hepatocyte-specific phase. With progressing dedifferentiation, the nodules lose their ability to take up the hepatocyte-specific contrast agent and appear hypointense in the hepatobiliary phase. These hepatobiliary hypointense dysplastic nodules may be mistaken for HCC. Dysplastic nodules may also instead lose the ability to excrete the hepatocyte-specific contrast agent and appear iso- or hyperintense on hepatobiliary phase images. Hypovascular cirrhotic nodules with hypointense appearance in the hepatobiliary phase carry a significant risk of transforming into hypervascular HCC with a pooled overall rate of 28% (95% CI, 22.7–33.6%). The size of the hypovascular nodule is a second risk factor for hypervascular transformation with nodules ≥9 mm in size showing a higher risk [14].

6.3.3 Malignant Lesions

Hepatocellular carcinoma (HCC) occurs as a solitary lesion (in half of the cases), as multiple lesions or diffuse. The vast majority of HCCs (90%) occur in cirrhotic livers. In this setting, HCCs can be commonly diagnosed based on imaging features alone without histological confirmation [15]. The second most common primary hepatic tumor is intrahepatic cholangiocarcinoma (ICC), which accounts for 10–20% of all primary hepatic tumors. Recently, cirrhosis and viral hepatitis C and B have been recognized as risk factors for cholangiocarcinoma, especially for the intrahepatic type [16]. Radiologic features of cholangiocarcinoma such as progressive contrast enhancement from arterial to venous and late phase, arterial rim enhancement, and peripheral washout can help differentiate ICC from HCC in the cirrhotic liver [17]. The imaging characteristics of focal HCC and ICC are discussed in the chapter on "Focal liver lesions."

A challenging diagnosis is the diagnosis of diffuse HCC, or also known as infiltrative HCC in a cirrhotic liver, which accounts for 7–20% of HCC cases. Diffuse HCC usually spreads over multiple liver segments and is frequently associated with portal vein tumor thrombosis. The tumor is often difficult to distinguish from background changes in cirrhosis at imaging and portal vein thrombosis may be the only obvious finding. The tumor often shows only minimal arterial enhancement and heterogeneous washout on contrast-enhanced CT or MRI. Diffusion-weighted MRI can be helpful as the tumor appears hyperintense compared to the cirrhotic liver [18].

6.3.4 Confluent Focal Fibrosis

In advanced stages of cirrhosis additional focal fibrosis can appear as wedge-shaped area from the porta hepatis to the liver surface. This so-called confluent focal fibrosis is typically located in segments 4, 7, or 8, leads to capsular retraction, and appears as hypointense area on T1-weighted MRI. It is slightly hyperintense on T2, shows late enhancement with extracellular contrast agents due to contrast accumulation in fibrotic tissue and hepatobiliary phase hypointensity (Fig. 6.8) [19].

6.3.5 Standardized Reporting with LI-RADS

Due to a great overlap in imaging features across the spectrum of cirrhotic nodules from regenerative nodules to poorly differentiated HCC, a definite diagnosis of a benign or malignant lesion is often not possible. Furthermore, a great variety in nomenclature of imaging features of cirrhotic nodules is used. To overcome these difficulties, the Liver Imaging-Reporting and Data System (LI-RADS) has been developed, which is a comprehensive system for standardized interpretation and reporting of computed tomography (CT) and magnetic resonance (MR) examinations performed in patients at risk for HCC. It uses a standardized nomenclature and provides a diagnostic algorithm that uses imaging features to categorize the observations seen in patients at risk for HCC along a spectrum from benign to malignant. Liver lesions in these patients are rated for their risk of being an HCC. LI-RADS 1 category observations demonstrate imaging features diagnostic of a benign entity, for example, cyst and hemangioma. LI-RADS 2 observations are probably benign, such as a hemangioma with an atypical enhancement pattern or a probably benign cirrhotic nodule. Major features including arterial-phase enhancement, lesion diameter, washout appearance, capsule appearance, and threshold growth are imaging features used to categorize LI-RADS 3

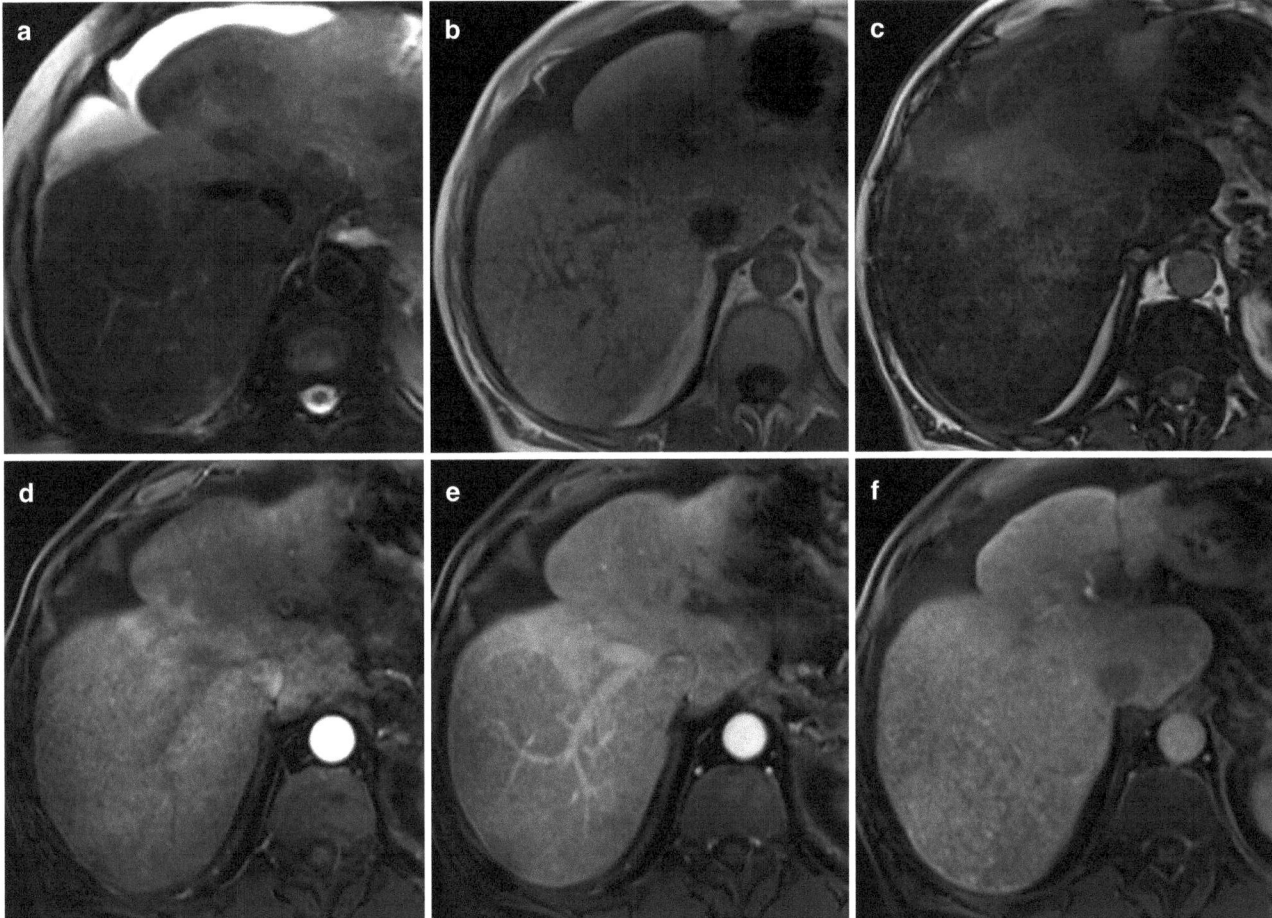

Fig. 6.8 Confluent focal fibrosis. A 62-year-old man with cirrhosis. (**a**) Axial T2-weighted fat saturated image with capsular retraction in liver segment VIII and adjacent focal hyperintense area. The liver parenchyma shows signal drop from in-phase (**b**) to opposed-phase (**c**) images corresponding to diffuse fat deposition with exception of the area in segment VIII. The area of focal fibrosis in segment VIII shows slight arterial (**d**) and portal venous (**e**) enhancement and subtle hypointensity in hepatobiliary phase (**f**)

(indeterminate probability of HCC), LI-RADS 4 (probably HCC), and LI-RADS 5 (definitely HCC) lesions. LI-RADS 5 lesions have typical imaging features diagnostic for HCC. To further refine and adjust LI-RADS categories ancillary imaging features favoring benignity or malignancy can be used [20].

> **Key Points**
> Regenerative and dysplastic nodules share overlapping imaging features and may be difficult to distinguish. LI-RADS helps in rating the risk of such a focal lesion in cirrhosis of being an HCC.

6.4 Diffuse Vascular Liver Disease

6.4.1 Arteriovenous Shunts

Intrahepatic arterioportal shunts are communications between the hepatic arterial system and a portal vein or between hepatic arteries and hepatic veins which can be either at the level of the trunk, sinusoids, or peribiliary venules. In a cirrhotic liver, they can occur spontaneously, represent pseudolesions and subsequently resolve. Secondary shunts may be posttraumatic, post biopsy, or instrumentation. On imaging, they appear as small, peripheral, nonspherical enhancing foci, which become isoattenuating to the liver in the portal venous phase. It may be difficult to distinguish an arterioportal shunt from a small hepatocellular carcinoma. Repeating imaging after 6 months usually helps distinguishing, these entities and demonstrates resolution or stability of an arterioportal shunt, or growth of an HCC.

6.4.2 Budd-Chiari Syndrome

Budd-Chiari syndrome is defined as lobar or segmental hepatic venous outflow obstruction at the level of the inferior vena cava (IVC, type 1), at the level of the hepatic veins (type 2) or occlusion of small centrilobular veins (type 3). The most common cause of hepatic vein obstruction is thrombosis, most commonly due to hypercoagulability (oral contraceptive use, pregnancy, polycythemia) or less common due to obstruction after chemotherapy or radiation. Other primary causes are webs and membranes in the hepatic veins or IVC either of congenital origin or after thrombosis. The outflow obstruction may also be due to extrinsic compression of the hepatic outflow by hepatic masses (malignant or non-malignant). The imaging findings in the acute phase differ from the chronic

phase. In the acute state, the inferior vena cava (IVC) and/or hepatic veins may appear hyperattenuating on unenhanced CT images because of the increased attenuation of a thrombus. On contrast-enhanced CT or MRI a vascular filling defect due to thrombotic material, reduction of hepatic vein caliber, missing connection between hepatic veins and IVC can be present or hepatic veins may not be visible at all. In the acute phase, hepatomegaly with diminished enhancement of the liver periphery and accentuated enhancement of central liver parts and caudate lobe is seen. Later on, peripheral liver enhancement becomes heterogeneous as disorganized, comma-shaped intrahepatic collateral veins, and systemic collateral veins develop. In chronic Budd-Chiari syndrome, fibrotic changes appear in the liver. Large regenerative nodules in a dysmorphic liver are frequent findings in longer standing venous outflow obstruction. These regenerative nodules appear hyperintense on hepatobiliary phase images after administration of a hepatocyte-specific contrast agent. Hypertrophy of the caudate lobe with variation in attenuation due to separate venous drainage should not be interpreted as a tumor [21]. In chronic Budd-Chiari syndrome not only benign regenerative nodules, but also HCC can develop, which may be difficult to differentiate since both can appear markedly hyperenhanced on arterial phase.

6.4.3 Sinusoidal Obstruction Syndrome

Hepatic sinusoidal obstruction syndrome (SOS) formerly known as "veno-occlusive disease" is characterized by a hepatic venous outflow obstruction in the intrahepatic sinusoidal venules. An injury to the hepatic venous endothelium leads to necrosis and obstruction of sinusoidal venules. SOS can present with severe complications, such as congestive hepatopathy, portal hypertension, impaired liver function, and acute liver failure, but can also remain asymptomatic. SOS can occur in the setting of hematopoietic stem cell transplantation and with different chemotherapeutic agents (mainly oxaliplatin-containing chemotherapies). An association of SOS with herbal remedies containing pyrrolizidine and nonpyrrolizidine alkaloids, consumption of bush tea, and oral contraceptives in women with antiphospholipid syndrome has been described. On CT and MR imaging heterogeneous, mosaic-like enhancement of the liver parenchyma usually located in the periphery of the right lobe is seen. On hepatobiliary phase MR images, liver parenchyma shows varying degrees of reticular hypointensities (Fig. 6.9), which is highly specific for SOS [22]. Indirect signs of severe SOS related to reduced liver outflow and portal hypertension include hepatomegaly, gallbladder wall thickening, peripor-

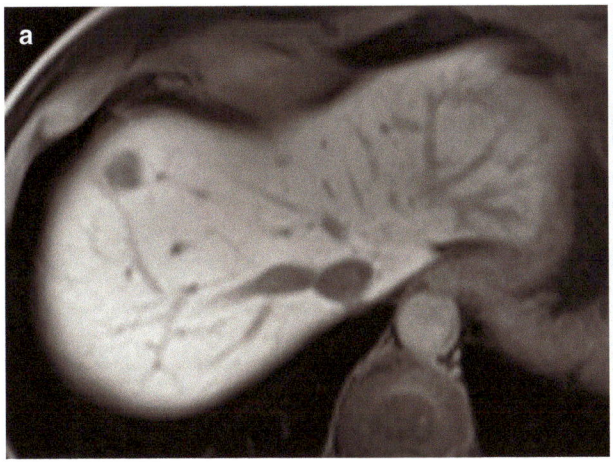 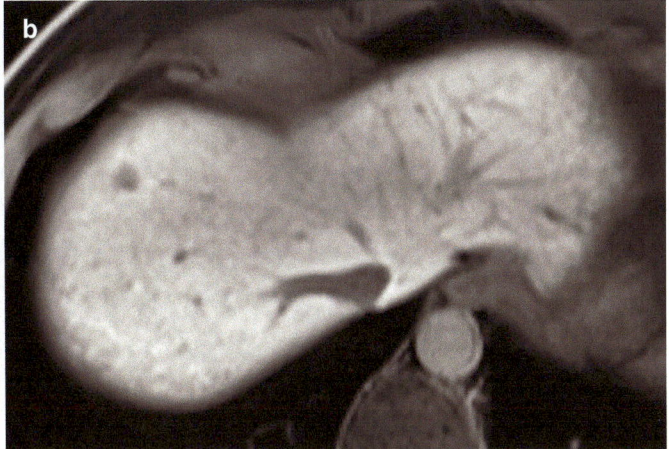

Fig. 6.9 Sinusoidal obstruction syndrome. A 62-year-old man with colorectal liver metastases. (**a**) Prior to chemotherapy axial hepatobiliary phase image shows a liver metastasis in segment VIII and homogeneous enhancement of the liver parenchyma. (**b**) After four cycles of capecitabine and oxaliplatin, the liver metastasis decreased in size. The liver parenchyma shows a reticular hypointense pattern on hepatobiliary phase corresponding to parenchymal changes due to sinusoidal obstruction syndrome

tal edema, splenomegaly, esophageal varices, umbilical vein patency, and ascites [23].

6.4.4 Passive Hepatic Congestion and Fontan-Associated Liver Disease

Passive hepatic congestion is due to chronic right-sided heart failure, which leads to stasis of blood within the liver parenchyma. An enlarged, heterogeneous liver may be seen as a manifestation of acute or early cardiac disease. Early arterial enhancement of the dilated IVC and central hepatic veins is caused by reflux of contrast material from the right atrium into the IVC. A heterogeneous, mottled mosaic pattern of enhancement is present in the parenchymal phase, a condition also known as "nutmeg" liver. In long standing disease, progressive cellular necrosis results in a small cirrhotic liver. Early changes of hepatic congestion are visible on MR Elastography, with a pattern of peripheral T2 hyperintensity (oedema) associated with matching raised parenchymal stiffness. An important patient group in whom this may be seen is those with the so-called Fontan circulation following correction of pediatric congenital heart disease in those born with a single ventricle physiology. As life expectancy has improved, an increasing number of adult patients are now seen in whom chronic hepatic congestion results in the early onset of fibrosis and cirrhosis—Fontan-Associated Liver Disease (FALD). While differentiation of fibrosis and congestion may be difficult or impossible in many cases, and often co-exist, typical patterns of elevated stiffness may provide a clue to the predominant etiology and facilitate appropriate treatment (Fig. 6.10) [24].

6.4.5 Hereditary Hemorrhagic Telangiectasia (HHT)

HHT is an autosomal dominant disorder characterized by vascular malformations (VM) in multiple organs, including the hepatobiliary and gastrointestinal tract. VMs occur in up to 74% of patients with HHT, increase in frequency with age and range from small telangiectasias (dilatation of postcapillary venules that communicate directly with arterioles) to larger shunts between arteries and hepatic or portal veins, as well as between portal and hepatic venous branches [25]. In severe cases, these may lead to significant shunting, portal hypertension, biliary ischemia, high output cardiac failure or hepatic encephalopathy. Dilatation of the common hepatic artery of more than 7 mm is frequently seen, as well as an increased incidence of visceral aneurysms (Fig. 6.11). The so-called confluent vascular masses may arise within the liver parenchyma from the fusion of multiple smaller telangiectasias, in addition to large regenerative nodules and focal nodular hyperplasia (FNH), the latter demonstrating typical arterial hyperenhancement with retention of hepatobiliary contrast agents in the delayed phase.

> **Key Points**
>
> Vascular disorders of the liver may be either congenital (e.g., HHT) or acquired, arising from prior intervention (e.g., adult congenital heart disease), drug-related toxicities (e.g., SOS) or from idiopathic thrombotic events (Budd-Chiari syndrome). In some cases, these may result in the formation of benign lesions which can be challenging to differentiate from malignancy.

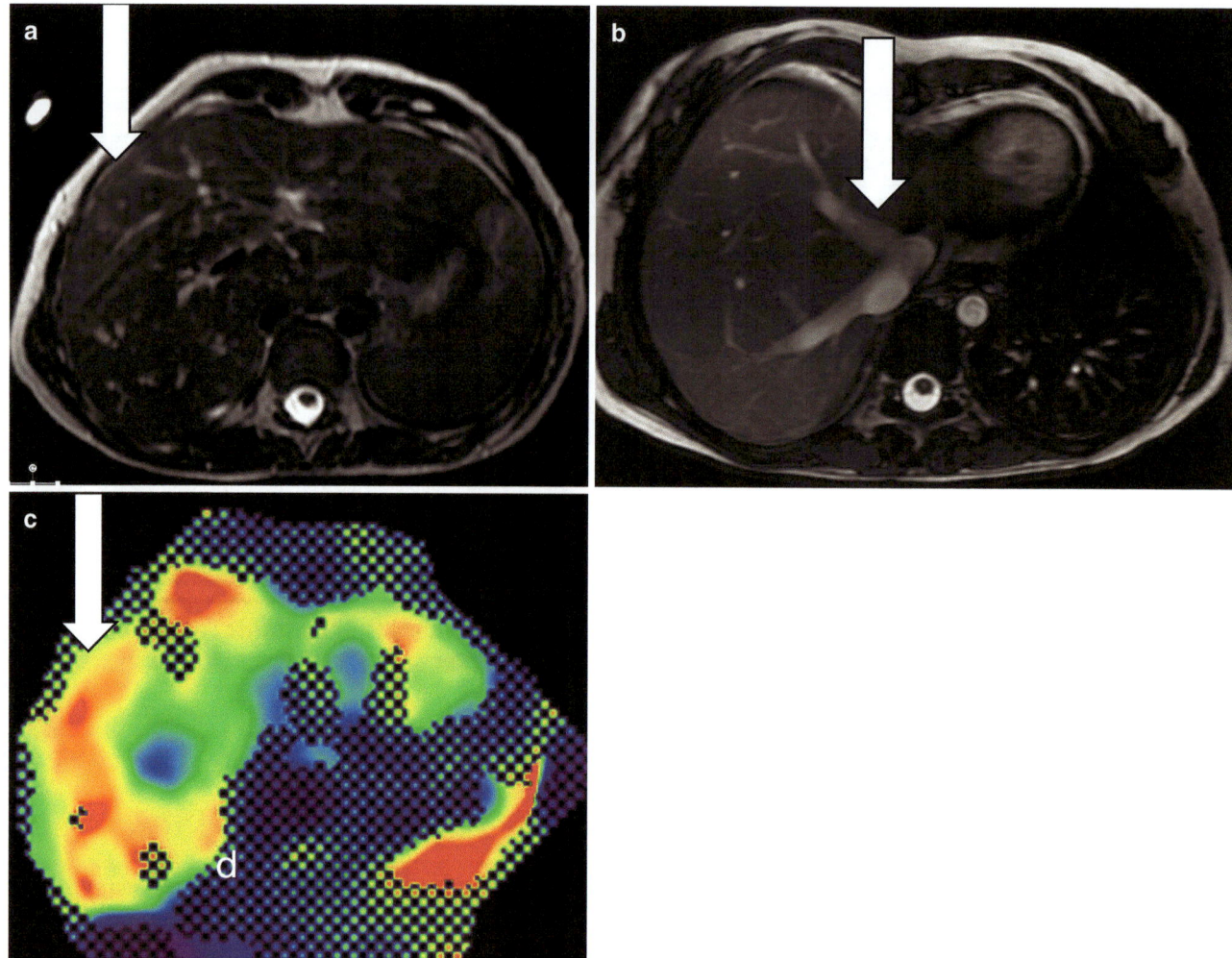

Fig. 6.10 Fontan-associated liver disease in a young adult patient 20 years following corrective surgery. (**a**) Axial T2-weighted image shows diffuse peripheral T2 hyperintensity (arrow), with dilated hepatic veins (**b**) in keeping with hepatic congestion. (**c**) Color MR elastogram demonstrates elevated stiffness within the periphery, supportive of congestion as the predominant pathology. Ultimately, there will be progression to fibrosis and cirrhosis in the absence of effective treatment

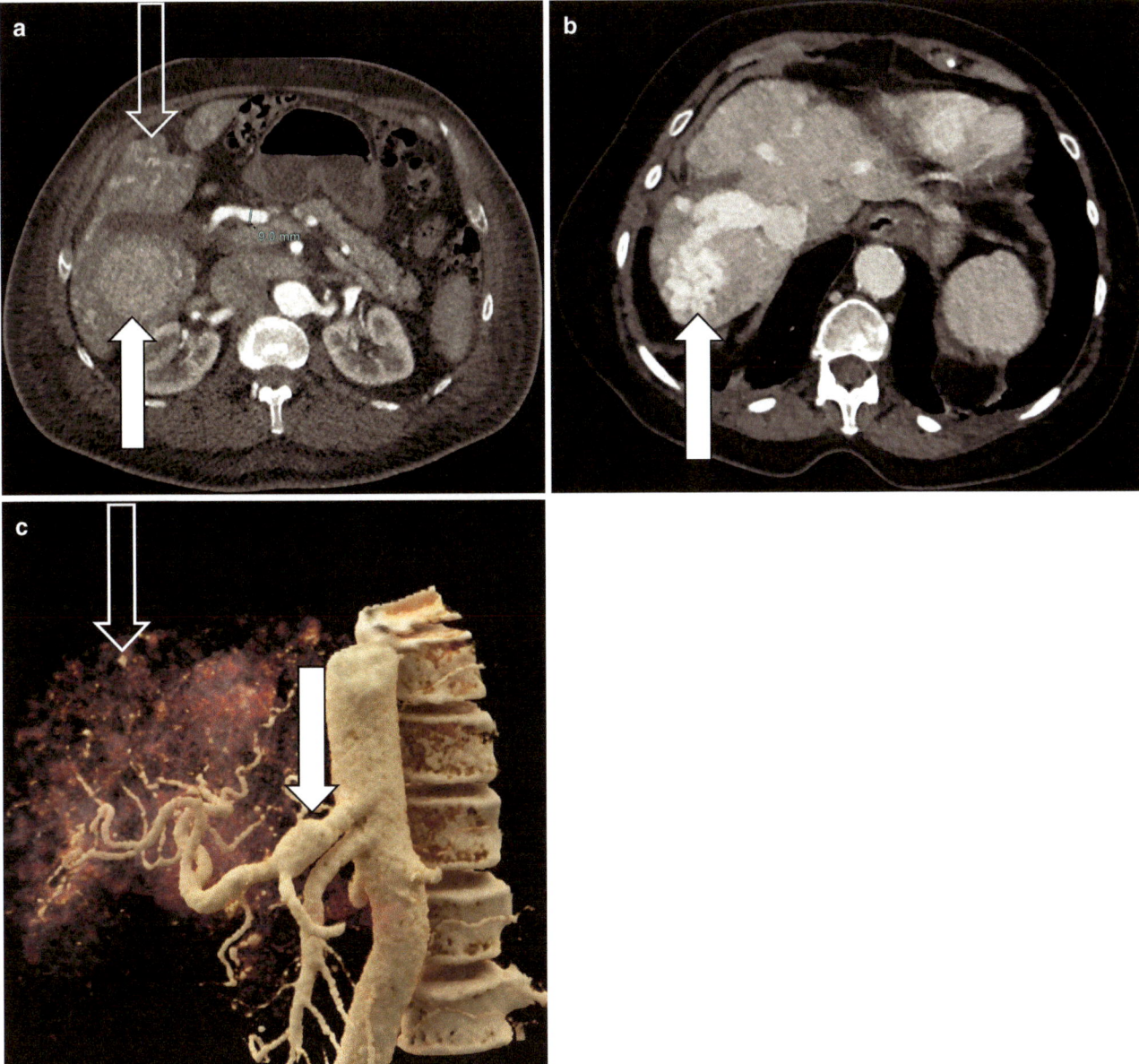

Fig. 6.11 Vascular findings in a patient with hereditary hemorrhagic telangiectasia. (**a**) Axial arterial phase CT image demonstrating dilatation of the common hepatic artery (9 mm), a large confluent vascular mass (white arrow) and multiple tiny telangiectasias (open arrow). (**b**) Axial portal venous phase CT image showing large portal to hepatic venous shunts, with resultant dilatation of the right hepatic vein. (**c**) Volume-rendered image of the same patient, demonstrating aneurysmal dilatation of the celiac axis (white arrow), a large caliber common hepatic artery and multiple tiny hepatic telangiectasias (open arrow)

6.5 Diffuse Metastatic Disease

Hepatic metastases may show an infiltrative growth pattern with intrasinusoidal spread of tumor cells, which has been reported in breast cancer, gastric cancer, urothelial, small cell lung cancer, and melanoma. The intrasinusoidal spread induces hepatic ischemia, necrosis, and tumoral portal vein thrombosis leading to acute liver failure. Imaging diagnosis is difficult as no typically focal liver metastases can be seen.

The diffusely infiltrated liver parenchyma can appear heterogeneous compared to normal parenchyma. MRI is helpful to identify diffuse metastatic spread showing marked hyperintensity on diffusion-weighted images and hypointensity on hepatobiliary phase images. The degree of enhancement is variable also depending on the underlying primary tumor. Definite diagnosis can only be made by biopsy.

Another rare type of diffuse liver parenchyma changes is the so-called pseudocirrhosis, which can appear with hepatic breast cancer metastases and less common in cancer of the gastrointestinal tract, ovarian, or thyroid cancer [26]. The liver shows a nodular contour, capsular retraction, and shrinkage. Even signs of portal hypertension can develop over time. The etiology of the pseudocirrhosis is not very clear; it can be seen after chemotherapy with capsular retractions at the site of the liver metastases as response to chemotherapy, but it can also result from desmoplastic reaction surrounding the liver metastases.

6.6 Concluding Remarks

Chronic liver disease, in particular cirrhosis, is an increasing global epidemic which has already resulted in a major burden on healthcare systems with an ever-increasing incidence of primary liver malignancies and hepatic decompensation. Early identification of those at risk using quantitative imaging techniques, in particular elastography, fat fraction assessment and iron quantification is therefore essential in order to reduce its impact. MR elastography has proven a robust and accurate methodology for the assessment of those in whom rapid clinic-based techniques are unreliable. While outside the scope of this review, future developments of this technology (e.g., 3D MRE) may provide additional valuable information that could, for example, enable the differentiation of fibrosis from congestion in patients with vascular disorders such as congestive heart failure. When assessing those with cirrhosis, a methodical and consistent approach is required in order to identify malignancies, and in particular HCC, at a sufficiently early stage to enable effective treatment.

> **Take Home Messages**
> - Metabolic disease and cirrhosis are frequently under-recognized.
> - Familiarity with the morphologic features of diffuse liver disease and current/emerging quantitative imaging techniques is key to its early identification.
> - A consistent, rigorous approach to the assessment of associated lesions (e.g., using the LiRADS system) is essential and aids communication between clinicians as well as improving consistency in reporting.
> - Vascular liver disease may lead to chronic liver damage and development of regenerative nodules, which need to be differentiated from HCC.

References

1. Sepanlou, et al. The global, regional, and national burden of cirrhosis by cause in 195 countries and territories, 1990–2017: a systematic analysis for the Global Burden of Disease Study 2017. Lancet Gastroenterol Hepatol. 5:245–66. https://doi.org/10.1016/S2468-1253(19)30349-8.
2. Pickhardt PJ, at al. Specificity of unenhanced CT for non-invasive diagnosis of hepatic steatosis: implications for the investigation of the natural history of incidental steatosis. Eur Radiol. 2012;22(5):1075–82. https://doi.org/10.1007/s00330-011-2349-2. Epub 2011 Dec 4.
3. Idilman IS, Aniktar H, Idilman R, et al. Hepatic steatosis: quantification by proton density fat fraction with MR imaging versus liver biopsy. Radiology. 2013;267(3):767–75.
4. Hernando D, Levin YS, Sirlin CB, Reeder SB. Quantification of liver iron with MRI: state of the art and remaining challenges. J Magn Reson Imaging. 2014 Nov;40(5):1003–21. https://doi.org/10.1002/jmri.24584.
5. Henninger B, et al. Performance of different Dixon-based methods for MR liver iron assessment in comparison to a biopsy-validated R2* relaxometry method. Eur Radiol. 2021;31(4):2252–62.
6. Akhan O, et al. Imaging findings of liver involvement of Wilson's disease. Eur J Radiol. 2009;69(1):147–55.
7. Venkatesh SK, Hoodeshenas S, Venkatesh SH, Dispenzieri A, Gertz MA, Torbenson MS, Ehman RL. Magnetic resonance elastography of liver in light chain amyloidosis. J Clin Med. 2019;8(5):739.
8. Regenboog M, et al. Hepatocellular carcinoma in Gaucher disease: an international case series. J Inherit Metab Dis. 2018;41(5):819–27.
9. Guglielmo FF, Venkatesh SK, Mitchell DG. Liver MR elastography technique and image interpretation: pearls and pitfalls. Radiographics. 2019;39(7):1983–2002.
10. Yin M, Glaser KJ, Talwalkar JA, Chen J, Manduca A, Ehman RL. Hepatic MR elastography: clinical performance in a series of 1377 consecutive examinations. Radiology. 2016;278(1):114–24.
11. Brancatelli G, Federle MP, Ambrosini R, et al. Cirrhosis: CT and MR imaging evaluation. Eur J Radiol. 2007;61(1):57–69.
12. Parente DB, Perez RM, Eiras-Araujo A, et al. MR imaging of hypervascular lesions in the cirrhotic liver: a diagnostic dilemma. Radiographics. 2012;32(3):767–87.
13. LeGout JD, Bolan CW, Bowman AW, Caserta MP, Chen FK, Cox KL, Sanyal R, Toskich BB, Lewis JT, Alexander LF. Focal nodular hyperplasia and focal nodular hyperplasia-like lesions. Radiographics. 2022;42(4):1043–61.
14. Suh CH, et al. Hypervascular transformation of hypovascular hypointense nodules in the hepatobiliary phase of gadoxetic acid-enhanced MRI: a systematic review and meta-analysis. AJR Am J Roentgenol. 2017;209(4):781–9.
15. McEvoy SH, et al. Hepatocellular carcinoma: illustrated guide to systematic radiologic diagnosis and staging according to guidelines of the American Association for the Study of Liver Diseases. Radiographics. 2013;33(6):1653–68.
16. Razumilava N, Gores GJ. Cholangiocarcinoma. Lancet. 2014;383(9935):2168–79.
17. Kim R, et al. Differentiation of intrahepatic mass-forming cholangiocarcinoma from hepatocellular carcinoma on gadoxetic acid-enhanced liver MR imaging. Eur Radiol. 2016;26(6):1808–17.
18. Reynolds AR, et al. Infiltrative hepatocellular carcinoma: what radiologists need to know. Radiographics. 2015;35(2):371–86.
19. Ronot M, et al. Focal lesions in cirrhosis: not always HCC. Eur J Radiol. 2017;93:157–68.

20. https://www.acr.org/Clinical-Resources/Reporting-and-Data-Systems/LI-RADS

21. Torabi M, Hosseinzadeh K, Federle MP. CT of nonneoplastic hepatic vascular and perfusion disorders. Radiographics. 2008;28(7):1967–82.

22. Shin NY, et al. Accuracy of gadoxetic acid-enhanced magnetic resonance imaging for the diagnosis of sinusoidal obstruction syndrome in patients with chemotherapy-treated colorectal liver metastases. Eur Radiol. 2012;22(4):864–71.

23. Elsayes KM, et al. A comprehensive approach to hepatic vascular disease. Radiographics. 2017;37(3):813–36.

24. Idilman IS, Li J, Yin M, Venkatesh SK. MR elastography of liver: current status and future perspectives. Abdom Radiol (NY). 2020;45(11):3444–62.

25. Buscarini E, Gandolfi S, Alicante S, Londoni C, Manfredi G. Liver involvement in hereditary hemorrhagic telangiectasia. Abdom Radiol (NY). 2018;43(8):1920–30.

26. Gopalakrishnan D, et al. Pseudocirrhosis in breast cancer—experience from an Academic Cancer Center. Front Oncol. 2021;11:679163.

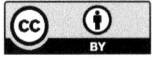

Focal Liver Lesions

7

Wolfgang Schima and Dow-Mu Koh

Learning Objectives
- To learn about the imaging protocol in MDCT and MRI for detection and characterization of focal liver lesions.
- To learn the typical and atypical imaging features of benign and malignant focal lesions.
- To understand the importance of knowledge about chronic liver disease because the presence of chronic liver disease alters the differential diagnosis and the diagnostic approach.

Contrast-enhanced MDCT remains the modality of choice for routine liver imaging. MR imaging is still used largely as a problem-solving tool, when MDCT or US are equivocal or if there is concern for malignancy in high-risk populations.

In this chapter, we will highlight imaging of focal liver lesions, focusing on the use of MDCT and MR imaging for disease detection and characterization. The reader should learn how to optimize CT and MR imaging in his/her own practice, understand how to apply and interpret CT and MR imaging for the management of focal liver lesions and appreciate the expanding role of liver-specific MR contrast agents for lesion characterization.

7.1 Introduction

Multidetector computed tomography (MDCT) and magnetic resonance (MR) imaging provide non-invasive insights into liver anatomy and the pathophysiology of liver diseases, which allows for better diagnosis of focal liver lesions, monitoring of disease evolution and treatment response, as well as for guiding treatment decisions. Understanding the application of different imaging techniques is critical for the management of focal liver lesions. In the current climate of challenging health economics, the most appropriate and cost-effective modality should be utilized. For liver imaging, ultrasonography (US) is widely available, non-invasive, and is often used in the community for disease screening but has unfortunately limited diagnostic sensitivity and specificity.

7.2 MDCT Imaging Techniques

Advantages of MDCT imaging in clinical practice are very rapid scan acquisition, which avoids motion artifacts, and the capability of multi-planar imaging. Using a state-of-the-art MDCT system, the entire liver can be scanned within 1-3 s using a sub-millimeter detector configuration allowing for high-quality 3D-reconstructions [1]. When viewed axially, reconstructed sections of 2.5–3 mm thickness with an overlap of 0.5–1 mm are usually used in clinical practice. Thinner slices do not improve lesion conspicuity because of increased image noise [2, 3] that can decrease diagnostic specificity [3]. The amount of contrast material administered should be adapted according to the patient's weight, with 0.5 g iodine/kg b.w. being a typical dosage (i.e., 1.7 mL/kg b.w. at 300 mg iodine/mL). The total amount of iodine administered determines the quality of the portal venous imaging phase, with the aim of increasing the liver attenuation by 50 HU after contrast injection [4]. To achieve good arterial-phase imaging, a relatively high contrast medium injection rate of 4–5 mL/s is recommended [5]. However, the weight-based adaptation of contrast media dosage should also go hand in hand with an adaptation of the contrast media injection rate. Accordingly, studies using a fixed injection duration of 30 s

W. Schima (✉)
Department of Diagnostic and Interventional Radiology, Goettlicher Heiland Krankenhaus, Barmherzige Schwestern Krankenhaus, and Sankt Josef Krankenhaus, Vinzenzgruppe, Vienna, Austria
e-mail: wolfgang.schima@khgh.at

D.-M. Koh
Department of Radiology, The Royal Marsden NHS Foundation Trust, Sutton, UK

© The Author(s) 2023
J. Hodler et al. (eds.), *Diseases of the Abdomen and Pelvis 2023-2026*, IDKD Springer Series,
https://doi.org/10.1007/978-3-031-27355-1_7

(meaning that the injection rate will differ according to patient's weight) have shown that this approach provides consistent image quality.

The timing of the image acquisition in relation to contrast media administration depends on whether imaging is required during early arterial phase (for arterial anatomy only), late arterial phase (for hypervascular tumor detection and characterization), or venous phase (for follow-up imaging and hypovascular tumor detection). For the detection and characterization of focal liver lesions, late arterial-phase imaging (scan delay of aortic transit time plus 15–18 s) [6, 7], and a venous phase scan (20–30 s interscan delay or with fixed delay of app. 60–70 s) are performed. In patients with chronic liver disease, a delayed phase (at app. 3 min post contrast) for better lesion characterization is recommended.

Automated methods of measuring arterial enhancement (aortic transit time) on CT, often termed bolus tracking, has largely replaced the use of fixed scan-delay times because it provides better coincidence of scanning with peak enhancement of liver tumors (in the late arterial phase) and the liver parenchyma (in the venous phase).

Different techniques for dose reduction and optimization of image quality are now widely in use: automatic exposure control by tube current (mA) modulation, selection of lower tube potential (kVp), and adaptive dose shielding to minimize overscanning in the z-axis, to name a few. Conventional filtered back projection (FBP), the standard CT image reconstruction technique for many years, has given way to iterative reconstruction (IR) techniques. IR allows for dose reduction by reconstruction low-noise image data from intrinsically noisy reduced-dose CT acquisitions, preserving imaging quality [8]. IR techniques can be either hybrid or model-based, with the latter being more advance, allowing for stronger dose reduction at the cost of slower images reconstruction. All major manufacturers now provide iterative reconstruction techniques (SAFIRE [hybrid], ADMIRE [model-based], Siemens; iDose [hybrid], IMR [model-based], Philips; ASIR [hybrid], MBIR [model-based], GE Healthcare; AIDR 3D [hybrid], FIRST [model-based],

Canon [8]. Stepwise IR reduces CT noise levels. However, (too) high levels of IR may produce an unfamiliar image texture that may render image quality unacceptable [9]. A substantial dose reduction of 38–55% is possible with IR without compromising image quality [10–12]. In recent years, dual energy and spectral CT technique has emerged, where different vendors use different concepts. Utilization of dual source or a split-beam (Siemens), kV-switching during scanning (GE healthcare, Canon) and the use of dual-layer CT detectors (Philips) provide the differential attenuation of X-ray beams of different kV when scanning different tissues. In clinical practice, spectral CT has found several applications in oncologic imaging: in the liver, it improves the detection of hypervascular hepatocellular carcinomas [13] or allows quantification of hepatic iron content [14]. More recently, the advent of photon-counting CT promises even further improvement in the spatial and contrast resolution of CT images. Photo-counting CT detectors can directly convert detected X-rays into electrical signal for image reconstruction, making it possible to use smaller detectors to improve spatial resolution and producing images at different keVs to improve contrast resolution (Fig. 7.1).

> **Key Points**
> - For detection and characterization of focal lesions at least a bi-phasic contrast-enhanced protocol is necessary, in patients with chronic liver disease (cirrhosis, chronic hepatitis B infection) a triple-phasic enhanced protocol is recommended.
> - Iterative reconstruction techniques are standard to reduce image noise and, thus, to reduce radiation dose.
> - Spectral CT is achieved by various technologies (dual source, rapid kV switching, dual layer detector) by different vendors. It may be particularly of help in oncologic imaging.

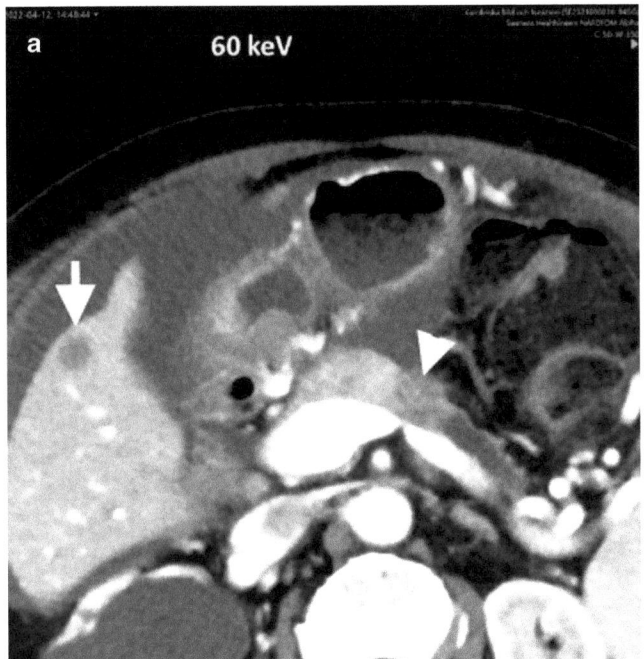

Fig. 7.1 A woman with pancreatic carcinoma evaluated using photon-counting CT in the upper abdomen. Images reconstructed at tube voltages of (**a**) 60 keV and (**b**) 40 keV. Both the primary tumor (arrowhead) and the liver metastasis (arrow) appear more conspicuous on the lower 40 keV image. The use of photon-counting CT can improve image spatial and contrast resolution of disease. [Images courtesy of Dr. Nikolaos Kartalis, Karolinska Institute, Sweden]

7.3 MR Imaging Technique

MR imaging of the liver can be performed at both 1.5 T and 3.0 T, the latter providing improved image quality due to increased signal-to-noise ratio. MR examination of the liver should include unenhanced T1-weighted and T2-weighted sequences, diffusion-weighted imaging as well as contrast-enhanced sequences. Specific acquisition sequences vary by manufacturer, patient compliance, and the clinical question being addressed.

T1-weighted MRI should be performed using a 3D DIXON technique, which can generate in-phase, opposed-phase (syn.: out-of-phase), water-only and fat-only images of the whole liver volume in a single breath-hold acquisition. In- and opposed-phase T1-weighted imaging is used for characterization of fat-containing tumors (e.g., adenoma, HCC) and the presence of steatosis. The resultant water-only images have been shown to improve the uniformity of fat-suppression at 3 T, compared with conventional spectral fat-suppression technique [15]. The use of the DIXON images for dynamic contrast-enhanced acquisition has also been shown to improve the detection of HCC compared with standard fat-suppressed sequences.

Another useful recent implementation is non-cartesian radial T1-weighted imaging, which allows 3D volume T1-weighted imaging of the liver to be performed in free

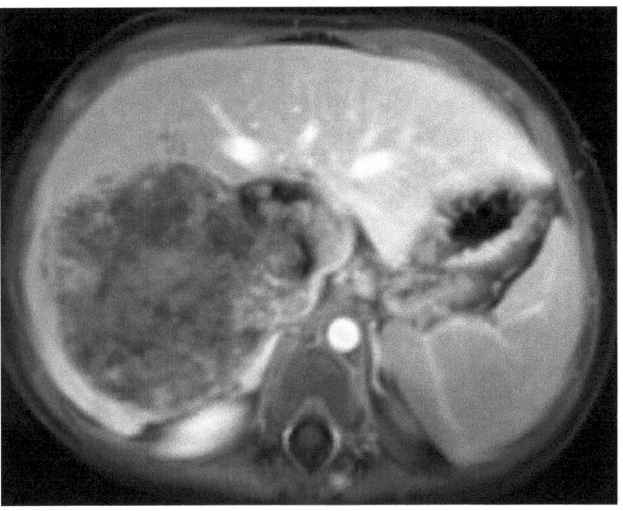

Fig. 7.2 Radial acquisition technique. Portal venous phase T1-weighted MRI in a child presenting with a liver metastasis from a rhabdomyosarcoma. In children and adults who are unable to breath-hold, the radial acquisition technique performed in free-breathing can overcome the effects of respiratory motion

breathing. This allows good quality T1-weighted GRE of the liver to be obtained in patients with poor breath holding (e.g., elderly patients in poor general condition or young children) (Fig. 7.2), especially during dynamic contrast-enhanced acquisitions [16]. T2-weighted pulse sequences with fat-suppression provide better lesion contrast than non-fat-suppressed sequences and are also widely used.

Diffusion-weighted imaging (DWI) is standard in liver imaging, and it is now available on all scanners. In general, DWI depends upon the microscopic mobility of water, called Brownian motion, in tissue. Water-molecule diffusion (and thus the measured signal intensity) depends on tissue cellularity, tissue organization, integrity of cellular membranes, and extracellular space tortuosity. Usually, lower water diffusion is found in most solid tumors, which is attributed to their high cellularity [17]. Thus, DWI is helpful for detecting liver solid focal liver lesions [18–20]. By performing diffusion-weighted imaging using two or more b-values, we can quantify the apparent diffusion coefficient (ADC) of liver tissues. Benign focal liver lesions have been shown to have higher ADC value than malignant liver lesions although there is significant overlap [20]. Nonetheless, quantitative ADC values may be useful to support lesion characterization and for identifying early tumor response to treatment.

Imaging after the administration of intravenous contrast agents remain the cornerstone for liver MR imaging. Of these, nonspecific extracellular gadolinium contrast medium is still most widely used. Following the intravenous (IV) bolus injection of an extracellular gadolinium-based contrast agents, dynamic imaging (using volumetric T1-weighted GRE) is performed for lesion characterization, lesion detection, evaluating tumor response to systemic therapy and detecting recurrence after locoregional therapy.

Liver-specific (or hepatobiliary) MR contrast agents are available and have specific roles in the management of focal liver lesions. These include gadobenate dimeglumine (MultiHance®, Bracco) and gadoxetic acid (Primovist® or Eovist®, Bayer Healthcare). Liver-specific MR contrast agents are also usually administered IV as a bolus, as with nonspecific gadolinium chelates for dynamic imaging. However, imaging is also performed at a delayed liver-specific or hepatobiliary phase, the timing of this differs according to the contrast agent. These liver-specific agents are taken up into hepatocytes to varying extent (gadobenate dimeglumine 4–5%; gadoxetic acid ~50%), resulting in avid T1 enhancement of the liver parenchyma in the hepatobiliary phase, which is performed at 20 min for gadoxetic acid and about 1–2 h for gadobenate dimeglumine after contrast administration. Liver-specific contrast agents have been shown to improve the detection of liver metastases [21–24], especially when used in combination with diffusion-weighted MR imaging.

7.4 Benign Hepatic Lesions

7.4.1 Cysts

Simple hepatic cysts are common, occurring in 5–14% of the general population. As they are usually asymptomatic, they are detected incidentally on US, CT, or MR imaging. On CT, hepatic cysts are well circumscribed and typically show attenuation values similar to water (0–15HU) although smaller cysts may show higher attenuation values due to partial volume effects. Cysts should not show mural thickening, nodularity, or contrast enhancement. Small cysts (≤ 3 mm in size) may pose a diagnostic challenge in the cancer patient on CT as they are too small to be fully characterized and stability on follow-up imaging is important to reassure. Nonetheless, the vast majority (>90%) of small hypodense liver lesions even in the oncology patient are benign. On MR imaging examinations, cysts are well-defined, homogeneous lesions that appear hypointense on T1-weighted images (unless hemorrhagic) and markedly hyperintense on T2-weighted images. Their marked hyperintensity on T2-weighted imaging (in comparison to solid lesions) provides greater confidence towards the diagnosis of small cysts on MRI.

7.4.2 Hemangioma

Hemangioma is the most common benign liver tumor. On US, liver hemangioma appears circumscribed, well-defined, and hyperechoic. Small hemangiomas usually appear homogeneous but larger hemangiomas (>4 cm) can show a heterogeneous appearance.

On CT, hemangiomas are well-defined hypodense masses. They are hypointense on T1-weighted and markedly hyperintense on T2-weighted imaging, sometimes with a lobular contour. Hyperintensity on T2-weighted MRI (especially on single-shot T2 TSE) helps to differentiate hemangiomas from other solid neoplasms [25, 26]. At a relatively long T2 echo time (140 ms or longer), a homogeneously bright lesion is characteristic of a benign lesion, such as a cyst or hemangioma. Exceptions (that can be quite bright on heavily T2-weighted sequences) include cystic or mucinous metasta-

ses, gastrointestinal stromal tumor (GIST), and neuroendocrine tumor metastases.

Hemangiomas show three distinctive patterns of enhancement at CT/MRI (Type I to III) [27]. Characteristically, there is enhancement that closely follows the enhancement of blood pool elsewhere [28]. Small lesions (up to ~2 cm) may show immediate and complete enhancement in the arterial phase, with sustained enhancement in the venous and delayed phases (type I, "flash filling" hemangioma) [29] (Fig. 7.3). On delayed imaging, the enhancement usually fades to a

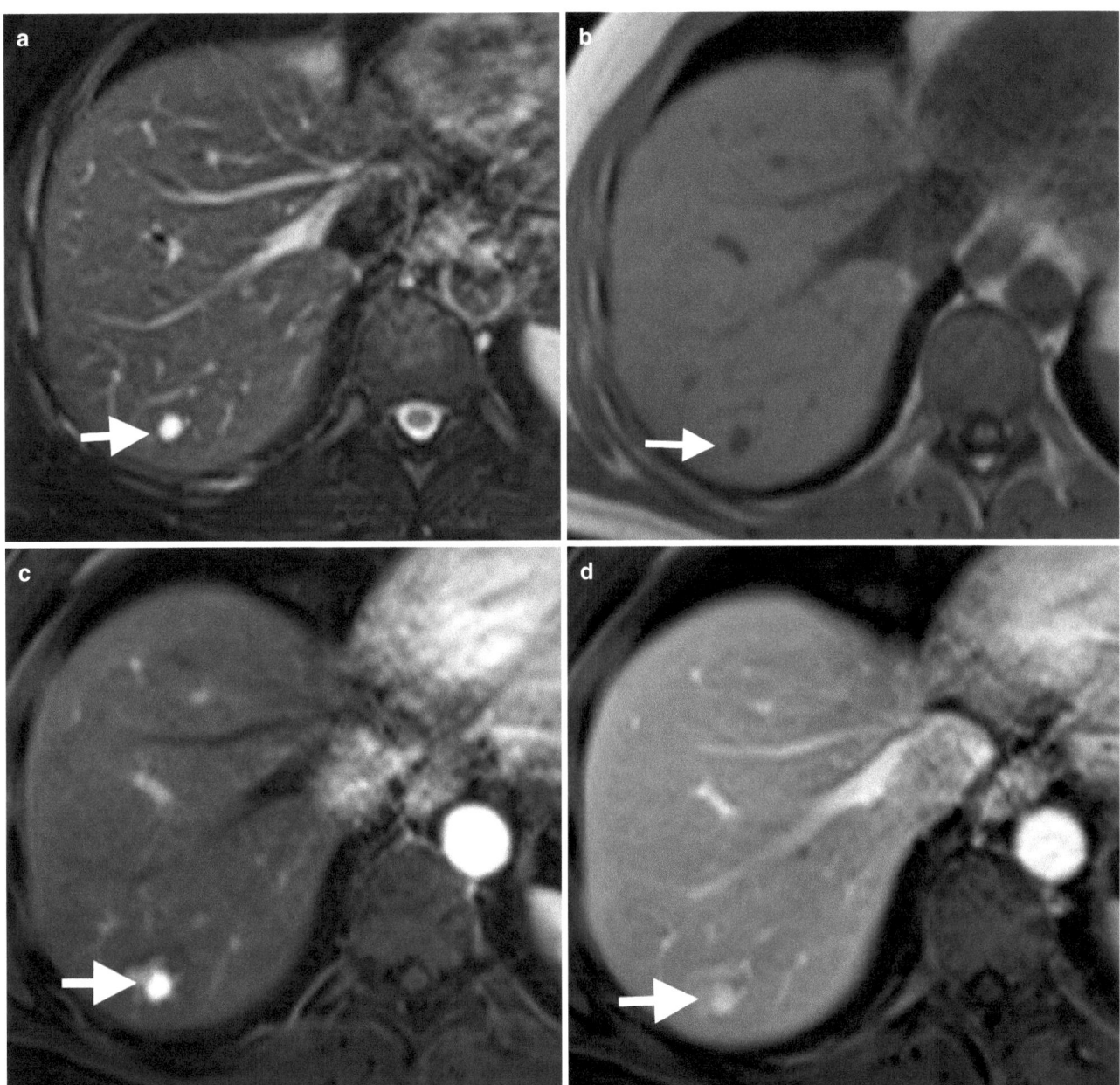

Fig. 7.3 Hemangioma type 1 with liver-specific MR contrast agent. A 45-year-old woman with incident lesion (arrows) in right lobe of liver. This appears (**a**) as high signal intensity on T2-weighted imaging, (**b**) as low signal intensity on T1-weighted imaging and (**c–e**) shows uniform enhancement on dynamic T1-weighted contrast-enhanced imaging, isointense to the arterial signal at all phases. The lesion appears (**f**) hypointense in the hepatobiliary phase of gadoxetic acid-enhanced MRI

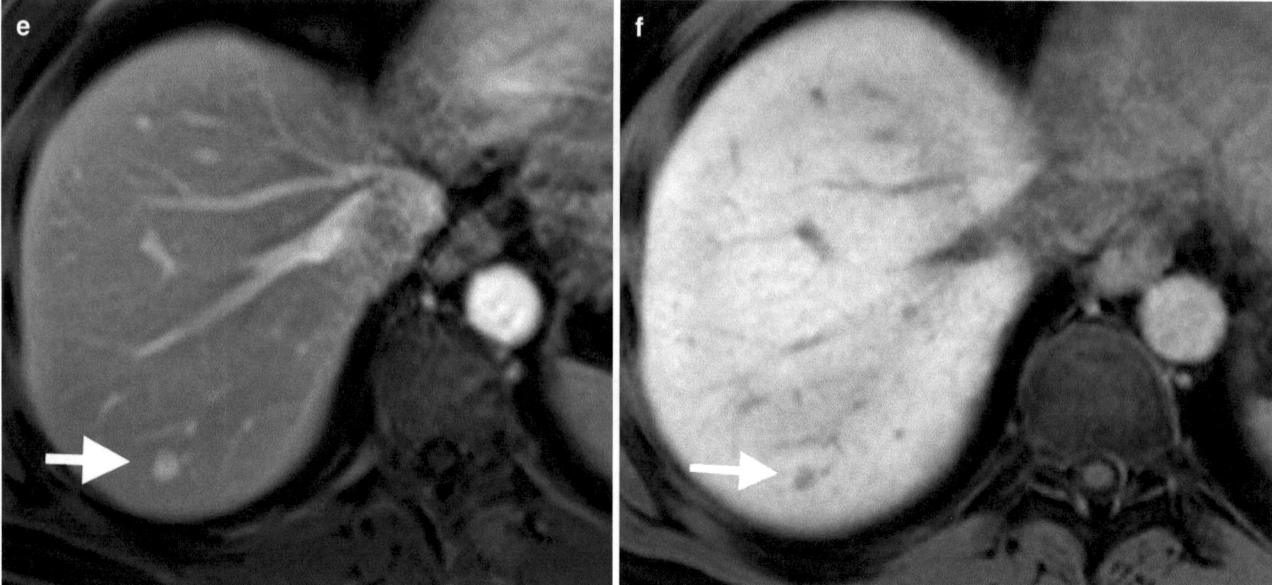

Fig. 7.3 (continued)

similar extent as the blood pool. The most common enhancement pattern is peripheral nodular discontinuous enhancement, with progressive fill-in over time (type II). Larger lesions (>5 cm) or lesions with central thrombosis/fibrosis may lack central fill-in (type III) (Fig. 7.4). Dynamic extracellular gadolinium chelate-enhanced MRI is superior to contrast-enhanced CT for characterization of small and slow-flow hemangioma, which start to show typical enhancement only in the delayed phase. When evaluated using liver-specific contrast agents, the appearance of hemangiomas in the dynamic arterial and venous phases is similar to that with extracellular gadolinium chelates. However, in the delayed phase (at 3 min post contrast), there may be "pseudowashout" (hypointensity) due to early hepatocellular enhancement of liver parenchyma (Fig. 7.5). In the hepatobiliary phase, hemangiomas may appear hypointense to the parenchyma, thus mimicking liver metastases. In this instance, DWI may help to differentiate between hemangioma and other solid lesions, as the apparent diffusion coefficient (ADC) of uncomplicated hemangiomas is significantly higher (typically $>1.70 \times 10^{-3}$ s/mm^2) than in malignant solid lesions [30, 31].

7.4.3 Focal Nodular Hyperplasia (FNH)

FNH is the second most common benign tumor, usually found in young women. It is a non-neoplastic lesion that can cause confusion when it is incidentally detected during imaging. At US the lesion is usually isoechoic or slightly hypoechoic [32] to liver, but it may appear hypoechoic in patients with diffuse hepatic steatosis. Typically, FNH dem-

onstrates a lobular contour, which is quite uncommon in malignant lesions. A central scar is present in about 67% of larger lesions, and about 33% of smaller lesions [33]. The central scar in FNH is usually hyperintense on T2-weighted images, with a comma-shaped or spoke-wheel appearance. This scar can be differentiated from fibrolamellar HCC, where a central scar is predominantly of low signal intensity on T2-weighted MRI due to fibrosis. Color/power Doppler US may show blood flow within the scar [34].

FNH is isodense or minimally hypodense on unenhanced and equilibrium-phase post-contrast CT and may be only suspected because of the presence of mass effect on adjacent vessels. On unenhanced T1- and T2-weighted MR images, FNH return signal intensity similar to hepatic parenchyma, but is usually slightly different on either T1-weighted or T2-weighted images. Due to the prominent arterial vascular supply, FNH demonstrates marked homogenous enhancement during the arterial phase of contrast-enhanced CT/MR imaging, which becomes rapidly isodense/isointense to liver parenchyma in the portal venous phase [33]. The comma-shaped or spoke-wheel central scar often showed delayed enhancement (Fig. 7.6) because of its vascular component [32]. Another key feature is that the scar in FNH is usually T2-weighted hyperintense in appearance compared with the heterogenous, low SI appearance encountered in fibrolamellar HCC.

Using liver-specific MR contrast agents, FNH frequently shows enhancement on delayed images after administration of hepatobiliary contrast agents (gadoxetic acid or gadobenate dimeglumine) because of the presence of normal biliary ductules within the lesion and the expression of OATP receptors (Fig. 7.6). However, the uptake of hepatobiliary contrast

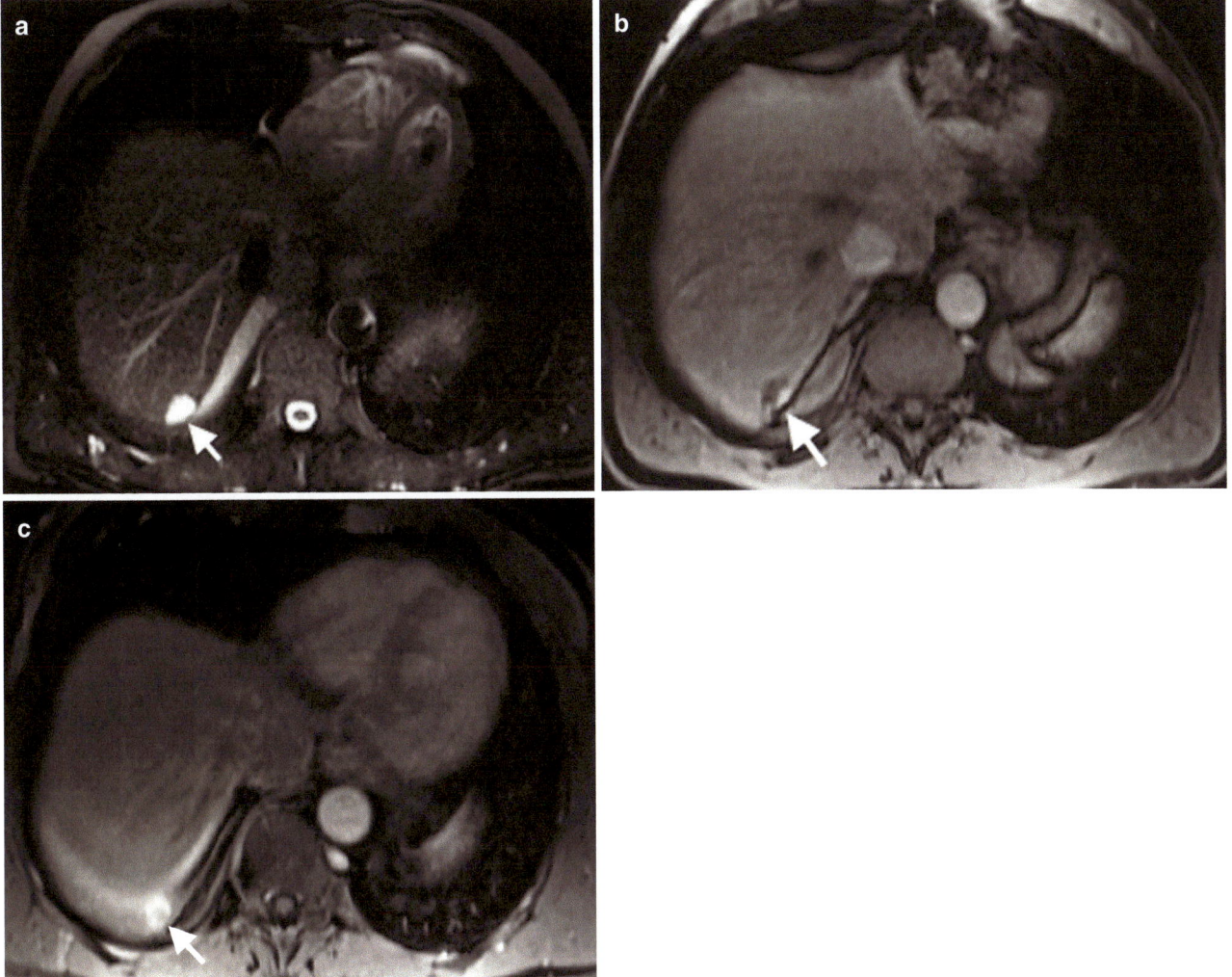

Fig. 7.4 Liver hemangioma with type 3 enhancement using extracellular gadolinium chelate. (**a**) Fat-suppressed T2-weighted image shows a high signal intensity lesion in the posterior right lobe typical for a hemangioma (arrow). Fat-suppressed contrast-enhanced T1-weighted image in the (**b**) arterial and (**c**) delayed phases of contrast enhancement, show initial nodular peripheral enhancement with progressive centripetal filling (arrows)

agents within FNH may be rarely heterogenous or absent [35]. The central scar is spared in the hepatobiliary phase, and a more ring-like enhancement in the hepatobiliary phase due to a very prominent non-enhancing scar can be seen (Fig. 7.6) [36]. Nonetheless, a recent meta-analysis showed that lesion T1 isointensity or hyperintensity at delayed hepatobiliary phase MRI has a high sensitivity (91–100%) and specificity (87–100%) for diagnosing FNH [35]. This feature can be helpful for differentiating FNH from hypervascular metastases or hepatic adenomas (HCA) and hepatocellular carcinomas (HCC) (which rarely take up liver-specific agents) [29, 37]. However, it should be noted that some HCAs (particularly inflammatory HCA) and HCC can appear isointense or hyperintense at delayed imaging after hepatobiliary contrast media administration. While differentiating FNH from variants of HCA remains challenging, characterization should never be based on the hepatobiliary phase appearance alone. Regarding HCC, the presence of contrast washout (i.e., lesion hypointensity compared to liver parenchyma) in the portal venous or transitional phase of dynamic contrast enhancement can be used to distinguish between HCC (that shows contrast uptake in the hepatobiliary phase) and FHN nodules. The majority of FNH tend to remain static in size although FNH may increase in size on follow-up oral contraceptives do not appear to stimulate FNH growth [38, 39].

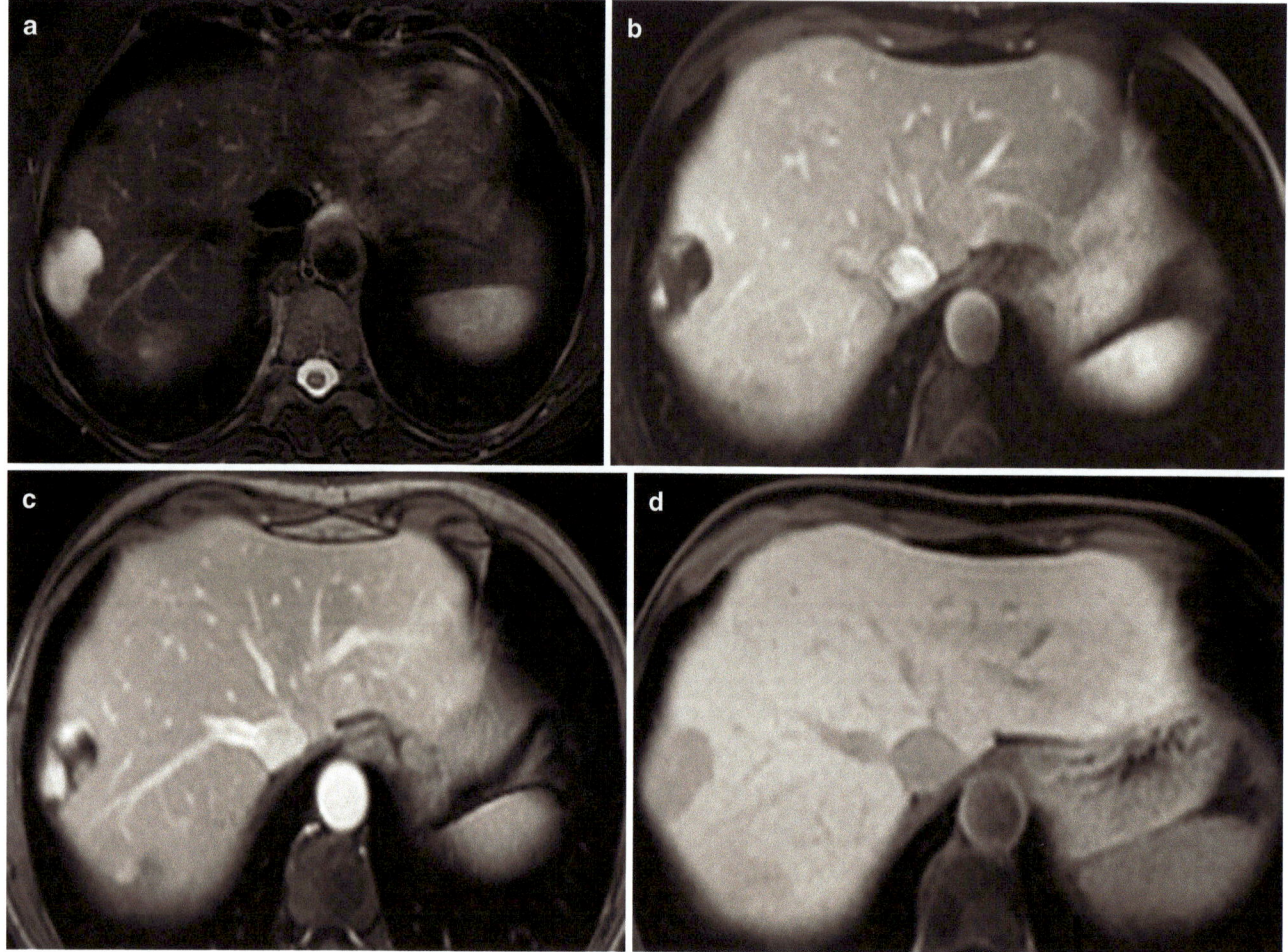

Fig. 7.5 Hemangioma type 3: liver-specific MR contrast agent. (**a**) T2-weighted TSE shows a large lobulated lesion of very high signal intensity. (**b–d**) Dynamic gadoxetic acid-enhanced imaging shows peripheral nodular enhancement in the arterial (**b**) and venous phases (**c**). In the hepatobiliary phase (**d**) there is hypointensity of the lesion due to lack of hepatocellular uptake in the lesion and marked enhancement of surrounding liver parenchyma. Please note there is some enhancement of the lesion because of vascular/extracellular pooling of contrast

Key Points
- FNH are usually (near) isointense on T1-weighted and T2-weighted images, with homogenous arterial-phase hyperenhancement.
- The central scar (seen in most FNH >3 cm) is hypoattenuating/hypointense in the early contrast phases, with delayed-phase enhancement.
- After liver-specific CM, FNH is almost always homogenously isointense/hyperintense in the hepatobiliary phase, with an hypointense central scar.

7.4.4 Hepatocellular Adenoma

Hepatocellular adenomas (HCA) are uncommon liver tumors, which occur more often in women of reproductive age. There is an association with oral contraceptives. Other risk factors include anabolic steroid usage, glycogen storage disease type, and obesity. Histologically, HCA is composed of cells resembling normal hepatocytes but lacking bile ducts, which distinguishes them from FNH [39].

In the last two decades, considerable progress has been made in the diagnosis of HCA, by establishment of molecular and immunohistological classification of HCA subtypes [40]. The molecular classification categorizes HCA into the following six sub-groups: HNF1A inactivated HCA (H-HCA), inflammatory HCA (I-HCA), beta-catenin activated HCA (b-HCA), sonic hedgehog HCA (shHCA), and unclassified HCA (UHCA) [41, 42]. The most common complications of HCA are bleeding and malignant transformation.

The imaging features of HCA are heterogeneous and varied and depend on the subtype. HCA are often hypervascular and may appear heterogenous due to the presence of fat,

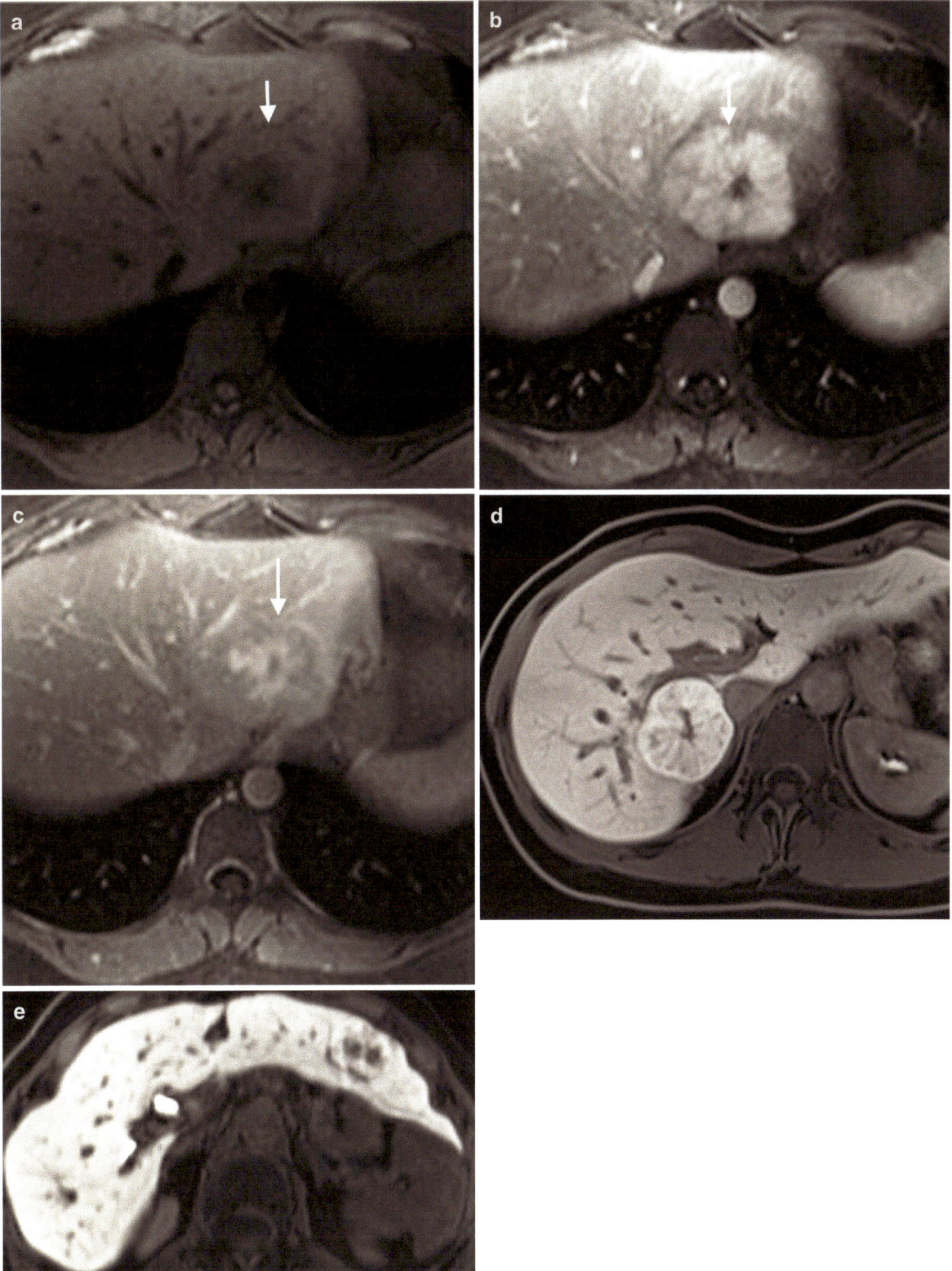

Fig. 7.6 FNH found incidentally (arrows). (**a**) Pre-contrast T1-weighted image shows an isointense lesion with a central hypointense scar, which shows minimal mass effect upon adjacent vasculature. (**b**) Arterial-phase T1-weighted contrast-enhanced image shows hypervascularity of the lesion. (**c**) T1-weighted delayed phase imaging after contrast shows that the lesion is now predominantly isointense to the liver, but with late enhancement of the (vascular) central scar. The enhancement pattern is typical for FNH. (**d, e**) Hepatobiliary phase imaging of FNH in 2 other patients: (**d**) homogenous uptake of the liver-specific MR contrast agent, the spoke-wheel central scar is typically not enhanced. (**e**) Ring-like contrast uptake by the lesion in the left lobe with large hypointensity due to a large central scar

necrosis, or hemorrhage [39, 43]. T1-weighted chemical shift or DIXON imaging is useful for detecting intratumoral fat, while the presence of high T1-signal before contrast administration will raise the suspicion of spontaneous hemorrhage. The reader should be familiar with the differential diagnoses of fat containing focal liver lesions on MRI, which include focal fat infiltration, HCA (particularly the HNF1A inactivating subtype), hepatocellular carcinoma (usually well-differentiated), angiomyolipoma, lipoma, teratoma and liver metastases from fat containing malignancies (e.g. liposarcomas). The presence of intratumoral fat helps to narrow the differential diagnosis of a hypervascular lesion, as hemangioma can be excluded and metastases and FNH rarely contain fat.

On dynamic contrast-enhanced CT or MR, adenomas usually show marked arterial-phase enhancement, with rapid transition to either iso- or hypoattenuating/intense to hepatic parenchyma on portal venous phase imaging. Our understanding of the molecular aberrations associated with HCA has improved our understanding of HCA subtypes, which is linked to risk factors, histological features, clinical presentation, and imaging appearances [44, 45].

What is important for radiologists [46]? Inactivating mutations of hepatocyte nuclear factor 1 alpha (HNF1A) are observed in approximately 30% of HCA. HNF1A-inactivated HCA usually contains fat as evidenced by diffuse and homogenous signal loss on chemical shift T1-weighted imaging (Fig. 7.7). They return variable T2 signal. At contrast-enhanced T1-weighted MRI, they are hypervascular, often with contrast washout in the portal venous or delayed phase. They are typically hypointense on hepatobiliary-phase MRI using liver-specific contrast medium. HNF1A-inactivated HCAs have a very low risk of malignant transformation.

Inflammatory HCA accounts for 40–50% of HCA cases. Obesity and a history of oral contraceptives intake are risk factors for their development. Inflammatory HCA appear strongly hyperintense on T2-weighted MRI, which may be diffuse or rim-like in the periphery of the lesion (atoll sign). Intralesional fat is uncommon, when present is often patchy or heterogeneous. On contrast-enhanced imaging, there is usually intense arterial enhancement, with persistent enhancement on delayed-phase imaging (Figs. 7.8 and 7.9). Although the majority of inflammatory HCA are hypointense on hepatobiliary phase using liver-specific contrast media, about 30% may appear iso- or hyperintense. Inflammatory HCA may also harbor activating mutations of b-catenin in exon 3 and are therefore at risk of malignant transformation.

Mutations of catenin b1 (CTNNB1) are seen in 10–15% of HCA. These are associated with a higher risk of malignant transformation. These variants of HCA do not have typical imaging features and may be difficult to differentiate from HCC or FNH. HCA with mutations of catenin b1 (b-catenin-HCA) may show gadoxetic acid uptake in the hepatobiliary phase of MRI in up to 80% of patients [47].

Activation of sonic hedgehog pathway occurs in approximately 5% of HCA. As these are relatively uncommon, the spectrum of imaging features associated with these is yet to be fully described. Nonetheless, these lesions have a higher propensity to undergo spontaneous hemorrhage. About 7% of HCA remains unclassified. These do not have typical clinical or imaging appearances. Overall, the imaging features at MRI, including their appearances are helpful in distinguishing between FNH and HCA. Early studies also reported on the high value of liver-specific MR contrast agent for differentiation between FNH and adenoma (with FNH being predominantly iso-hyperintense in the hepatobiliary phase and HCA most often hypointense). [48, 42]. A recent meta-analysis on the value of hepatobiliary phase gadoxetic acid-enhanced MRI showed that HA subtypes other than H-HCA demonstrated proportions of iso- to hyperintensity on hepatobiliary phases images ranging from 11% to 59% [49]. Radiologists should thus recognize the low specificity hepatobiliary phase iso-hyperintensity for differentiating FNH from HCA subtypes other than H-HCA [49]. Of note is that diffusion-weighted MRI has little value in helping to distinguish between HCA and FNH or HCC because of the substantial overlap in the ADC values.

Key Points
- Adenomas are uncommon benign tumors, most often in women. Risk factors include oral contraceptives, anabolic steroid usage, glycogen storage disease type, and obesity.
- Several subtypes, with distinctive molecular and immunohistological features have been identified (e.g., HNF1A-inactivated HCA, inflammatory HCA, beta-catenin activated HCA, sonic hedgehog HCA, and unclassified HCA), with distinctive risk profiles (bleeding and malignant degeneration).
- Imaging features are heterogenous vary depending on subtype, but arterial-phase hypervascularity is common.

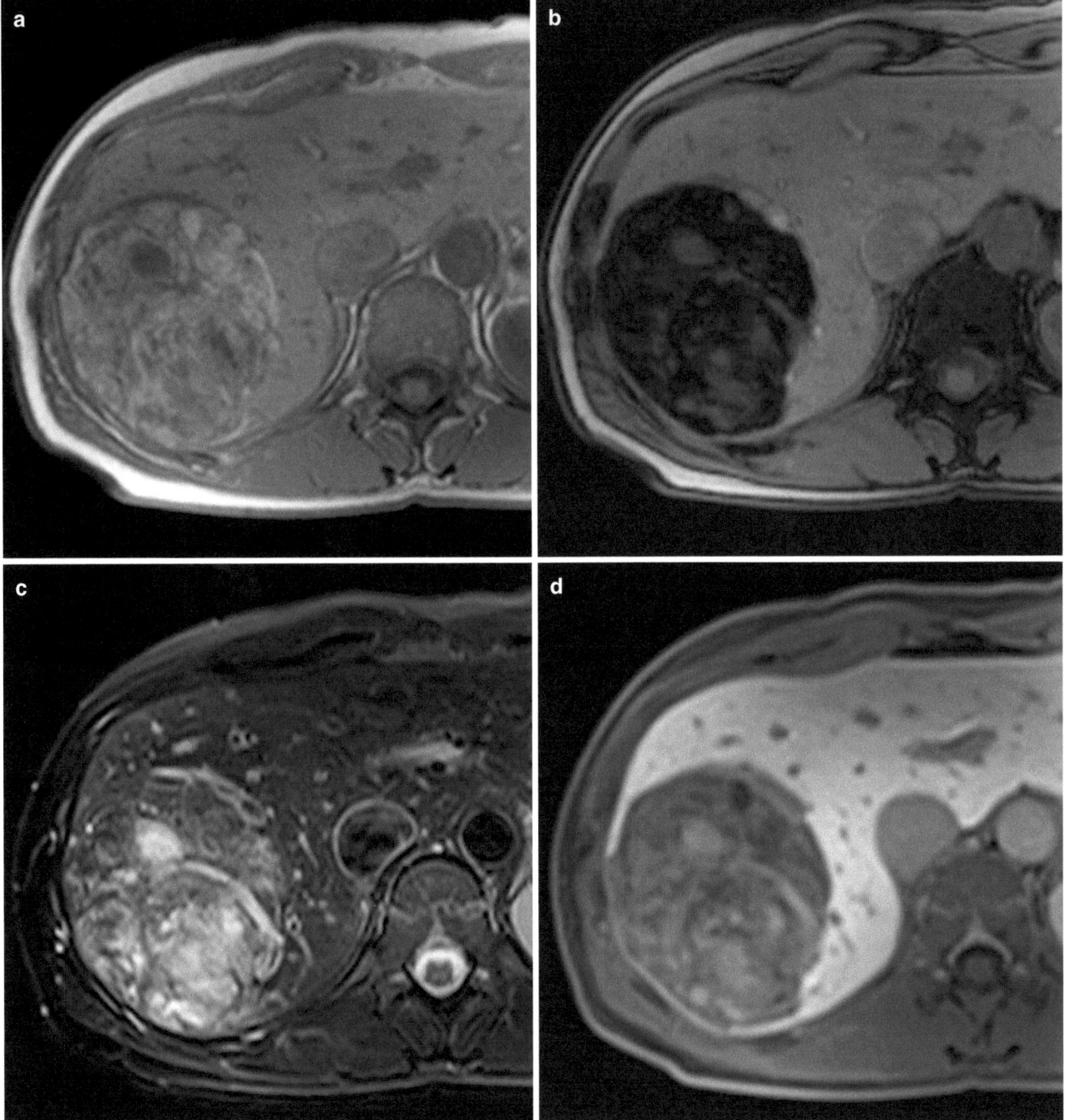

Fig. 7.7 Adenoma (HNF1A subtype). (**a**) T1-weighted in-phase GRE image demonstrates a very large mass in a young woman. The mass is inhomogenous and shows bright spots. (**b**) There is typical signal intensity drop on the opposed-phase image indicative of intratumoral fat. (**c**) T2-weighted TSE image shows moderate hyperintensity. (**d**) On gadoxetic acid-enhanced image (hepatobiliary phase), there is little to no enhancement

7.4.5   Biliary Hamartomas (von Meyenburg Complex)

Bile duct hamartomas are congenital malformations of the ductal plate without connections to the bile ducts. They are usually incidentally discovered at abdominal imaging. Although of no clinical significance, they can mimic disseminated small liver metastases in the patient with cancer. Biliary hamartomas are typically small (5–10 mm in size) and diffusely spread in both lobes of the liver. On ultrasound, they appear as small hyperechoic or hypoechoic lesions and can demonstrate ringing artifacts (comet tail appearance).

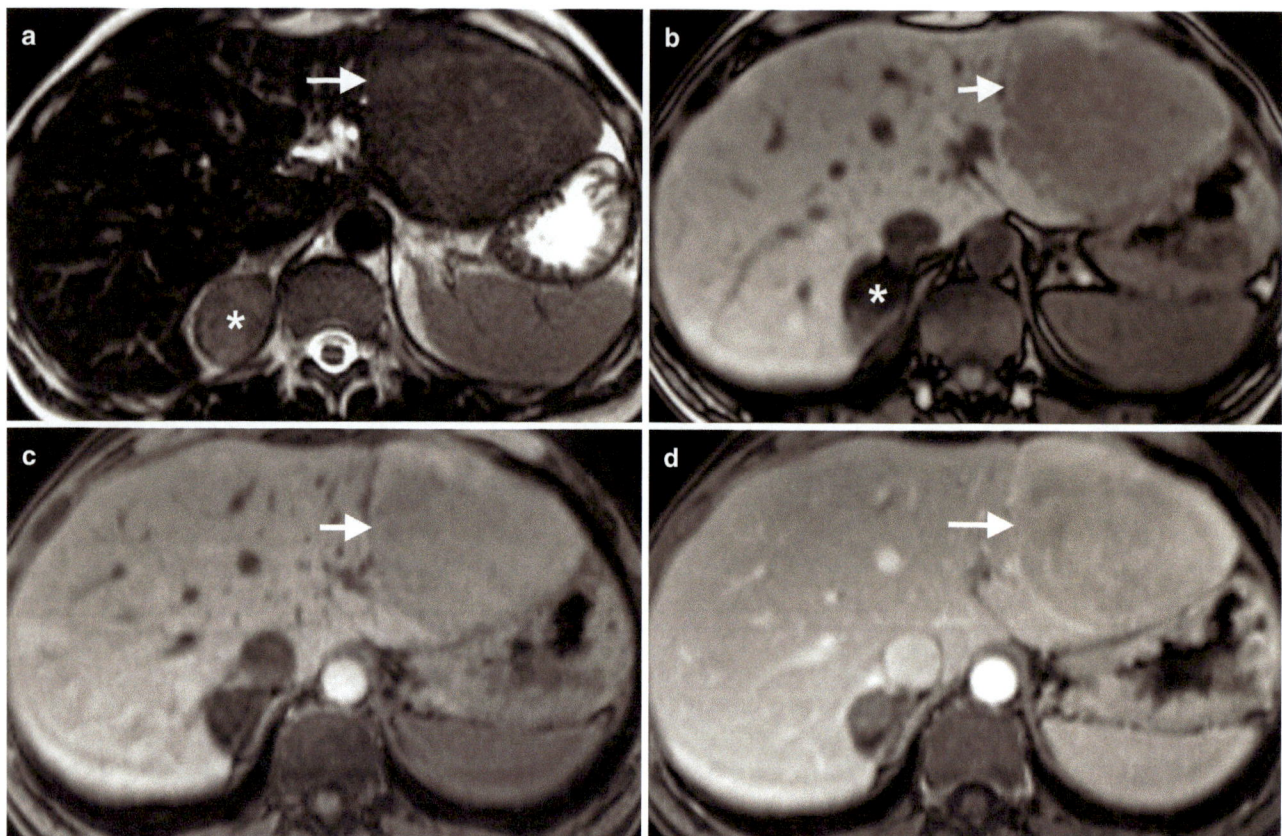

Fig. 7.8 Adenoma: inflammatory type. (**a**) T2-weighted TSE shows a large circumscribed mildly hyperintense mass in the left hepatic lobe (arrow) with an incidental right adrenal adenoma (*). (**b**) On opposed-phase T1-weighted GE image, the mass (arrow) is mildly hypointense. Note signal loss in the adrenal adenoma indicating intratumoral fat. (**c**) Pre-contrast and (**d**) portal venous phase post-contrast T1-weighted GRE show mild internal enhancement of the lesion (arrows)

On CT, they appear as small cystic lesions of round, oval, or irregular shape without contrast enhancement although thin rim enhancement may sometimes be present, thus mimicking hypovascular liver metastases [43]. When enhancement is present, it is usually very thin (≤2 mm) and observed only on equilibrium-phase images, related to the fibrous component of the lesions [50]. On MRI, biliary hamartomas appear as low signal intensity on T1-weighted imaging, and high signal intensity on T2-weighted imaging (Fig. 7.10). They are best observed on maximum intensity projections MRCP sequences as high signal intensity foci without connection to or associated abnormalities of the intra-hepatic ducts. Occasionally, bile duct hamartomas can be very large, up to 20 cm, and be symptomatic from internal hemorrhage or pressure on adjacent structures [51]. Differential diagnosis of biliary hamartomas includes peribiliary cysts (predominantly perihilar distribution in patients with liver parenchymal disease), polycystic disease, and Caroli's disease (cysts communicate with bile ducts and are associated with bile duct abnormalities).

7.4.6 Hepatic Abscess and Echinococcus

The appearances of hepatic abscesses on imaging depend on etiology (cholangitic abscesses tend to be small and scattered adjacent to the biliary tree; hematogenous distribution via the hepatic artery or via the portal vein in appendicitis or diverticulitis tends to lead to larger lesions diffusely spread in the liver). US reveals a cystic lesion with internal echoes. On CT, hepatic abscesses are hypodense lesions with capsules that may show enhancement (Fig. 7.11); clustering may be noted when multiple abscesses are present [52]. CT appearance of hepatic abscess is nonspecific and can be mimicked by cystic or necrotic metastases. Hence, appropriate clinical and laboratory corroboration is vital towards making the right radiological diagnosis. However, the distribution of abscesses in the liver may hint at the etiology (Fig. 7.11). Though present in only a small minority of cases, central gas is highly specific for abscess. On MR imaging, hepatic abscesses are hypointense relative to liver parenchyma on T1-weighted

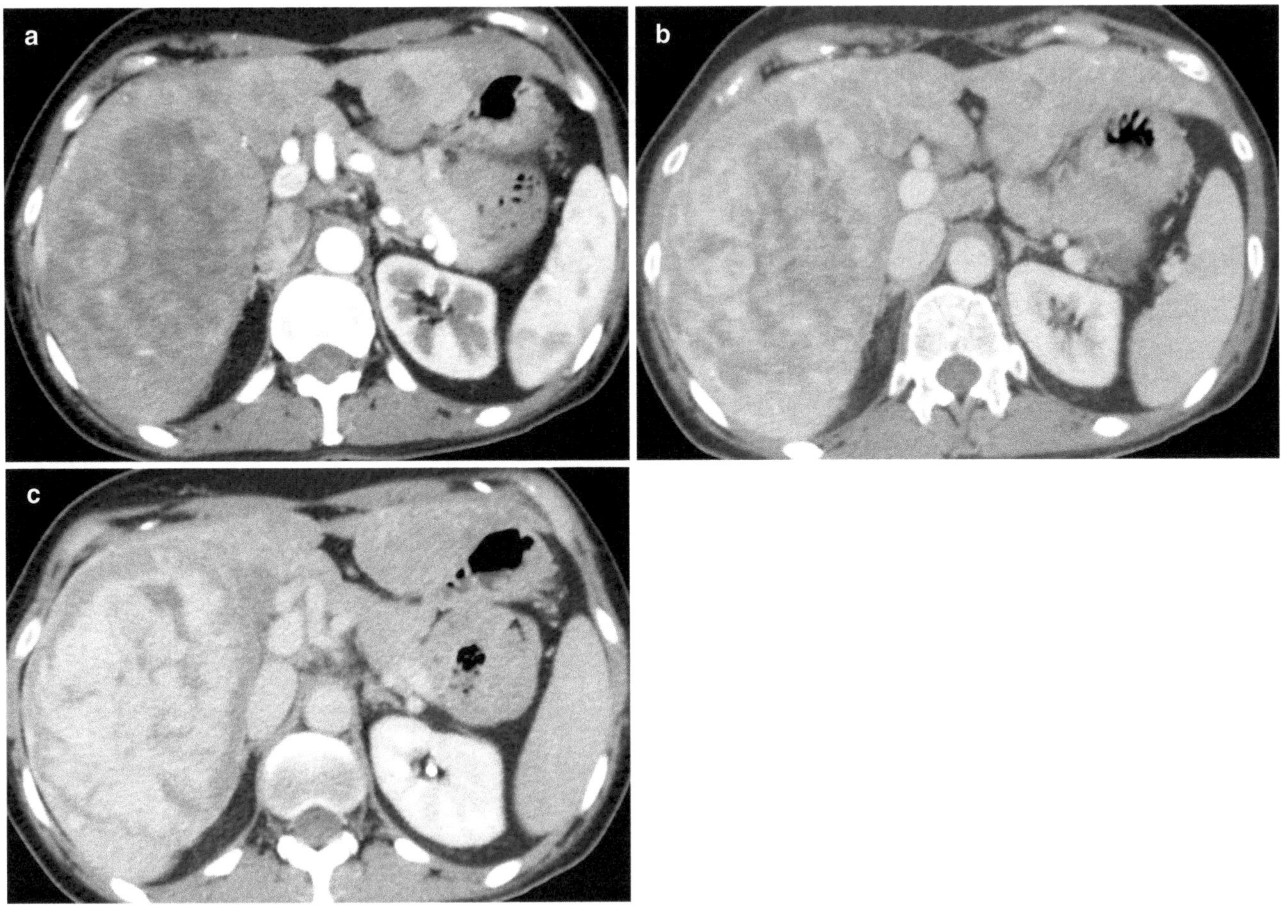

Fig. 7.9 Adenoma: inflammatory type. (**a–c**) Arterial (**a**) venous (**b**) phase CT show strong and progressive contrast enhancement of the lesion, which retains enhancement in the delayed phase (**c**), typical for peliotic changes in inflammatory adenoma

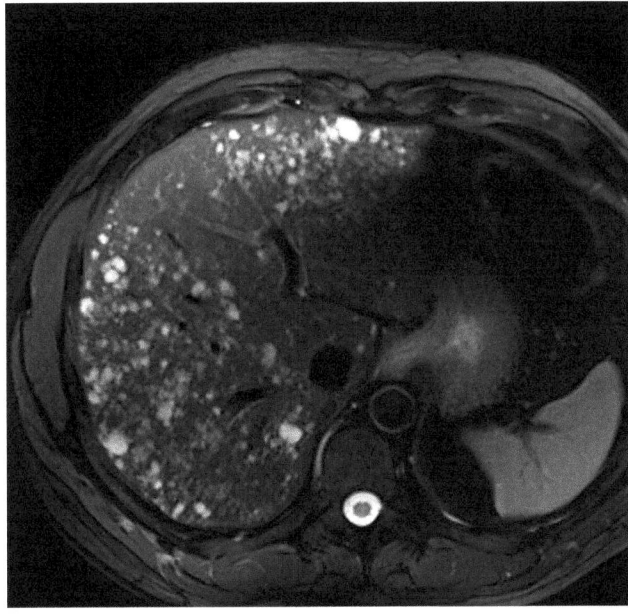

Fig. 7.10 Biliary hamartomas (von Meyenburg complexes). A middle-aged man was referred to MRI following an equivocal ultrasound examination. There are multiple foci of high T2-weighted signal (of variable size and shape) spread throughout the liver, suggestive of biliary hamartomas

images and markedly hyperintense on T2-weighted images, often surrounded by an area of slight T2 hyperintensity representing perilesional edema, which may also show increased enhancement after contrast administration. On DWI, there is marked diffusion restriction, best seen as hypointensity on the ADC map.

Amebic liver abscess is nonspecific. It usually appears as a solitary, hypodense lesion, with an enhancing wall that may be smooth or nodular and is often associated with an incomplete rim of edema. Like any bacterial abscess, lesions are hypointense on T1-weighted images and heterogeneously hyperintense on T2-weighted images [53].

On CT scan, involvement of liver by echinococcus granulosus (hydatid cyst) can manifest as unilocular or multilocular cysts with thin or thick walls and calcifications, usually with smaller daughter cysts with/without septations at the margin of or inside the mother cyst (i.e., this appearance is quite different from a "usual" multi-cystic tumor). On MR imaging, diagnostic features are the presence of a hypointense (i.e., densely fibrotic or even calcified) rim on T1-weighted and T2-weighted images and a multiloculated appearance.

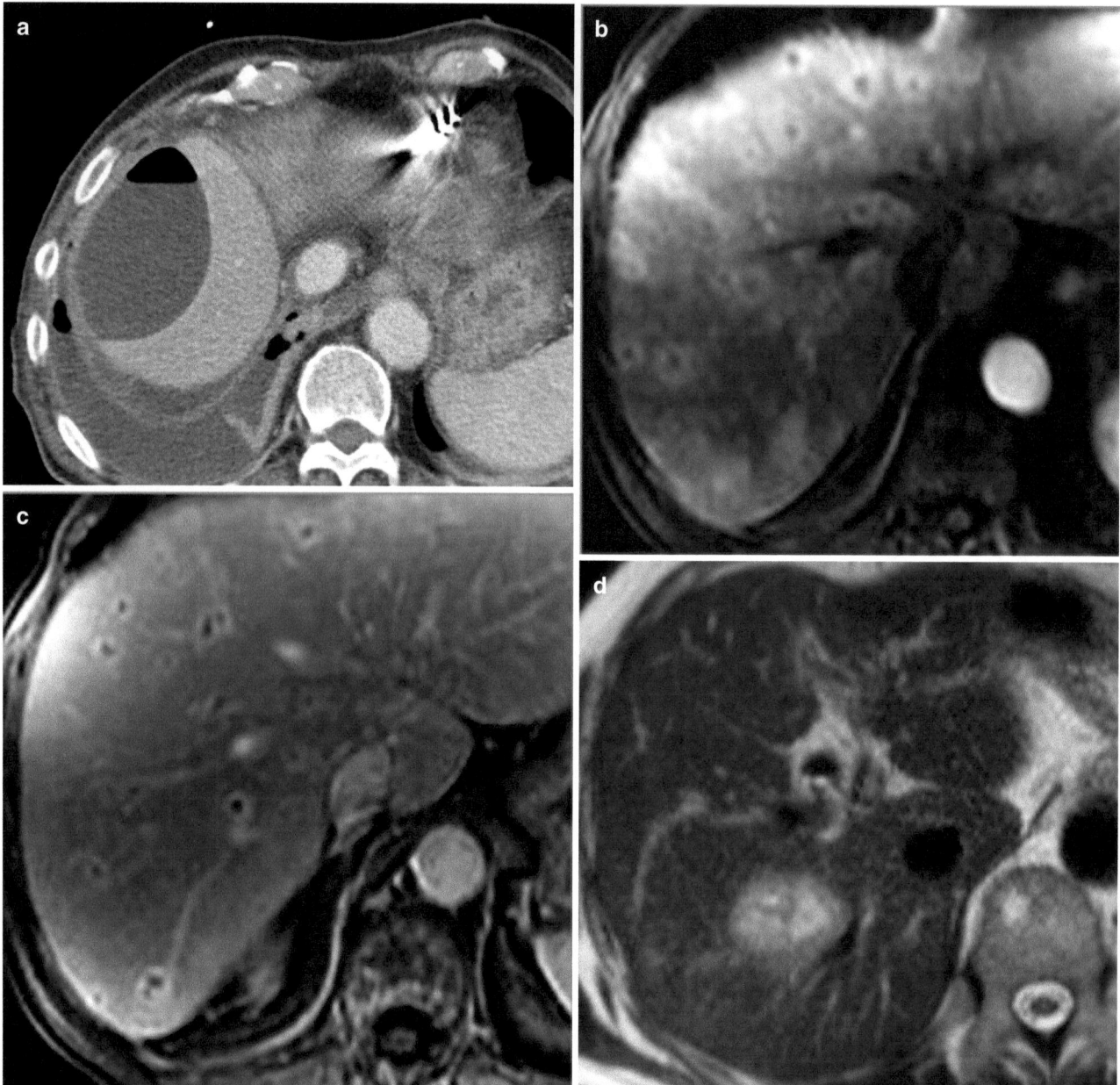

Fig. 7.11 Abscesses. (**a**) Typical large subcapsular (postoperative) abscess with an air-fluid level and a reactive pleural effusion. (**b**, **c**) Hematogenous abscesses in another patient with fever and right upper quadrant pain. T1-weighted contrast-enhanced images in the (**b**) arterial and (**c**) portal venous phase demonstrate multiple ring-enhancing lesions in both lobes of the liver. In the arterial phase, there is also associated increased parenchyma enhancement surrounding many of the lesions. The appearance is consistent with multiple septic abscesses. (**d**) Cholangitis abscess: T2-weighted MRI shows a solitary heterogeneous high signal lesion in the right hepatic lobe with (**e**) impeded diffusion at DWI (b750) with higher signal centrally. (**f**) T1-weighted contrast-enhanced image shows a serpiginous and thick rim enhancement pattern in keeping with a hepatic abscess

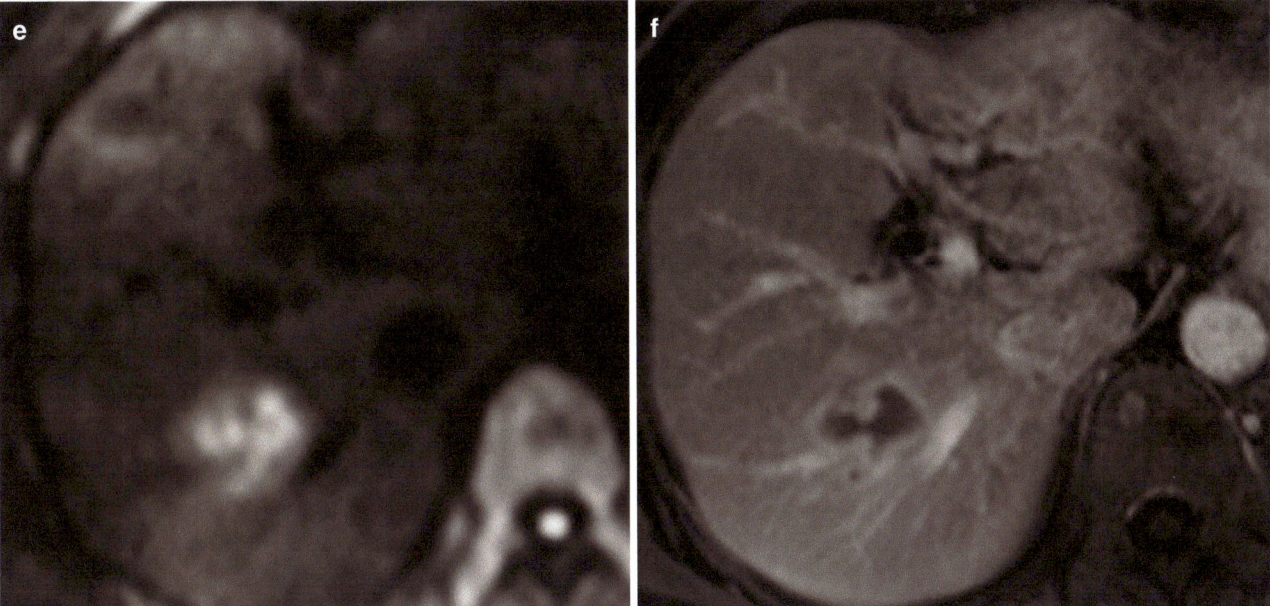

Fig. 7.11 (continued)

7.5 Malignant Primary Tumors

7.5.1 Hepatocellular Carcinoma

HCC is the most common primary liver cancer, with the highest incidence in Asia and the Mediterranean. In European countries, HCC is found mostly in patients with chronic liver disease (e.g., liver cirrhosis due to HBV or HCV, alcohol abuse, metabolic syndrome or hemochromatosis, or due to chronic hepatitis B infection). At histopathology, HCC is characterized by abnormal hepatocytes arranged in trabecular and sinusoidal patterns. Lesions may be solitary, multifocal, or diffusely infiltrating.

There are wide varying appearances of HCC on imaging. An early HCC within at-risk population is typically small (<3 cm) and has a homogenous appearance. By contrast, late presentation disease (including tumor in non-cirrhotic patients) is characterized by more advanced disease, presenting as a larger heterogeneous lesion. US is frequently used for disease screening and surveillance of cirrhosis patients. The appearance of HCC on US is variable, with iso-, hypo-, or hyper-echogenicity (increased echogenicity is often due to intratumoral fat). Smaller lesions are typically homogeneous and larger lesions heterogeneous. A surrounding fibrous capsule is often present and characteristic for HCC, appearing as a hypoechoic rim surrounding the lesion.

On unenhanced CT images, most HCCs are hypo- or isodense (the latter particularly if small). The presence of intratumoral fat can lower CT attenuation and is suggestive of primary hepatocellular tumors in the appropriate clinical settings. Due to their altered and predominant arterial supply,

HCCs enhance avidly in the arterial phase of contrast enhancement, becoming iso- or hypodense with the liver parenchyma in the portal venous phase of enhancement. Delayed-phase images show most HCC lesions as hypodense compared with surrounding liver. The washout of contrast in these tumors is a diagnostic characteristic of HCC (Fig. 7.12). Small HCCs may have a nodule-in-nodule appearance on CT and MR images, especially when the disease develops within a regenerative or dysplastic nodule (Fig. 7.13). At MR imaging, such a nodule can exhibit higher signal intensity on T2-weighted images and display hypervascularity on arterial-phase images.

Multi-phase imaging after contrast administration on CT helps to optimize the detection and characterization of HCC. Late arterial-phase imaging is the most sensitive for detecting small lesions [6, 54, 55]. A venous phase is always necessary for tumor detection/characterization and assessment of venous structures (Fig. 7.12), as well as other abdominal organs. The delayed-phase imaging (e.g., at 2–3 min) can occasionally help to detect a lesion that may be missed [56]. Much more important it can help to make a firm diagnosis of HCC by showing typical lesion contrast washout, if it had not been present in the portal venous phase [57]. Unenhanced images are important for identifying hyperdense siderotic nodules and for detecting hypodense intratumoral fat. Unenhanced images are also useful for tumor follow-up after chemoembolization or after tumor ablation. For these reasons, a three- to four-phasic MDCT protocol is utilized at most centers to evaluate HCC.

The reliance on focal hypervascularity in the arterial phase can lead to false-positive diagnosis of HCC [58].

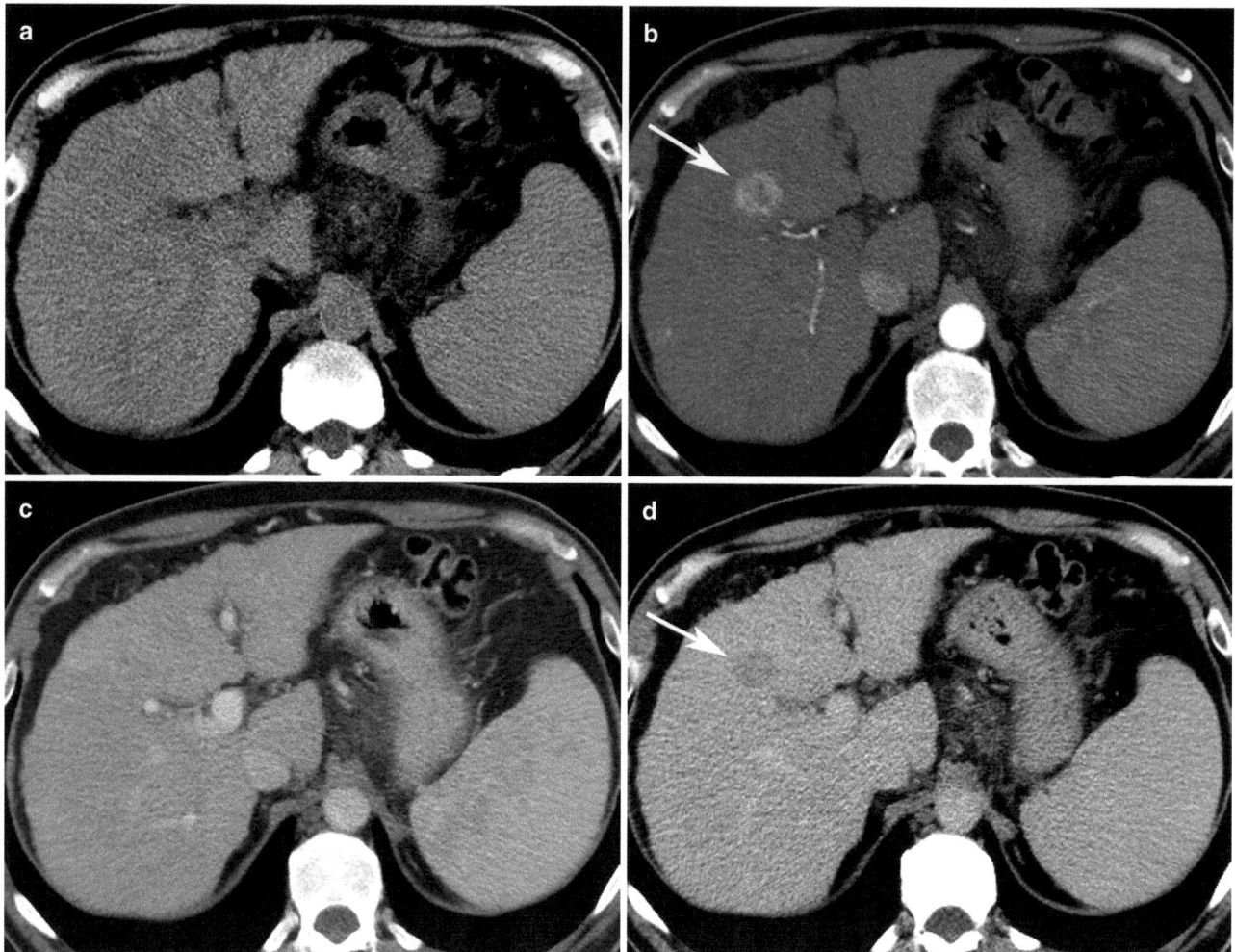

Fig. 7.12 HCC: Quadruple-phasic CT for detection and characterization. (**a**) Non-contrast CT shows liver cirrhosis and splenomegaly. In segment 4 a lesion is only faintly seen. (**b**) In the late arterial phase, a hypervascular HCC is depicted in segment 4 (arrow). (**c**) In the portal venous phase, the lesion is not visible. (**d**) Delayed phase scan reveals wash-out of the lesion, which is now hypoattenuating (arrow). The combination of arterial hypervascularity and wash-out is specific for HCC in the context of liver cirrhosis or chronic hepatitis B infection

Transient focal enhancement of liver parenchyma during arterial phase, also termed transient hepatic attenuation differences (THAD), can lead to a false diagnosis of HCC. In cirrhotic patients, transient focal enhancement is often related to arterial-portal shunting, resulting in early focal areas of portal venous distribution enhancement in the liver. THAD are usually peripherally located in the liver, appear wedge shaped and may be poorly circumscribed. Subcapsular lesions that do not exhibit mass effect or a round nature should be carefully evaluated before suggesting the diagnosis of HCC. THAD are not associated with lesion hypodensity in the portal venous or delayed phases of contrast enhancement. The combination of hyperdensity on arterial-phase images combined with washout to hypodensity on venous- or delayed-phase images, although not sensitive (33%), is highly specific (100%) for the diagnosis of HCC

[59] (Fig. 7.12). However, a small proportion of HCC is iso-attenuating or hypoattenuating compared with the liver, which can be difficult to diagnose.

The typical MR imaging features of larger HCC include a fibrous capsule, intratumoral septa, daughter nodules, and tumor thrombus (Fig. 7.14) [60]. These lesions are often heterogeneous in appearances (mosaic architecture) on both CT and MR [61]. Whereas most large HCC are hyperintense on T2-weighted images, smaller lesions, but some even measuring 3–4 cm, can appear isointense or hypointense. On T1-weighted images, HCC shows variable signal intensity relative to hepatic parenchyma. A tumor capsule may be seen on T1-weighted and less commonly, as hypointensity on T2-weighted imaging.

Dynamic extracellular gadolinium-enhanced imaging in HCC parallels the features described for CT, with character-

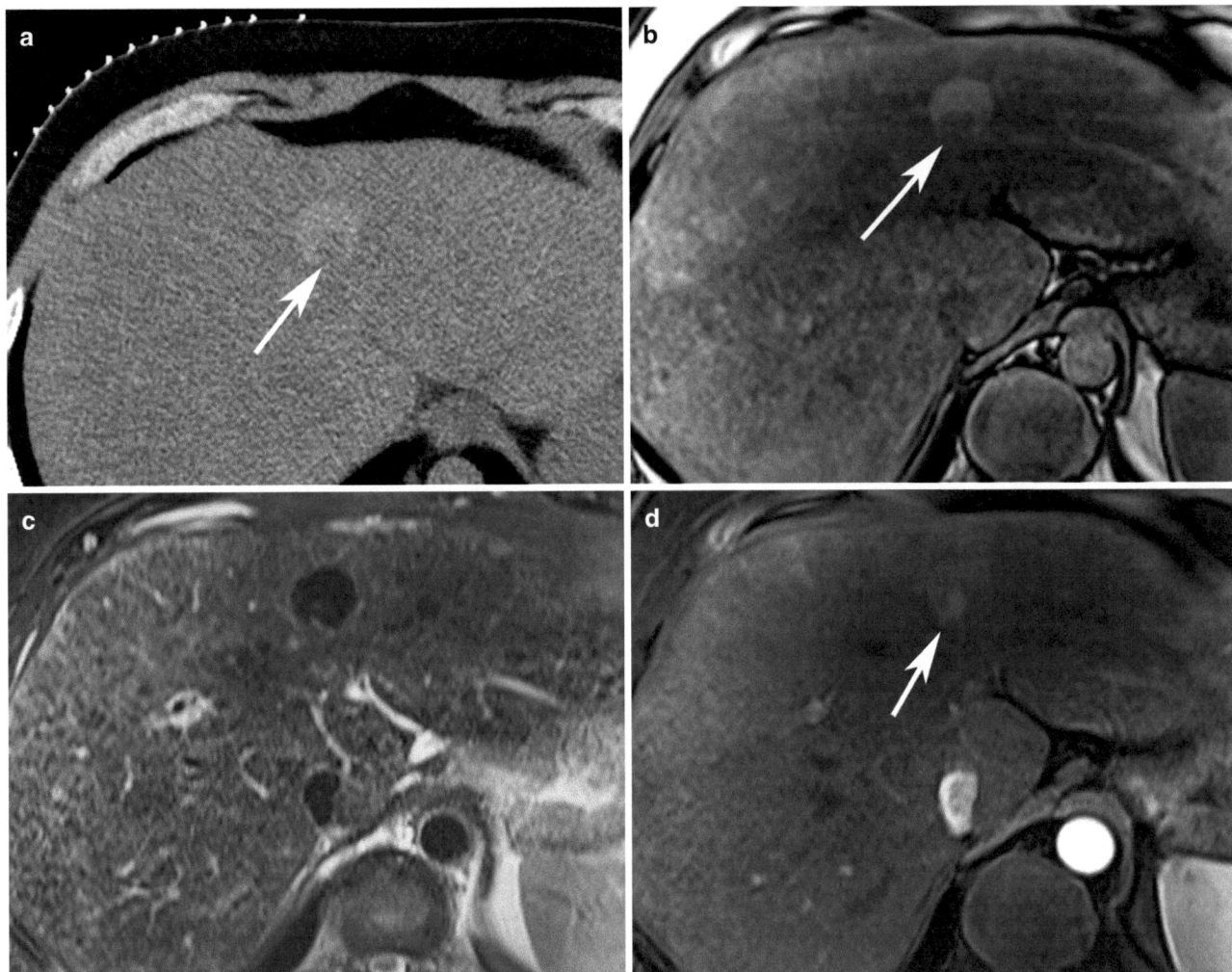

Fig. 7.13 HCC with nodule-in-nodule appearance. (**a**) Unenhanced CT show a siderotic (hyperattenuating) large nodule, which contains a low-density (non-siderotic) focus (arrow). (**b**) On T1-weighted GRE opposed-phase image, the marginal nodule shows low signal intensity (arrow). (**c**) The large nodule shows siderosis on T2-weighted TSE images, but the marginal focus displays higher SI. (**d**) Dynamic gadolinium-enhanced T1-weighted GRE images show (**d**) arterial hypervascularity of the malignant focus (arrow)

istic early peak contrast enhancement and delayed-phase tumor contrast washout of the nodular solid components; as well as T1 enhancement of the capsule. Liver-specific MR contrast agents (gadoxetic acid; Primovist, Bayer Healthcare or gadobenate dimeglumine, MultiHance, Bracco) can be administered to provide arterial, portal venous, and equilibrium-phase imaging, but has the added advantage of revealing additional characteristics at the delayed hepatobiliary phase of contrast enhancement. HCC typically do not show uptake of liver-specific contrast medium in the hepatobiliary phase, which can add confidence towards the detection and characterization of HCC (Fig. 7.15) [62]. It has been shown that using gadoxetic acid-enhanced MRI can improve the detection of small or early HCCs, as it is superior for detecting HCC measuring up to 2 cm in size compared with

CT [63]. In addition, sub-centimeter lesions detected by gadoxetic acid-enhanced MRI are likely to be or can transform to become HCC within a short interval [64]. Hence, several evolving guidelines for the imaging evaluation of HCC are incorporating the role of liver-specific contrast media for the diagnosis of sub-centimeter HCC. However, there is currently a lack of standardization across HCC guidelines on the target populations for surveillance, diagnosis, staging, or monitoring; the imaging modalities and imaging criteria to be applied; or recommended treatment [65].

It is important to recognize the pitfalls of using liver-specific contrast media for HCC evaluation. Benign regenerating nodules may appear hypointense at the hepatobiliary phase of contrast enhancement although the majority appears isointense of the liver [66]. In addition, some well-

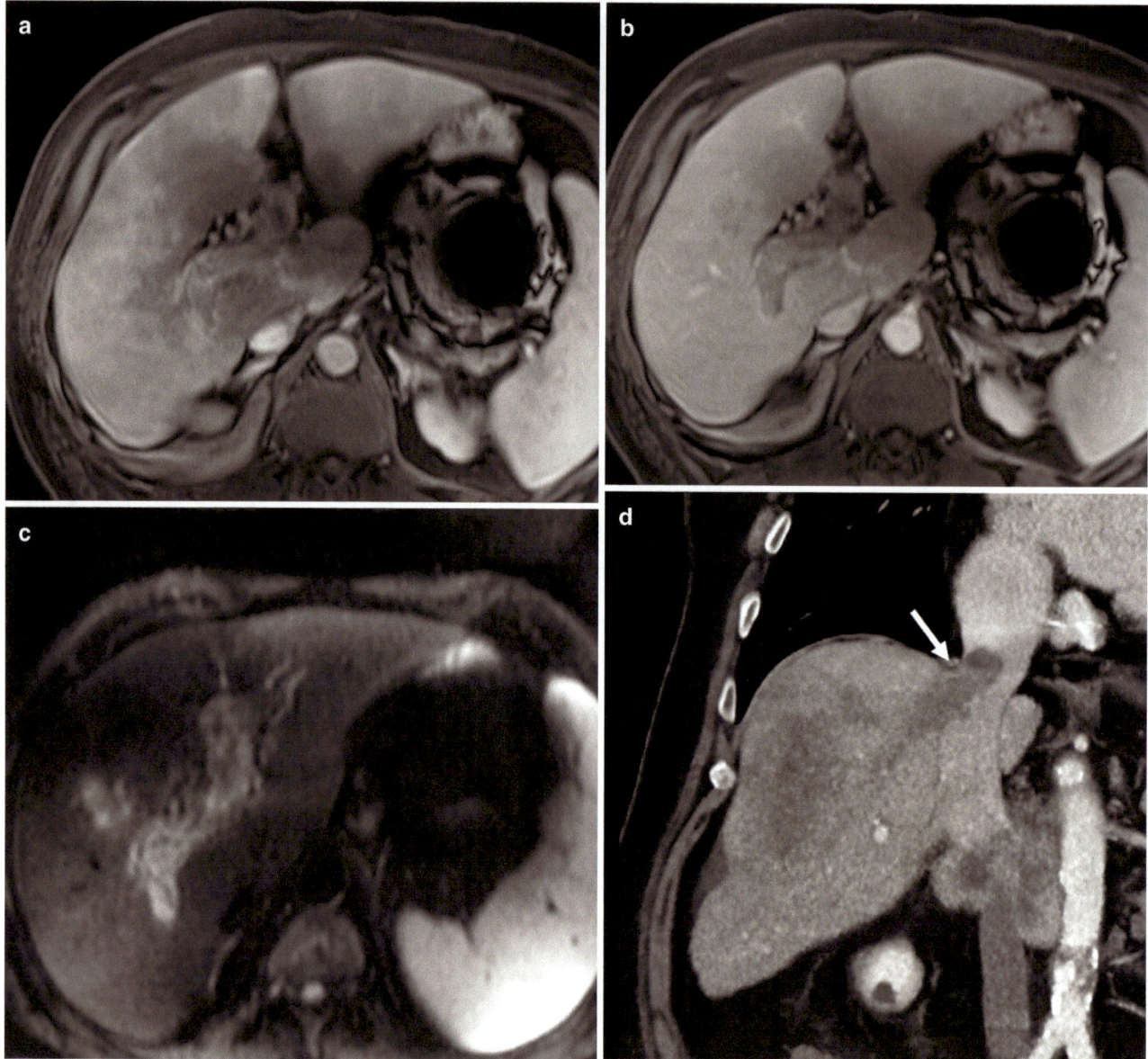

Fig. 7.14 HCC in the right lobe with tumor thrombus. (**a**) Late arterial and (**b**) portal venous phase T1-weighted GRE show inhomogenous enhancement and expansion of the portal vein. There is inhomogenous enhancement of the right lobe, but no definite tumor is seen. (**c**) DWI shows a solid mass in the entire intrahepatic portal vein and part of the tumor in the right lobe. (**d**) In another patient with a large HCC in the right lobe, tumor extension into the right hepatic vein (arrow) and the inferior vena cava are seen

differentiated or moderately differentiated HCC may appear isointense or hyperintense due to higher levels of OATP1B3 and MRP3 receptor expression. For this reason, the use of ancillary imaging features at MRI can improve the confidence of HCC diagnosis. These include mild to high T2 signal intensity and impeded diffusion on high b-value DWI. The use of liver-specific contrast agents may also help towards the identification of isoenhancing or hypoenhancing HCC that do not show typical arterial-phase hyperenhancement. With regard to the use of diffusion-weighted MRI for HCC evaluation, a higher b-value (e.g., 800 s/mm²) DWI may help in the identification of disease, particularly if the

suspected nodule also demonstrates typical vascularity pattern at contrast-enhanced MRI. Higher grade/poorly differentiated HCC are more likely to show impeded diffusion and lower ADC values compared with well-differentiated HCC.

To summarize, many MR characteristics are often as associated with HCC (arterial-phase hyperenhancement, portal venous or delayed-phase washout, lack of liver-specific MR contrast agent uptake on hepatobiliary phase images, moderate T2 hyperintensity, and restricted diffusion on high-b-value DWI). However, for each of these findings, there is only ~60–80% sensitivity, and benign lesions can also show these findings, depending on finding, contrast

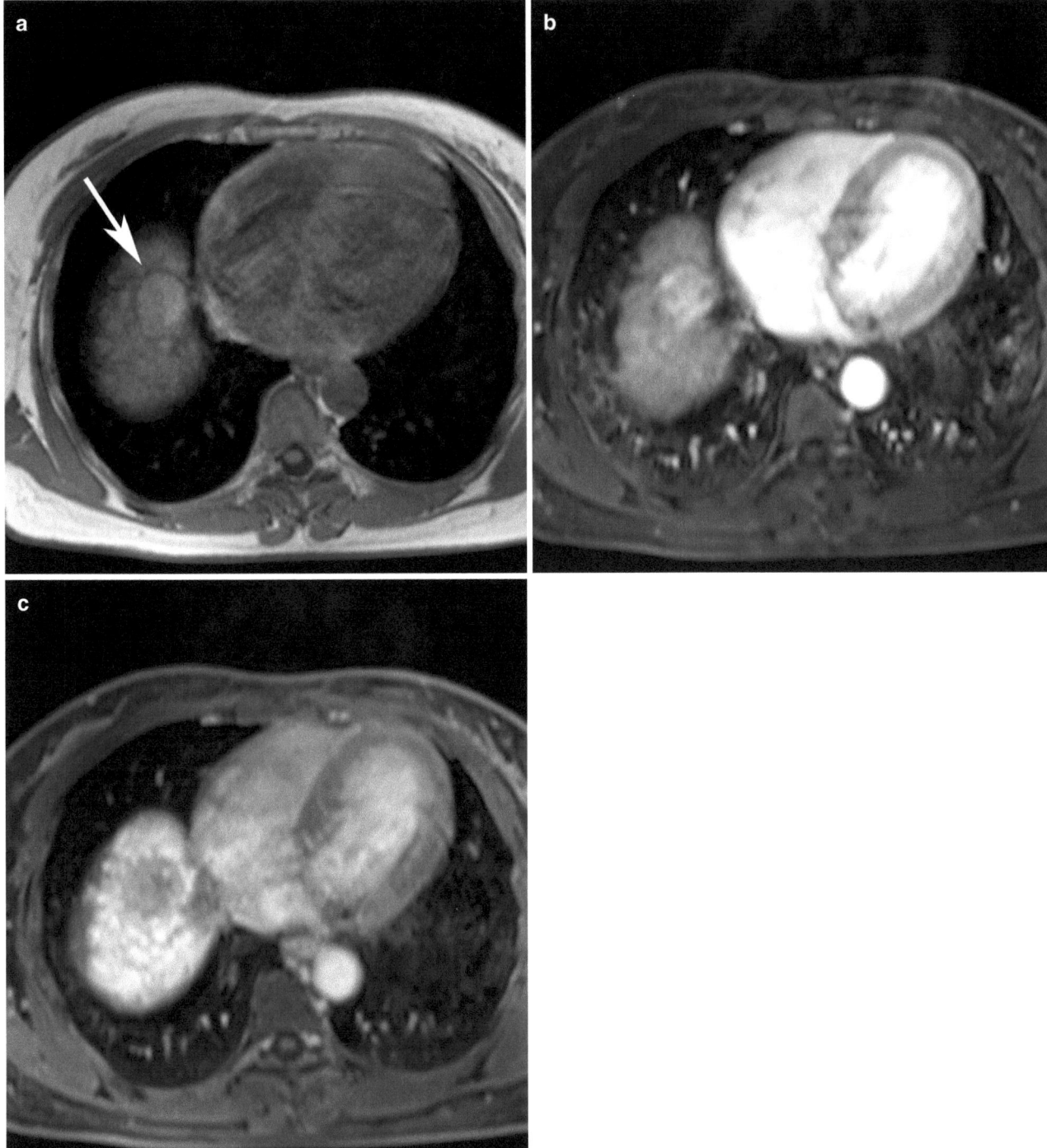

Fig. 7.15 HCC: MRI with liver-specific contrast agent (gadoxetic acid). (**a**) Axial T1-weighted GRE shows an encapsulated slightly hyperintense mass in the dome of the liver. (**b**) Gadoxetic acid-enhanced image shows strong enhancement in the arterial phase. (**c**) In the hepatobiliary phase the lesion shows hypointensity due to lack of hepatocellular uptake

agent used, and series reported [66, 67]. Furthermore, depending on the guidelines (EASL, AASLD, APASL, JSH, or KLCA-NCC) applied, this can lead to different diagnostic accuracies for the diagnoses of HCC [66]. To overcome the problems with inconsistent terminology and different imaging criteria, the American College of Radiology developed

the Liver Imaging Reporting and Data System (LI-RADS®), with a standardized lexicon of terminology. The LIRADS CT/MRI guideline has been revised several times (now in its v2018) [68]. This guideline is applicable in adult patients (≥18 years) with liver cirrhosis or chronic hepatitis B. In general, focal liver lesions (called "observations" are categorized as LR-1 through LR-5, depending on the probability of HCC. For probably or definitely malignant lesions not necessarily HCC, the category of LR-M is appropriate, and LR-TIV for malignant tumors extending into the veins (Fig. 7.14). LI-RADS® uses major and ancillary imaging features to categorize observations. The validity of these imaging features has been proven in several study.

Key Points

- Risk factors for HCC include liver cirrhosis (of various etiologies) and chronic hepatitis B infection.
- The key imaging features at contrast-enhanced MDCT and MRI are arterial-phase hyperenhancement and washout (to hypoattenuation/hypointensity) in the portal venous phase and/or the 3-min delayed phase.
- The CT/MRI LI-RADS® v2018 Guideline by the American College of Radiology is an excellent tool, which provides standard terminology, an imaging feature lexicon, and a diagnostic algorithm to classify focal lesions ("observations") in patients at risk for HCC.

7.5.2   Fibrolamellar HCC

Fibrolamellar HCC (FL-HCC) typically affects young patients without chronic liver disease On CT, FL-HCC appears as a large, hypervascular mass with a central scar and calcifications in up to 70% of cases [69, 70]. It often shows aggressive features: vascular invasion, biliary obstruction, satellite lesions, and lymph node metastases [71]. On MR imaging, FL-HCC are typically hypointense on

T1-weighted and hyperintense on T2-weighted images, with T1-weighted and T2-weighted hypointense central scar (Fig. 7.16). This is in contrast to the scar of FNH, which is most often hyperintense on T2-weighted images. The fibrous central zone FL-HCC may show delayed retention of CT and extracellular gadolinium MR contrast agents. In contrast to FNH, the contrast enhancement in FL-HCC is usually heterogeneous compared with the homogenous enhancement pattern of FNH.

7.5.3   Cholangiocellular Carcinoma

Cholangiocellular carcinoma (CCC) is the second most common primary malignancy of the liver. Intrahepatic CCC originates from the intralobular bile ducts (in contrast to hilar CCC, which arises from a main hepatic duct or from the bifurcation) (Fig. 7.17). Intrahepatic CCC often presents late as a large mass [72]. According to the growth characteristics, CCC is classified as mass forming, periductal infiltrating, or intraductal growing, with the mass-forming type being most common in intrahepatic CCC [72]. At CT and MR imaging, lesions tend to be hypodense at unenhanced CT and hypointense on T1-weighted images, with peripheral enhancement at dynamic contrast-enhanced studies [73]. Delayed-phase CT/MR imaging (after 5–15 min) may show enhancement homogeneously or in the center of the lesion due to its rich fibrous stroma, which is suggestive of the diagnosis of CCC (Fig. 7.18) [74]. CCC shows a target appearance on DWI, with the central fibrotic stroma often shows signal suppression on diffusion-weighted MRI compared with the cellular rim and return relatively high ADC value. More recently, the intrahepatic CCC can also be classified into the "large duct type" or the "small duct type" depending on the cell of origin, which are associated with different imaging appear-

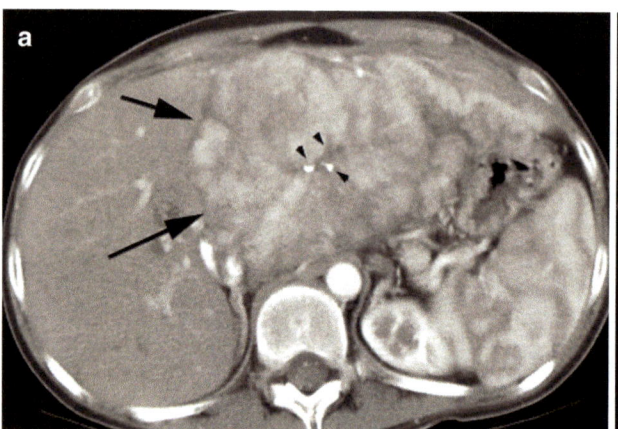
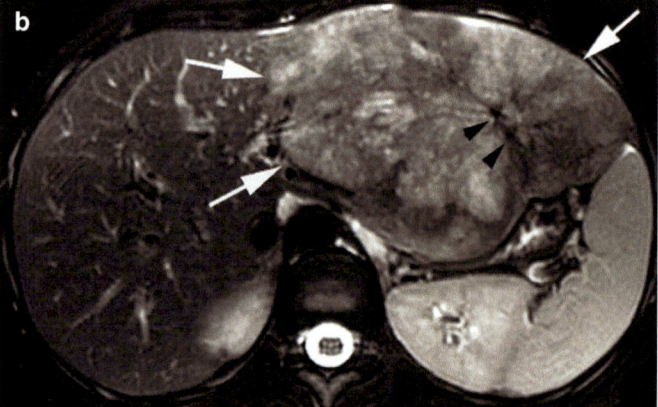
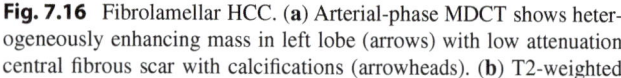

Fig. 7.16 Fibrolamellar HCC. (**a**) Arterial-phase MDCT shows heterogeneously enhancing mass in left lobe (arrows) with low attenuation central fibrous scar with calcifications (arrowheads). (**b**) T2-weighted MRI shows large left lobe mass (arrows) with heterogeneous appearance and mild to moderately increased signal intensity. Fibrous central scar is of very low signal intensity (arrowheads)

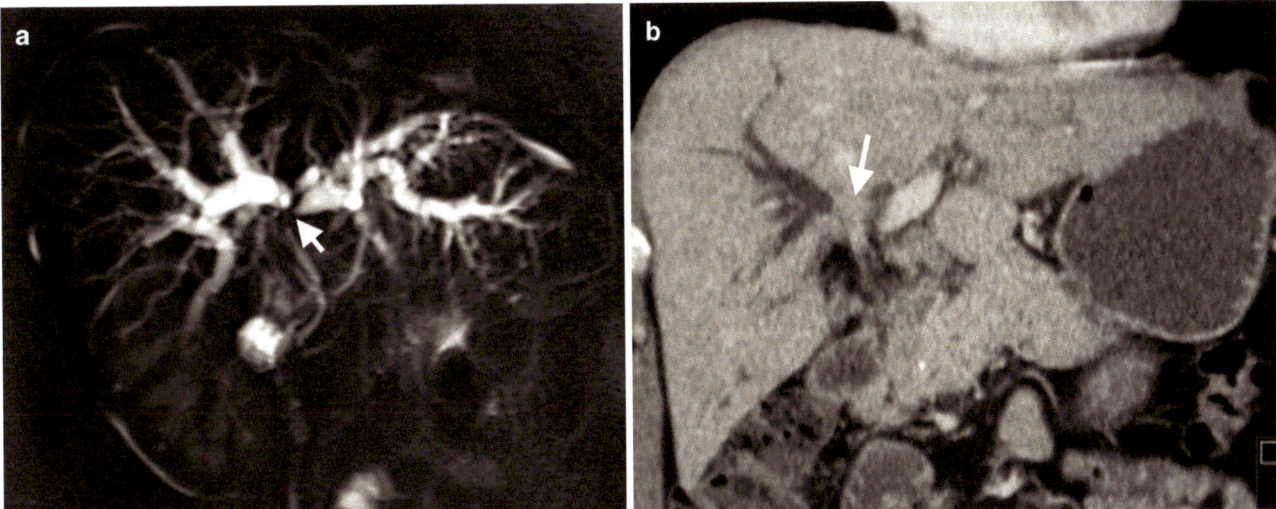

Fig. 7.17 Hilar cholangiocarcinoma in a man with jaundice. (**a**) MRCP (maximum intensity projection) shows dilated right and left intrahepatic ducts, which can be traced to their confluence (arrow). The common bile duct and pancreatic duct are not dilated. (**b**) Delayed post-contrast coronal CT reformation shows enhancing soft tissue at the confluence of the right and left hepatic ducts typical of perihilar cholangiocarcinoma

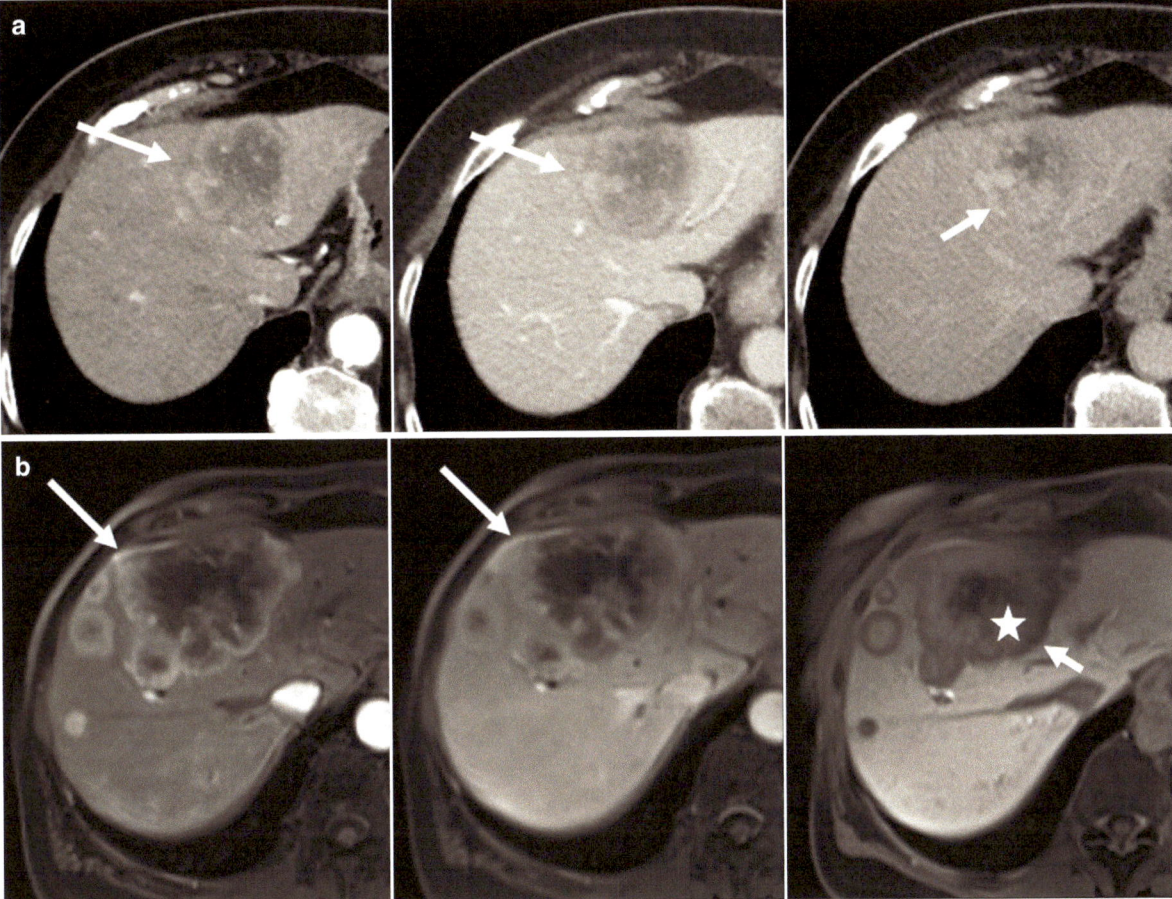

Fig. 7.18 Peripheral cholangiocarcinoma: contrast enhancement characteristics in 2 patients. (**a**) Contrast-enhanced CT in the arterial, portal venous, and delayed phases demonstrate thick irregular rim enhancement (arrows) with delayed central enhancement due to the fibrotic matrix (small arrow). (**b**) Gadoxetic-acid-enhanced MRI in the arterial, portal venous, and hepatobiliary phases show a mass with satellite nodules and thick irregular rim enhancement (arrows), progressing over time. In the hepatobiliary phase there is central retention of contrast material (asterisk) due to fibrous matrix, which should not be confused with hepatocellular uptake of a hepatocellular lesion. In CCC, quite often peripheral wash-out of contrast is seen in late phases (small arrow)

ances. Large duct type tumor has a worse prognosis and are found to be more likely to show infiltrative contours, diffuse biliary dilatation, vascular invasion, and absence of arterial enhancement [75]. Periductal infiltrative CCC causes early segmental dilatation of bile ducts in a stage when the tumor itself may be difficult to discern [73]. In addition, there are morphologic features that can suggest the diagnosis of CCC. Peripheral lesions often demonstrate overlying capsular retraction due to their scirrhous, fibrous matrix. Dilated intrahepatic bile ducts proximal to an intrahepatic CCC can also provide clues to the diagnosis, as biliary obstruction is unusual with intrahepatic metastases (with the exception of colorectal cancer [76].

7.6 Rare Primary Liver Tumors

7.6.1 Biliary Cystadenoma/ Cystadenocarcinomas

These tumors present a similar appearance and morphology as their mucinous counterparts in the pancreas and occur usually in women. Even when benign, these tumors have a propensity for malignant degeneration, and any such tumor should be considered potentially malignant. They appear as unilocular or septated cystic masses, with the typical anechoic and hypoechoic US appearance and near water-like attenuation contents on CT. For differentiation between simple cyst and cystadenoma, the assessment of septations is helpful: in cystadenoma, the septa usually arise from a smooth cyst wall, whereas in simple cysts the septa there are indentations of the cyst wall at the origin of the septa [77]. The presence of papillary excrescences, soft-tissue nodularity or septations are associated with a higher risk of malignancy in cystadenoma [78]. The cystic areas show variable signal intensity at T1-weighted MRI, including being hyperintense to liver related to its proteinaceous content. Coarse calcifications may be observed at US and CT in both cystadenoma and cystadenocarcinoma and is not a sign of benignity.

7.6.2 Hepatic Angiosarcoma

Hepatic angiosarcoma is a rare tumor. There is a strong association with prior exposure to carcinogens such as vinyl chloride and Thorotrast, as well as in patients with hemo-

chromatosis. However, in the majority, the tumor is idiopathic. Pathologically, angiosarcoma presents as large, solitary masses or with multiple tumor nodules with blurred lesion margins [79]. The imaging appearance of angiosarcoma is often nonspecific, appearing hypodense on unenhanced CT, hypointense on T1-weighted MR imaging, and mildly hyperintense on T2-weighted imaging (although if prominent sinusoidal vascular spaces are present, these can appear of homogeneous and very high T2-weighted signal intensity). Following iodine or gadolinium-based contrast administration, most lesions show nonspecific heterogeneous enhancement or even centripetal enhancement. Potentially problematic are those tumors with prominent sinusoidal vascular spaces, because they can mimic the appearance of benign hemangioma on CT and MRI. The high T2-weighted MR signal in such lesions further compounds this problem. In most such cases, however, careful evaluation will show that the tumoral enhancement does not follow characteristics of blood pool at all phases, or that there are other features, such as multiple lesions, that makes the diagnosis of hemangioma unlikely [80, 81].

7.6.3 Epithelioid Hemangioendothelioma

Epithelioid hemangioendothelioma (EHE) is a rare tumor of vascular origin, not to be confused with infantile hemangioendothelioma, which is a very different tumor. These hepatic tumors are characterized by multiple, peripherally located lesions that progressively become confluent masses (Fig. 7.19). In addition to the unusual peripheral liver distribution, a key characteristic feature is the presence of overlying capsular retraction, due to the presence of fibrosis and scarring [82]. The CT attenuation or MR signal intensity characteristics are nonspecific, although occasional tumoral calcifications may be seen. Contrast enhancement with CT or MR gadolinium chelates often shows a central zone of decreased enhancement with marked rim enhancement (Fig. 7.19) [79]: The reverse pattern has also been observed with a central area of increased enhancement and peripheral decreased enhancement. Concentric zones of marked enhancement have also been reported. A visible branch of the portal or hepatic vein terminating at the periphery of these lesions (lollipop sign) has also been described, although this is not pathognomonic of the disease [83]. Lesions often become confluent and may grow large enough to replace nearly the entire liver parenchyma.

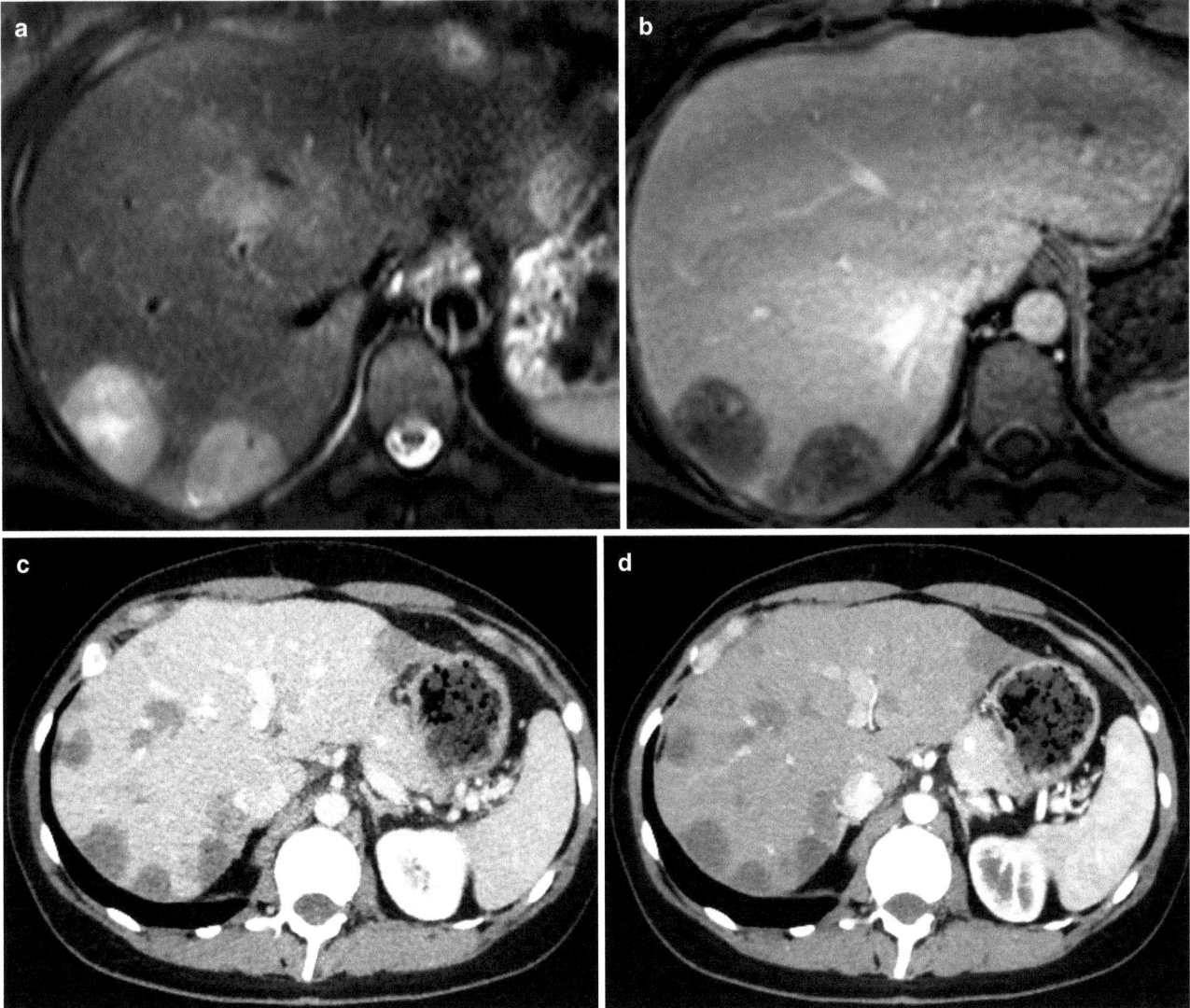

Fig. 7.19 Epithelioid hemangioendothelioma. (**a**) Fat-suppressed T2-weighted TSE shows multiple subcapsular hyperintense lesions, some showing biphasic pattern with central higher T2 signal core compared with the periphery. (**b**) Portal venous phase fat-suppressed T1-weighted MRI shows mild enhancement in the periphery of these overall hypointense lesions. (**c, d**) Contrast-enhanced MDCT in the arterial and portal venous phases typically shows multiple subcapsular lesions in both lobes

7.7 Hepatic Metastases

At US, liver metastases can appear hypoechoic, isoechoic, or hyperechoic. On dynamic contrast-enhanced CT, most metastases appear hypovascular and hypodense relative to liver parenchyma on the portal venous phase (Fig. 7.20). Hypervascular metastases are most commonly seen in renal cell carcinoma, neuroendocrine tumors, sarcomas, and breast tumor patients (Fig. 7.20). These tumors are best seen in the arterial phase and may become isodense and difficult to detect at the later phases of contrast enhancement. At MR, metastases are usually hypointense on T1-weighted and moderately hyperintense on T2-weighted images [84]. Peritumoral edema makes lesions appear larger on T2-weighted images and is highly suggestive of a malignant mass [85]. High signal intensity on T1-weighted sequences is typical for melanoma metastases due to the paramagnetic nature of melanin. It can also be seen in and around metastases after tumor ablation due to coagulation necrosis. Some lesions may have a central area of hyperintensity (target sign) on T2-weighted images, which corresponds to central necrosis. DWI with high b-values (e.g., 600–800) is very helpful for detecting small liver metastases, which may otherwise escape detection (Fig. 7.21). On dynamic contrast-enhanced MR imaging, metastases demonstrate enhancement characteristics similar to those

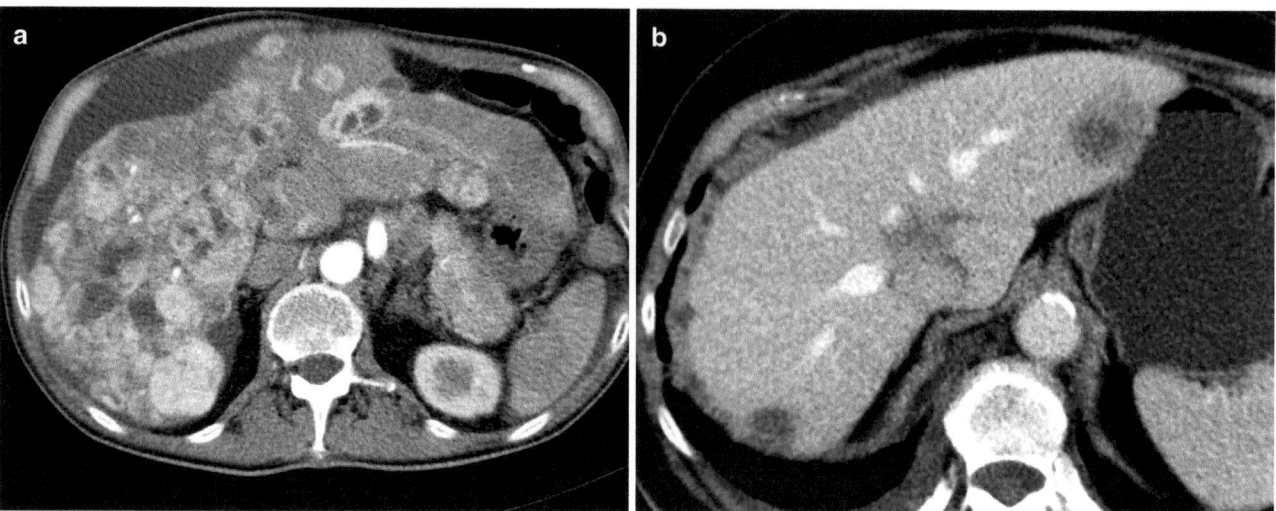

Fig. 7.20 Metastases. (**a**) Contrast-enhanced MDCT in the arterial phase demonstrates several predominantly hypervascular liver metastases of neuroendocrine cancer of the pancreas. (**b**) Contrast-enhanced MDCT in the venous phase shows typical hypovascular colorectal metastases

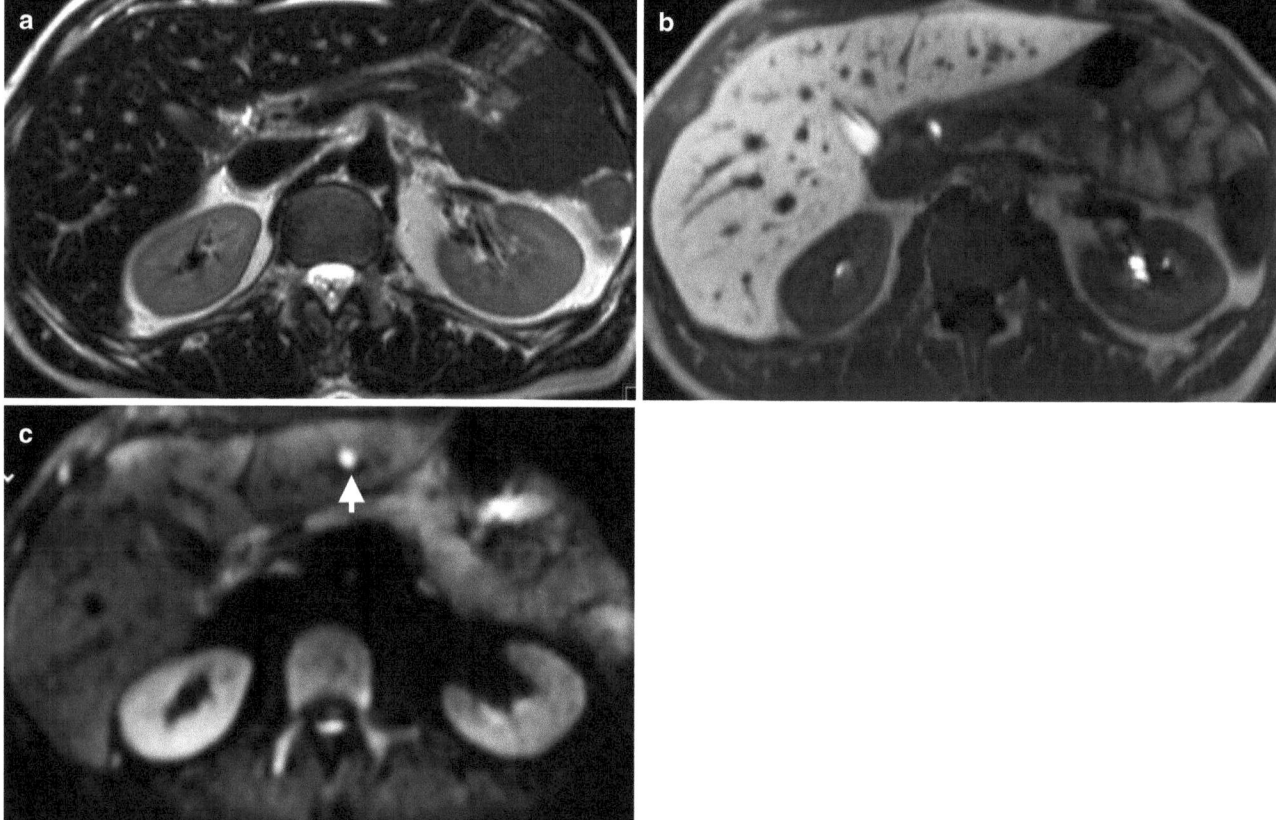

Fig. 7.21 Value of diffusion-weighted MRI for detection of small metastases. (**a**) T2-weighted MRI and (**b**) Gadoxetic acid-enhanced T1-weighted MRI (hepatobiliary phase) shows no apparent lesions within the liver. (**c**) DWI (b750 image) clearly shows a small metastasis in the left hepatic lobe (arrow). The lesion was also not visualized on a contemporaneous FDG PET/CT examination

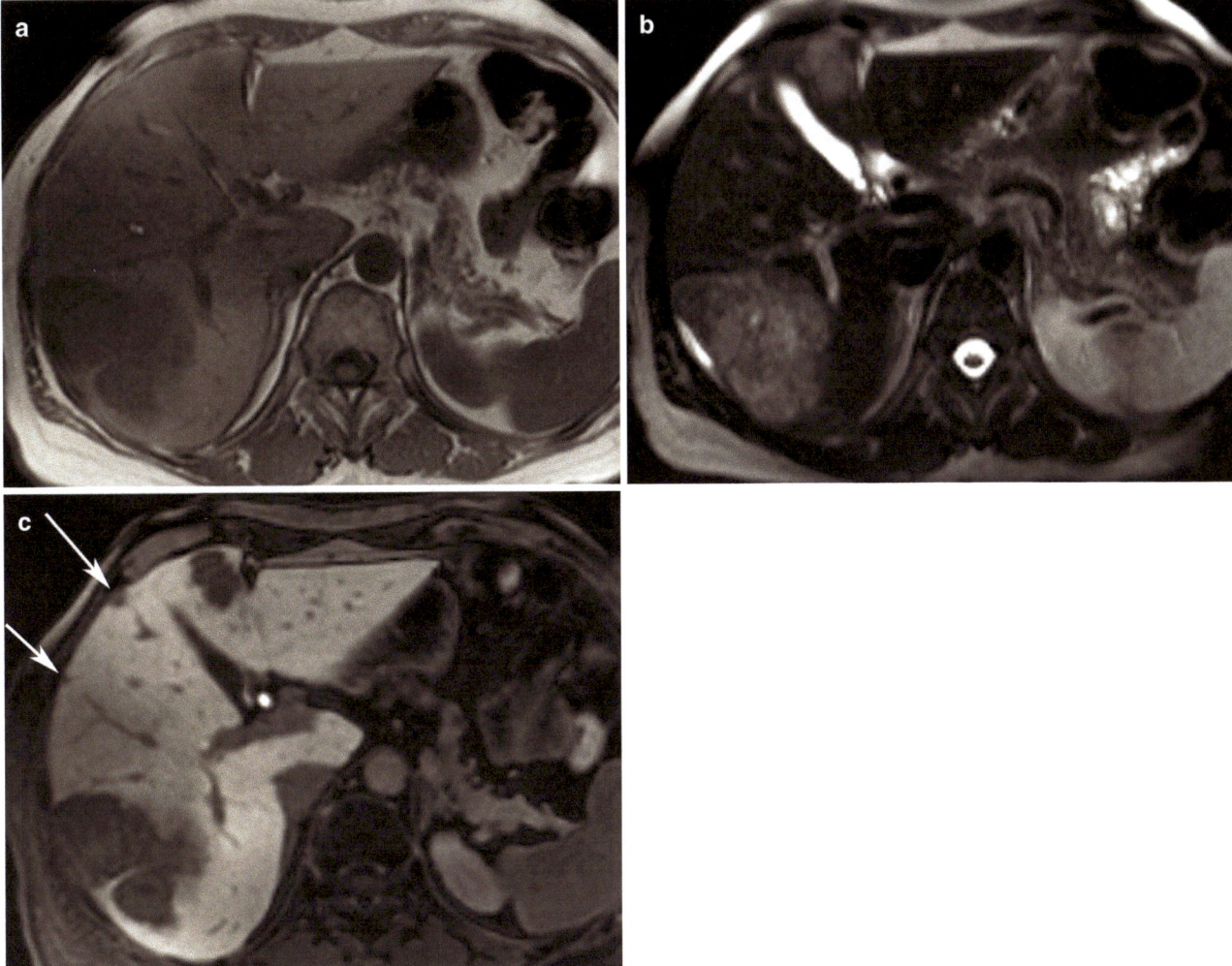

Fig. 7.22 Colorectal liver metastases at gadoxetic acid-enhanced MRI. (**a**) Unenhanced T1-weighted MRI shows two hypointense lesions in segments 6/7 and 4. (**b**) T2-weighted TSE image shows the lesions to be moderately hyperintense. (**c**) Gadoxetic acid-enhanced MRI in the hep- atobiliary phase shows two additional small subcapsular metastases (arrows) not seen on unenhanced MRI or MDCT (not shown)

described for CT. Metastases may demonstrate a hypoin- tense rim compared with the center of the lesion on delayed images (peripheral washout sign), which is highly specific for malignancy. It has been shown in colorectal cancer, that the combination of using DWI, together with liver-specific contrast media-enhanced MRI results in the highest diag- nostic accuracy for the detection of liver metastases (Fig. 7.22) [86]. The role of liver-specific MR contrast agents in patients with suspected liver metastases is still under discussion. However, liver-specific MR contrast agents are undoubtedly the preferred imaging method for pre-surgical or pre-interventional planning for liver metas- tases [65].

> **Key Points**
> - Liver metastases of extrahepatic primaries are much more common than primary cancers of the liver.
> - Most metastases (of adenocarcinoma or squamous cell cancer origin) are hypovascular.
> - Renal cell cancer, neuroendocrine tumors, sarco- mas, melanoma, and occasionally breast cancer may seed hypervascular metastases.
> - At MRI the combination of DWI and liver-specific MR contrast agents yields the best results regarding detection of metastases.

7.8 Differential Diagnosis of Focal Liver Lesions

The approach to characterizing a focal liver lesion seen on MDCT begins with determining its density. If the lesion shows near water attenuation, is homogenous in character, and has sharp margins, then a cyst should be considered and can be confirmed with US in almost all cases. However, the radiologist should be familiar with the imaging features of other cystic lesions that can mimic simple cysts. When evaluating solid focal liver lesions, disease characterization is largely reliant on observing the rate and pattern of contrast enhancement. If a lesion shows peripheral and nodular enhancement, with the density of enhancing portions showing the same general levels of blood vessels in the arterial, venous, and delayed phases, a hemangioma can be confidently diagnosed. Arterially hypervascular enhancing lesions include FNH, HCA, HCC, and metastases from neuroendocrine tumors, melanoma, renal cell carcinoma, and breast cancer. In general, HCC is considered in a setting of cirrhosis or chronic liver disease. The CT/MRI LI-RADS® guideline of the American College of Radiology has undergone several revisions since its release in 2011 [87–89]. It provides standard terminology, an imaging feature lexicon, and a validated classification system for focal lesions found in patients at risk for HCC (adults with cirrhosis or chronic hepatitis B). LI-RADS terminology should be implemented in clinical practice to improve communication between radiologists and referring hepatologists, oncologists, and surgeons.

FNH is most likely in young women with a non-cirrhotic liver and if the lesion is homogeneous and near isodense/isointense on unenhanced CT/MR imaging with a central T2-weighted hyperintense scar. By comparison, thick, irregular, heterogeneous enhancement or the presence of peripheral washout at the delayed phase suggests a malignant mass, such as metastases, CCC, or even HCC. In particular, delayed enhancement is a feature of CC due to is fibrotic stroma.

Liver-specific MR contrast has been shown to improve the characterization of FNH and HCA. They are recommended in the preoperative assessment of patients with potentially resectable liver metastases (from colorectal cancer). DWI is also now routinely performed in liver imaging. Its main clinical benefit is the detection of focal liver lesions, which may be missed on conventional and contrast-enhanced imaging sequences. Quantitative ADC measurements can support the characterization of focal liver lesions, with higher ADC values favoring benign lesions. However, the use of ADC value should be made considering all other imaging findings because of the significant overlap of ADC values between benign and malignant lesions.

7.9 Concluding Remarks

Contrast-enhanced liver MDCT for detection and characterization of focal masses should be at least bi-phasic. A triple-phasic contrast-enhanced protocol is recommended in the LI-RADS® guideline for HCC detection and characterization in high-risk patients. The MRI protocol should routinely include T1-weighted GRE DIXON, T2-weighted TSE (with or without fatsat), DWI, and dynamic-contrast-enhanced pulse sequences. Liver-specific MR contrast agents are recommended for evaluation of patients with potentially resectable colorectal liver metastases. Liver-specific MR contrast agents are also helpful for characterization of hepatocellular lesions (especially FNH vs. adenoma).

Take-Home Messages
- Contrast-enhanced liver MDCT for detection and characterization of focal masses should be at least bi-phasic. A triple-phasic contrast-enhanced protocol is recommended in the LI-RADS® guideline for HCC detection and characterization in high-risk patients.
- MRI protocol should routinely include T1-weighted GRE DIXON, T2-weighted TSE (with or without fatsat), DWI, and dynamic-contrast-enhanced pulse sequences.
- Liver-specific MR contrast agents are recommended for evaluation of patients with potentially resectable colorectal liver metastases.
- Liver-specific MR contrast agents are helpful for characterization of FNH and adenoma.

References

1. Laghi A, Multidetector CT (64 Slices) of the liver: examination techniques. Eur Radiol. 2007;17:675–83.
2. Weg N, Scheer MR, Gabor MP. Liver lesions: improved detection with dual-detector-array CT and routine 2.5-mm thin collimation. Radiology. 1998;209:417–26.
3. Ichikawa T, Nakajima H, Nanbu A, Hori M, Araki T. Effect of injection rate of contrast material on CT of hepatocellular carcinoma. AJR Am J Roentgenol. 2006;186:1413–8.
4. Foley WD, Hoffmann RG, Quiroz FA, Kahn CE Jr, Perret RS. Hepatic helical CT: contrast material injection protocol. Radiology. 1994;192:367–71.
5. Kim T, Murakami T, Takahashi S, Tsuda K, Tomoda K, Narumi Y, et al. Effects of injection rates of contrast material on arterial phase hepatic CT. AJR Am J Roentgenol. 1998;171:429–32.
6. Schima W, Hammerstingl R, Catalano C, Marti-Bonmati L, Rummeny EJ, Montero FT, et al. Quadruple-phase MDCT of the liver in patients with suspected hepatocellular carcinoma: effect of contrast material flow rate. AJR Am J Roentgenol. 2006;186:1571–9.

7. Sultana S, Awai K, Nakayama Y, Nakaura T, Liu D, Hatemura M, et al. Hypervascular hepatocellular carcinomas: bolus tracking with a 40-detector CT scanner to time arterial phase imaging. Radiology. 2007;243:140–7.

8. Stiller W. Basics of iterative reconstruction methods in computed tomography: a vendor-independent overview. Eur J Radiol. 2018;109:147–54.

9. Singh S, Kalra MK, Hsieh J, Licato PE, Do S, Pien HH, et al. Abdominal CT: comparison of adaptive statistical iterative and filtered back projection reconstruction techniques. Radiology. 2010;257:373–83.

10. May MS, Wüst W, Brand M, Stahl C, Allmendinger T, Schmidt B, et al. Dose reduction in abdominal computed tomography: intra-individual comparison of image quality of full-dose standard and half-dose iterative reconstructions with dual-source computed tomography. Investig Radiol. 2011;46:465–70.

11. Gonzalez-Guindalini FD, Ferreira Botelho MP, Töre HG, Ahn RW, Gordon LI, Yaghmai V. MDCT of chest, abdomen, and pelvis using attenuation-based automated tube voltage selection in combination with iterative reconstruction: an intrapatient study of radiation dose and image quality. AJR Am J Roentgenol. 2013;201:1075–82.

12. Fuentes-Orrego JM, Hayano K, Kambadakone AR, Hahn PF, Sahani DV. Dose-modified 256-MDCT of the abdomen using low tube current and hybrid iterative reconstruction. Acad Radiol. 2013;20:1405–12.

13. Altenbernd J, Heusner TA, Ringelstein A, Ladd SC, Forsting M, Antoch G. Dual-energy-CT of hypervascular liver lesions in patients with HCC: investigation of image quality and sensitivity. Eur Radiol. 2011;21:738–43.

14. Luo XF, Xie XQ, Cheng S, Yang Y, Yan J, Zhang H, et al. Dual-energy CT for patients suspected of having liver iron overload: can virtual iron content imaging accurately quantify liver iron content? Radiology. 2015;277:95–103.

15. Lee MH, Kim YK, Park MJ, Hwang J, Kim SH, Lee WJ, et al. Gadoxetic acid-enhanced fat suppressed three-dimensional T1-weighted MRI using a multiecho Dixon technique at 3 tesla: emphasis on image quality and hepatocellular carcinoma detection. J Magn Reson Imaging. 2013;38:401–10.

16. Chandarana H, Block KT, Winfeld MJ, Lala SV, Mazori D, Giuffrida E, et al. Free-breathing contrast-enhanced T1-weighted gradient-echo imaging with radial k-space sampling for paediatric abdominopelvic MRI. Eur Radiol. 2014;24:320–6.

17. Padhani AR, Liu G, Koh DM, Chenevert TL, Thoeny HC, Takahara T, et al. Diffusion-weighted magnetic resonance imaging as a cancer biomarker: consensus and recommendations. Neoplasia. 2009;11:102–25.

18. Koh DM, Brown G, Riddell AM, Scurr E, Collins DJ, Allen SD, et al. Detection of colorectal hepatic metastases using MnDPDP MR imaging and diffusion-weighted imaging (DWI) alone and in combination. Eur Radiol. 2008;18:903–10.

19. Holzapfel K, Reiser-Erkan C, Fingerle AA, Erkan M, Eiber MJ, Rummeny EJ, et al. Comparison of diffusion-weighted MR imaging and multidetector-row CT in the detection of liver metastases in patients operated for pancreatic cancer. Abdom Imaging. 2011;36:179–84.

20. Vandecaveye V, De Keyzer F, Verslype C, Op de Beeck K, Komuta M, Topal B, et al. Diffusion-weighted MRI provides additional value to conventional dynamic contrast-enhanced MRI for detection of hepatocellular carcinoma. Eur Radiol. 2009;19:2456–66.

21. Oudkerk M, Torres CG, Song B, König M, Grimm J, Fernandez-Cuadrado J, et al. Characterization of liver lesions with mangafodipir trisodium-enhanced MR imaging: multicenter study comparing MR and dual-phase spiral CT. Radiology. 2002;223:517–24.

22. Scharitzer M, Schima W, Schober E, Reimer P, Helmberger TK, Holzknecht N, et al. Characterization of hepatocellular tumors: value of mangafodipir-enhanced magnetic resonance imaging. J Comput Assist Tomogr. 2005;29:181–90.

23. Ward J, Robinson PJ, Guthrie JA, Downing S, Wilson D, Lodge JP, et al. Liver metastases in candidates for hepatic resection: comparison of helical CT and gadolinium- and SPIO-enhanced MR imaging. Radiology. 2005;237:170–80.

24. Hammerstingl R, Huppertz A, Breuer J, Balzer T, Blakeborough A, Carter R, et al. Diagnostic efficacy of gadoxetic acid (Primovist)-enhanced MRI and spiral CT for a therapeutic strategy: comparison with intraoperative and histopathologic findings in focal liver lesions. Eur Radiol. 2008;18:457–67.

25. Schima W, Saini S, Echeverri JA, Hahn PF, Harisinghani M, Mueller PR. Focal liver lesions: characterization with conventional spin-echo versus fast spin-echo T2-weighted MR imaging. Radiology. 1997;202:389–93.

26. Farraher SW, Jara H, Chang KJ, Ozonoff A, Soto JA. Differentiation of hepatocellular carcinoma and hepatic metastasis from cysts and hemangiomas with calculated T2 relaxation times and the T1/T2 relaxation times ratio. J Magn Reson Imaging. 2006;24:1333–41.

27. Semelka RC, Brown ED, Ascher SM, Patt RH, Bagley AS, Li W, et al. Hepatic hemangiomas: a multi-institutional study of appearance on T2-weighted and serial gadolinium-enhanced gradient-echo MR images. Radiology. 1994;192:401–6.

28. Oto A, Kulkarni K, Nishikawa R, Baron RL. Contrast enhancement of hepatic hemangiomas on multiphase MDCT: can we diagnose hepatic hemangiomas by comparing enhancement with blood pool? AJR Am J Roentgenol. 2010;195:381–6.

29. Ba-Ssalamah A, Uffmann M, Saini S, Bastati N, Herold C, Schima W. Clinical value of MRI liver-specific contrast agents: a tailored examination for a confident non-invasive diagnosis of focal liver lesions. Eur Radiol. 2009;19:342–57.

30. Taouli B, Koh DM. Diffusion-weighted MR imaging of the liver. Radiology. 2010;254:47–66.

31. Vossen JA, Buijs M, Liapi E, Eng J, Bluemke DA, Kamel IR. Receiver operating characteristic analysis of diffusion-weighted magnetic resonance imaging in differentiating hepatic hemangioma from other hypervascular liver lesions. J Comput Assist Tomogr. 2008;32:750–6.

32. Kehagias D, Moulopoulos L, Antoniou A, Hatziioannou A, Smyrniotis V, Trakadas S, et al. Focal nodular hyperplasia: imaging findings. Eur Radiol. 2001;11:202–12.

33. Brancatelli G, Federle MP, Grazioli L, Blachar A, Peterson MS, Thaete L. Focal nodular hyperplasia: CT findings with emphasis on multiphasic helical CT in 78 patients. Radiology. 2001;219:61–8.

34. Uggowitzer MM, Kugler C, Mischinger HJ, Gröll R, Ruppert-Kohlmayr A, Preidler KW, et al. Echo-enhanced doppler sonography of focal nodular hyperplasia of the liver. J Ultrasound Med. 1999;18:445–51; quiz 53–4.

35. McInnes MD, Hibbert RM, Inácio JR, Schieda N. Focal nodular hyperplasia and hepatocellular adenoma: accuracy of gadoxetic acid-enhanced mr imaging—a systematic review. Radiology. 2015;277:413–23.

36. Fujiwara H, Sekine S, Onaya H, Shimada K, Mikata R, Arai Y. Ring-like enhancement of focal nodular hyperplasia with hepatobiliary-phase Gd-EOB-DTPA-enhanced magnetic resonance imaging: radiological-pathological correlation. Jpn J Radiol. 2011;29:739–43.

37. Purysko AS, Remer EM, Coppa CP, Obuchowski NA, Schneider E, Veniero JC. Characteristics and distinguishing features of hepatocellular adenoma and focal nodular hyperplasia on gadoxetate disodium-enhanced MRI. AJR Am J Roentgenol. 2012;198:115–23.

38. Leconte I, Van Beers BE, Lacrosse M, Sempoux C, Jamart J, Materne R, et al. Focal nodular hyperplasia: natural course observed with CT and MRI. J Comput Assist Tomogr. 2000;24:61–6.

39. Mathieu D, Kobeiter H, Maison P, Rahmouni A, Cherqui D, Zafrani ES, et al. Oral contraceptive use and focal nodular hyperplasia of the liver. Gastroenterology. 2000;118:560–4.
40. Bioulac-Sage P, Gouw ASH, Balabaud C, Sempoux C. Hepatocellular adenoma: what we know, what we do not know, and why it matters. Histopathology. 2022;80:878–97.
41. Blanc JF, Frulio N, Chiche L, Sempoux C, Annet L, Hubert C, et al. Hepatocellular adenoma management: call for shared guidelines and multidisciplinary approach. Clin Res Hepatol Gastroenterol. 2015;39:180–7.
42. Nault JC, Paradis V, Cherqui D, Vilgrain V, Zucman-Rossi J. Molecular classification of hepatocellular adenoma in clinical practice. J Hepatol. 2017;67:1074–83.
43. Prasad SR, Sahani DV, Mino-Kenudson M, Narra VR, Menias C, Wang HL, et al. Benign hepatic neoplasms: an update on cross-sectional imaging spectrum. J Comput Assist Tomogr. 2008;32:829–40.
44. Katabathina VS, Menias CO, Shanbhogue AK, Jagirdar J, Paspulati RM, Prasad SR. Genetics and imaging of hepatocellular adenomas: 2011 update. Radiographics. 2011;31:1529–43.
45. van Aalten SM, Thomeer MG, Terkivatan T, Dwarkasing RS, Verheij J, de Man RA, et al. Hepatocellular adenomas: correlation of MR imaging findings with pathologic subtype classification. Radiology. 2011;261:172–81.
46. Wong VK, Fung AW, Elsayes KM. Magnetic resonance imaging of hepatic adenoma subtypes. Clin Liver Dis (Hoboken). 2021;17:113–8.
47. Katabathina VS, Khanna L, Surabhi VR, Minervini M, Shanbhogue K, Dasyam AK, et al. Morphomolecular classification update on hepatocellular adenoma, hepatocellular carcinoma, and intrahepatic cholangiocarcinoma. Radiographics. 2022;42:1338–57.
48. Grazioli L, Bondioni MP, Haradome H, Motosugi U, Tinti R, Frittoli B, et al. Hepatocellular adenoma and focal nodular hyperplasia: value of gadoxetic acid-enhanced MR imaging in differential diagnosis. Radiology. 2012;262:520–9.
49. Kim TH, Woo S, Ebrahimzadeh S, McLnnes MDF, Gerst SR, Do RK. Hepatic adenoma subtypes on hepatobiliary phase of Gadoxetic acid-enhanced MRI: systematic review and meta-analysis. AJR Am J Roentgenol. 2022;
50. Semelka RC, Hussain SM, Marcos HB, Woosley JT. Biliary hamartomas: solitary and multiple lesions shown on current MR techniques including gadolinium enhancement. J Magn Reson Imaging. 1999;10:196–201.
51. Martin DR, Kalb B, Sarmiento JM, Heffron TG, Coban I, Adsay NV. Giant and complicated variants of cystic bile duct hamartomas of the liver: MRI findings and pathological correlations. J Magn Reson Imaging. 2010;31:903–11.
52. Jeffrey RB Jr, Tolentino CS, Chang FC, Federle MP. CT of small pyogenic hepatic abscesses: the cluster sign. AJR Am J Roentgenol. 1988;151:487–9.
53. Barreda R, Ros PR. Diagnostic imaging of liver abscess. Crit Rev Diagn Imaging. 1992;33:29–58.
54. Laghi A, Iannaccone R, Rossi P, Carbone I, Ferrari R, Mangiapane F, et al. Hepatocellular carcinoma: detection with triple-phase multi-detector row helical CT in patients with chronic hepatitis. Radiology. 2003;226:543–9.
55. Ichikawa T, Kitamura T, Nakajima H, Sou H, Tsukamoto T, Ikenaga S, et al. Hypervascular hepatocellular carcinoma: can double arterial phase imaging with multidetector CT improve tumor depiction in the cirrhotic liver? AJR Am J Roentgenol. 2002;179:751–8.
56. Monzawa S, Ichikawa T, Nakajima H, Kitanaka Y, Omata K, Araki T. Dynamic CT for detecting small hepatocellular carcinoma: usefulness of delayed phase imaging. AJR Am J Roentgenol. 2007;188:147–53.
57. Iannaccone R, Laghi A, Catalano C, Rossi P, Mangiapane F, Murakami T, et al. Hepatocellular carcinoma: role of unenhanced and delayed phase multi-detector row helical CT in patients with cirrhosis. Radiology. 2005;234:460–7.
58. Baron RL, Brancatelli G. Computed tomographic imaging of hepatocellular carcinoma. Gastroenterology. 2004;127:S133–43.
59. Forner A, Vilana R, Ayuso C, Bianchi L, Solé M, Ayuso JR, et al. Diagnosis of hepatic nodules 20 mm or smaller in cirrhosis: prospective validation of the noninvasive diagnostic criteria for hepatocellular carcinoma. Hepatology. 2008;47:97–104.
60. Tublin ME, Dodd GD 3rd, Baron RL. Benign and malignant portal vein thrombosis: differentiation by CT characteristics. AJR Am J Roentgenol. 1997;168:719–23.
61. Stevens WR, Gulino SP, Batts KP, Stephens DH, Johnson CD. Mosaic pattern of hepatocellular carcinoma: histologic basis for a characteristic CT appearance. J Comput Assist Tomogr. 1996;20:337–42.
62. Kim TK, Lee KH, Jang HJ, Haider MA, Jacks LM, Menezes RJ, et al. Analysis of gadobenate dimeglumine-enhanced MR findings for characterizing small (1-2-cm) hepatic nodules in patients at high risk for hepatocellular carcinoma. Radiology. 2011;259:730–8.
63. Choi JW, Lee JM, Kim SJ, Yoon JH, Baek JH, Han JK, et al. Hepatocellular carcinoma: imaging patterns on gadoxetic acid-enhanced MR images and their value as an imaging biomarker. Radiology. 2013;267:776–86.
64. Chen L, Zhang L, Bao J, Zhang J, Li C, Xia Y, et al. Comparison of MRI with liver-specific contrast agents and multidetector row CT for the detection of hepatocellular carcinoma: a meta-analysis of 15 direct comparative studies. Gut. 2013;62:1520–1.
65. Koh DM, Ba-Ssalamah A, Brancatelli G, Fananapazir G, Fiel MI, Goshima S, et al. Consensus report from the 9(th) international forum for liver magnetic resonance imaging: applications of gadoxetic acid-enhanced imaging. Eur Radiol. 2021;31:5615–28.
66. Song KD, Kim SH, Lim HK, Jung SH, Sohn I, Kim HS. Subcentimeter hypervascular nodule with typical imaging findings of hepatocellular carcinoma in patients with history of hepatocellular carcinoma: natural course on serial gadoxetic acid-enhanced MRI and diffusion-weighted imaging. Eur Radiol. 2015;25:2789–96.
67. Lee MH, Kim SH, Park MJ, Park CK, Rhim H. Gadoxetic acid-enhanced hepatobiliary phase MRI and high-b-value diffusion-weighted imaging to distinguish well-differentiated hepatocellular carcinomas from benign nodules in patients with chronic liver disease. AJR Am J Roentgenol. 2011;197:W868–75.
68. Liver Reporting & Data System (LI-RADS®) https://www.acr.org/Clinical-Resources/Reporting-and-Data-Systems/LI-RADS. Accessed 2022-10-15.
69. Ichikawa T, Federle MP, Grazioli L, Madariaga J, Nalesnik M, Marsh W. Fibrolamellar hepatocellular carcinoma: imaging and pathologic findings in 31 recent cases. Radiology. 1999;213:352–61.
70. Ichikawa T, Federle MP, Grazioli L, Marsh W. Fibrolamellar hepatocellular carcinoma: pre- and posttherapy evaluation with CT and MR imaging. Radiology. 2000;217:145–51.
71. Yoon JK, Choi JY, Rhee H, Park YN. MRI features of histologic subtypes of hepatocellular carcinoma: correlation with histologic, genetic, and molecular biologic classification. Eur Radiol. 2022;32:5119–33.
72. Lim JH. Cholangiocarcinoma: morphologic classification according to growth pattern and imaging findings. AJR Am J Roentgenol. 2003;181(3):819–27.
73. Han JK, Choi BI, Kim AY, An SK, Lee JW, Kim TK, et al. Cholangiocarcinoma: pictorial essay of CT and cholangiographic findings. Radiographics. 2002;22:173–87.

74. Jhaveri KS, Halankar J, Aguirre D, Haider M, Lockwood G, Guindi M, et al. Intrahepatic bile duct dilatation due to liver metastases from colorectal carcinoma. AJR Am J Roentgenol. 2009;193:752–6.

75. Park S, Lee Y, Kim H, Yu MH, Lee ES, Yoon JH, et al. Subtype classification of intrahepatic cholangiocarcinoma using liver MR imaging features and its prognostic value. Liver Cancer. 2022;11:233–46.

76. Lee WJ, Lim HK, Jang KM, Kim SH, Lee SJ, Lim JH, et al. Radiologic spectrum of cholangiocarcinoma: emphasis on unusual manifestations and differential diagnoses. Radiographics. 2001;21 Spec No:S97–s116.

77. McIntyre CA, Girshman J, Goldman DA, Gonen M, Soares KC, Wei AC, et al. Differentiation of mucinous cysts and simple cysts of the liver using preoperative imaging. Abdom Radiol (NY). 2022;47:1333–40.

78. Buetow PC, Buck JL, Pantongrag-Brown L, Ros PR, Devaney K, Goodman ZD, et al. Biliary cystadenoma and cystadenocarcinoma: clinical-imaging-pathologic correlations with emphasis on the importance of ovarian stroma. Radiology. 1995;196:805–10.

79. Liu Z, Yi L, Chen J, Li R, Liang K, Chen X, et al. Comparison of the clinical and MRI features of patients with hepatic hemangioma, epithelioid hemangioendothelioma, or angiosarcoma. BMC Med Imaging. 2020;20:71.

80. Peterson MS, Baron RL, Rankin SC. Hepatic angiosarcoma: findings on multiphasic contrast-enhanced helical CT do not mimic hepatic hemangioma. AJR Am J Roentgenol. 2000;175:165–70.

81. Koyama T, Fletcher JG, Johnson CD, Kuo MS, Notohara K, Burgart LJ. Primary hepatic angiosarcoma: findings at CT and MR imaging. Radiology. 2002;222(3):667–73.

82. Miller WJ, Dodd GD 3rd, Federle MP, Baron RL. Epithelioid hemangioendothelioma of the liver: imaging findings with pathologic correlation. AJR Am J Roentgenol. 1992;159:53–7.

83. Alomari AI. The lollipop sign: a new cross-sectional sign of hepatic epithelioid hemangioendothelioma. Eur J Radiol. 2006;59:460–4.

84. Schima W, Kulinna C, Langenberger H, Ba-Ssalamah A. Liver metastases of colorectal cancer: US, CT or MR? Cancer Imaging. 2005, 5 Spec No A:S149–56.

85. Vilgrain V, Esvan M, Ronot M, Caumont-Prim A, Aubé C, Chatellier G. A meta-analysis of diffusion-weighted and gadoxetic acid-enhanced MR imaging for the detection of liver metastases. Eur Radiol. 2016;26:4595–615.

86. Lee MJ, Saini S, Compton CC, Malt RA. MR demonstration of edema adjacent to a liver metastasis: pathologic correlation. AJR Am J Roentgenol. 1991;157:499–501.

87. Elsayes KM, Kielar AZ, Agrons MM, et al. Liver imaging reporting and data system: an expert consensus statement. J Hepatocell Carcinoma. 2017;4:29–39.

88. Schima W, Heiken J. LI-RADS v2017 for liver nodules: how we read and report. Cancer Imaging. 2018;18:14.

89. Kielar AZ, Chernyak V, Bashir MR, et al. An update for LI-RADS: Version 2018. Why so soon after version 2017? J Magn Reson Imaging. 2019(50):1990–1.

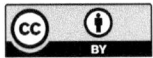

Diseases of the Gallbladder and the Biliary Tree

8

Richard K. Do and Daniel T. Boll

Learning Objectives
- To discuss typical imaging features of common cholangiopathies.
- To discuss the imaging diagnosis of premalignant tumors of the gallbladder and bile duct.
- To explain classification systems of cholangiocarcinoma.
- To discuss the strengths and weaknesses of imaging modalities in the diagnostic work-up of biliary malignancies.

Key Points
- Cross-sectional imaging of biliary disease often requires a multimodality imaging approach.
- Sclerosing cholangitis represents a diseases spectrum disease of inflammation, fibrosis, and doctoral strictures, which can be classified as primary and secondary sclerosing cholangitis.
- Although tissue biopsy needed for the definitive diagnosis of many of biliary strictures or mass -like lesions, certain imaging characteristics such as thickened wall, long-segment involvement, asymmetry, indistinct outer margin, luminal irregularity, hyperenhancement relative to the liver parenchyma may favor a malignant cause.

- Biliary malignancies demonstrate arterial phase enhancement with persistent enhancement into the portal venous phase, due greater proportion of fibrotic tissue within these neoplasms.

8.1 Biliary Tract

Richard K. G. Do

The biliary tree is a common site of both benign diseases, such as choledocholithiasis or congenital malformations, and malignant diseases predominantly in the form of cholangiocarcinoma (CCA). Since benign diseases are often predisposing factors for the development of malignancy, especially if accompanied by chronic biliary inflammation, this chapter will emphasize benign entities that may require further long-term surveillance or surgical intervention. When repeated bouts of inflammation occur in the biliary tree, chronic injury leads to cellular proliferation and eventual survival of mutated cells and eventually bile duct neoplasia and malignancy [1]. While CCA can arise from epithelial cells anywhere along the biliary tree, they are most common at sites that harbor the highest density of peribiliary glands, which contain hepatic stem/progenitor cells (HPCs). These are located at branching points including the cystic duct, biliary confluence, and periampullary region [2, 3].

8.1.1 Normal Anatomy and Variants

The biliary tree is divided into intrahepatic and extrahepatic segments, with the right and left hepatic ducts usually draining the right and left hepatic lobes. The right and left ducts join at the biliary confluence, which forms the superior por-

R. K. Do
Department of Radiology, Memorial Sloan Kettering Cancer Center, New York, NY, USA
e-mail: dok@mskcc.org

D. T. Boll (✉)
Radiology and Nuclear Medicine, University Hospital of Basel, Basel, Switzerland
e-mail: daniel.boll@usb.ch

© The Author(s) 2023
J. Hodler et al. (eds.), *Diseases of the Abdomen and Pelvis 2023-2026*, IDKD Springer Series,
https://doi.org/10.1007/978-3-031-27355-1_8

tion of the extrahepatic biliary tree. The common hepatic duct extends below the biliary confluence while the common bile duct starts below the insertion of the cystic duct. On imaging, when the insertion of the cystic duct is not visible, the extrahepatic duct is simply referred to as the common duct.

The right hepatic duct is usually formed as the confluence of the right anterior and right posterior ducts, which drain the anterior and posterior sectors respectively. The most common variant biliary anatomy consists of the posterior right hepatic duct draining into the left hepatic duct [4]. If this variant is not recognized, it can be led to bile duct injury for a living donor or during hepatic tumor resections. A biliary trifurcation is another common variant, with the posterior right, anterior right, and left hepatic duct joining at the confluence.

8.1.2 Congenital Biliary Anomalies

8.1.2.1 Choledochal Cysts and Anomalous Pancreatobiliary Ductal Junction

Choledochal cysts describe pathologic dilatations of the biliary tract and are classified by their anatomic location [5]. MRCP is the imaging modality of choice to identify choledochal cysts and the exact type of abnormality. The incidence of biliary malignancy, most commonly adenocarcinoma, varies with the type of choledochal cyst, with the highest among Todani Type I at 68%, followed by Type IV (21%), and below 10% for the remaining [6]. Surgical resection is thus indicated whenever possible, to reduce the risk of malignancy. Cholangiocarcinoma in the setting of a choledochal cyst presents as an intracystic soft tissue mass or irregular thickening of the cyst wall (Fig. 8.1).

Anomalous pancreaticobiliary ductal junction describes a congenital anomaly where the common bile duct and pancreatic duct join before the duodenal wall, leading to abnormal outflow of bile and pancreatic secretions. The abnormal flow of secretions leads to chronic inflammation of the biliary epithelium and a higher predisposition to bile duct malignancy [7]. The risk of malignancy from pancreaticobiliary maljunction varies with the presence or absence of biliary dilatation [8]. While choledochal cysts frequently coexist with a pancreaticobiliary maljunction, the latter is not always present.

8.1.3 Pathologic Conditions

8.1.3.1 Choledocholithiasis

Ultrasound is often used as a first line imaging modality for assessment of right upper quadrant pain, but its sensitivity for biliary stones is only 21–63%, due to challenges in

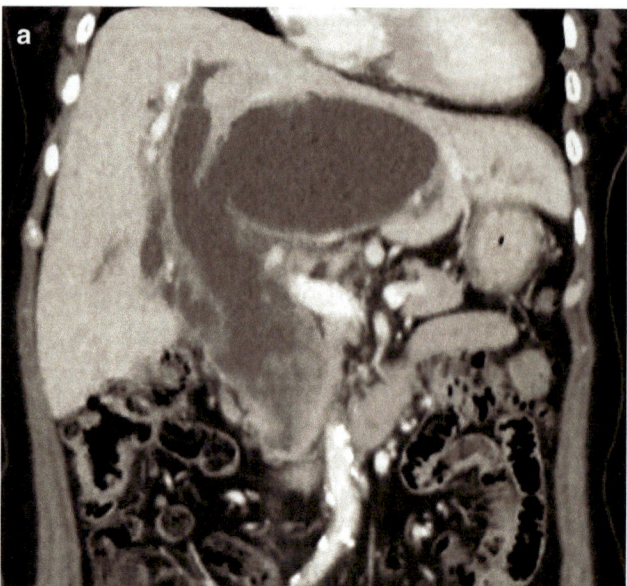
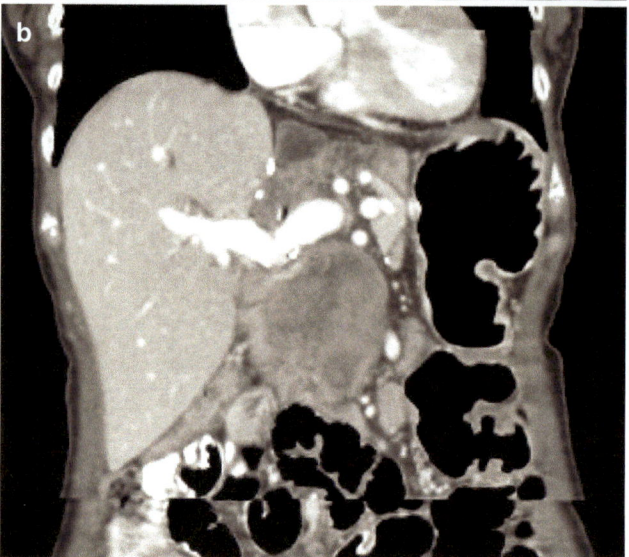

Fig. 8.1 (**a**) A 64-year-old female with Type IV choledochal cyst with enhancing soft tissue in the common bile duct consistent with malignant degeneration. (**b**) The extrahepatic bile duct was resected along with a left hepatectomy, but tumor recurred 4 years later in the retroperitoneum

obtaining an acoustic window, especially for the common bile duct [9]. CT is also commonly used for assessment of right upper quadrant pain, but its sensitivity for bile duct stones varies depending on their composition. Calcified gallstones are easiest to detect on CT (Fig. 8.2) while radiolucent stones are hard to distinguish from surrounding bile. Biliary stones are better detected by MR cholangiography, which has a very high sensitivity, especially for detection of stones in the common bile duct. On MRCP, stones are dark on T2 and have variable T1 signal, often appearing T1 hyperintense.

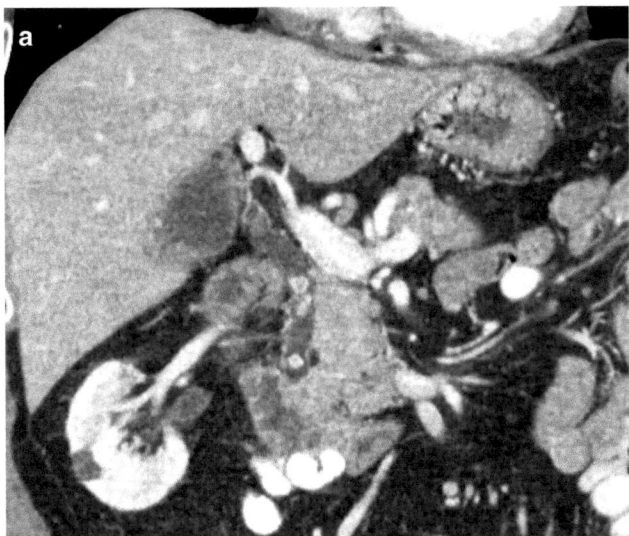

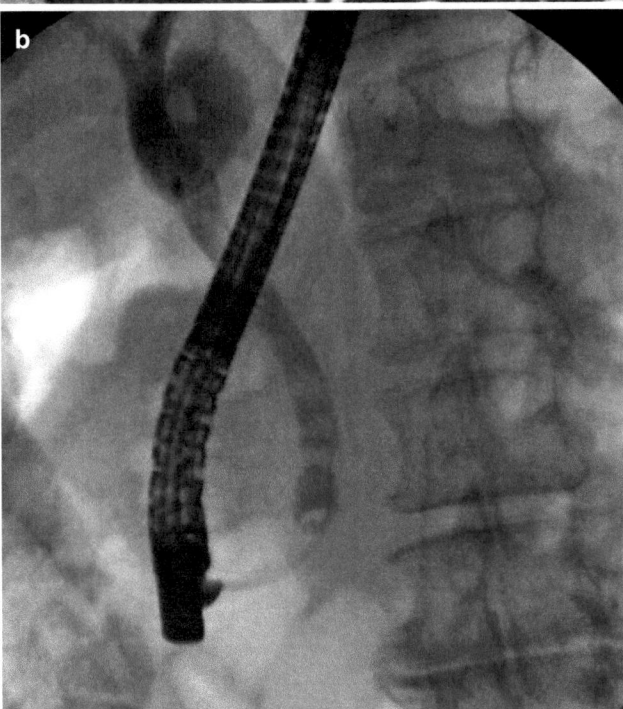

Fig. 8.2 Choledocholithiasis. (**a**) A 80-year-old male with calcified stones in the common duct. (**b**) Fluoroscopic image obtained during endoscopic retrograde cholangiogram showing filling defects in the common duct consistent with stones

8.1.3.2 Cholangitis

Suppurative Cholangitis

Choledocholithiasis can lead to acute bacterial cholangitis, which is demonstrated on imaging by diffuse concentric wall thickening of the bile duct with associated periductal edema and mural enhancement. Arterial phase hyperenhancement of the adjacent parenchyma is often seen and reflects inflammation of the affected liver.

Pyogenic Cholangitis

In endemic areas, such as Southeast Asia, recurrent pyogenic cholangitis (RPC) is a manifestation of chronic parasitic infections in the bile ducts from parasites, including Clonorchis sinensis and Ascaris lumbricoides. The repeated bouts of cholangitis lead to multifocal strictures and superinfection with bacteria, and subsequent stone formation. A characteristic "arrowhead" appearance has been described, due to abrupt tapering of the peripheral ducts [10]. The risk of CCA is increased, given the chronic inflammatory milieu, and tends to arise in atrophic segments or ducts with heavy stone burden.

Primary Sclerosing Cholangitis

Primary sclerosing cholangitis (PSC) is an idiopathic and chronic inflammatory disease of the bile ducts, is presumed to be autoimmune and has a strong association with inflammatory bowel disease. On imaging, multifocal areas of bile duct narrowing are identified, with intervening normal or mildly dilated ducts, yielding an overall beaded appearance of the bile ducts [11]. Given the presence of chronic inflammation and high likelihood of developing bile duct malignancy, these patients are followed by MRCP to identify new or worsening irregular high-grade stricture. Because these malignancies are often periductal infiltrating CCA, imaging may not demonstrate an obvious mass, but focal biliary wall thickening is present. Intrahepatic mass-forming CCA can also occur in PSC, and the appearance and contrast to periductal infiltrating CCA is further described below.

8.1.3.3 IgG4 Cholangitis

IgG4 sclerosing cholangitis (SC) is commonly found in association with autoimmune pancreatitis (AIP), occurring in about 60–80% of patients with AIP [12]. In these cases, the most commonly involved segment is in the pancreatic head. IgG4 SC can also occur without concurrent AIP. On imaging, the bile duct can be focally or diffusely thickened, with upstream biliary dilatation (Fig. 8.3). PSC occurs more commonly in younger patients and is more often multifocal. When a single extrahepatic bile duct stricture is present, it can be challenging to distinguish from cholangiocarcinoma. Radiologists should seek concurrent pancreatic or extrapancreatic diseases to raise the possibility of IgG4 SC.

8.1.3.4 Neoplasms of the Biliary System

Benign Tumors of the Bile Ducts

Hamartomas and adenomas

Biliary hamartomas, which are also known as von Meyenburg complexes, are benign tumor composed of disorganized bile

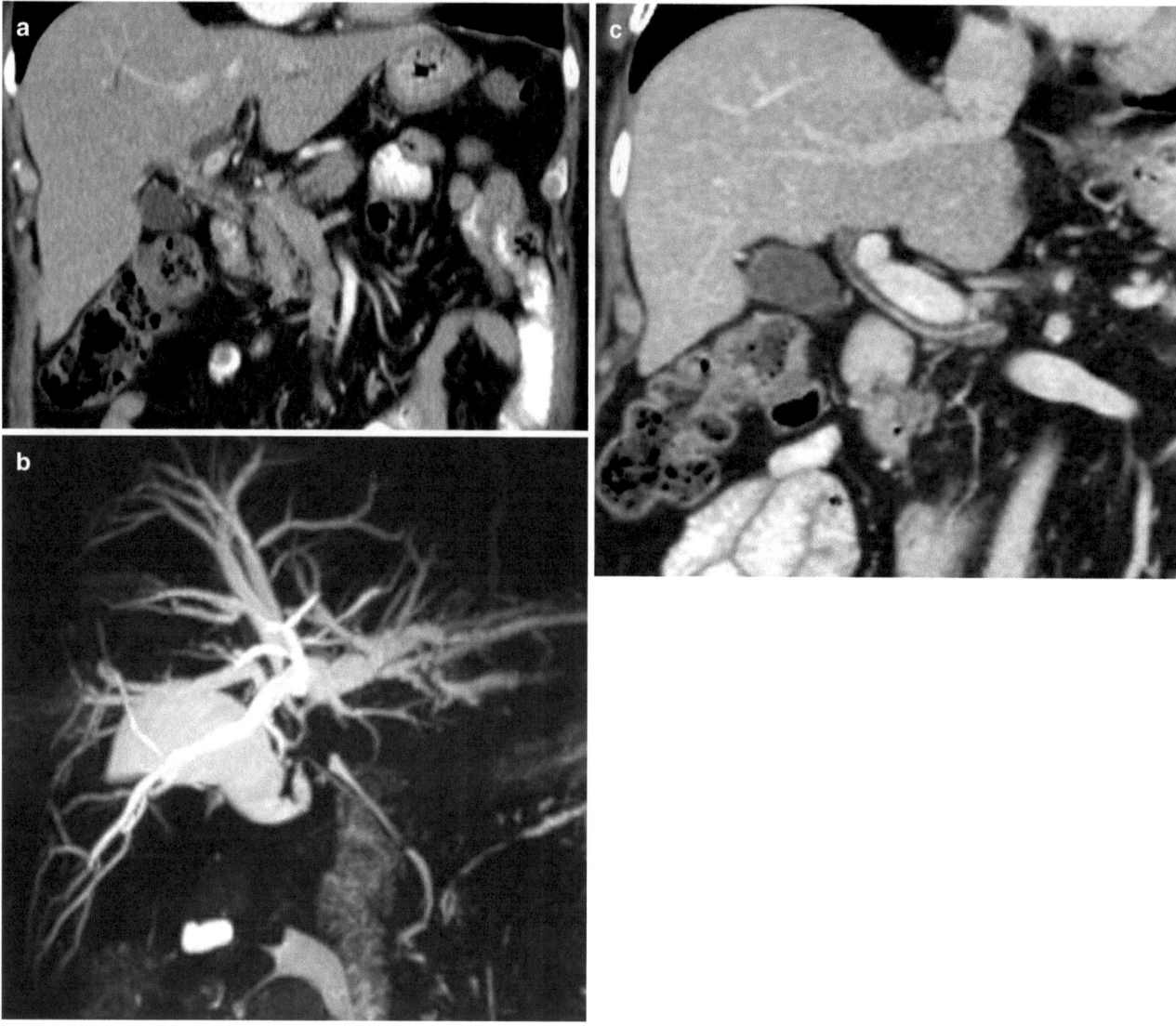

Fig. 8.3 IgG4 sclerosing cholangitis. (**a**) A 60-year-old male with irregularly thickened extrahepatic bile duct on coronal CT with contrast. (**b**) 3D MRCP MIP image of narrowed common hepatic duct and moderate intrahepatic biliary dilatation. (**c**) Resolved bile duct wall thickening and biliary dilatation after treatment with steroids

ducts and ductules best seen on T2-weighted imaging as innumerable cystic appearing T2 hyperintense lesions throughout the liver, usually between 1 and 5 mm [13]. On CT, these are usually too small to characterize as cystic and can mimic metastatic disease. Bile duct adenomas are usually indistinguishable from hamartomas but are usually encountered as a solitary subcentimeter hypodense lesion.

Biliary Intraepithelial Neoplasm and Intraductal Papillary Neoplasms of the Bile Ducts

Chronic inflammation can lead to the appearance of biliary intraepithelial neoplasm (BilIN), a precursor lesion often found in association with RPC and PSC. It is also present in a majority of cases of CCA and is particularly common with extrahepatic CCA [14]. As a microscopic lesion, it is gener-
ally not seen on imaging. On the other hand, intraductal papillary neoplasms of the bile duct (IPNB) can appear as a macroscopic lesion on imaging, with variable appearance depending on the tumor growth, its location, and the degree of mucin production [8]. A papillary mass can be visible once the tumor grows to a sufficient size. On T2-weighted MRCP sequences, a papillary lesion appears dark compared to the surrounding T2 hyperintense bile; pre and post contrast imaging, however, shows clear enhancement, distinguishing these from biliary stones or sludge. When mucin production is high, the bile ducts may appear dilated either focally or throughout a segment, both above and below the level of the tumor. This is a distinguishing characteristic that is a result of excess mucin production. An alternative appearance of IPNB is the cystic form, due to focal aneurysmal

dilatation of the involved bile duct, also due to excessive mucin production. IPNB can progress to an intraductal growing CCA, as described below [15].

Mucinous Cystic Neoplasms

According to WHO classification (5th edition), mucinous cystic neoplasms (MCNs), formerly referred to as biliary cystadenomas/cystadenocarcinomas, are cyst-forming epithelial neoplasms lined by cuboidal, columnar, or flattened mucin-producing epithelium overlying ovarian like-stroma (OLS), without biliary communication. The presence of OLS is the key distinguishing feature [16]. These tumors occur almost exclusively in mildly aged women. The vast majority of MCNs are benign, and malignant ones tend to occur in older patients. On imaging, they tend to by multi-locular with associated septations and calcifications and are more common in the left hepatic lobe. On MRI, they are T2 hyperintense similar to cysts, but have more variable T1 internal signal due to the presence of hemorrhage or protein-aceous contents. While calcifications and mural nodules are associated with malignancy, imaging cannot reliably distin-guish between from malignant MCNs, so these tumors are often resected when the diagnosis is suspected.

Malignant Tumors of the Bile Ducts

Cholangiocarcinoma

CCA are categorized by their location as either intrahepatic or extrahepatic, with the latter beginning at the biliary con-fluence. For radiologists, the morphologic classification as mass-forming, periductal infiltrating, or intraductal growing is more helpful because of their distinct imaging patterns on cross-sectional imaging.

Mass-forming CCA arise more commonly in patients with chronic hepatitis, especially those with cirrhosis and hepatitis B [17]. They form the majority of intrahepatic CCA and pres-ent as a lobulated mass, often with a targeted enhancement pattern, as defined by the American College of Radiology Liver Imaging Reporting and Data Systems. This pattern cor-responds pathologically to the presence of a cellular periphery in the tumor that often show arterial phase hyperenhancement and washout, along with a fibrotic/desmoplastic center that shows delayed hyperenhancement (Fig. 8.4). While capsular retraction and peripheral biliary dilatation are distinguishing features of mass-forming CCA, these features are not always present [18]. Some mass-forming CCA are predominantly hypovascular and may overlap in appearance with metastatic disease from a gastrointestinal primary malignancy. A domi-nant liver mass with satellite lesions may help clue the radiolo-gist to the possibility of a primary liver tumor.

Periductal infiltrating CCA are usually extrahepatic in location. They are referred to as Klatskin tumors if they involve the biliary confluence. The tumors cause biliary dila-

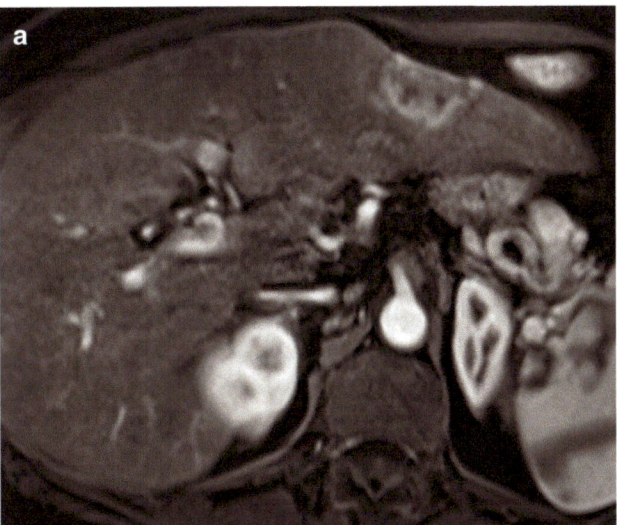
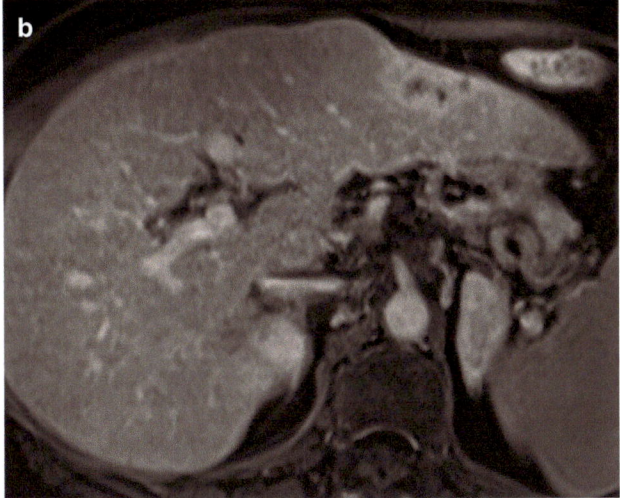

Fig. 8.4 Intrahepatic mass-forming cholangiocarcinoma. (**a**) A 78-year-old female with left intrahepatic cholangiocarcinoma on T1-weighted fat saturated imaging showing rim arterial phase hyperen-hancement, a targeted imaging feature. (**b**) Persistent hyperenhance-ment on delayed hepatobiliary phase with capsular retraction along the anterior liver surface

tation upstream above the level of biliary stricture, which is accompanied by focal bile duct wall thickening (Fig. 8.5). However, the tumors are often ill-defined and hard to delin-eate in their entirety, even with optimal CT and MR tech-niques. As a result, the degree of ductal involvement is often underestimated. For radiologists, reporting the degree of vas-cular involvement is just as critical, with contact of the hepatic arterial and portal venous anatomy often determining the likelihood of resectability. Vascular contact can be described as absent, abutment (up to 180°), or encasement (180° or more). A structured reporting form has been pro-posed by the Korean Society of Abdominal Radiology to describe relevant preoperative findings for CCA with the goal of future validation [19].

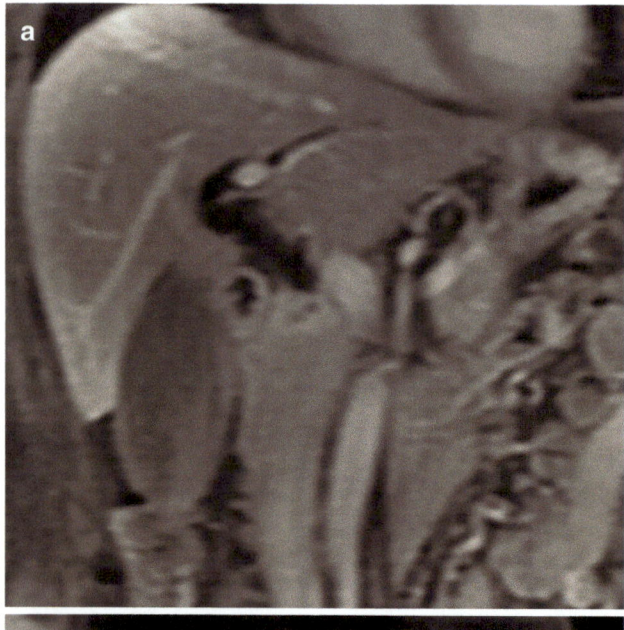

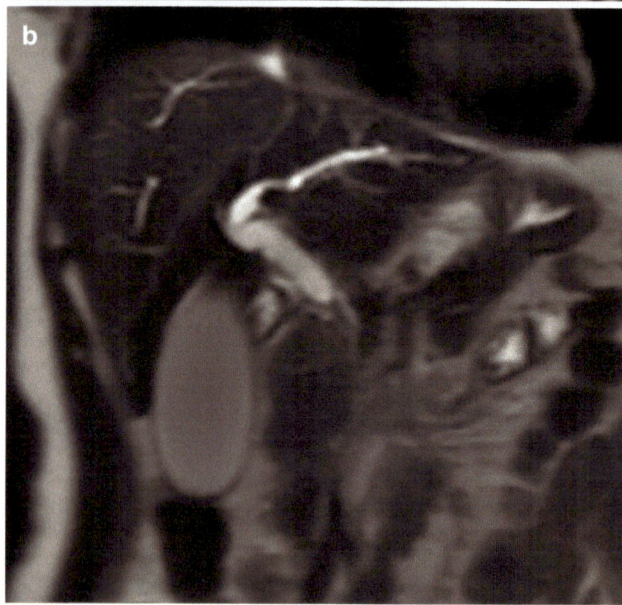

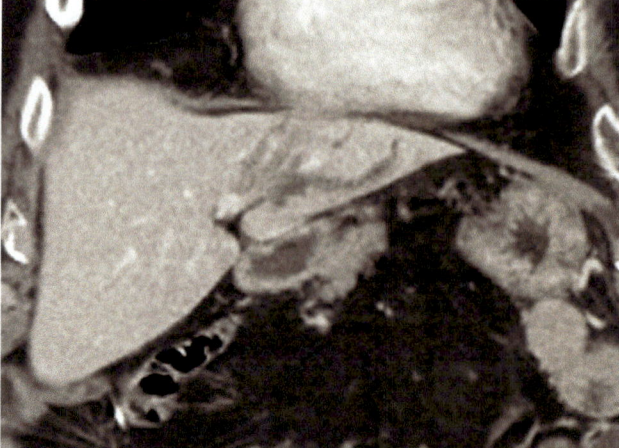

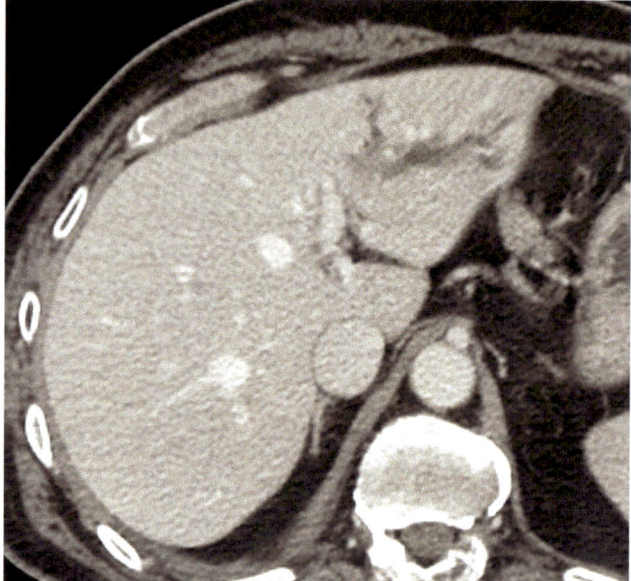

Fig. 8.6 Colorectal metastasis to left intrahepatic bile duct

Fig. 8.5 Extrahepatic cholangiocarcinoma. (**a**)A 53-year-old female with a lower extrahepatic bile duct stricture with thickened wall on post contrast T1-weighted imaging. (**b**) Biliary ductal dilatation with abrupt cutoff on T2 coronal single shot fast spin echo

Metastatic Disease

Metastatic disease to the bile ducts is extremely rare, with colorectal cancer being more common than other cancers such as lung, breast, gallbladder, testicular, prostate, pancreas, melanoma, and lymphoma [20] (Fig. 8.6).

8.2   Gallbladder

Daniel T. Boll

8.2.1   Normal Anatomy

Being positioned along the undersurface of the liver in the plane of the interlobar fissure between the right and left hepatic lobes, the gallbladder is physiologically tubular in structure with a cross-sectional diameter of up to 5 cm and a normal wall thickness of 1–3.5 mm, dependent on luminal distention [21, 22].

The bile-filled lumen of the gallbladder measures water-isodensity (0–20 Hounsfield Units) on CT and water-isointense signal characteristics on T2-weighted MR imaging; formation and retention of sludge may create layering or smooth gradients of MR intensity/CT attenuation, resulting in a parfait-like appearance. Vicarious excretion of CT contrast material from prior contrast-enhanced CT imaging through gastrointestinal uptake as well as utilization of hepatocyte-specific contrast materials in hepatic MR imaging may alter the imaging appearance of bilious fluid on contrast-enhanced CT as well as MR imaging [23, 24].

8.2.2 Congenital Variants and Anomalies

8.2.2.1 Agenesis of the Gallbladder

Agenesis of the gallbladder, a rare malformation (0.01–0.2% in autopsy series), results from a developmental failure of the caudal division of the primitive hepatic diverticulum or failure of vacuolization. It may result in formation of extrahepatic and intrahepatic gallstones in up to 50% of patients [21, 25].

8.2.2.2 Duplication of the Gallbladder

Duplication of the gallbladder, an equally rare malformation (0.02% in autopsy series), is characterized by a longitudinal septum, dividing the gallbladder cavity, and each cavity draining through its own cystic duct. Developmental it is the consequence of an incomplete revacuolization of the primitive gallbladder and has to be differentiated from gallbladder folds, a bilobed gallbladder, a choledochal cysts, or a gallbladder diverticulum [26].

8.2.2.3 Phrygian Cap of the Gallbladder

The most common anomaly of the gallbladder is a Phrygian cap configuration through septations of body and the distal fundus and may be seen in up to 6% of patients [21, 27].

8.2.2.4 Diverticula of the Gallbladder, Multiseptate Gallbladder, and Ectopic Gallbladder

True gallbladder diverticula are congenital in nature and contain all three muscle layers; pseudodiverticula are usually associated with adenomyomatosis and contain little or no smooth muscle layers in their walls. (Pseudo)Diverticula can occur throughout the gallbladder wall [21, 29].

Septations throughout the gallbladder creating communicating chambers may lead to stasis of bile and formation of gallstones [28].

Various locations of the gallbladder have been described, in particular an intrahepatic location of the gallbladder, which is entirely surrounded by hepatic parenchyma.

Intrahepatic subcapsular locations may particularly complicate the diagnosis of an acute cholecystitis as secondary signs of inflammation may be subtle or masked entirely. Shrinkage of the liver in patients with cirrhosis, as well as patients with chronic obstructive pulmonary disease may show gallbladders interposed between liver surface and diaphragm [21, 30].

8.2.3 Pathologic Conditions

8.2.3.1 Gallstones

In cross-sectional imaging, the appearance of gallstones is primarily based on composition and size; most gallstones contain various admixtures of bile pigment, cholesterol, and calcium. Larger proportions of calcium may render gallstones radiodense on CT imaging, while less calcium may potentially lead to entirely radiolucent gallstones. While pure cholesterol stones may be lower in CT density than surrounding bile, central inclusions may contain gas mostly consist of nitrogen.

The high signal intensity of bile on T2-weighted images allows the better delineation of hypointense gallstones compared to T1-weighted sequences. While cholesterol stones are usually hypointense in appearance on T1-weighted images, pigment stones tend to have higher signal intensities; central areas of T2 hyperintensity usually corresponds to fluid-filled clefts [21, 31, 32].

8.2.3.2 Acute Cholecystitis

An obstruction of either the gallbladder neck or the cystic duct may lead to increased intraluminal pressures and eventually results in an inflammation of the gallbladder wall. Gallstones lodged in the neck of the gallbladder or the cystic duct leading to biliodynamic obstruction as well as pressure-induced mucosa ischemia and mucosal injury are the pre-eminent reason for acute cholecystitis. Ultrasound, CT, and MRI may show distinct features of acute calculous cholecystitis, such as cholecystolithiasis, gallbladder wall thickening, the pericholecystic fluid and inflammation, thickened bile, an indistinct interface between gallbladder wall and liver capsule and potentially gallbladder perforation. Gallbladder perforations can be subdivided into acute, subacute, and chronic scenarios; a subacute perforation with surrounding abscess is the most frequently encountered type of gallbladder perforation. The use of hepatobiliary contrast agents in MR imaging may provide additional functional information about cystic duct patency [21, 33, 34].

In emphysematous cholecystitis and additional vascular compromise of the cystic artery is hypothesized to accelerate the development of gas-forming organisms in the resultant anaerobic environment with eventual penetration of gas into the gallbladder wall. A more frequent occurrence in diabetic patients, as well as the male population with an acalculous gallbladder potentially hints at a separate pathogenesis in contrast to calculous cholecystitis [35].

Inflammation causing ulceration of the mucosal lining and subsequent necrosis may lead to hemorrhagic cholecystitis. The intraluminal hematoma may be seen on CT and MRI may, however, be difficult to differentiate from high intensity/density bile. An accompanying perforation of the gallbladder wall may lead to hemoperitoneum [36].

Coexisting cardiovascular disease predispositions patients with acute cholecystitis to develop gangrenous wall segments. Intraluminal membranes and irregularity of the gallbladder wall intermittently perforated and potentially surrounded by a pericholecystic abscess are key imaging features.

8.2.3.3 Acalculous Cholecystitis

In approximately 5% of all patients with acute cholecystitis, no intraluminal stones can be found. Long stays in intensive care units and abdominal trauma may lead to increased viscosity and subsequent stasis of bile eventually leading to obstruction and mucosa ischemia [21, 37].

8.2.3.4 Chronic Cholecystitis

Repetitive mucosal trauma through pre-existing gallstones as well as recurrent episodes of acute cholecystitis events may contribute to the poorly understood pathogenesis of this fairly common disease. A florid inflammatory response to irritations may also indicate a genetic predisposition. While cross-sectional imaging of chronic cholecystitis may not substantially differ from acute cholecystitis, the greatest difference appears to be a contracted state of the gallbladder in chronic cholecystitis compared to the acute scenario. A decreased gallbladder ejection fraction is oftentimes associated with chronic cholecystitis [21].

Microperforations through mucosal ulcerations as well as ruptured Rokitansky-Aschoff sinuses may lead to penetration of bile into the gallbladder wall, resulting in the formation of xanthogranulomas representing the hallmark of xanthogranulomatous cholecystitis. Gallstones are almost always present, and an irregular configuration of the gallbladder wall is frequently observed. Xanthogranulomatous lesions in the wall may potentially also lead to abscess formations. These may appear hypodense on contrast-enhanced CT imaging as well as hyperintense nodules on T2-weighted MR imaging. Differentiation from gallbladder cancer may be challenging; however, a patent mucosal lining/luminal surface is more indicative of xanthogranulomatous cholecystitis [21].

Impaction of gallstones inside the cystic duct with subsequent compression of the common hepatic duct, and resultant inflammation are mechanisms leading to Mirizzi syndrome. A fairly low insertion of the cystic duct into the common hepatic duct may represent a predisposition.

Differentiating the inflammatory origin of the stricture of the common hepatic duct from a neoplastic process may be challenging, the lack of lymphadenopathy, as well as a distinct focal mass may be helpful secondary signs. Erosion of gallstones through the gallbladder wall directly into the adjacent bowel via a cholecystoenteric fistula is the most common mechanism to form a gallstone ileus, in particular, involving the distal ileum [21, 38].

Chronic inflammatory changes of the gallbladder wall may lead to dystrophic calcifications associated with thick fibrous tissue layers of the gallbladder wall, indicating a porcelain gallbladder. The porcelain gallbladder is frequently associated with gallbladder carcinoma [39].

8.2.3.5 Hyperplastic Cholecystosis

A benign proliferation of normal gallbladder wall tissue characterizes this non-inflammatory condition. A deposition of cholesterol-laden macrophages into the lamina propria of the gallbladder wall may lead to the formation of cholesterol polyps and cholesterolosis. Due to their small size, these polyps are best seen on ultrasound imaging [21, 40].

A hypertrophy of the muscular wall with corresponding mucosal overgrowth, formation of intramural diverticula and sinus tracts, then called Rokitansky-Aschoff sinuses, is the hallmark of this disease. Detection of a thickened gallbladder wall in addition to small cystic spaces on CT and MR imaging helps to differentiate adenomyomatosis from gallbladder cancer [40].

8.2.3.6 Gallbladder Neoplasms

Benign neoplasms of the gallbladder are rare and usually represent adenomas, which are incidentally, (0.3–0.5%) found during cholecystectomies [21].

During the 6th or 7th decades of life with a female predilection of up to 3:1, gallbladder carcinomas, histopathologically usually presenting as adenocarcinomas; however, adenosquamous, squamous, or neuroendocrine carcinomas can also be found may arise from the gallbladder wall. Predisposing factors associated with gallbladder carcinoma are gallstones (75% of patients with gallbladder carcinomas have gallstones), porcelain gallbladder, genetic factors as well as pancreatobiliary ductal unions (reflux of pancreatic juice into the common bile duct leading to chronic inflammation). On cross-sectional imaging, either a mass is visualized invading the gallbladder fossa or the mass is noted to fill most of the enlarged and deformed gallbladder. Invasion of surrounding structures, in particular the liver, the hepatoduodenal ligament, the right hepatic flexure, or the duodenum is frequently observed. Lymphatic spread to the regional and distant lymph nodes is very common; hematogenous metastasis are usually found in the liver, peritoneal seeding is also fairly common. Biliary obstruction may be observed in up to 50% of patients [21, 41, 42].

Secondary lymphoma to the gallbladder may be seen in disseminated lymphomatous stages, lymphoma involving the gallbladder is extremely rare [43].

Metastases to the gallbladder have been described, malignant melanoma being the most common cause of metastatic tumors, accounting for more than 50% of all cases of gallbladder metastases [44].

8.3 Conclusion

Knowledge of various diseases of the gallbladder and biliary tract in combination with careful inspection of the imaging appearances is of paramount importance for correct interpretation of biliary studies. Offering a succinct set of differential diagnoses for various cholangiopathies is important because specific management pathways exist and prognosis can differ according to the type of underlying disease. Cross-sectional imaging studies play an essential roles in the diagnosis and treatment planning as well as visualization of disease evolution of patients with biliary malignancies and multimodality and multiparametric imaging approaches can provide complementary information in evaluating the tumor extent and resectability.

Take-Home Messages
- An appreciation of the pathologic basis of diseases of the gallbladder and biliary tract, combined with careful inspection of the imaging appearances, is vital for the correct interpretation of biliary studies.
- Differential diagnosis of various cholangiopathies is important because specific management exists and prognosis can differ according to the type of disease.
- Cross-sectional imaging studies play an essential role in the diagnosis and treatment planning as well as visualization of disease evolution of patients with biliary malignancies and multimodality and multiparametric imaging approaches can provide complementary information in evaluating the tumor extent and resectability.

References

1. Labib PL, Goodchild G, Pereira SP. Molecular pathogenesis of cholangiocarcinoma. BMC Cancer. 2019;19(1):185.
2. Cardinale V, Carpino G, Reid L, Gaudio E, Alvaro D. Multiple cells of origin in cholangiocarcinoma underlie biological, epidemiological and clinical heterogeneity. World J Gastrointest Oncol. 2012;4(5):94–102.
3. Alpini G, McGill JM, Larusso NF. The pathobiology of biliary epithelia. Hepatology. 2002;35(5):1256–68.
4. Catalano OA, Singh AH, Uppot RN, Hahn PF, Ferrone CR, Sahani DV. Vascular and biliary variants in the liver: implications for liver surgery. Radiographics. 2008;28(2):359–78.
5. Kim OH, Chung HJ, Choi BG. Imaging of the choledochal cyst. Radiographics. 1995;15(1):69–88.
6. Todani T, Tabuchi K, Watanabe Y, Kobayashi T. Carcinoma arising in the wall of congenital bile duct cysts. Cancer. 1979;44(3):1134–41.
7. Kamisawa T, Kuruma S, Chiba K, Tabata T, Koizumi S, Kikuyama M. Biliary carcinogenesis in pancreaticobiliary maljunction. J Gastroenterol. 2017;52(2):158–63.
8. Zulfiqar M, Chatterjee D, Yoneda N, Hoegger MJ, Ronot M, Hecht EM, Bastati N, Ba-Ssalamah A, Bashir MR, Fowler K. Imaging features of premalignant biliary lesions and predisposing conditions with pathologic correlation. Radiographics. 2022;42(5):1320–37.
9. Yeh BM, Liu PS, Soto JA, Corvera CA, Hussain HK. MR imaging and ct of the biliary tract. RadioGraphics. 2009;29(6):1669–88.
10. Seo N, Kim SY, Lee SS, et al. Sclerosing cholangitis: clinicopathologic features, imaging spectrum, and systemic approach to differential diagnosis. Korean J Radiol. 2016;17:25–38.
11. Venkatesh SK, Welle CL, Miller FH, Jhaveri K, Ringe KI, Eaton JE, Bungay H, Arrivé L, Ba-Ssalamah A, Grigoriadis A, Schramm C, Fulcher AS, IPSCSG. Reporting standards for primary sclerosing cholangitis using MRI and MR cholangiopancreatography: guidelines from MR Working Group of the International Primary Sclerosing Cholangitis Study Group. Eur Radiol. 2022;32(2):923–37.
12. Martínez-de-Alegría A, Baleato-González S, García-Figueiras R, Bermúdez-Naveira A, Abdulkader-Nallib I, Díaz-Peromingo JA, Villalba-Martín C. IgG4-related disease from head to toe. Radiographics. 2015;35(7):2007–25.
13. Horton KM, Bluemke DA, Hruban RH, Soyer P, Fishman EK. CT and MR imaging of benign hepatic and biliary tumors. Radiographics. 1999;19(2):431–51.
14. Sibulesky L, Nguyen J, Patel T. Preneoplastic conditions underlying bile duct cancer. Langenbecks Arch Surg. 2012;397(6):861–7.
15. Park HJ, Kim SY, Kim HJ, Lee SS, Hong GS, Byun JH, Hong SM, Lee MG. Intraductal papillary neoplasm of the bile duct: clinical, imaging, and pathologic features. AJR Am J Roentgenol. 2018;211(1):67–75.
16. Lee MH, Katabathina VS, Lubner MG, Shah HU, Prasad SR, Matkowskyj KA, Pickhardt PJ. Mucin-producing cystic hepatobiliary neoplasms: updated nomenclature and clinical, pathologic, and imaging features. Radiographics. 2021;41(6):1592–610.
17. Lee CH, Chang CJ, Lin YJ, Yeh CN, Chen MF, Hsieh SY. Viral hepatitis-associated intrahepatic cholangiocarcinoma shares common disease processes with hepatocellular carcinoma. Br J Cancer. 2009;100(11):1765–70.
18. Horvat N, Nikolovski I, Long N, Gerst S, Zheng J, Pak LM, Simpson A, Zheng J, Capanu M, Jarnagin WR, Mannelli L, Do RKG. Imaging features of hepatocellular carcinoma compared to intrahepatic cholangiocarcinoma and combined tumor on MRI using liver imaging and data system (LI-RADS) version 2014. Abdom Radiol (NY). 2018;43(1):169–78.
19. Lee DH, Kim B, Lee ES, Kim HJ, Min JH, Lee JM, Choi MH, Seo N, Choi SH, Kim SH, Lee SS, Park YS, Chung YE. Korean Society of Abdominal Radiology. Radiologic evaluation and structured reporting form for extrahepatic bile duct cancer: 2019 consensus recommendations from the Korean Society of Abdominal Radiology. Korean J Radiol. 2021;22(1):41–62.
20. Riopel MA, Klimstra DS, Godellas CV, Blumgart LH, Westra WH. Intrabiliary growth of metastatic colonic adenocarcinoma: a pattern of intrahepatic spread easily confused with primary neoplasia of the biliary tract. Am J Surg Pathol. 1997;21(9):1030–6.

21. Lim JH, Kim KW, Choi D-i. Biliary tract and gallbladder. In: Haaga JR, Boll DT, editors. CT and MRI of the whole body. 6th ed. Philadelphia: Elsevier; 2017. p. 1192–267.

22. Smathers RL, Lee JK, Heiken JP. Differentiation of complicated cholecystitis from gallbladder carcinoma by computed tomography. AJR Am J Roentgenol. 1984;143:255–9.

23. Havrilla TR, Reich NE, Haaga JR, Seidelmann FE, Cooperman AM, Alfidi RJ. Computed tomography of the gallbladder. AJR Am J Roentgenol. 1978;130:1059–67.

24. Strax R, Toombs BD, Kam J, Rauschkolb EN, Patel S, Sandler CM. Gallbladder enhancement following angiography: a normal CT finding. J Comput Assist Tomogr. 1982;6:766–8.

25. Al-Fallouji MA. Perforated posterior peptic ulcer associated with gallbladder agenesis and midgut malrotation. Br J Clin Pract. 1983;37:353–6, 358.

26. Sheng H, Chen G, Yang M, Guan H. A proposed feasible classification of common bile duct duplications based on a newly described variant and review of existing literature. BMC Pediatr. 2022;22(1):647.

27. Chen X, Yi B. Triple gallbladder. J Pediatr. 2022;247:173–4.

28. Hopmann P, Tan E, Lo D. Multiseptate gallbladder presenting with biliary colic. J Surg Case Rep. 2022;2022(9):rjac417.

29. Kochhar R, Nagi B, Mehta SK, Gupta NM. ERCP diagnosis of a gallbladder diverticulum. Gastrointest Endosc. 1988;34:150–1.

30. Gore RM, Ghahremani GG, Joseph AE, Nemcek AA Jr, Marn CS, Vogelzang RL. Acquired malposition of the colon and gallbladder in patients with cirrhosis: CT findings and clinical implications. Radiology. 1989;171:739–42.

31. Brink JA, Ferrucci JT. Use of CT for predicting gallstone composition: a dissenting view. Radiology. 1991;178:633–4.

32. Tsai HM, Lin XZ, Chen CY, Lin PW, Lin JC. MRI of gallstones with different compositions. AJR Am J Roentgenol. 2004;182:1513–9.

33. Bennett GL, Balthazar EJ. Ultrasound and CT evaluation of emergent gallbladder pathology. Radiol Clin North Am. 2003;41:1203–16.

34. Paulson EK. Acute cholecystitis: CT findings. Semin Ultrasound CT MR. 2000;21:56–63.

35. Jacob H, Appelman R, Stein HD. Emphysematous cholecystitis. Am J Gastroenterol. 1979;71:325–30.

36. Jenkins M, Golding RH, Cooperberg PL. Sonography and computed tomography of hemorrhagic cholecystitis. AJR Am J Roentgenol. 1983;140:1197–8.

37. Mirvis SE, Vainright JR, Nelson AW, et al. The diagnosis of acute acalculous cholecystitis: a comparison of sonography, scintigraphy, and CT. AJR Am J Roentgenol. 1986;147:1171–5.

38. Koehler RE, Melson GL, Lee JK, Long J. Common hepatic duct obstruction by cystic duct stone: Mirizzi syndrome. AJR Am J Roentgenol. 1979;132:1007–9.

39. Kane RA, Jacobs R, Katz J, Costello P. Porcelain gallbladder: ultrasound and CT appearance. Radiology. 1984;152:137–41.

40. Jutras JA. Hyperplastic cholecystoses; Hickey lecture, 1960. Am J Roentgenol Radium Ther Nucl Med. 1960;83:795–827.

41. Hamrick RE Jr, Liner FJ, Hastings PR, Cohn I Jr. Primary carcinoma of the gallbladder. Ann Surg. 1982;195:270–3.

42. Yoshimitsu K, Honda H, Shinozaki K, et al. Helical CT of the local spread of carcinoma of the gallbladder: evaluation according to the TNM system in patients who underwent surgical resection. AJR Am J Roentgenol. 2002;179:423–8.

43. Mitropoulos FA, Angelopoulou MK, Siakantaris MP, et al. Primary non-Hodgkin's lymphoma of the gall bladder. Leuk Lymphoma. 2000;40:123–31.

44. Guida M, Cramarossa A, Gentile A, et al. Metastatic malignant melanoma of the gallbladder: a case report and review of the literature. Melanoma Res. 2002;12:619–25.

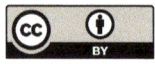

Diseases of the Pancreas

9

Thomas K. Helmberger and Riccardo Manfredi

Learning Objectives

- To understand typical imaging criteria to identify and differentiate solid and cystic pancreatic structural changes and neoplasia.
- To understand the limitations of imaging in complex pancreatic diseases and
- To appreciate the importance of additional clinical information.

Modern cross-sectional imaging with high spatial and contrast resolution allows a perfect delineation of the pancreas in its retroperitoneal home. The organ typically presents itself with a length between 12 and 15 cm and a diameter at the head area of about 2.5 cm, at the body of about 2 cm, and at the tip of the pancreatic tale of about 1.5 cm. Anatomically, the pancreatic head is defined as the area to the right of the left border of the superior mesenteric vein, the body as the area between the left border of the superior mesenteric vein and the left border of the aorta, and the tail as the area between left border of the aorta and the hilum of the spleen. The normal pancreatic duct ranges between 1.5 mm at the tail to 3 mm at the head.

Usually (ca. 60% of cases) the pancreatic main duct (duct of Wirsung), the duct of Santorini, and the common bile duct

The original version of the chapter has been revised. A correction to this chapter can be found at https://doi.org/10.1007/978-3-031-27355-1_22

T. K. Helmberger (✉)
Institute of Radiology, Neuroradiology and Minimal-Invasive Therapy, Muenchen Klinikum Bogenhausen, Academic Teaching Hospital, Technical University Munich, Munich, Germany
e-mail: thomas.helmberger@muenchen-klink.de

R. Manfredi (✉)
Diagnostic Radiology and General Interventional Radiology at Diagnostic Imaging, Oncological Radiotherapy and Haematology, Fondazione Policlinico Universitario "A. Gemelli"—IRCCS Università Cattolica del Sacro Cuore, Rome, Italy
e-mail: riccardo.manfredi@unicatt.it

join together within the pancreatic head, entering the duodenum via the papilla of Vater.

Several conditions that affect the function and integrity of the pancreas, as developmental anomalies, neoplastic and inflammatory diseases will be discussed.

9.1 Developmental Anomalies of the Pancreas

During embryogenesis, the pancreas is formed from a larger, dorsal bud (tail, body, parts of the head) and a small, ventral bud (rest of the head). The ventral bud migrates downwards dorsal from the dorsal bud. During the union of both the buds, the main pancreatic duct within the ventral bud ends via the duct of Santorini in the minor papilla. This duct gets then reduced to an accessory duct, whereas the main pancreatic duct of the dorsal bud merges with the duct of the former ventral bud ending in the major papilla [1, 2]. The disturbed union of the two buds can cause three major anomalies.

Pancreas divisum, a non-union anomaly of the pancreas is found in autopsy studies with a frequency of 1 to 14%, and is characterized by the separate drainage of the main pancreatic duct via the duct of Santorini into the minor papilla, and of the duct of Wirsung into the major papilla. Only 1% of individuals with pancreas divisum will develop unspecific abdominal symptoms (abdominal discomfort, most likely caused by recurrent episodes of mild pancreatitis). Therefore—without real proof—some authors consider pancreas divisum a promoting factor for pancreatic tumors based on recurrent and lately chronic focal pancreatitis [3].

In pancreas annulare, the-non-migration of the ventral bud of the pancreas causes the ventral and dorsal bud forming a ring around the duodenum. This rare anomaly (estimated prevalence 0.01%) can be associated with other birth deformities as congenital duodenal atresia, mesenterium commune, oral facial defects, and Down's syndrome. Clinical signs are determined by stenosis and occlusion of the duodenum.

To reveal a union/migration anomaly of the pancreas, in most of the cases MRCP will add the crucial information of the distorted duct configuration.

The generally asymptomatic ectopic pancreatic tissue can be found in the stomach, duodenum, and ileum, very rarely in Meckel's diverticulum, gall bladder, bile duct, and spleen, whereas autopsy studies reveal a frequency between 0.6 and 15%. Typically, pancreatic ectopic tissue is detected by endoscopy.

Total agenesis of the pancreatic gland, hypoplasia of the pancreas (partial agenesis), congenital pancreatic cysts (dysontogenetic cysts, hamartosis), multiple congenital cysts associated with von Hippel-Lindau disease (cysts also in the liver and kidneys), and also cystic degenerative transformation of the pancreas in cystic fibrosis are in general rare and are identified by MRI, as well as by sonography and CT, based on the partial or complete missing of the organ or by solitary or multiple cysts [2, 4].

> **Key Point**
> The majority of pancreatic anomalies are asymptomatic. MRI and MRCP are superior in identifying the structural variants and to exclude suspected neoplastic conditions.

9.2   Pancreatic Neoplasms

Pancreatic tumors can be classified according to their cellular origin, enzymatic activity, and their benign or malignant potential. The most recent WHO classification (2010, revised 2012 und 2017) divides pancreatic tumors into primary epithelial and mesenchymal tumors, lymphomas, and secondary tumors; from a clinical-practical point of view tumor like lesions can be added (Table 9.1). In clinical reality, many of the rare and very rare tumors have no specific imaging appearance and can be differentiated only pathologically.

9.2.1   Pancreatic Carcinoma

Exocrine pancreatic carcinoma arising from ductal, acinar, and their stem cells accounts for 85–95% of all malignant pancreatic tumors (15–20% in gastrointestinal malignancies, 3% in all carcinomas), whereas most of the various subtypes of pancreatic carcinoma can be differentiated only by histo- and immunopathology. In general, the tumors are located predominantly in the pancreatic head (60–70%; body: 15% and tail: 5%). A multifocal or diffuse tumor spread is uncommon. The prognosis is poor—slightly better in mucinous, non-cystic CA, and worse in adenosquamous CA—since

Table 9.1 Classification of pancreatic lesions modified according to WHO classification, Pancreas (modified according to [5] and the 2017 update for neuroendocrine tumors [6])

Epithelial tumors	
Benign	Acinar cell cystadenoma **Serous cystadenoma**, not otherwise specified (NOS)
Premalignant lesions	Pancreatic intraepithelial neoplasia, grade 3 (PanIN-3) Intraductal papillary mucinous neoplasm (IPMN) with low- or intermediate-grade dysplasia Intraductal papillary mucinous neoplasm (IPMN) with high-grade dysplasia Intraductal tubulopapillary neoplasm (ITPN) Mucinous cystic neoplasm (MCN) with low- or intermediate-grade dysplasia Mucinous cystic neoplasm (MCN) with high-grade dysplasia

Malignant lesions	**Ductal adenocarcinoma**
	    Adenosquamous carcinoma
	    Mucinous adenocarcinoma (colloid, non-cystic)
	    Hepatoid carcinoma
	    Medullary carcinoma, NOS
	    Signet ring cell carcinoma
	    Undifferentiated carcinoma
	    Undifferentiated carcinoma with osteoclast-like cells
	Acinar cell carcinoma
	Acinar cell cystadenocarcinoma
	Intraductal papillary mucinous carcinoma (IPMN) with an associated invasive carcinoma
	Mixed acinar-ductal carcinoma
	Mixed acinar-neuroendocrine carcinoma
	Mixed acinar-neuroendocrine-ductal carcinoma
	Mixed ductal-neuroendocrine carcinoma
	Mucinous cystic neoplasm (MCN) with an associated invasive carcinoma
	Pancreatoblastoma
	Serous cystadenocarcinoma, NOS
	Solid-pseudopapillary neoplasm

Neuroendocrine neoplasms	Nonfunctioning (nonsyndromic) neuroendocrine tumors (PanNEN G1/G2/G3)
	    Pancreatic neuroendocrine microadenoma
	    Non-functioning pancreatic neuroendocrine tumor
	Functioning (syndromic) neuroendocrine tumors (PanNEN G1/G2/G3)
	    Insulinoma
	    Glucagonoma
	    Somatostatinoma
	    Gastrinoma
	    VIPoma
	    Serotonin-producing tumors with and without carcinoid syndrome
	    ACTH-producing tumor with Cushing syndrome
	Pancreatic neuroendocrine carcinoma (PanNEC G3, poorly differentiated neuroendocrine neoplasm)
	Mixed neuroendocrine non-neuroendocrine neoplasms (MiNEN)
	    Mixed ductal neuroendocrine carcinoma
	    Mixed acinar neuroendocrine carcinoma

Table 9.1 (continued)

Epithelial tumors	
Mesenchymal tumors	Lymphangioma, NOS
	Lipoma, NOS
	Solitary fibrous tumor
	Ewing sarcoma
	Desmoplastic small round cell tumor
	Perivascular epithelioid cell neoplasm
Lymphomas	Diffuse large B-cell lymphoma (DLBCL), NOS
Secondary tumors	Metastases
Tumor-like lesions	Acute pancreatitis
	Chronic pancreatitis
	Groove pancreatitis
	Autoimmune pancreatitis
	Cystic lesions
	Pancreas divisum
	Pancreas annulare

most tumors are detected late in an advanced stage of spread. An early metastatic spread along perivascular, ductal, lymphatic, and perineural pathways is promoted by the absence of a true capsule around the organ.

For detection, staging and follow-up after treatment endoscopic ultrasound, contrast-enhanced CT, MRI, and FDG-PET may be applied, whereas endoscopic ultrasound presents the highest accuracy in detecting small pancreatic head and periampullary tumors, and FDG-PET in detecting distant metastatic spread. Nevertheless, CECT and MRI provide a sufficient and comprehensive display of the primary tumor and its sequalae with an accuracy of about 90% and even more [7–9].

The imaging appearance of common pancreatic adenocarcinoma is determined by its typically dense, fibrous, low vascularized stroma resulting in low soft-tissue density in CT and low signal on T1-weighted and T2-weighted in MRI, and no or only minor contrast enhancement (Fig. 9.1) what makes the tumors best delineable to the normal glandular parenchyma on CE-imaging.

The pancreatic duct maybe involved depending on the primary tumor localization within the pancreas ranging from no duct involvement at all in peripheral tumors, over segmental obstruction due to intraductal tumor invasion (duct penetrating sign), to obstruction of both pancreatic and common bile duct (double duct sign) in pancreatic head tumors.

The relation between tumor and ducts is non-invasively seen best on MRCP.

Assessing potential invasive local growth, metastatic spread to local and regional lymph nodes, to the liver, and vascular invasion, completes staging of pancreatic malignancies (Fig. 9.1).

Not well-defined tumor margins and blurred surroundings are still a challenge for every imaging modality since microscopic local invasive peritumoral spread and an inflammatory desmoplastic reaction can often not be differentiated causing over- or underestimation of the T-stage of the tumor [10].

At the time of diagnosis of the primary, about two thirds of the patients will present distant metastases (lymph node metastases 40%, hematogenous metastases to the liver 40%, peritoneal metastases 35%) which will be detected with accuracies above 90% by CE-MRI and FDG-PET-CT [11, 12]. Non-resectability in pancreatic cancer is determined by vascular encasement of the superior mesenteric artery, the celiac trunk, hepatic or splenic artery, and peripancreatic veins which is very likely if a vessel circumference is encased more than 50% (typical signs: decreased vessel caliber, dilated peripancreatic veins, teardrop shape of superior mesenteric vein present).

9.2.2 Other Tumors of Ductal Origin

This heterogeneous group of tumors embrace cystic neoplasms, tumors neuroendocrine components, and a variety of very rare tumors as pancreatoblastoma and solid-pseudopapillary neoplasm.

> **Key Point**
> Pancreatic adenocarcinoma is the most common malignancy of the pancreas. CT and MRI are the established imaging tools for diagnosing the primary, staging the extent of the disease and to establish operability.

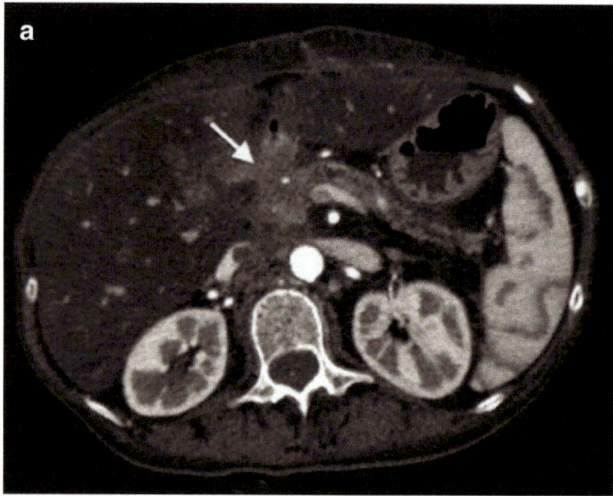 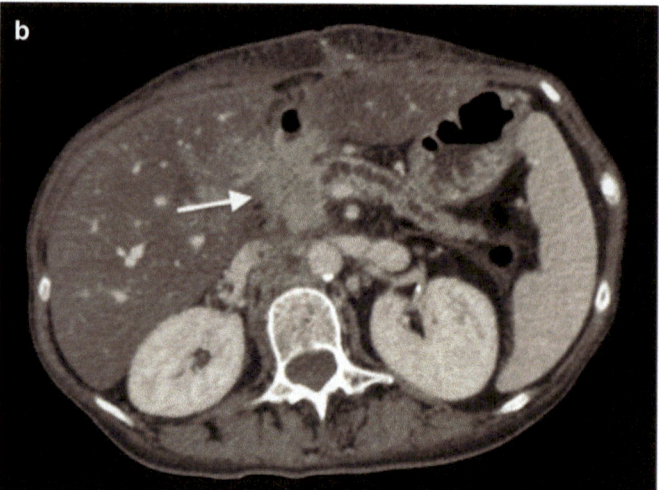

Fig. 9.1 (**a, b**) Adenocarcinoma of the head of the pancreas locally invasive. (**a**) Axial contrast-enhanced Computed Tomography (CT) during the pancreatic phase shows a hypovascular focal pancreatic lesion of the head, responsible of infiltration of the main pancreatic duct with obstructive chronic pancreatitis and infiltration of the peripancreatic fat (arrow). (**b**) Axial contrast-enhanced Computed Tomography (CT) during the portal venous phase shows infiltration of the posterior peripancreatic fat

9.3   Cystic Neoplasm

In modern high-resolution imaging, pancreatic cysts are a common finding by MRI (~20%) and CT (~3%). Due to the slightly increased risk of malignancy in incidental cysts, mainly in the younger than 65 of years, incidentally found pancreatic cysts have to be assessed carefully without exaggerating unnecessary therapeutical consequences [13, 14].

9.3.1   Serous Cystadenoma

Serous cystic neoplasms are accounting for about 50% of all cystic tumors including serous cystadenomas, serous oligocystic adenomas, cystic lesions in von Hippel-Lindau syndrome, and rarely serous cystadenocarcinomas [15, 16].

The most common subtype is the benign serous cystadenoma (microcystic type), typically in elderly women (60–80 years of age). In most cases, the lesion is located in the pancreatic head, composed of multiple tiny cysts, separated by thin septae. Spotty calcifications and a central stellate nidus might be present (Fig. 9.2).

About 10% of all serous cystic tumors present as an oligocystic variant with only a few cysts of 2 to 20 mm diameter and a higher prevalence in men (30–40 years).

The rare cystadenocarcinomas are usually large at clinical presentation already with local invasive growth and metastases to lymph nodes and liver.

The diagnosis of serous cystic lesions of the pancreas by imaging is ruled by the proportion of small cysts and septae without contrast enhancement what may create an almost solid impression in CT, whereas the cystic components still can be best appreciated by MRI. Even if the tumors can grow rather large the mismatch of tumor size, missing both ductal involvement and secondary signs of malignancy will direct to the right diagnosis.

For the differentiation of oligocystic adenomas from mucinous cystic tumors, IPMN or walled-off cysts tumor localization, an "empty" clinical history, and normal ducts in MRCP can be helpful [17, 18].

9.3.2   Mucinous Cystic Neoplasm (MCN)

Mucin-producing cystic tumors, typically in middle-aged women (f:m = 19:1), are characterized by a missing connection to the pancreatic ducts and the histological presence of an ovarian-like stroma. In comparison to SCN, MCN are less frequent (10% of all cystic pancreatic lesions), in general asymptomatic, detected as solitary, large lesions arising in the body and tail of the pancreas (95%), and composed of only few cysts with pronounced septae. Since the cysts may contain mucinous, hemorrhagic, necrotic, jelly-like content they may present intermediate and higher densities and signal intensities on CT and MRI whereas T2-weighted MRI displays the true cystic structure of the tumor the best. Nodular enhancement of

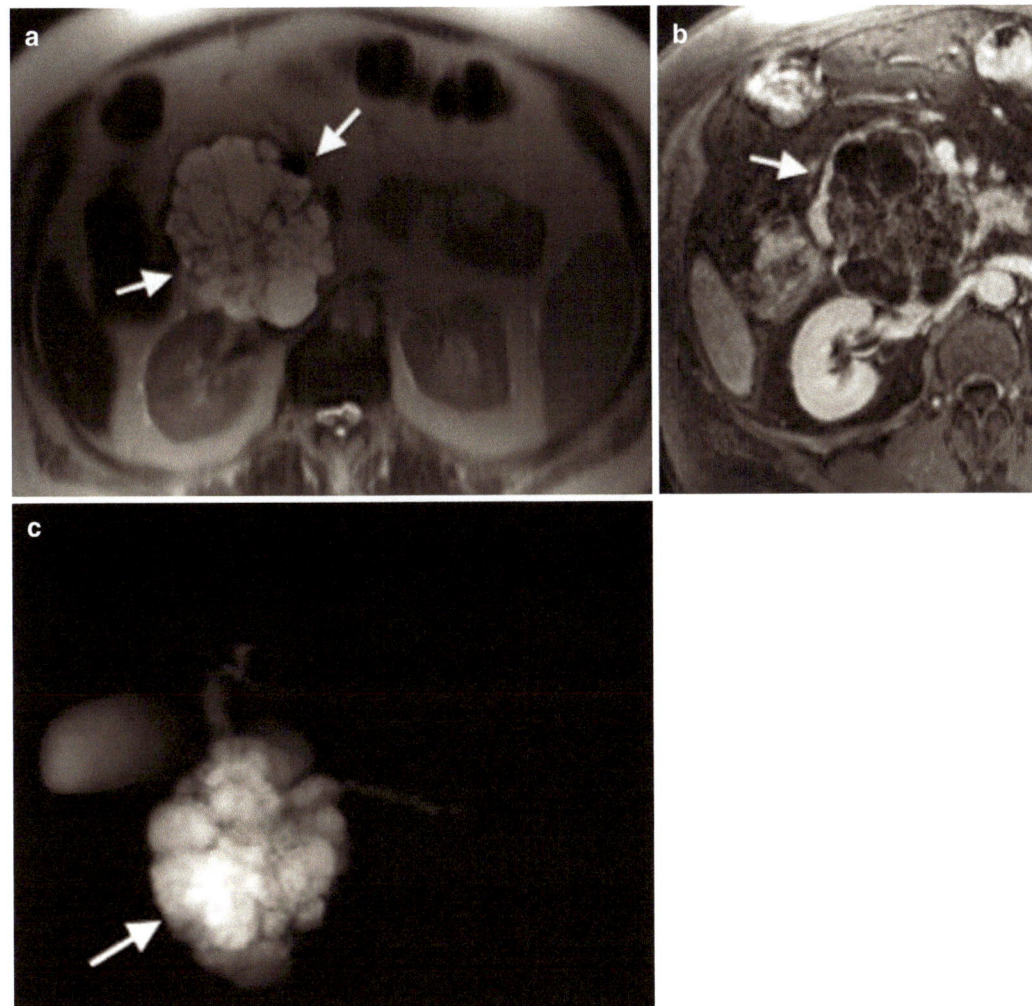

Fig. 9.2 (**a–c**) Serous cystadenoma. A) Axial T2-weighted Turbo Spin Echo image (TR/TE 4500/102) shows a multicystic microcystic neoplasm of the head of the pancreas (arrows). (**b**) On axial fat-saturated volumetric T1-weighted Gradient Echo image (TR/TE 4.86/1.87 ms) during the portal venous phase of the dynamic study following Gd-chelates administration serous cystadenoma shows enhancement of the internal septa and lack of a peripheral wall. (**c**) On the coronal MRCP image, single shot RARE (TR/TE ∞/110 ms), serous cystadenoma is responsible of compression of the main pancreatic duct with upstream dilatation

the septae is indicating potential malignancy which occurs in up to 30% of MCN [17–19].

9.3.3 Intraductal Papillary Mucinous Neoplasm (IPMN)

Due to increased detection rates by high-resolution imaging IPMN is considered the most common cystic neoplasm of the pancreas, seen more often in men than in women.

IPMNs may affect the main duct (28%), side branches (46%), or both duct components (26%) based on a mucin-producing neoplasm arising from the ductal epithelium. The side branch type can be found as a solitary or multifocal duct dilatation all over the pancreas and may also form a system of cystic dilated ducts that may mimic a microcystic appearance as in SCN. Segmental or general dilatation is typical for the main duct type creating a chronic pancreatitis like appearance. In such cases, patients' history is the crucial differential diagnostic information.

Since main duct type IPMN and MCN have a low malignant potential a thorough follow-up regimen should be recommend in non-surgical cases (Table 9.2).

Key Point
MRI is the superior imaging method allowing the detailed characterization of cystic lesions and neoplasia of the pancreas.

Table 9.2 Guideline recommendations for stratifying treatment and surveillance in pancreatic cystic lesions [20–25]

Guideline	High-risk stigmata indicating surgery in fit patients					Surveillance (in patients without worrisome features)	
	Symptoms	Size	Mural nodule	MPD	Cytology	Follow-up	Surveillance
WGO 2019 [25]	Jaundice, pancreatitis	≥3 cm growth rate ≥3 mm/year	Any	≥10 mm	+ high CA19.9	6–12 months for 1 year, then every 2 years, after 5 years, annually, if resources allow. Consider closer intervals for cysts >2 cm or if changes occur	As long as fit for surgery
Eu 2018 [24]	Jaundice, pancreatitis new diabetes mell.	≥4 cm growth rate ≥5 mm/year	>5 mm	≥10 mm	+ high CA19.9	EUS/MRI and CA 19-9 after 6 months then EUS/MRI and CA 19-9 yearly	Lifelong as long as fit for surgery
ACG 2018 [21]	Jaundice, pancreatitis new diabetes mell.	≥3 cm growth rate ≥3 mm/year	Any	≥5 mm	+ high CA19.9	Similar to ICG	Lifelong as long as fit for surgery. Not in older than 75 years
ICG 2017 [26]	Jaundice	Size alone is not appropriate	>5 mm	≥10 mm	+	<1 cm—CT/MRI in 2-3 years 1-2 cm—CT/MRI yearly × 2 then lengthen as appropriate *2–3 cm— EUS in 3–6 months then lengthen as appropriate *>3 cm—MRI/EUS every 3–6 months up to 1 year	Lifelong as long as fit for surgery
ACR 2017 [20]	Jaundice	Size-dependent growth rate of 50-100% in cysts ≤15 mm, of 20% in cysts >15 mm	Any	>7 mm	+	Similar to ICG	If stable up to 10 years or patient older than 80 years
AGA 2015 [22]	Na	Na	Any	Dilated	+	MRI after 1 year then MRI every 2 years	If stable up to 5 years

9.4 Other Neoplasm

9.4.1 Neuroendocrine Tumors

The WHO (2010, last modification 2017, unchanged in 2019) classified these tumors mainly according to their grading (well—moderately—poor differentiated) and their hormonal activity (PanNEN: pancreatic neuroendocrine neoplasm), as well as the Ki67 proliferative index.

In general, these tumors are rare and account for about 5–7% of all pancreatic tumors with the most common subtypes being insulinoma, glucagonoma, and nonhormonal active tumors. If a specific hormone release is not the leading clinical sign, also imaging features of various PanNEN are often rather similar what makes immuno-histochemical staining a crucial issue (Fig. 9.3) [27, 28].

9.4.1.1 Insulinoma

The presentation of insulinomas—the most common PanNEN (60%)—is determined by hyperinsulinism (Whipple triad: starvation attack, hypoglycemia after fasting, and relief by i.v. dextrose). The majority of tumors are solitary (95%), small (<2 cm), hypervascularized with a peripherally pronounced enhancement, and localized in the pancreatic body and tail [29].

9.4.1.2 Gastrinoma

Gastrinoma is the second most common PanNEN (20–30%) clinically associated with the Zollinger—Ellison syndrome (peptic ulcer disease, diarrhea) due to the massively elevated gastrin blood levels. At detection, the tumors usually present with a moderate size (mean 3 cm, ranging from 0.1–20 cm) and in half of the cases with multiple nodules. The vast majority of gastrinomas will arise within the gastrinoma triangle determined by the confluence of the cystic and common bile duct, the junction of the second and third portions of the duodenum, and the junction of the neck and body of the pancreas. On imaging, gastrinomas are revealed as mainly solid tumors with intermediate densities and signal intensities on both CT and MRI with moderate to strong contrast enhancement. Even if about 60% of the tumors are malignant, extensive metastatic spread is rare [30].

9.4.2 Other Rare Pancreatic Neoplasm

Beside the above displayed neoplasms, there is still a wide variety of pancreatic tumors which—in general—can be differentiated only by specific immunohistologic staining. This rare tumors comprise a number of variably differentiated neuroendocrine tumors inclusively mixed neuroendocrine non-

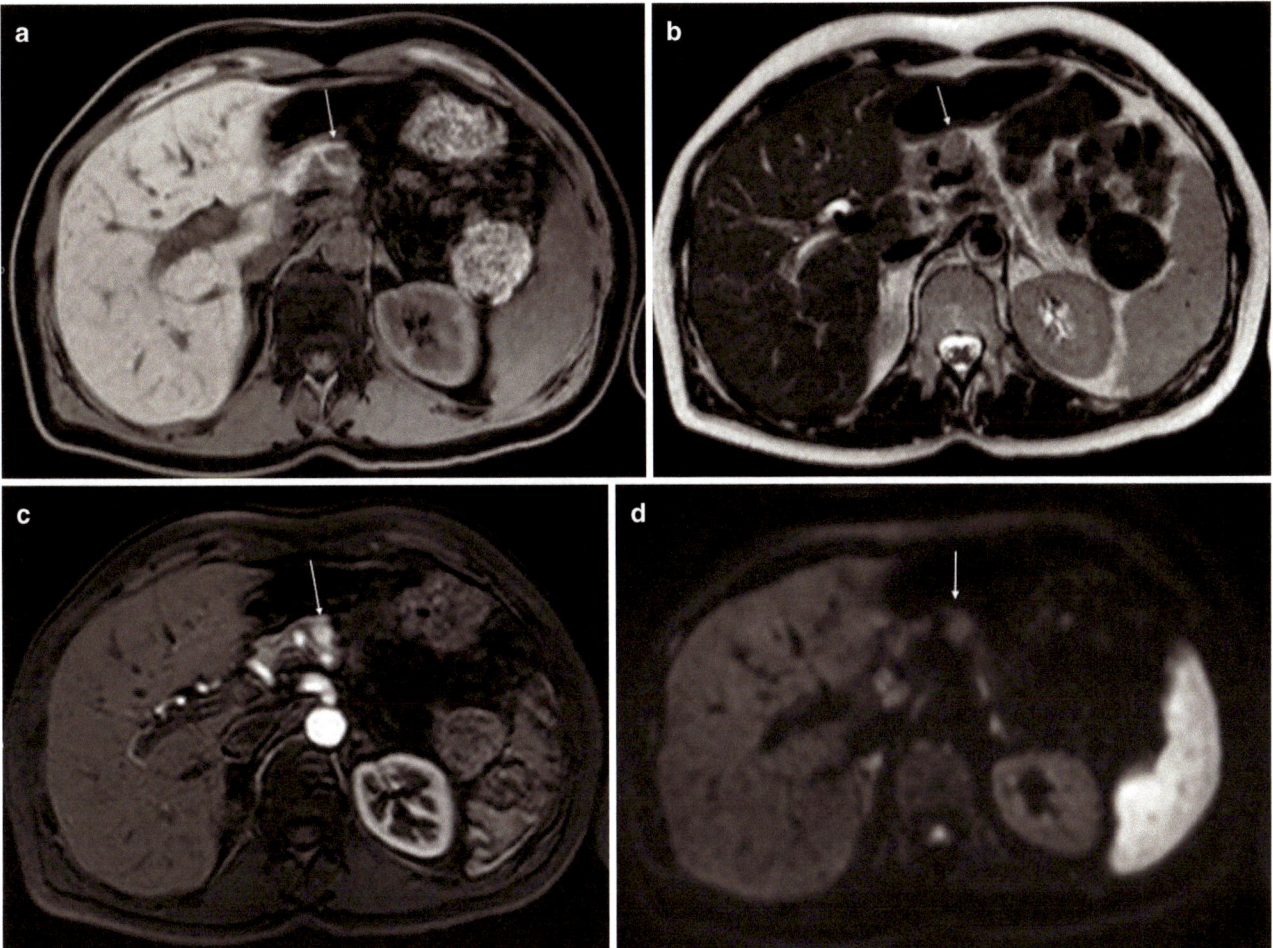

Fig. 9.3 (a–d) Small neuroendocrine neoplasm. (a) Axial T1-weighted Gradient Echo image (TR/TE 180/4.66 ms) with fat saturation shows a neuroendocrine neoplasm that appears hypointense compared to adjacent pancreatic parenchyma (arrow). (b) Axial T2-weighted Turbo Spin Echo image (TR/TE 4500/102) shows a small neuroendocrine neoplasm that appears hyperintense compared to adjacent parenchyma (arrow). (c) On the axial fat-saturated volumetric T1-weighted Gradient Echo image (TR/TE 4.86/1.87 ms) during the pancreatic phase of the dynamic study following Gd-chelates administration, the neuroendocrine neoplasms appear hyperintense compared to adjacent pancreatic parenchyma (arrow). (d) On axial diffusion-weighted image ($b = 1000$), the neuroendocrine neoplasms show restricted diffusion (arrow)

neuroendocrine tumors, mostly without functional activity, rare malignant pancreatoblastoma in children (a large, encapsulated tumor in the pancreatic head often associated with elevated alpha-fetoprotein levels and metastases to liver and lymph nodes), acinar cell carcinoma (relatively large tumors in elderly men with an imaging appearance similar to pancreatic adenocarcinomas and potential excessive release of serum lipase followed by focal panniculitis and polyarthritis as diagnostic hint), and solid pseudopapillary tumor (of mainly young women (frequently incidental tumor in women 20–30 years of age; m:f = 1:10; large, heterogenous tumor of uncertain dignity) and occasionally children) [31].

Mesenchymal tumors (sarcoma, cystic dermoid, lymphangioma, leiomyosarcoma, hemangiopericytoma, hemangioma, malignant fibrous histiocytoma, lymphoepithelial cysts, primary lymphoma) and secondary tumors (secondary lymphoma, metastases) of the pancreas are very rare and may be identified due to specific imaging features as peripheral nodular enhancement on dynamic imaging or high signal intensity in T1- and T2-weighted imaging as, for example, hemangioma or lipoma; otherwise, clinical context and histopathological proof will determine the diagnosis.

> **Key Point**
>
> PanNEN comprises a complex group of neoplasia which can be identified usually by imaging—beside very small tumors. Nevertheless, without clinical information and immune-histopathological correlation a precise diagnosis is not possible. In malignant transformation, the mismatch between tumor size and missing secondary signs of malignant spread as common in pancreatic cancer can be helpful.

9.5   Inflammatory Diseases of the Pancreas

9.5.1   Acute and Chronic Pancreatitis

Especially in the Western world the incidence of inflammatory diseases of the pancreas is increasing. The most common causes are biliary stone disease and alcohol abuse; nevertheless, a heterogenous variety of other causes as metabolic syndrome (hyperlipidemia types I, IV, V; hypercalcemia), drugs, infections, trauma (e.g., post surgery), and very rare conditions as alpha-1-antitrypsin deficiency, or mutations of protease serine (PRSS) and serine protease inhibitor Kazal type (SPINK1) has been identified as promoting factor. Depending on the type and severity of the

inflammatory process no, mild or extensive morphological and functional deterioration is seen.

In general, the task of imaging is to monitor substantial structural changes and complications in acute pancreatitis, as parenchymal integrity vs. necrosis, peripancreatic inflammation, subtle and substantial fluid collections, formation of pseudo cysts and walled-off cysts, vascular and ductal affections (Fig. 9.4), and to assist in the clinical outcome prognosis together with the clinical assessment [32–36].

In chronic pancreatitis differentiation of long-term parenchymal and ductal changes from similar changes caused by neoplasms—e.g., focal or complete duct dilation, focal parenchymal lesions, and cystic degeneration—is mandatory to rule out complications and potential pancreatic cancer (Fig. 9.5). Perfusion MRI, DWI, and FDG-PET can be helpful in such cases. Nevertheless, the common clinical presenta-

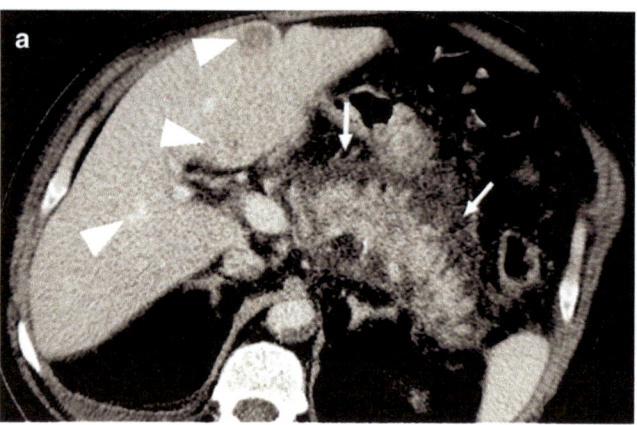
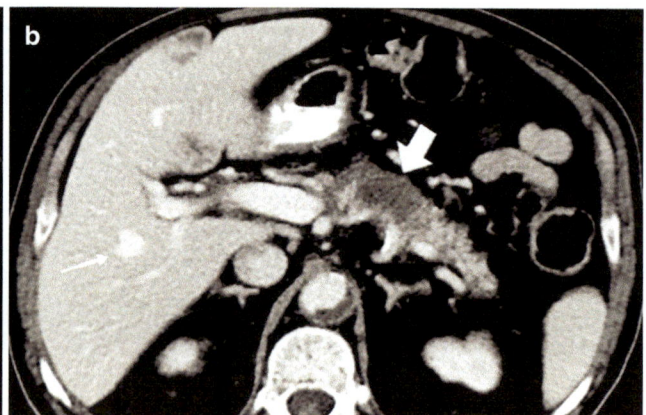
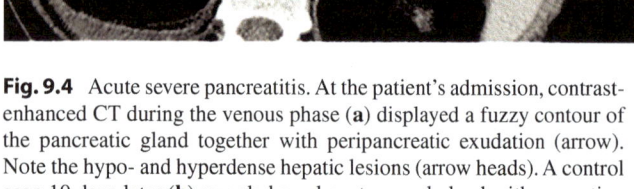

Fig. 9.4 Acute severe pancreatitis. At the patient's admission, contrast-enhanced CT during the venous phase (**a**) displayed a fuzzy contour of the pancreatic gland together with peripancreatic exudation (arrow). Note the hypo- and hyperdense hepatic lesions (arrow heads). A control scan 10 days later (**b**) revealed an almost normal gland with resorption

of the peripancreatic fluid. However, there was an area with a lack of enhancement representing focal necrosis (large arrow). In the liver, one lesion turned out to be a hemangioma (arrow) while the other two lesions were small abscesses

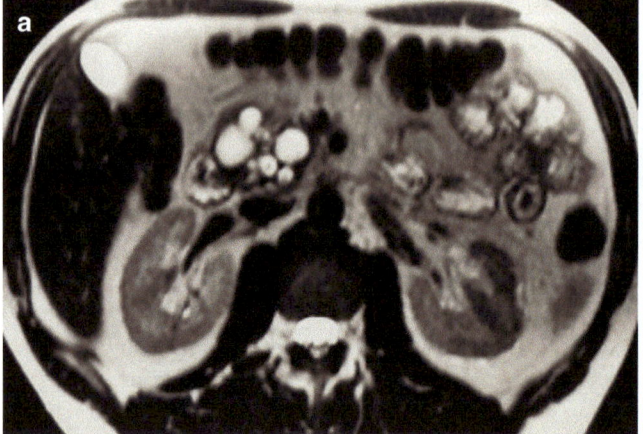
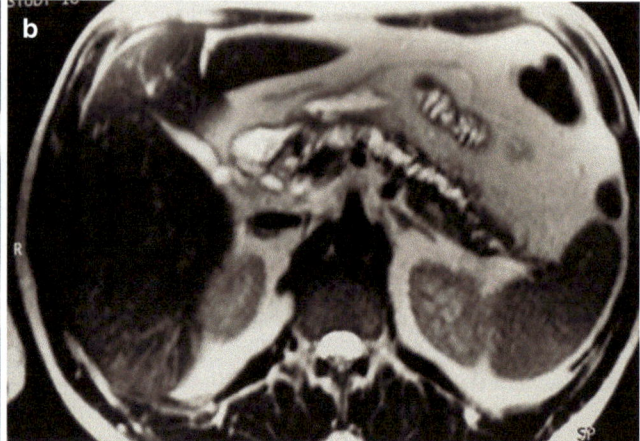

Fig. 9.5 Chronic pancreatitis. Cystic degeneration of the pancreatic head (**a**) together with irregular dilatation of the pancreatic main duct (**b**) in MRI (fastSE T2). Note the similar imaging appearance to other cystic lesions of the pancreas

tion with chronic abdominal pain in chronic pancreatitis does not correlate very well with imaging findings [35, 37–42].

9.5.2 Autoimmune Pancreatitis

In comparison to gall stone or alcohol-associated pancreatitis, autoimmune pancreatitis (AIP) is a rare disease in which the pathophysiological understanding has evolved significantly over the last years. The most common form, type 1 AIP is associated with IgG4-related diseases. Type 2 AIP is a different, even rarer entity and may be associated to chronic inflammatory bowel disease [43–45].

Both diseases have a similar clinical presentation with unspecific upper abdominal pain, obstructive jaundice, furthermore weight loss, and endo- and/or exocrine pancreatic insufficiency. Clinically, there is an overlap with pancreatic carcinoma, which cannot be solved by imaging alone since AIP may provide diffuse ("sausage" like) or focal ("mass forming") enlargement of the gland together with segmental or focal duct strictures or dilatation. In consequence, the task of imaging and further parameters as serology and histology is the differentiation of both entities to guide each to the appropriate therapy and to avoid the small number, but unnecessary pancreatectomies (Fig. 9.6).

The International Association of Pancreatology defined diagnostic consensus criteria (Table 9.3) which provide a high accuracy in identifying an AIP. Both types of AIP usually present an excellent response to steroid therapy, however, in Type 1 AIP 60% of patients will have relapse. Over the last years the body of knowledge in AIP was growing significantly, identifying also AIP not otherwise specified (NOS) not meeting the criteria for Type 1 or 2 AIP, and AIP in the context of IgG4-related disease (IgG4-RD) characterized by immune-mediated fibroinflammatory multi-organ involvement [46, 47].

> **Key Point**
> Acute and chronic pancreatitis are common diseases, whereas the diagnosis is ruled by the clinical history and/or presentation. Imaging adds the crucial information on the severity and complications of the disease. In AIP imaging findings contribute to the cardinal criteria, however, imaging alone is not suitable to establish the diagnosis in AIP.

> **Take-Home Message**
> Pancreatic lesions encompass a wide variety of anatomical variants as well as benign and malignant neoplastic, and inflammatory diseases. The specific anatomical position of the gland and patient-specific conditions allows often only limited insight by ultrasound and endoscopy. Therefore, cross-sectional imaging by CT and MRI is of ample importance in assessing the pancreas and related disorders, allowing for a very high accuracy in depicting structural alterations of the parenchymal and ductal components of the gland. In the majority of clinical-diagnostic situations, there is no significant difference between the two imaging modalities with respect to diagnostic efficacy. However, MRI will reveal its superiority particularly in conditions where the assessment of ductal and intra- and peripancreatic cystic structures as well as subtle parenchymal changes is pivotal.

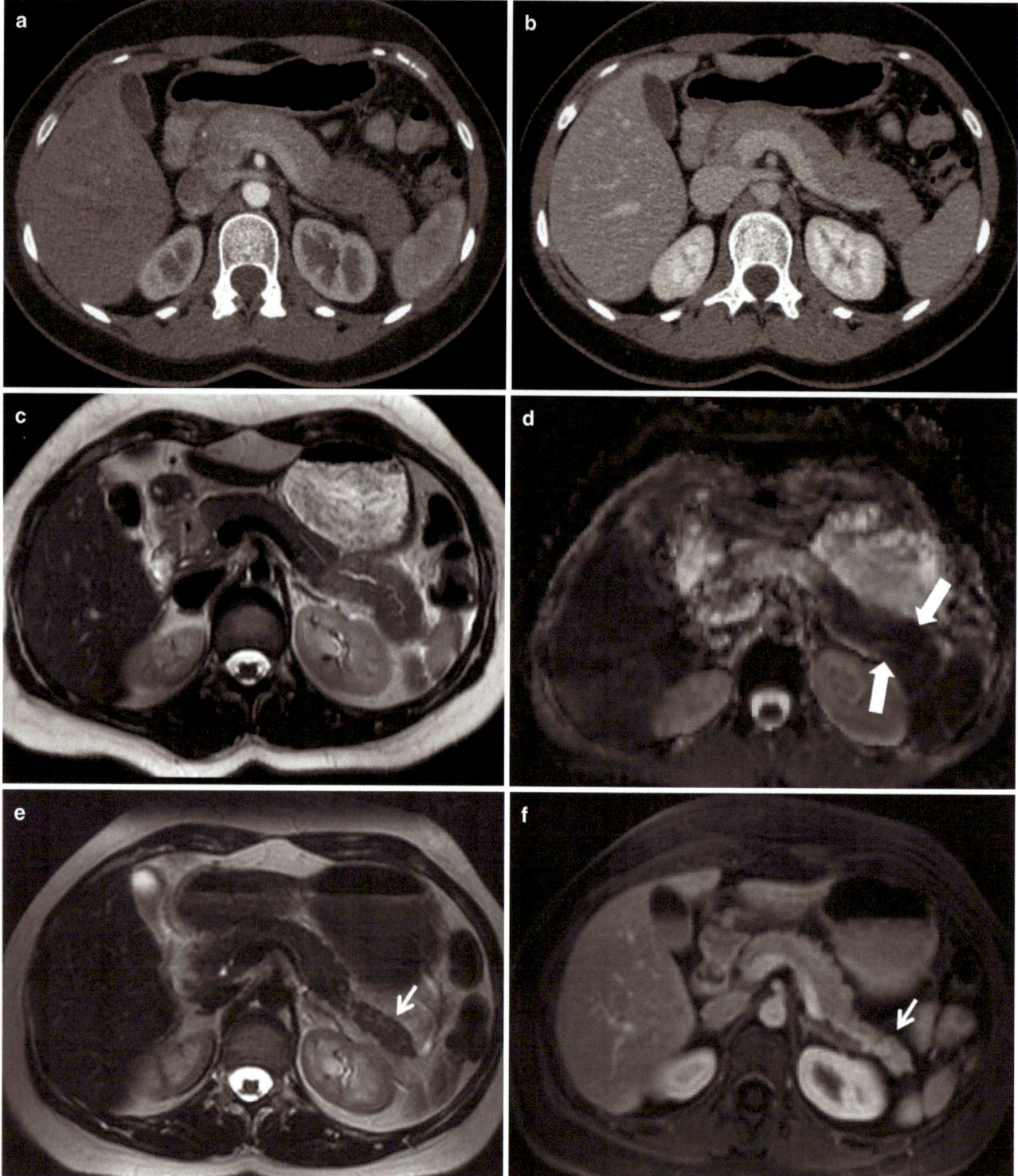

Fig. 9.6 AIP type 1. Well-demarcated focal enlargement of the pancreatic tail on CT (**a**, **b**). Note the slightly reduced perfusion in the early parenchymal phase (**a**). Low signal intensity on T2-weighted MRI (**c**) and diffusion restriction on DWI ADC Map (**d**) reveals the lymphoplasmatic infiltration with fibrotic components in contrast to edema in "usual" pancreatitis. After 6 weeks therapy with steroids, note the significant atrophy of the pancreatic tail on T2-weighted (**e**) and CE T1-weighted MRI (**f**)

Table 9.3 Revised consensus criteria in type 1 and type 2 AIP ([48–50] modified acc. to Shimosegawa et al. [51], and O'Reilly et al. [52]; L level, ERP endoscopic retrograde pancreatography, IgG4-RD IgG4-related disease, IBD inflammatory bowel disease, GEL granulocytic epithelial lesions)

	Type 1 AIP		Type 2 AIP	
Synonym	Lymphoplasmacellular sclerosing pancreatitis (LPSP)		Idiopathic ductal-centric pancreatitis (IDCP)	
Incidence	0.9/100.000			
Geographic frequency seiche	EU/USA 50%, Asia 95%		EU/USA 50%	
Age (years)	50–70		30–50	
Sex	M (75%) ≫ F		M = F	
Consensus Criteria of the International Association of Pancreatology [51]				
Cardinal criteria	Level 1	Level 2	Level 1	Level 2
Imaging: Parenchyma (P)	Typical: diffuse enlargement ("sausage sign"), delayed (interstitial) enhancement (sometimes capsule-like, nodular enhancement)	Indeterminate:: focal enlargement with delayed enhancement	Typical: diffuse enlargement ("sausage sign"), delayed (interstitial) enhancement (sometimes capsule-like, nodular enhancement)	Indeterminate:: focal enlargement with delayed enhancement atypical: hypodense in CT, duct dilatations, atrophy
Imaging: Pancreatic duct (D), validated for ERP; analogue interpretation in MRCP	Long (>1/3 of duct length) or multiple strictures (skip lesions) without proximal (upstream) dilatation, duct penetrating sign	Segmental/focal strictures with proximal (upstream) dilatation (<5 mm)	Long (>1/3 of duct length) or multiple strictures (skip lesions) without proximal (upstream) dilatation, duct penetrating sign	Segmental/focal strictures with proximal (upstream) dilatation (<5 mm)
Serology (S)	IgG4 >2 × upper limit	IgG4 1–2 × upper limit	–	–
Other organ involvement (OOI)	IgG4-related disease (RD) (50%) ≥3 histological findings in other organs: – Lymphoplasmatic cellular infiltrates and fibrosis without granulocytes – Storiform fibrosis – Obliterating phlebitis – IgG4-positive cells (>10/HPF) ≥1 radiological finding: – Segmental/multiple bile duct strictures – Retroperitoneal fibrosis IgG4-RD (ca. 60%) – Chronic-sclerosing sialadenitis (14–39%) – IgG4-assoc cholangitis (IAC) (12–47%) – IgG4-assoc tubulointerstitial nephritis and renal parenchymal lesions (35%) – Enlarged hilar pulmonary LN (8–13%) – Retroperitoneal fibrosis – Chronic thyroiditis – Prostatitis – Chronic inflammatory bowel disease (0.1–6%)	Bile duct involvement plus both – Lymphoplasmatic cellular infiltrates without granulocytes – IgG4-positive cells (>10/HPF) Or ≥1 criterion (imaging or clinical exam) – symmetric enlarged salivary glands – renal involvement	No association with IgG4-RD – Histological and/or clinical diagnosis of inflammatory bowel disease (16%) – Involvement of proximal bile duct possible – Involvement of thyroid possible	

(continued)

Table 9.3 (continued)

	Type 1 AIP		Type 2 AIP	
Histology (H), TruCut-biopsy or resection, EUS-FNB not suitable	Periductal lymphoplasmacellular infiltrations, inflammatory, cell-rich stroma			
	3 of 4 criteria – Storiform fibrosis – Obliterative phlebitis – Prominent lymphatic follicles – IgG4-positive plasma cell – No neoplastic cells detected and no signs of malignancy in imaging – No neoplastic cells detected by EUS-FNA	2 of 4 criteria – Storiform fibrosis – Obliterative phlebitis – Prominent lymphatic follicles – IgG4-positive plasma cells – No neoplastic cells detected and no signs of malignancy in imaging	– GEL with or without granulocytic acinar infiltration – No or few (10 <10 HPF) IgG4-positive plasma cells – No neoplastic cells detected and no signs of malignancy in imaging	– Granulocytic and lymphoplasmatic acinar infiltrate – No or few (>10 HPF) IgG4-positive plasma cells – No neoplastic cells detected and no signs of malignancy in imaging
Response to steroids (Rt)	Rapid ($\leq$2 weeks) response to therapy with significant improvement in imaging			
Relapse post steroids	20–60%		<10%	
Diagnosis based on criteria	Type 1 AIP		Type 2 AIP	
Definitive	Histo L1 + imaging L1/2 Imaging L1 + other criteria L1/2 Imaging L2 + $\geq$ 2 criteria L1 Steroid Response + Bildgebung L2 + 3 Kriterien L1 oder 4 Kriterien L2		Imaging L1/2 + Histo L1 or IBD + Histo L2 + response to steroids	
Probable	Imaging L2 + other criteria L2		Imaging L1/2 + Histo L2 + IBD + response to steroids	

References

1. Anupindi SA. Pancreatic and biliary anomalies: imaging in 2008. Pediatr Radiol. 2008;38(Suppl 2):S267–71.
2. Yu J, Turner MA, Fulcher AS, Halvorsen RA. Congenital anomalies and normal variants of the pancreaticobiliary tract and the pancreas in adults: part 1, biliary tract. AJR Am J Roentgenol. 2006;187(6):1536–43.
3. Nishino T, Toki F, Oi I, Oyama H, Hatori T, Shiratori K. Prevalence of pancreatic and biliary tract tumors in pancreas divisum. J Gastroenterol. 2006;41(11):1088–93.
4. Yu J, Turner MA, Fulcher AS, Halvorsen RA. Congenital anomalies and normal variants of the pancreaticobiliary tract and the pancreas in adults: part 2, pancreatic duct and pancreas. AJR Am J Roentgenol. 2006;187(6):1544–53.
5. Flejou JF. WHO classification of digestive tumors: the fourth edition. Ann Pathol. 2011;31(5 Suppl):S27–31.
6. Kim JY, Hong SM, Ro JY. Recent updates on grading and classification of neuroendocrine tumors. Ann Diagn Pathol. 2017;29:11–6.
7. Best LM, Rawji V, Pereira SP, Davidson BR, Gurusamy KS. Imaging modalities for characterising focal pancreatic lesions. Cochrane Database Syst Rev. 2017;4:CD010213.
8. Krishna SG, Rao BB, Ugbarugba E, Shah ZK, Blaszczak A, Hinton A, et al. Diagnostic performance of endoscopic ultrasound for detection of pancreatic malignancy following an indeterminate multidetector CT scan: a systemic review and meta-analysis. Surg Endosc. 2017;31(11):4558–67.
9. Xu MM, Sethi A. Imaging of the pancreas. Gastroenterol Clin N Am. 2016;45(1):101–16.
10. Swords DS, Firpo MA, Johnson KM, Boucher KM, Scaife CL, Mulvihill SJ. Implications of inaccurate clinical nodal staging in pancreatic adenocarcinoma. Surgery. 2017;162(1):104–11.
11. Allen PJ, Kuk D, Castillo CF, Basturk O, Wolfgang CL, Cameron JL, et al. Multi-institutional validation study of the American Joint Commission on Cancer (8th edition) changes for T and N staging in patients with pancreatic adenocarcinoma. Ann Surg. 2017;265(1):185–91.
12. Joo I, Lee JM, Lee DH, Lee ES, Paeng JC, Lee SJ, et al. Preoperative assessment of pancreatic cancer with FDG PET/MR imaging versus FDG PET/CT plus contrast-enhanced multidetector CT: a prospective preliminary study. Radiology. 2017;282(1):149–59.
13. Chiang AL, Lee LS. Clinical approach to incidental pancreatic cysts. World J Gastroenterol. 2016;22(3):1236–45.
14. Del Chiaro M, Verbeke C. Cystic tumors of the pancreas: opportunities and risks. World J Gastrointest Pathophysiol. 2015;6(2):29–32.
15. Doulamis IP, Mylonas KS, Kalfountzos CE, Mou D, Haj-Ibrahim H, Nasioudis D. Pancreatic mucinous cystadenocarcinoma: epidemiology and outcomes. Int J Surg. 2016;35:76–82.
16. Reid MD, Choi HJ, Memis B, Krasinskas AM, Jang KT, Akkas G, et al. Serous neoplasms of the pancreas: a clinicopathologic analysis of 193 cases and literature review with new insights on macrocystic and solid variants and critical reappraisal of so-called "serous cystadenocarcinoma". Am J Surg Pathol. 2015;39(12):1597–610.
17. Esposito I, Schlitter AM, Sipos B, Kloppel G. Classification and malignant potential of pancreatic cystic tumors. Pathologe. 2015;36(1):99–112; quiz 3–4.
18. Ketwaroo GA, Mortele KJ, Sawhney MS. Pancreatic cystic neoplasms: an update. Gastroenterol Clin N Am. 2016;45(1):67–81.
19. Manfredi R, Ventriglia A, Mantovani W, Mehrabi S, Boninsegna E, Zamboni G, et al. Mucinous cystic neoplasms and serous cystadenomas arising in the body-tail of the pancreas: MR imaging characterization. Eur Radiol. 2015;25(4):940–9.
20. Megibow AJ, Baker ME, Morgan DE, Kamel IR, Sahani DV, Newman E, et al. Management of Incidental Pancreatic Cysts: a white paper of the ACR incidental findings committee. J Am Coll Radiol. 2017;14(7):911–23.

21. Elta GH, Enestvedt BK, Sauer BG, Lennon AM. ACG clinical guideline: diagnosis and management of pancreatic cysts. Am J Gastroenterol. 2018;113(4):464–79.

22. Tanaka M. International consensus on the management of intraductal papillary mucinous neoplasm of the pancreas. Ann Transl Med. 2015;3(19):286.

23. Adamova D, Aggarwal MM, Aglieri Rinella G, Agnello M, Agrawal N, Ahammed Z, et al. Production of sigma (1385)± and theta (1530)0 in p–pb collisions at $\sqrt{s_{NN}}$ = 5.02 TeV. Eur Phys J C Part Fields. 2017;77(6):389.

24. European study group on cystic tumours of the P. European evidence-based guidelines on pancreatic cystic neoplasms. Gut. 2018;67(5):789–804.

25. WGO practice guideline: pancreatic cystic lesions; 2019. https://www.worldgastroenterology.org/guidelines/pancreatic-cystic-lesions/pancreatic-cystic-lesions-english

26. Tanaka M, Fernandez-Del Castillo C, Kamisawa T, Jang JY, Levy P, Ohtsuka T, et al. Revisions of international consensus Fukuoka guidelines for the management of IPMN of the pancreas. Pancreatology. 2017;17(5):738–53.

27. Manfredi R, Bonatti M, Mantovani W, Graziani R, Segala D, Capelli P, et al. Non-hyperfunctioning neuroendocrine tumours of the pancreas: MR imaging appearance and correlation with their biological behaviour. Eur Radiol. 2013;23(11):3029–39.

28. De Robertis R, Cingarlini S, Tinazzi Martini P, Ortolani S, Butturini G, Landoni L, et al. Pancreatic neuroendocrine neoplasms: magnetic resonance imaging features according to grade and stage. World J Gastroenterol. 2017;23(2):275–85.

29. Dromain C, Deandreis D, Scoazec JY, Goere D, Ducreux M, Baudin E, et al. Imaging of neuroendocrine tumors of the pancreas. Diagn Interv Imaging. 2016;97(12):1241–57.

30. Tamm EP, Bhosale P, Lee JH, Rohren EM. State-of-the-art imaging of pancreatic neuroendocrine tumors. Surg Oncol Clin N Am. 2016;25(2):375–400.

31. Barral M, Faraoun SA, Fishman EK, Dohan A, Pozzessere C, Berthelin MA, et al. Imaging features of rare pancreatic tumors. Diagn Interv Imaging. 2016;97(12):1259–73.

32. Banks PA. Acute pancreatitis: landmark studies, management decisions, and the future. Pancreas. 2016;45(5):633–40.

33. Sahu B, Abbey P, Anand R, Kumar A, Tomer S, Malik E. Severity assessment of acute pancreatitis using CT severity index and modified CT severity index: correlation with clinical outcomes and severity grading as per the revised Atlanta classification. Indian J Radiol Imaging. 2017;27(2):152–60.

34. Tyberg A, Karia K, Gabr M, Desai A, Doshi R, Gaidhane M, et al. Management of pancreatic fluid collections: a comprehensive review of the literature. World J Gastroenterol. 2016;22(7):2256–70.

35. Gupta P, Dawra S, Chandel K, Samanta J, Mandavdhare H, Sharma V, et al. Fat-modified computed tomography severity index (CTSI) is a better predictor of severity and outcome in patients with acute pancreatitis compared with modified CTSI. Abdom Radiol (NY). 2020;45(5):1350–8.

36. Gupta P, Kumar MP, Verma M, Sharma V, Samanta J, Mandavdhare H, et al. Development and validation of a computed tomography index for assessing outcomes in patients with acute pancreatitis: "SMART-CT" index. Abdom Radiol (NY). 2021;46(4):1618–28.

37. Anaizi A, Hart PA, Conwell DL. Diagnosing chronic pancreatitis. Dig Dis Sci. 2017;62(7):1713–20.

38. DiMagno EP, DiMagno MJ. Chronic pancreatitis: landmark papers, management decisions, and future. Pancreas. 2016;45(5):641–50.

39. Dominguez-Munoz JE, Drewes AM, Lindkvist B, Ewald N, Czako L, Rosendahl J, et al. Recommendations from the united European gastroenterology evidence-based guidelines for the diagnosis and therapy of chronic pancreatitis. Pancreatology. 2018;18(8):847–54.

40. Dominguez-Munoz JE, Drewes AM, Lindkvist B, Ewald N, Czako L, Rosendahl J, et al. Corrigendum to "Recommendations from the United European Gastroenterology evidence-based guidelines for the diagnosis and therapy of chronic pancreatitis" [Pancreatology 18(8) (2018) 847–854]. Pancreatology. 2020;20(1):148.

41. Lohr JM, Dominguez-Munoz E, Rosendahl J, Besselink M, Mayerle J, Lerch MM, et al. United European gastroenterology evidence-based guidelines for the diagnosis and therapy of chronic pancreatitis (HaPanEU). United European Gastroenterol J. 2017;5(2):153–99.

42. Park WG. Clinical chronic pancreatitis. Curr Opin Gastroenterol. 2016;32(5):415–21.

43. Manfredi R, Frulloni L, Mantovani W, Bonatti M, Graziani R, Pozzi MR. Autoimmune pancreatitis: pancreatic and extrapancreatic MR imaging-MR cholangiopancreatography findings at diagnosis, after steroid therapy, and at recurrence. Radiology. 2011;260(2):428–36.

44. Madhani K, Farrell JJ. Autoimmune pancreatitis: an update on diagnosis and management. Gastroenterol Clin N Am. 2016;45(1):29–43.

45. Vasaitis L. IgG4-related disease: a relatively new concept for clinicians. Eur J Intern Med. 2016;27:1–9.

46. de Pretis N, Vieceli F, Brandolese A, Brozzi L, Amodio A, Frulloni L. Autoimmune pancreatitis not otherwise specified (NOS): clinical features and outcomes of the forgotten type. Hepatobiliary Pancreat Dis Int. 2019;18(6):576–9.

47. Yoo BW, Song JJ, Park YB, Lee SW. 2019 American College of Rheumatology/European league against rheumatism classification criteria for IgG4-related disease by Wallace et al. Ann Rheum Dis. 2020;

48. Okazaki K, Kawa S, Kamisawa T, Ikeura T, Itoi T, Ito T, et al. Amendment of the Japanese consensus guidelines for autoimmune pancreatitis, 2020. J Gastroenterol. 2022;57(4):225–45.

49. Kawa S, Kamisawa T, Notohara K, Fujinaga Y, Inoue D, Koyama T, et al. Japanese clinical diagnostic criteria for autoimmune pancreatitis, 2018: revision of Japanese clinical diagnostic criteria for autoimmune pancreatitis, 2011. Pancreas. 2020;49(1):e13–e4.

50. Umehara H, Okazaki K, Kawa S, Takahashi H, Goto H, Matsui S, et al. The 2020 revised comprehensive diagnostic (RCD) criteria for IgG4-RD. Mod Rheumatol. 2021;31(3):529–33.

51. Shimosegawa T, Chari ST, Frulloni L, Kamisawa T, Kawa S, Mino-Kenudson M, et al. International consensus diagnostic criteria for autoimmune pancreatitis: guidelines of the International Association of Pancreatology. Pancreas. 2011;40(3):352–8.

52. O'Reilly DA, Malde DJ, Duncan T, Rao M, Filobbos R. Review of the diagnosis, classification and management of autoimmune pancreatitis. World J Gastrointest Pathophysiol. 2014;5(2):71–81.

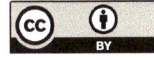

Adrenal Diseases

10

Isaac R. Francis and William W. Mayo-Smith

10.1 Introduction

Learning Objectives
- Provide an overview for the evaluation of an adrenal mass in various clinical scenarios
- Provide an understanding of the different imaging techniques and procedures available for the detection and characterization of adrenal masses
- Understand the differentiating features between benign and malignant adrenal masses
- Outline the current recommendations and limitations of European and US clinical practice guidelines for incidental adrenal masses, including treatment options

In this chapter, we will define an adrenal "incidentaloma," describe imaging techniques and procedures used to evaluate adrenal masses, discuss hyperfunctioning lesions/tumors of the gland, and illustrate these with examples, as well as outline current clinical practice guidelines for incidental and functioning adrenal masses including treatment options.

When an adrenal nodule/mass is detected on imaging, its appearance as well as some detailed history as listed below may help at arriving at an initial list of diagnoses.

1. Presence of morphological/internal features such as presence of macroscopic fat, fluid density, or other specific features?

I. R. Francis (✉)
Department of Radiology, Michigan Medicine,
Ann Arbor, MI, USA
e-mail: ifrancis@umich.edu

W. W. Mayo-Smith
Department of Radiology, Brigham and Women's Hospital,
Boston, MA, USA
e-mail: wmayo-smith@bwh.harvard.edu

2. Known underlying or history of a prior malignancy?
3. Stability of adrenal mass compared to prior imaging exams
4. Adrenal hyperfunction

This chapter will be divided into:

(1) The incidental adrenal mass in non-oncology, (2) the adrenal mass detected in patients with an underlying malignancy, and (3) Imaging evaluation in patients suspected of harboring hyperfunctioning adrenal lesions.

10.2 Incidental Adrenal Mass: No Underlying Malignancy

An adrenal incidentaloma can be defined as "an unsuspected and asymptomatic mass (measuring ≥1 cm in short axis) detected on imaging exams obtained for purposes other than detection of adrenal disease."

The overwhelming majority of incidentalomas are benign, i.e., non-functioning adrenal cortical adenomas [1, 2]. Other common benign adrenal masses include myelolipoma, cyst, and adrenal hemorrhage, neurogenic tumors among other rare lesions. If an adrenal incidentaloma has >50% of macroscopic fat [myelolipoma as shown in Fig. 10.1a, b] or features of a simple cyst (≤20 HU increase on enhanced CT compared to unenhanced CT), these are specific diagnosis, for which no additional workup or follow-up imaging is needed, except in cases of large myelolipomas which are being managed conservatively, some of which may grow and undergo hemorrhage, and therefore need follow-up imaging. Variable amounts of macroscopic fat can be seen in myelolipomas, with a small amount also seen in degenerated adenomas and rarely in adrenal cancers [3–4]. If an adrenal mass is of high density (higher than that of paraspinal musculature) on unenhanced images and shows <10 HU change between

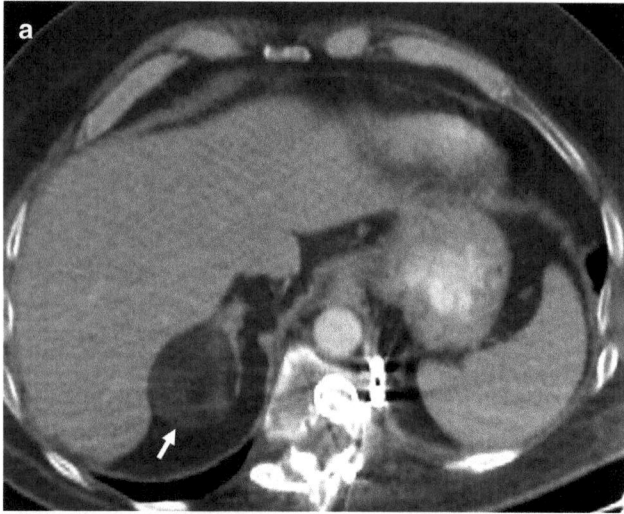

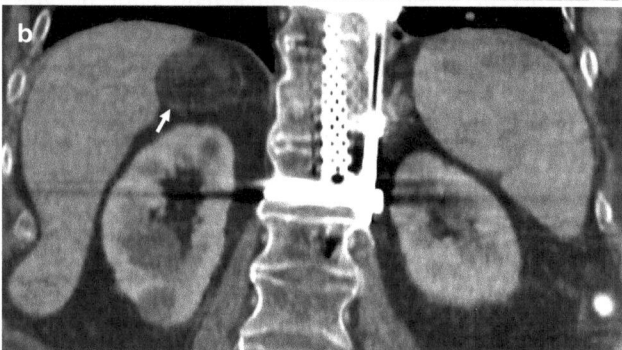

Fig. 10.1 (**a, b**) Contrast-enhanced CT image shows heterogenous mass (arrow) containing macroscopic fat diagnostic of a myelolipoma

pre- and post-contrast enhanced images, the possibility of adrenal hemorrhage should be suspected in the appropriate clinical setting. Follow-up imaging is essential to exclude hemorrhage into an underlying tumor, except when the hemorrhage is due to trauma or stress such as surgery [5].

There are two features of adenomas that are helpful in their characterization on CT and MRI: (1) the presence of intracellular lipid—low density on unenhanced CT, and loss of signal intensity and chemical shift (CSI) out-of-phase (OOP) MRI and (2) CT contrast washout features—rapid washout on contrast-enhanced CT.

10.2.1 Unenhanced CT

Most incidental adenomas are lipid-rich adenomas (measuring ≤10 HU on unenhanced CT) although between 20%–30%, are lipid-poor adenomas measuring >10 HU [6, 7]. Unenhanced CT density measurement of ≤10HU is highly specific (>95%) for the diagnosis of adenoma; however, some studies have shown that even higher density numbers could be used to diagnose benign adrenal lesions [8, 9]. In a recent study of 250 patients with incidental adrenal masses,

who either underwent surgery or follow-up for at least 1 year, it was shown that even if the density threshold on unenhanced CT was raised to <20 HU for lesions <3 cm, and <15 HU for lesions <4 cm, a specificity of 100% for predicting benign lesions could be achieved [8]. However, this threshold, currently lacks sufficient evidence for routine clinical use.

10.2.2 CT Contrast-Washout

Although a threshold of ≤10 HU is used to diagnose lipid-rich adenomas, lipid-poor adenomas do not contain adequate lipid and cannot be diagnosed by non-contrast CT using this threshold as there is overlap in density with primary malignancies and metastases.

As an alternative imaging strategy, differences in CT contrast enhancement and washout, can be used to diagnose non-hypervascular adenomas and differentiate them from metastases. Lipid-rich and lipid-poor adenomas both have rapid washout with intravenous contrast (iodinated CT contrast or MR gadolinium chelates) whereas most metastases do not [7, 10, 11]. Using density measurements, from images obtained at various time points after injection of intravenous contrast, washout calculations can be performed.

Absolute percent washout (APW) % values are calculated by the formula:

$$\frac{HU\ at\ dynamic\left(60-70\ s\right)CT - HU\ at\ non\ contrast\ CT}{HU\ at\ 15\ min\ delayed\ CT - HU\ at\ non\ contrast\ CT} \times 100$$

A threshold washout value ≥60% is diagnostic of an adenoma.

Relative percent washout (RPW) % can be used when a non-contrast CT is not available, and the dynamic enhanced values are compared to 15-min delayed scans. RPW % is calculated by the formula:

$$\frac{HU\ dynamic\ CT\left(60-70\ s\right) - HU\ 15\ min\ delayed\ CT}{HU\ dynamic\ CT} \times 100$$

A threshold washout value ≥40% is diagnostic of adenoma.

Specificity for adenoma diagnosis using these washout threshold values was >90%, when first reported in a few small studies that compared adenomas with small numbers of metastases and other malignant lesions, i.e., not incidentalomas [7, 10, 11]. A more recent study of 336 incidentalomas in 299 patients, however showed that for differentiating benign from malignant adrenal nodules (including pheochromocytomas) absolute CT contrast-washout % had a sensitivity of only 77.5% and specificity of 70% [12, 13], as some metastatic hypervascular nodules such as from clear cell renal cell cancer (CCRCC) and hepatocellular carcinoma

(HCC), as well approximately 20–30% pheochromocytomas had washout values like adenomas [14, 15]. So, the routine use of CT washout to distinguish between benign and malignant adrenal nodules in incidentally discovered adrenal lesions has limitations but may still be useful in the setting of oncology patients.

10.2.3 Dual Energy CT

Dual energy CT has also been used to characterize lipid-rich adenomas using density measurements from virtual unenhanced images, but this has slightly lower specificity than conventional unenhanced density measurements, as there is a tendency for the technique to overestimate the native unenhanced attenuation values due to incomplete iodine subtraction [16].

10.2.4 MRI

Chemical-shift MRI[CSI-MRI] or out-of-phase (OOP) images can detect of intracellular lipid and diagnose lipid-rich adenomas with a high degree of specificity, demonstrating loss of signal intensity on OOP images as shown in Fig. 10.2a, b. In a meta-analysis study of 1280 adrenal nodules, CSI-MRI, had a pooled sensitivity of 94% and specificity of 95% [17]. However, this high specificity diminishes with lipid-poor adenomas, especially those whose unenhanced CT density exceeds 30 HU [18]. Intracellular lipid-containing metastases from clear cell renal cell carcinoma (CCRCC) and some hepatocellular carcinomas [HCC] [19], can mimic adenomas on CSI-MRI. But imaging characteristics on other sequences, such as increased signal intensity

and lesion heterogeneity on T2 images can be used to distinguish these metastases from adenomas [20]. Importantly, these two primary neoplasms (CCRCC, HCC) often have a known primary and other coexisting metastatic disease.

More recently diffusion-weighted imaging has been used to try and differentiate between adenomas and malignant masses, but with limited success [21].

10.2.5 FDG PET/CT

FDG-PET/CT is used as a secondary tool to exclude adrenal malignancy using the SUV max tumor/liver ratio and based on the results of a study of non-cancerous patients found that a threshold of less than 1.5, was suggestive of a benign lesion [22, 23]. Adrenal metastases tend to demonstrate increased metabolic activity, with higher tracer uptake relative to the liver or background, while most benign adenomas do not. This imaging technique has extremely high sensitivity, but the specificity is lower (87–97%), as few adenomas can have mildly increased FDG uptake, mimicking malignant lesions [22, 23].

10.2.6 Lesion Morphology

Risk factors for malignancy include lesion size, and characteristics such as enhancement, heterogeneity, irregular margins, interval change in size, as well as prior a history of malignancy. Current management guidelines used data that suggested the risk of adrenal cortical carcinoma (ACC) based on size was 2%, 6%, and 24% for lesions <4 cm, 4–6 cm, and >6 cm, respectively [24–26]. But a recent study of risk assessment in 2219 patients found that the risk is much lower being

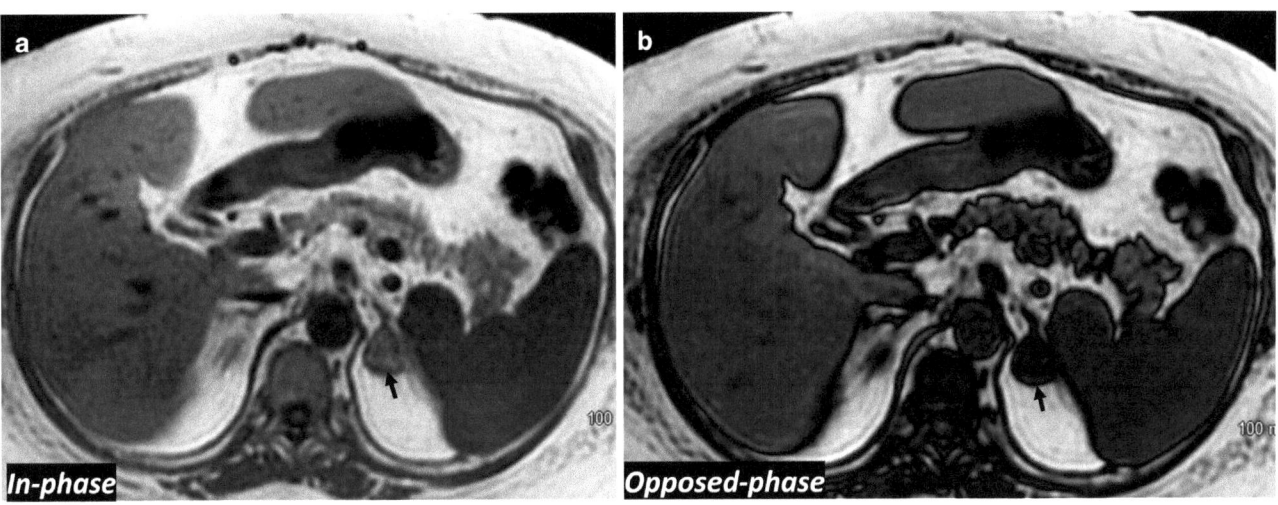

Fig. 10.2 (**a**) MR in-phase image shows a small homogeneous left adrenal mass (arrow). (**b**) Opposed-phase MR image shows diffuse loss of signal in left adrenal mass (arrow) diagnostic of a lipid-rich adenoma

0.1%, 2.4%, and 19.5% risk for lesions <4 cm, between 4 and 6 cm, and >6 cm, respectively [27]. However, in addition to size, a patient's age should also be taken into consideration when risk of ACC is assessed, as incidentalomas are uncommon in patients <40 years. of age and in these patients, additional evaluation to exclude a malignancy is warranted. Lesion characteristics such as margin, heterogeneity, contrast enhancement, have high specificity for the diagnosis of malignant lesions, but the low sensitivity precludes routine application in clinical practice [28].

10.2.7 Adrenal Biopsy

Non-invasive imaging as described above has been employed to successfully characterize most incidentally discovered adrenal masses. Adrenal biopsy is usually employed to definitively diagnose metastatic disease and stage patients with suspected malignancy. It is not recommended in patients with incidental indeterminate adrenal masses, as (1) the diagnosis of adrenal cortical cancer cannot be made definitively with percutaneous needle biopsies, and (2) in cases, where a pheochromocytoma has not been excluded by biochemical evaluation, a biopsy can precipitate an adrenal crisis. CT-guided adrenal biopsy has however been shown to be a safe procedure, with a diagnostic accuracy of 96% and a 3% complication rate although it has a non-diagnostic rate of between 3% and 8.7% [29].

10.2.8 Management

The American College of Radiology Whitepaper on incidental adrenal nodules recommends no further imaging follow-up for patients with no history of malignancy, and small (<4 cm) incidentally discovered homogeneous adrenal masses, measuring <10 HU on unenhanced images, and for other benign lesions such as small myelolipomas and adrenal cysts [30]. The American and European Endocrine Societies, however both recommend a biochemical workup to exclude mild autonomously functioning adrenal lesions, for all adrenal incidentalomas [2, 31]. In many centers in the USA, biochemical evaluation is not routinely performed in asymptomatic patients with small incidental adrenal adenomas. The European Society of Endocrinologists have recently changed their previous guidelines and now do not recommend routine follow-up imaging, for incidental adrenal adenomas, as several recent studies have shown that these lesions rarely grew or became malignant tumors such as an adrenocortical carcinoma [32–36]. The need for follow-up biochemical evaluation is also controversial, and the European Society of Endocrinology now recommends no routine follow-up biochemical evaluation, unless new clini-

cal signs of endocrine activity or comorbidities develop. Patients with mild autonomous cortisol secretion, at initial evaluation, however, do need clinical follow-up evaluation, as they are at risk for developing significant comorbidities of cortisol excess such as hypertension, stress fractures, and diabetes [33–35]. In patients with mild autonomous cortisol excess, an adrenalectomy is usually not felt to be necessary. But in the rare circumstance, when an adrenalectomy is thought to be beneficial, and is planned, a follow-up biochemical evaluation is recommended to confirm autonomous cortisol excess prior to surgery.

The American College of Radiology Whitepaper on incidental adrenal masses [30], and the European Society of Endocrinology recommend that if a known adrenal lesion is enlarging or develops a change in morphology or internal features such as necrosis, degeneration, or hemorrhage, then suspicion for malignancy should be raised, and additional biochemical and imaging workup is needed.

In patients with no history of cancer and an indeterminate adrenal mass >4 cm in size, resection should be considered and although this is the current standard, in both Europe and the USA, some recent studies suggest that this should be re-evaluated as the risk of adrenal cancer in masses of this size may have been overestimated. If there is a history of prior cancer, then a PET/CT scan and as indicated, an adrenal biopsy could be performed to exclude metastases [30].

10.3 Evaluation of Adrenal Mass in Patient with Known Extra-Adrenal Malignancy

Evaluation of adrenal gland masses in the oncology patient is problematic because it is not only a frequent site of adenomas but also metastases [estimated risk of metastases is between 26% and 36%] [34, 36]. CT, MRI, PET-FDG, and adrenal biopsy can be used to evaluate adrenal masses in these patients to diagnose adenomas and differentiate them from metastases, as described in the above sections.

Key Points
- All incidental adrenal nodules/masses should undergo biochemical evaluation (In the absence of clinical symptoms, patients with small incidental adenomas do not undergo biochemical evaluation in many centers in the USA)
- Lipid-rich adenomas can be differentiated from many metastases using unenhanced CT and CSI-MRI
- CT washout calculations helpful to distinguish lipid-poor adenomas from non-hypervascular

metastases, but limited role in distinguishing lipid-poor adenomas from some metastases and some pheochromocytomas.

- Majority of non-functioning adenomas (especially small) usually need no follow-up imaging or biochemical evaluation.
- In patients with mild autonomous cortisol excess, a follow-up biochemical evaluation is needed only if new clinical signs of endocrine activity or comorbidities develop.
- In oncology patients with indeterminate adrenal imaging findings, on CT and MRI, a PET-FDG and/or adrenal biopsy may be required to accurately stage the patient to help determine optimal treatment.
- Current guidelines both in the USA and in Europe suggest that indeterminate masses >4 cm in patients, and with no history of a malignancy, should be surgically removed.

10.4 Evaluation of Patient with Suspected Adrenal Hyperfunction

10.4.1 Adrenal Cortical Hyperfunction

Cushing's syndrome results from an overproduction of cortisol by the adrenal cortex and can be broadly divided into (1) ACTH-dependent and (2) ACTH-independent causes, resulting in elevated serum cortisol levels. Approximately 80% of Cushing's is due to ACTH-dependent cause of overstimulation of the adrenal glands by a pituitary adenoma. Primary adrenal cortical tumors: adenoma and adrenal cortical carci-

noma [ACC] are ACTH-independent cause of Cushing's and account for approximately 20% of cases, with <1% being due to ectopic production of ACTH by a neoplasm, located either in the chest, abdomen, or pelvis.

Adrenal cortical carcinomas are large, heterogeneous, and may have areas of calcification. On contrast-enhanced imaging (CT and MRI), they have heterogenous regions of enhancement as shown in Fig. 10.3a, b, and also show increased uptake on FDG-PET imaging [37, 38]. Functioning adenomas causing Cushing's are smaller in size than ACCs and have an imaging appearance like that of non-functioning adenomas.

Hyperaldosteronism or Conn's syndrome is suspected in a hypertensive patient with low serum potassium and is confirmed by measuring the serum aldosterone to renin ratio [39]. When the diagnosis is suspected based on biochemical assays, a CT scan is performed to exclude adrenal cortical carcinoma, as the etiology. In younger patients (<40 years), a CT may detect a unilateral small adrenal mass, and if the contralateral adrenal gland appears normal, a diagnosis of aldosterone-producing adenoma can be made with moderate accuracy. If CT findings are normal or equivocal for the detection of an adenoma, as is often the case especially in the older populations, patients with suspected hyperaldosteronism, undergo adrenal venous sampling to localize and lateralize the side of elevated aldosterone production is performed, prior to deciding further management [39].

10.4.2 Adrenal Medullary Hyperfunction

Pheochromocytomas originate from the adrenal medulla and are usually solitary and occur sporadically. Extra-adrenal paragangliomas can occur anywhere along the sympathetic chain. These tumors are seen in subjects with various syndromes such as MEN Type II, von Hippel-Lindau [vHL], and neurofibroma-

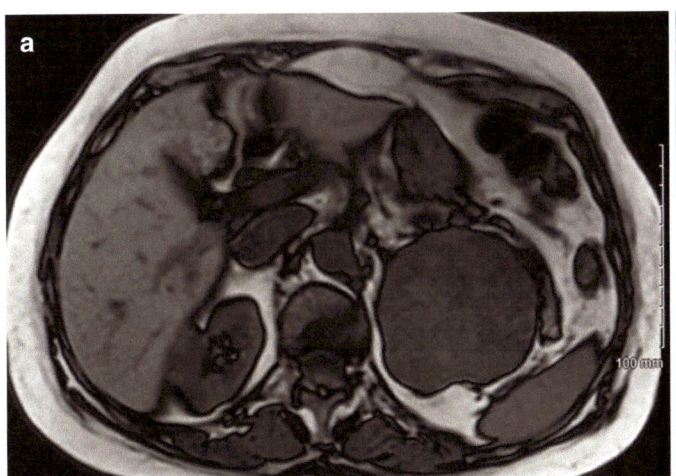
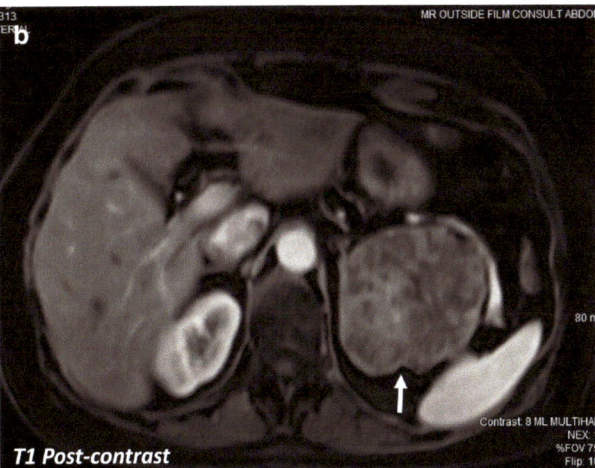

Fig. 10.3 (**a**) Axial T1 pre-contrast MR image shows large adrenal mass subsequently proven to be an adrenal carcinoma(arrow). (**b**) Post-contrast enhanced MR image shows the mass (arrow) has heterogenous enhancement, proven to be an adrenal carcinoma

tosis type I. More recent studies show that about 25% of pheochromocytomas may be familial. Subjects with mutations in the succinate dehydrogenase subunits are also at risk of developing pheochromocytomas and paragangliomas [38, 40].

The most appropriate first-line test is the measurement of plasma free or and urinary fractionated metanephrines. As >95% of pheochromocytomas originate in the adrenal glands, CT is the main modality that has been recommended. MRI examination can be performed when radiation dose is a consideration or if metastatic disease is suspected [11–14, 38, 40]. Most pheochromocytomas are moderate-sized tumors and have imaging appearances that overlap with that of other solid tumors such as ACC and metastases as shown in Fig. 10.4a [15, 38]. In patients with MEN and vHL, the tumors are small and multicentric [38].

While meta-iodobenzyl-guanidine (MIBG) scintigraphy has high specificity (>95%) for the diagnosis of pheochromocytoma, as shown in Fig. 10.4b, but its sensitivity only moderate, ranging between 77–90%. Recent studies have suggested that MIBG scintigraphy should be used selectively and only in patients with familial or hereditary disorders, in the detection of metastatic disease, and in patients with biochemical evidence for pheochromocytoma and negative CT or MRI. These studies also concluded that MIBG scintigraphy does not offer any added advantage in patients with biochemical evidence for a pheochromocytoma, and have an adrenal mass detected by CT or MRI but have no hereditary or familial diseases [40, 41].

The standard treatment of a biochemically active adrenal cortical and medullary tumors is laparoscopic or open surgical resection [34, 38].

Key Points
- In patients with suspected biochemically active adrenal tumors, the role of imaging is primarily to detect the tumor and exclude malignancy (exception pheochromocytoma).
- In patients with Conn's syndrome adrenal venous sampling (AVS) is required to lateralize the side of hyperfunction, after a malignant adrenal lesion has been excluded by CT or MRI.
- Adrenal cortical carcinomas are large heterogeneously enhancing masses.
- MIBG-scintigraphy is not 100% accurate in detecting pheochromocytomas, but is useful in detecting pheochromocytomas and paragangliomas, in patients with hereditary or familial diseases and detecting metastases.

10.5 Future Directions

There has been a high degree of variability in both radiologist detection of adrenal masses and an even greater variation in radiologist and endocrinologist recommendations for management of incidentally discovered adrenal masses. The American College of Radiology (ACR) Whitepaper for adrenal masses and European Guidelines for management of the incidentally discovered adrenal mass have been published to reduce practice variation and create best practices. The ACR is also developing "at the elbow" tools to standardize reporting for incidental findings and a reporting tool for adrenal masses to assist the radiologist at their workstation is underway. Artificial Intelligence and Machine Learning have been applied in many areas of radiology and hold promise to aid in both the detection of abnormalities and consistent charac-

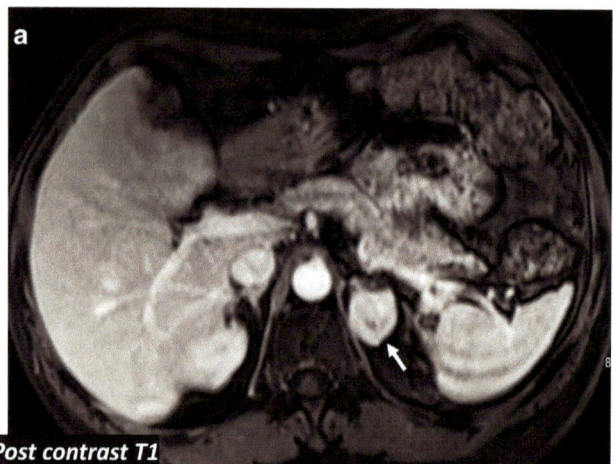

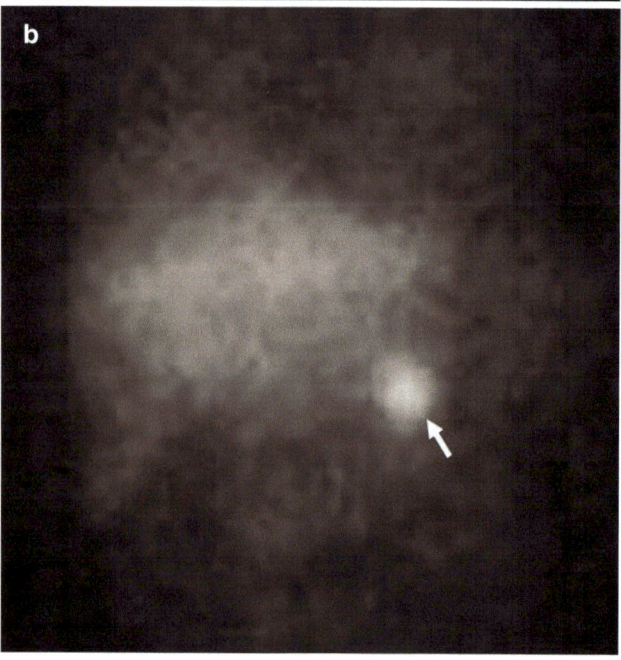

Fig. 10.4 (a) MR post-contrast image shows moderate-sized briskly enhancing left adrenal mass (arrow). (b) MIBG image shows uptake within the left adrenal mass (arrow), a pheochromocytoma

terization of these imaging findings. A recent publication has shown that machine learning algorithms can accurately segment (find) the adrenal glands on abdominal CT and differentiate adrenal masses from normal glands [42]. This may assist busy radiologists faced with high workloads and provide more consistent care for our patients.

10.6 Concluding Remarks

Most incidentally discovered adrenal masses are benign. But in the setting of a known malignancy, differentiation between a metastases and adenoma is essential to guide management. CT, MRI, and PET-FDG imaging are the main imaging tools available currently in the evaluation and characterization of adrenal masses.

Functioning adrenal lesions can be detected by CT, MRI, and MIBG scintigraphy and in patients with suspected hyperaldosteronism, additional invasive testing with AVS.

Take-Home Messages
- Incidental adrenal masses are common.
- Most incidental adrenal masses are benign, non-functioning adenomas.
- Current guidelines suggest biochemical evaluation for all incidentally discovered adrenal masses with a caveat for small lesions in asymptomatic patients.
- Unenhanced CT is the most used first line imaging modality used worldwide to characterize incidental adrenal lesions.
- Chemical shift MRI, CT washout, and PET-FDG are other imaging techniques used.
- Adrenal venous sampling is used to lateralize the side of hyperfunction in patients with suspected hyperaldosteronism.
- Pheochromocytomas can overlap the imaging appearance of other adrenal masses such as adrenal cortical carcinomas and metastases.
- MIBG scintigraphy in the setting of the hereditary and familial diseases is useful in the detection of primary tumors and metastases.

References

1. Song JH, Chaudhry FS, Mayo-Smith WW. The incidental adrenal mass on CT: prevalence of adrenal disease in 1049 consecutive adrenal masses in patients with no known malignancy. Am J Roentgenol. 2008;190:1163–8.
2. Fassnacht M, Arlt W, Bancos I, Dralle H, Newell-Price J, Sahdev A, Tabarin A, Terzolo M, Tsagarkis S, Dekkers OM. Management of adrenal incidentalomas: European Society of Endocrinology Clinical Practice guideline in collaboration with the European Network for the study of adrenal tumors. Eur J Endocrinol. 2016;175:G1–G34.
3. Sahdev A. Imaging incidental adrenal lesions. Br J Radiol. 2022;95:20220281.
4. Elsayes KM, Mukundan G, Narra V, et al. Adrenal masses: MR imaging features with pathological correlation. Radiographics. 2004;24:S73–86.
5. Jordan E, Poder L, Courtier J, et al. Imaging of non-traumatic adrenal hemorrhage. Am J Roentgenol. 2012;199:W91–8.
6. Korobkin M, Giordano TJ, Brodeur FJ. Adrenal adenomas: relationship between histologic lipid and CT and MR findings. Radiology. 1996;200:743–7.
7. Caoili EM, Korobkin M, Francis IR, et al. Adrenal masses: characterization with combined unenhanced and delayed enhanced CT. Radiology. 2002;222:629–33.
8. Marty M, Gaye D, Perez P, et al. Diagnostic accuracy of computed tomography to identify adenomas among adrenal incidentalomas in an endocrinological population. Eur J Endocrinol. 2018;178:439–46.
9. Hong AR, Kim JH, Park KS, et al. Optimal follow-up strategies for adrenal incidentalomas: reappraisal of 2016 ENSAT guidelines in real clinical practice. Eur J Endocrinol. 2017;177:475–83.
10. Korobkin M, Brodeur FJ, Francis IR, et al. CT time-attenuation washout curves of adrenal adenomas and nonadenomas. Am J Roentgenol. 1998;170:747–52.
11. Boland GW, Blake MA, Hahn PF, Mayo-Smith WW. Imaging characterization of adrenal incidentalomas: principles, techniques, and algorithms. Radiology. 2008;249:756–75.
12. Corwin MT, Badawy M, Elaine M Caoili EM et al. Incidental adrenal nodules in patients without known malignancy: prevalence of malignancy and utility of washout CT for characterization-A multi-institutional study. Am J Roentgenol 2022; 219:1–10.
13. Schloetelburg W, Ebert I, Petritsch B, et al. Adrenal wash-out CT: moderate diagnostic value in distinguishing benign from malignant adrenal masses. Eur J Endocrinol. 2021;186:183–93.
14. Choi YA, Kim CK, Park BK, et al. Evaluation of adrenal metastases from RCC and HCC. Radiology. 2013;266:514–20.
15. Woo S, Suh CH, Kim SY, et al. Pheochromocytoma as a frequent false positive in adrenal washout CT; a systematic review and meta-analysis. Eur Radiol. 2018;28(3):1027–36.
16. Nagayama Y, Inoue T, Oda S, et al. Adrenal adenomas versus metastases: diagnostic performance of dual-energy spectral CT virtual non-contrast imaging and iodine maps. Radiology. 2020;296(2):324–32.
17. Platzek I, Sieron D, Plodeck V, et al. Chemical shift imaging for evaluation of adrenal masses: a systematic review and meta-analysis. Eur Radiol. 2019;29(2):806–17.
18. Seo JM, Park BK, Park SY, et al. Characterization of lipid-poor adrenal adenoma: chemical shift MRI and washout CT. Am J Roentgenol. 2014;202(5):1043–50.
19. Tariq U, Poder L, Carlson D, Courtier J, Joe BN, Coakley FV. Multimodality imaging of fat-containing adrenal metastasis from hepatocellular carcinoma. Clin Nucl Med. 2012;37:e157–9.
20. Schieda N, Krishna S, McInnes MDF, et al. Utility of MRI to differentiate clear cell renal cell carcinoma adrenal metastases from adrenal adenomas. Am J Roentgenol. 2017;209(3):W152–9.
21. Sandrasegaran K, Patel AA, Ramaswamy R, et al. Characterization of adrenal masses with diffusion weighted imaging. Am J Roentgenol. 2011;197(1):132–8.
22. Guerin C, Pattou F, Brunaud L, et al. Performance of F-FDG PET/CT in the characterization of adrenal masses in non-cancer patients: a prospective study. J Clin Endocrinol Metab. 2017;102:2465–72.
23. Boland GW, Blake MA, Holalkere NS, Hahn PF. PET/CT for the characterization of adrenal masses in patients with cancer: qualita-

tive versus quantitative accuracy in 150 consecutive patients. Am J Roentgenol. 2009;192:956–62.

24. Barzon L, Sonino N, Fallo F, et al. Prevalence and natural history of adrenal incidentalomas. Eur J Endocrinol. 2003;149:273–85.

25. Mansmann G, Lau J, Balk E, et al. The clinically inapparent adrenal mass: update in diagnosis and management. Endocr Rev. 2004;25:309–40.

26. Cawood TJ, Hunt PJ, O'Shea D, et al. Recommended evaluation of adrenal incidentalomas is costly, has high false-positive rates and confers a risk of fatal cancer that is like the risk of the adrenal lesion becoming malignant; time for a rethink. Eur J Endocrinol. 2009;161:513–27.

27. Kahramangil B, Kose E, Remer EK, et al. A modern assessment of cancer risk in adrenal incidentalomas. Analysis of 2219 patients. Ann Surg. 2022;275(1):e238–44.

28. Song JH, Grand DJ, Beland MD, et al. Morphologic features of 211 adrenal masses at initial contrast-enhanced CT: can we differentiate benign from malignant lesions using imaging features alone? Am J Roentgenol. 2013;201:1248–53.

29. Bancos I, Tamhane S, Shah M, et al. Diagnosis of endocrine disease: the diagnostic performance of adrenal biopsy: a systematic review and meta-analysis. Eur J Endocrinol. 2016;175(2): R65–80.

30. Mayo-Smith WW, Song JH, Boland GL, et al. Management of Incidental adrenal masses: a white paper of the ACR incidental findings committee. Am Coll Radiol. 2017;14:1038–44.

31. Zeiger MA, Thompson GB, Duh QY, et al. American Association of Clinical Endocrinologists and American Association of Endocrine Surgeons: medical guidelines for the management of adrenal incidentalomas. Endocr Pract. 2009;15(Suppl 1)

32. Vaidya A, Hamrahian A, Bancos I, et al. The evaluation of incidentally discovered adrenal masses. Endocr Pract. 2019;25(2):178–92.

33. Cambos S, Tabarin A. Management of adrenal incidentalomas: working through uncertainty. Best Pract Res Clin Endocrinol Metab. 2020;34:101427.

34. Bancos I, Prete A. Approach to the patient with adrenal incidentaloma. J Clin Endocrinol Metab. 2021;106(11):3331–53.

35. Elhassan YS, Alahdab F, Prete A, et al. Natural history of adrenal incidentalomas with and without mild autonomous cortisol excess. Ann Intern Med. 2019;171:107–11.

36. Mao JJ, Dages KN, Suresh M, et al. Presentation, disease progression and outcomes of adrenal gland metastases. Clin Endocrinol. 2020;93(5):546–54.

37. Bharwani N, Rockall AG, Sahdev A, et al. Adrenocortical carcinoma: the range of appearances on CT and MRI. AJR Am J Roentgenol. 2011;196(6):W706–14.

38. Fassnacht M, Assie G, Baudin G, et al. Adrenocortical carcinomas and malignant phaeochromocytomas: ESMO-EURACAN clinical practice guidelines for diagnosis, treatment and follow up. Ann Oncol. 2020;31(11):1476–90.

39. Funder JW, Carey RM, Mantero F, et al. The management of primary aldosteronism: case detection, diagnosis, and treatment: an endocrine society clinical practice guideline. J Clin Endocrinol Metab. 2016;101(5):1889–196.

40. Lenders JWM, Duh QY, EIsenhofer G et al. Pheochromocytoma and paraganglioma: an Endocrine Society clinical practice guideline. J Clin Endocrinol Metab 2014; 99(6):1915–1942.

41. Greenblatt DY, Shenker Y, Chen H. The utility of meta-iodobenzylguanidine (MIBG) scintigraphy in patients with pheochromocytoma. Ann Surg Oncol. 2008;15:900–5.

42. Robinson-Weiss C, Patel J, Bizzo BC, et al. Machine learning for adrenal gland segmentation and classification of normal and adrenal masses at CT. Radiology. 2023;306:e220101. Published online September 2022.

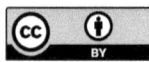

Benign and Malignant Renal Disease

11

Lejla Aganovic and Dominik Nörenberg

Learning Objectives

- To learn when very small renal masses can be ignored and when they should be followed.
- To learn about imaging features of AMLs and non-macroscopic fat-containing solid renal masses.
- To be familiar with the updated Bosniak cystic renal mass classification (version 2019).
- To be familiar with renal cancer staging including the use of the RENAL nephrometry score.
- To be knowledgeable of the emerging role of advanced imaging and multidisciplinary approaches for the management of RCC including renal mass biopsy, surgery, local ablation, active surveillance, SABR, and the imaging appearance of patients after treatment of RCC (including immunotherapy).

11.1 Introduction

Over the last decades, there have been several exciting developments in imaging assessment of renal masses, utilizing a multimodality imaging approach for the differential diagnosis and risk stratification of renal masses. The value of imaging for differential diagnosis of renal masses, local staging, risk stratification, and subsequent renal mass management will be discussed in the following paragraphs.

11.2 Modalities for Imaging Renal Masses

11.2.1 Ultrasound (US) and Contrast-Enhanced US (CEUS)

Although non-contrast US evaluates the internal morphology of cystic lesions with more detail than CT, it is not as sensitive in detecting or accurate in characterizing renal masses as CT or MRI. Most consider non-contrast US to be diagnostically definitive only when it identifies a renal mass as a simple cyst. On the other hand, CEUS using intravenous microbubbles as contrast agent allows a dynamic assessment of the microvasculature of renal masses [1]. Similarly to CT and MRI, CEUS can differentiate between cystic and solid renal lesions and is also beneficial for the characterization of complex cystic lesions. Therefore, CEUS is increasingly used as a diagnostic tool for secondary correlation of indeterminate renal lesions or in patients with contraindications to CT or MRI contrast agents [2].

11.2.2 Computed Tomography (CT) and Magnetic Resonance Imaging (MRI)

Multidetector CT can provide high spatial resolution images of the kidneys and renal vessels, respectively. MRI provides a higher signal-to-noise ratio and higher spatial as well as temporal resolution with a large spectrum of imaging sequences for a more detailed characterization of renal lesions. MRI is often considered as a "problem solver" in renal mass imaging, lesion classification, and staging (e.g., for the assessment of venous extension). The usage of contrast agents for renal MRI can now also be considered in patients with chronic and/or end-stage kidney disease according to the latest AUA guidelines [3, 4]. With the increasing use of cross-sectional imaging, the rate of incidentally detected indeterminate renal masses continues to increase [5]. On CT, it is quite common for only contrast-

L. Aganovic
Department of Radiology, University of California, San Diego Medical Center, San Diego, CA, USA

D. Nörenberg (✉)
Department of Radiology and Nuclear Medicine, University Medical Center Mannheim, Heidelberg University, Mannheim, Baden-Württemberg, Germany
e-mail: Dominik.Noerenberg@medma.uni-heidelberg.de

© The Author(s) 2023
J. Hodler et al. (eds.), *Diseases of the Abdomen and Pelvis 2023-2026*, IDKD Springer Series,
https://doi.org/10.1007/978-3-031-27355-1_11

enhanced images to have been obtained, in which case assessment of mass enhancement is limited. When only contrast-enhanced CT images are available, it may be difficult to distinguish hyperdense cysts from solid hypoenhancing renal lesions. Renal cell cancers (RCCs) are unlikely to measure >70 HU on unenhanced CT and <40 HU on contrast-enhanced CT [6].

> **Key Point**
>
> Multiphase renal CT or MRI in patients with normal renal function is the most appropriate imaging modality for renal mass characterization. Patients should be evaluated with unenhanced and at least one contrast-enhanced series (with the unenhanced MRI sequences including T1-weighted, fat-suppressed, T2-weighted, in- and out-of-phase gradient echo, diffusion-weighted images).

11.3 Very Small Renal Masses (<1–1.5 cm)

Very small renal masses (<1.0–1.5 cm in maximal diameter) are detected on nearly half of all adult patients undergoing CT scans [7]. Many very small renal masses detected with CT and MRI cannot be sufficiently characterized due to their size. In general, one in five detected small renal masses is histologically benign and may not benefit from aggressive treatment regimes. Accurate attenuation measurements in these very small lesions are problematic, due to volume averaging and "pseudoenhancement." Fortunately, the likelihood of any one of these lesions being malignant is exceedingly low [6, 8, 9].

> **Key Point**
>
> Follow-up imaging of very small renal masses should be performed only when they subjectively appear to be complex with evidence of heterogeneity, internal septations, mural nodules, wall thickening, or heterogeneity.

Some homogeneous low attenuation lesions can be considered suspicious if they appear in high-risk patients, such as those with known or suspected hereditary cancer syndromes (such as von Hippel Lindau (associated with clear cell RCC), hereditary papillary renal cell cancer (associated with type I papillary RCC), Birt–Hogg–Dube (associated with chromophobe RCC and oncocytoma) or hereditary leiomyomatosis-renal cancer syndrome (associated with type II papillary

RCC) [10]. Over the last years, there has been increasing knowledge of hereditary renal cancers, which account for approximately 8% of RCCs due to improved genotyping. When a very small renal mass is deemed suspicious, further evaluation should be performed within 6–12 months. Suspicious masses should be followed for at least 5 years. While follow-up can be obtained with CT or MRI, MRI is more accurate. Even small cysts have characteristic high T2 signal intensity. MRI is also much more sensitive to contrast enhancement than CT and not compromised by "pseudoenhancement" [9].

> **Key Point**
>
> Most benign and malignant very small renal masses grow at comparable slow rates, with many of these masses enlarging at a rate of no more than 3–5 mm in maximal diameter per year [11]. As a result, interval enlargement of a renal mass cannot be used to predict that the mass being followed is malignant. Instead, masses should be assessed for changes in morphology, increasing heterogeneity, or progression of other complicating features [9].

11.4 Cystic Renal Masses

To date, cystic renal lesions are classified using the Bosniak classification system, which was first proposed in 1986 [12] and was last revised in 2019 [8]. This system classifies cystic renal masses into five categories based upon their likelihood of being malignant. It is important to emphasize that the initial Bosniak classification system was designed for use with dedicated renal mass CT and not for ultrasound or MRI, respectively. The updated Bosniak classification (2019) includes clear definitions for several imaging terms (e.g., definition of cystic lesions, enhancement, thin vs. thick septa, etc.) to improve the clarity of radiology reporting and incorporates newly defined MRI criteria for the classification of cystic renal lesions. Because the updated Bosniak classification has been adopted for the use of CT, MRI, and CEUS, the presence and thickness of calcifications is neglected for lesion classification. Enhancement is defined as either clearly visible on cross-sectional imaging or non-visible based on established quantitative criteria. This includes an increase of 20 HU (or more) on contrast-enhanced CT in comparison to the native scan. On MRI, a signal intensity increase of 15% (or more) in comparison to non-contrast imaging is considered as an enhancement. The five updated Bosniak categories of cystic renal masses are as follows [8]:

- *Bosniak category I lesions* are simple cysts that constitute most cystic renal masses. They are homogeneous fluid-filled cystic lesions, anechoic on ultrasound and of water attenuation on CT or water signal intensity on MRI. They have smooth, thin walls (less or equal to 2 mm) that may enhance, but they do not contain nodules, septa, solid components, or calcifications. They do not enhance when contrast material is administered. Bosniak category I lesions are always benign; no follow-up is needed.

- *Bosniak category II lesions* are either "minimally complicated" cysts or "benign hyperattenuating" cysts and do not enhance on (multiphase) renal mass imaging. They may contain few (less or equal to 3) and thin (less or equal to 2 mm) septations with or without any type of calcifications. On CT, hyperdense renal cysts smaller than 3 cm in diameter with >70 HU or between −9 and 20 HU (on unenhanced CT) or between 21 and 30 HU (on portal venous phase) are also classified as category II lesions. The attenuation threshold signifying the need for additional imaging was recently changed from >20 HU to >30 HU [6, 8]. On MRI, incompletely characterized cystic renal lesions with T2 signal intensities of CSF or hyperintense lesions on unenhanced T1 images which are with approximately 2.5 times renal parenchymal signal intensity fall into the category of Bosniak II lesions. Additionally, hypoattenuating lesions that are too small to characterize are also classified as Bosniak category II lesions. All of them are considered as (likely) benign (chance of malignancy less than 1%); no follow-up is needed.

Key Point

Incidental detection of small homogeneous renal masses measuring 21–30 HU at portal venous phase CT imaging as well as the detection of incompletely characterized hypoattenuating lesions that are too small to characterize are classified as Bosniak II cystic renal masses. They do not require further imaging evaluation and no follow-up is needed.

- **Bosniak category IIF lesions** are well-defined renal masses and contain more than a few (greater than four) septa or septa with "minimal thickening" (3 mm or less). The wall or septa of Bosniak IIF cysts must enhance. On MRI, cystic masses which are heterogeneously hyperintense on fat-saturated T1-weighted imaging without contrast enhancement—a feature of pRCCs—also fall into the category Bosniak IIF lesions. On CT, heterogeneous masses without enhancement are considered as "incompletely characterized" and require further evaluation (e.g., with MRI or CEUS).

Key Point

Most Bosniak IIF cystic renal masses are benign, only 5–11% have been found to represent cancers or progress to become cancers and if, they are all indolent without locally recurrent or metastatic disease. For this reason, Bosniak IIF cystic renal masses must be followed, with repeated imaging studies performed at 6 months and 12 months, and then annually for at least 5 years. Cancer should be suspected, not when these lesions grow over time, but instead if they become increasingly complex.

- **Bosniak category III lesions** include cystic renal masses with thickened (greater than 4 mm) walls or septa and irregular enhancing walls or septa (focal or diffuse convex protrusion measuring 3 mm or less with obtuse margins with the walls or septa). Bosniak III cystic renal masses have a likelihood of malignancy in about 50–60% of the time and require treatment. When malignant, they tend to be less aggressive than other (predominantly solid) renal cancers (Fig. 11.1).

- **Bosniak category IV lesions** include cystic renal masses with enhancing nodules. "Nodules" are defined as "focal or diffuse convex protrusion of any size that has acute margins with the wall or septa, or a convex protrusion that is 4 mm or greater and has obtuse margins with the wall or septa lesions that have irregular enhancing walls or enhancing nodules." Bosniak IV cystic renal masses are nearly always (>90%) malignant, so treatment is warranted.

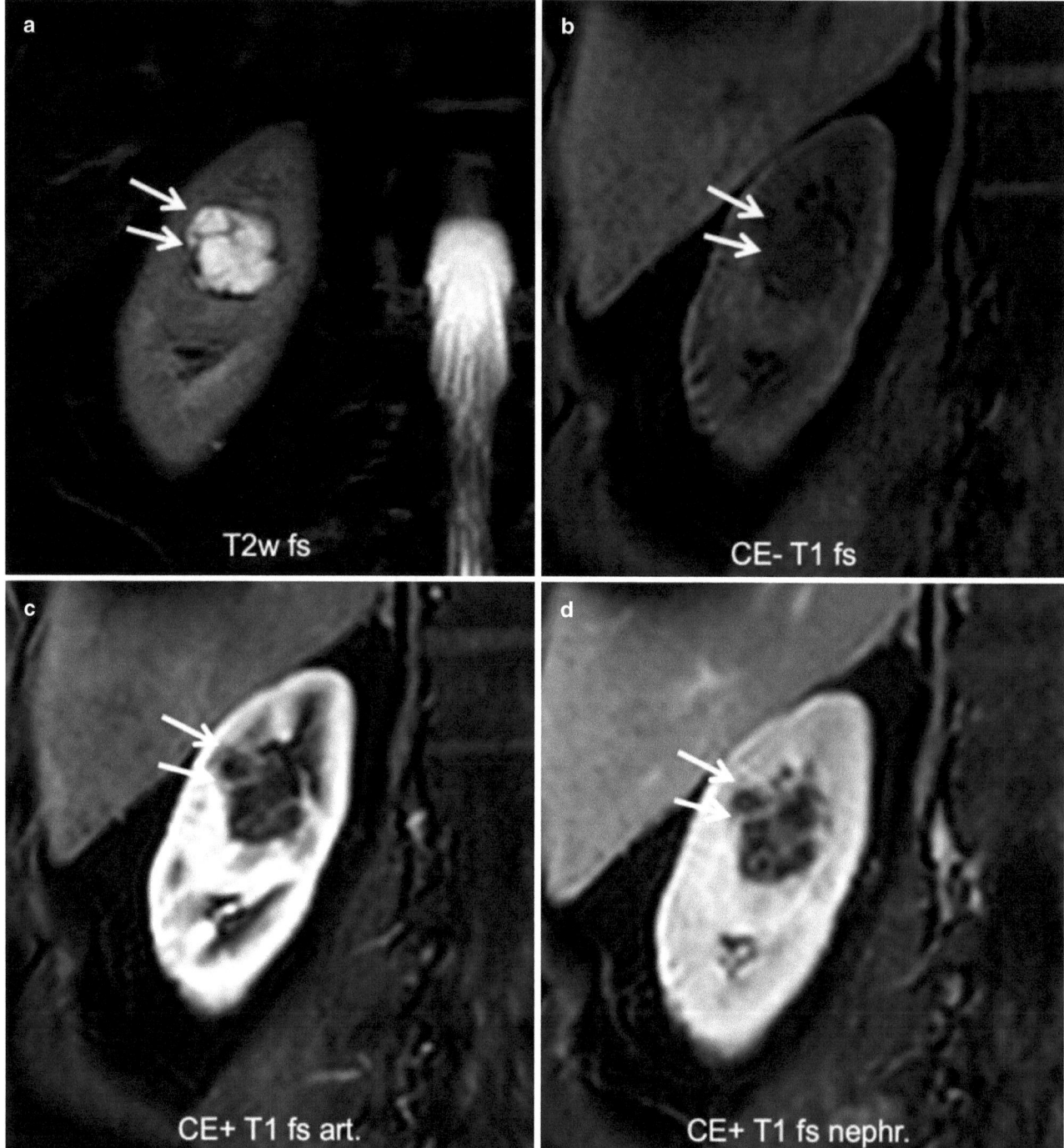

Fig. 11.1 Bosniak III cystic renal mass of the right kidney. (**a**) Coronal fs T2-weighted MR image shows a small hyperintense cystic mass (2.1 cm) in the upper pole of the right kidney with more than a few (>4) septa. (**b**) Coronal unenhanced fs T1-weighted MR image shows T1 hypointensity of the mass without hemorrhagic components. (**c, d**) Coronal contrast-enhanced fs T1-weighted MR images confirm enhancement of the lesion wall as well as septal enhancement both with "minimal thickening" (less or equal than 3 mm), no solid "nodules" are noted. Imaging findings are consistent with Bosniak III category of cystic renal masses. Postoperative histopathology confirmed the presence of a cystic ccRCC

11.5 Angiomyolipoma (AML)

AMLs are the most common benign solid renal neoplasms. Eighty percent of AMLs occur sporadically, are most diagnosed in middle-aged females, and are often associated with hereditary syndromes (tuberous sclerosis or lymphangioleiomyomatosis) [13]. AMLs are composed of angiomatous, myomatous, and fatty elements. While nearly all AMLs are echogenic on ultrasound, so are some small renal cancers. Echogenic masses detected on US are often further evaluated with CT or MRI to determine if macroscopic fat is present in the mass. If macroscopic fat is identified on CT or MRI, then the mass can be diagnosed as an AML (with only case reportable exceptions).

> **Key Point**
> On CT, visualization of at least some small areas of macroscopic fat within a renal mass (measuring 10 HU or less, predominantly with negative HU values) is considered diagnostic of macroscopic fat and thus, of an AML [14]. In contrast, the co-existence of macroscopic fat and calcifications within a lesion points toward malignancy (chromophobe or clear cell renal cancer) and requires further clarification.

> **Key Point**
> On MRI, such fat typically has high T1 and T2 signals and loses signal with fat suppression. On opposed-phase chemical-shift imaging, there is a characteristic "India ink" artifact at fat–water interfaces in the AML and between the AML and adjacent renal tissue (Fig. 11.2).

Some AMLs do not contain easily identifiable macroscopic fat. These AMLs are referred to as fat-poor AMLs (fpAMLs) and include fpAMLs that have the same or higher attenuation than normal renal parenchyma on unenhanced CT and AMLs with epithelial cysts (AMLEC), which can appear as solid masses with small cystic areas or multilocular cystic lesions [13]. Many studies have attempted to identify small foci of fat or other imaging features that might permit fpAMLs to be correctly distinguished from other solid renal neoplasms. These features have included assessing unenhanced CT mass attenuation, CT histograms, quantitatively assessed fat on MRI, and the degree and homogeneity of mass of enhancement [13, 15]. Results have been mixed. For example, some fpAMLs have higher unenhanced attenuation than normal renal parenchyma, but papillary renal cancers can also demonstrate

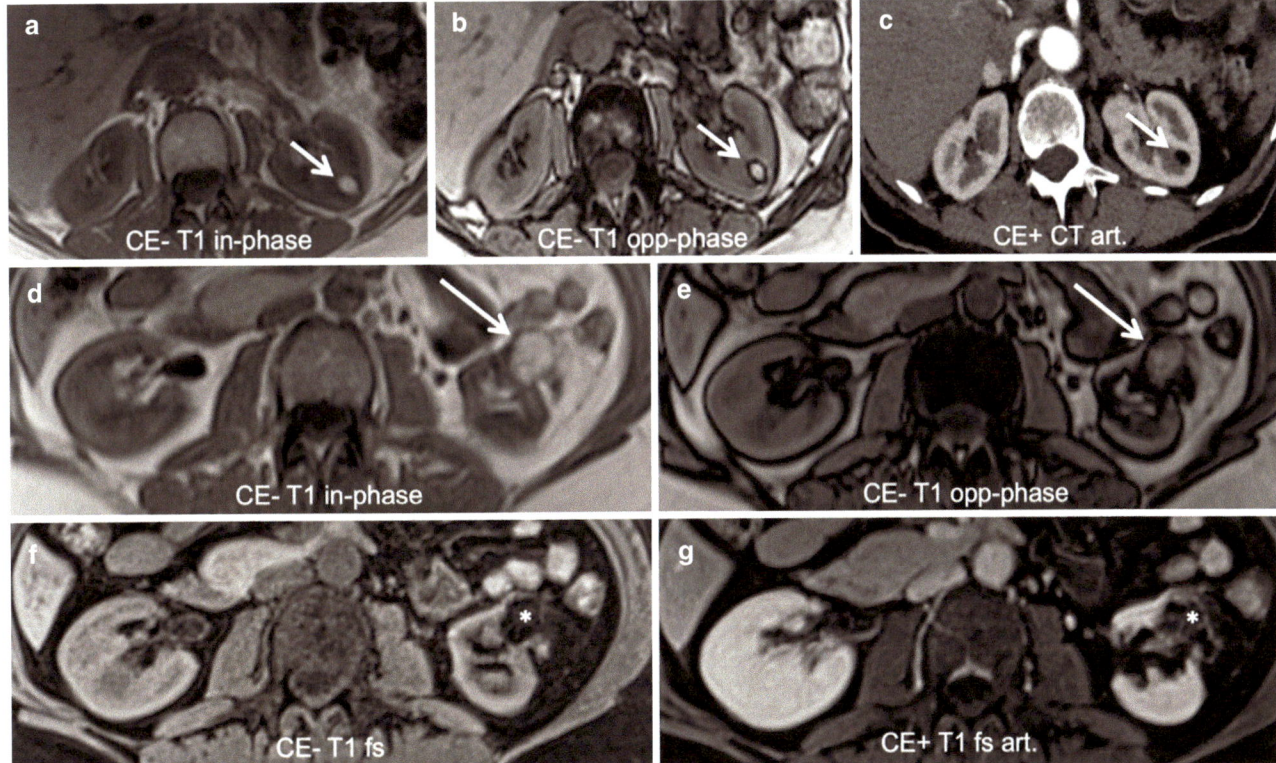

Fig. 11.2 Two solid renal masses with macroscopic fat consistent with AML (arrows) in two different patients (**a–c** and **d–g**). (**a**) axial in-phase T1-weighted MR image of the first patient shows a very small hyperintense mass (1 cm) of the left kidney. (**b**) opposed-phase MR image demonstrates "India ink" artifact at the interface of the renal mass with the kidney. (**c**) axial CT confirms intralesional macroscopic fat, confirming the diagnosis. (**d–g**) 2.5 cm AML of the left kidney in another patient with macroscopic fat (hyperintensity) on T1-weighted in-phase images without contrast (**d**), signal loss on T1-weighted opposed-phase images and (**e**) heterogenous, hypervascular enhancement on arterial phase imaging in comparison to non-contrast fs T1 imaging (*) (**f, g**)

this feature [16]. Some fpAMLs have low signal intensity on T2-weighted MR images, but papillary renal cancers may also demonstrate this behavior. Fortunately, fpAMLs usually demonstrate more MR contrast enhancement than do papillary renal neoplasms, so a hypervascular lesion that demonstrates a combination of high attenuation on unenhanced CT or low-T2 signal intensity on MRI is most likely to be an AML.

11.6 Other Solid Renal Masses and Cancer Mimics

Other solid renal masses without macroscopic fat include oncocytomas, renal cell cancers, lymphoproliferative neoplasms, and metastases. Many studies attempted to distinguish among the various non-fat or minimal fat-containing solid renal masses on CT and MRI and have met with limited success; however, a few occasionally suggestive imaging features have been described.

11.6.1 Oncocytomas

Oncocytomas are benign solid renal tumors. They may contain central scars that can be detected on imaging studies. However, necrosis in renal cancers is indistinguishable from scars in oncocytomas [17, 18]. In fact, differentiating oncocytomas from RCCs on imaging is not possible which is further supported by overlapping histopathological features [19].

11.6.2 Renal Cell Cancers (RCCs)

Chromosomal analysis has demonstrated that there are at least 13 distinct types of renal cancer of which the most common are clear cell (about 70–80%), papillary (10–15%), and chromophobe (less than 10%) renal cell cancer. Sarcomatoid renal cancer is no longer believed to be a distinct cell type. Instead, any type of primary renal neoplasm can dedifferentiate and develop sarcomatoid features with infiltrative behavior on imaging.

11.6.2.1 Clear Cell Renal Cell Cancer (ccRCC)

Clear cell renal cancers account for 70% of RCCs and have the highest metastatic potential and poorest survival of the major histologic RCC subtypes. They are usually heterogeneous renal cortical masses, and high-grade tumors may already present with renal vein invasion or perinephric fat infiltration on diagnosis. On unenhanced MRI, most ccRCCs demonstrate hyperintensity on T2-weighted images (Fig. 11.3) and a rather low amount of diffusion restriction. Due to abundant intracellular fat, clear cell cancers can lose signal on opposed-phase gradient echo T1-weighted images. Macroscopic fat within ccRCCs is very rare; however, this tends to occur with accompanying calcifications. Clear cell RCCs are hypervascular lesions and usually demonstrate heterogeneous enhancement, with peak enhancement occurring early on CMP images (Fig. 11.3):

11.6.2.2 Papillary Renal Cell Cancer (pRCC)

Papillary RCC accounts for 10–15% of RCCs and is the most common multifocal renal cancer subtype in up to 20–25% of the cases and bilaterally in up to 10% of the cases [20]. Papillary RCCs behave less aggressively than ccRCCs and are often less than 3 cm in size, rarely contain fat, are predominantly peripherally located, and show only indeterminate enhancement (between 10 and 20 HU). In these cases, further examination with CEUS or MRI is recommended [17]. On contrast-enhanced CT or MRI, papillary cancers tend to be homogeneous. On unenhanced CT, they may have higher attenuation than adjacent renal parenchyma and may be misdiagnosed as hemorrhagic cysts. A key feature on unenhanced MRI is low T2 signal intensity although this characteristic is unspecific and may be displayed as well by fat-poor AML or cysts with hemorrhagic components. In

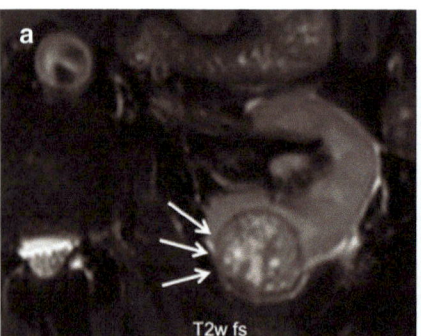 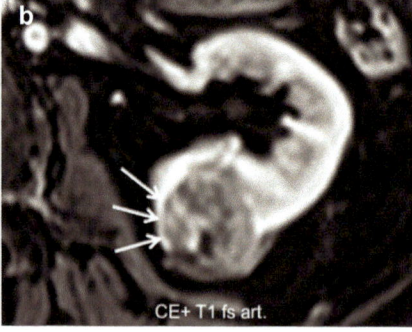 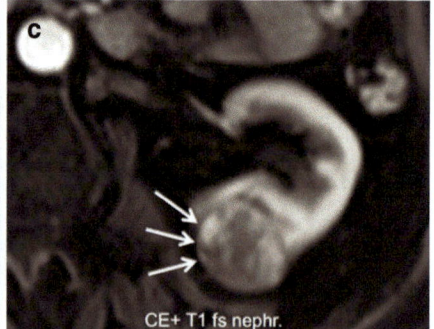

Fig. 11.3 Organ-confined clear cell renal cell carcinoma of the left kidney (arrows). (**a**) Axial fs T2-weighted image shows a lesion with smooth margins and moderate, heterogenous signal hyperintensity. (**b**, **c**) Axial fs T1-weighted arterial and nephrographic phase images show a hypervascular renal mass with heterogenous enhancement, subsequently confirmed to be ccRCC

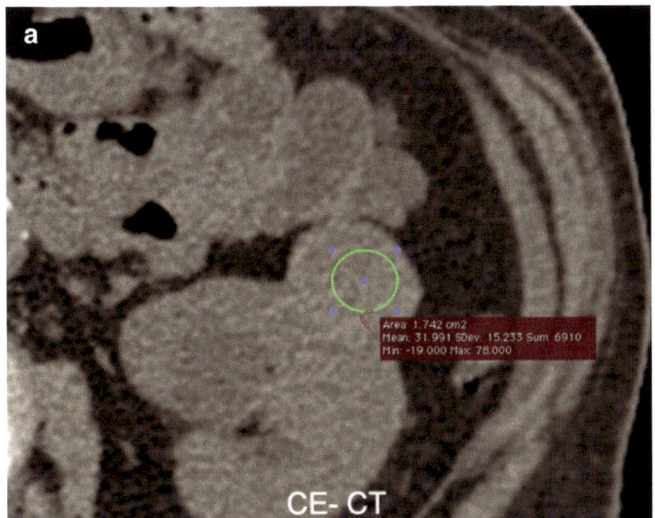
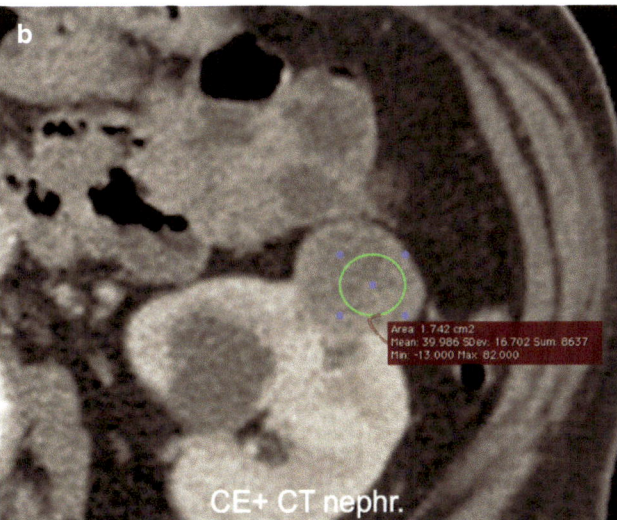

Fig. 11.4 Papillary renal cell carcinoma of the left kidney. Axial unenhanced CT (**a**) and contrast-enhanced CT (nephrographic phase) (**b**) demonstrate a homogenous hypoenhancing mass (ROI) measuring 2.4 cm in size in the anterior aspect of the mid-left kidney. Increase in HU density from 31 to 39 HU classifies this lesion as indeterminate. Subsequent CEUS and postoperative histopathology confirmed the presence of a pRCC

addition, they can lose signal on in-phase relative to out-of-phase T1 images due to hemosiderin content. They usually enhance homogeneously, more slowly, and to a lesser extent in comparison to other renal cancers, with peak enhancement not occurring until the NP or even the EP (Fig. 11.4):

11.6.2.3 Chromophobe Renal Cell Cancer (chRCC)

Chromophobe renal cell cancers account for 5% of renal malignancies and are less malignant than ccRCCs (with 5-year survival rates of 80–90%) [20]. chRCCs are generally well-differentiated cancers and, if they do not have sarcomatoid differentiation, are slow growing, show moderate, relatively uniform enhancement on CT- and MR imaging and may show areas of focal calcification. Even though some chRCCs may show "spoke-wheel enhancement" comparable to oncocytoma, they also do not have a definite characteristic appearance on imaging studies and cannot be reliably distinguished from other solid renal masses that do not contain macroscopic fat.

11.6.2.4 Uncommon Renal Cancer Cell Types

Many of the uncommon renal cancers do not have suggestive imaging appearances. Renal medullary, collecting duct, and XP11.2 translocation cancers generally arise in the renal medulla. Collecting duct cancers frequently occur in older adults, renal medullary and XP11.2 cancers are usually encountered in young patients [21]. The (rare) combination of an infiltrative renal lesion, African American race, sickle cell trait and metastases at baseline presentation points toward renal medullary cancer [22].

11.6.3 Urothelial Neoplasms and Lymphoma

It can occasionally be difficult to distinguish centrally located infiltrative RCC from urothelial cancers [23]. However, the correct etiology may be predicted in many instances, especially an additional lesion within the upper urinary tract or bladder points toward urothelial cancer. Upper tract urothelial cancer (UTUC) represents about 15% of all renal tumors, whereas simultaneous cancer of the bladder is present in 15–20% of UTUCs. Most UTUCs are low-grade tumors, only approximately 15% show infiltrative behavior. Unlike RCCs, UTUCs have an epicenter in the renal collecting system, can produce renal pelvic filling defects, and tend to preserve the normal renal contour. They also rarely contain cystic or necrotic areas seen in many, but not all, RCCs. Renal mass biopsy (RMB) is recommended when imaging findings are indeterminate. Another often centrally located and infiltrative renal mass that can be encountered and that can occasionally mimic infiltrative RCC (or UTUC) includes renal lymphoma.

In lymphomas, kidney involvement is rare and occurs most often in advanced disease stages with an established diagnosis at the time of imaging (typically for B-cell NHL subtypes). In addition, primary renal lymphoma is an extremely rare condition that accounts for less than 1% of the cases. On imaging, renal lymphomas present as hypovascular masses, and the renal veins/arteries remain patent despite extensive encasement. In parallel, there is often the presence of lymphadenopathy and splenomegaly. RMB may be recommended due to unspecific findings.

11.6.4 Other Non-neoplastic and Vascular Lesions

Other non-neoplastic lesions for the differential diagnosis of RCC include infective, inflammatory, and vascular entities such as renal artery aneurysms, xanthogranulomatous pyelonephritis (XGP) and post-transplant lymphoproliferative disease (PTLD).

Renal artery aneurysms are an extremely rare condition with a prevalence of <1% [24]. Risk factors include fibromuscular dysplasia and atherosclerosis and only 10% of renal artery aneurysms occur intraparenchymal, thereby mimicking solid or cystic renal lesions on US. CT- or MR-imaging should support definitive diagnostic characterization.

In the context of inflammatory cancer mimics, XGP is considered as a chronic inflammatory, destructive granulomatous kidney disease (accounting for 0.5–1% of histologically documented cases of pyelonephritis) [25]. XGP has a female predominance and is associated on imaging with renal calculi (either calyceal or staghorn), marked dilatation of the calyces, cortical thinning as well as reniform enlargement of the kidney. XGP can display features of (inflammatory) soft tissue proliferation that may extend into the perinephric space potentially mimicking infiltrative malignancy and/or lymphoproliferative disease.

Regarding lymphoproliferative cancer mimics, PTLD develops after solid organ or stem cell transplantation [26]. PTLD ranges from benign lymphoid hyperplasia to lymphoid hyperplasia with malignant potential and may mimic UTUC, lymphoma or solid renal cell cancer. Of note, PTLD occurs most frequently within 12 months after transplantation with a predominance in pediatric patients (or allograft PTLD in patients with renal transplants). On imaging, PTLD presents as heterogenous hilar mass and may encase vessels; additionally, it can present with multiple hypovascular lesions. RMB is required to confirm definitive diagnosis.

11.7 Solid Renal Mass Growth Rates

Both benign and malignant solid renal masses can remain stable in size or enlarge over time, with growth rates of both types of lesions usually being similarly slow. It has been suggested that a small solid mass that has an average growth rate of <3 mm per year over at least a 5-year period and that has not changed in morphology should be considered stable. Such a lesion, even if malignant, is exceedingly unlikely to metastasize. Conversely, rapid growth of a mass (>5 mm in 12 months) may indicate aggressiveness and/or malignant potential [27].

11.8 Radiomics

In recent years, there has been increasing interest in the utility of computer-assisted diagnosis (CAD) systems and advanced deep/machine-learning techniques such as "radiomics" in detecting and characterizing genitourinary abnormalities. With respect to renal masses, this has centered on the ability of computer-assisted techniques to differentiate among different types of solid and cystic renal masses [28–30]. For example, studies using computer-assisted diagnosis have demonstrated clear cell renal cancers to have greater objective heterogeneity (pixel standard deviation, entropy, and uniformity) than papillary renal cancers or AMLs [31]. CAD detection of differences in peak lesion attenuation has also been used to differentiate clear-cell renal cancers from other renal neoplasms with some success [32]. Renal mass perfusion parameters have been employed to distinguish some renal cancers of higher Fuhrman grade from those of lower grade [33]. These results are promising, but preliminary and currently still subjected to academic research.

11.9 Use of Imaging for Solid Renal Mass Differentiation

Over the past decades, there have been significant paradigm shifts in the treatment of renal masses, including active surveillance (AS), minimal-invasive ablations, and improvements in RMB accuracy. Additionally, the effects of neoadjuvant therapy for patients with advanced localized disease are under investigation [34]. Many of incidentally detected renal masses will remain indolent with either no or very slow growth and require no therapeutic intervention. Accordingly, the US and European guidelines for the management of clinical stage 1 renal masses include active surveillance (AS) as a valid option for patients with comorbidities and T1a (≤4 cm) or T1b (4–7 cm) tumors [35]. The reported metastatic risk is very low even for larger tumors (cT1b/T2, >4 cm) in patients undergoing AS, but varies significantly by histologic subtype whereas ccRCC has the worst prognosis and a higher risk of metastatic disease [36]. To date, there is no clear beneficial effect on reducing renal cancer-specific mortality after aggressive treatment of small renal tumors. This may suggest that many renal cancers have indolent oncologic behavior. Although active surveillance is increasingly recognized as a treatment option for some patients, the lack of reliable predictive biomarkers limits its use in clinical practice. The multiparametric MRI-derived clear cell likelihood score (ccLS), based on a Likert scale, is useful for identifying clear cell renal carcinoma as the most common and aggressive subtype that can be used in clinical practice [37].

The ccLS provides a framework for standardized multiparametric MRI evaluation of small solid renal masses with moderate diagnostic accuracy for ccRCC classification. The ccLS was shown to be associated with lesion growth of small renal masses and may be considered as useful tool for therapy guidance (e.g., AS selection for lesions with a low ccLS or early treatment for lesions with a high ccLS) [38].

> **Key Point**
>
> The MRI-derived clear cell likelihood score (ccLS) may provide useful information for identifying aggressive small renal masses such as ccRCC and is positively correlated with lesion growth; however, the ccLS is not intended to classify tumors as malignant versus benign.

11.10 Renal Mass Biopsy (RMB)

RMB can be performed accurately and safely, and the risk of needle tract seeding is minimal [39, 40]. The updated AUA guideline defines indications for RMBs more clearly following a "utility-based" approach whenever it may influence patient management [3, 41]. Given the substantial overlap in the imaging features of many renal lesions, percutaneous renal mass biopsy can be necessary for determining the nature of renal masses prior to treatment. Thus, RMB has an emerging role to guide the management of renal masses, to limit invasiveness and overtreatment as well as to support patient risk stratification (e.g., in cases prior ablation, prior active surveillance, with infiltrative or metastatic renal disease to allow subtyping for potential systemic therapy or to detect an underlying hereditary condition).

11.11 Pretreatment Assessment of Renal Cancer

11.11.1 Staging and Diagnostic Workup

CT and MRI (obtained during the portal venous phase of enhancement) are at least 90% accurate in renal cancer staging, with the AJCC TNM staging system for renal cancer as follows [42] (Table 11.1):

The most substantial limitation of imaging for renal cancer staging results from the fact that both CT and MRI have difficulties in determining whether renal cancer has invaded the renal capsule and spread into the perirenal or renal sinus fat (differentiating T2 from T3 cancers). Perinephric soft tissue stranding can be produced by tumor, edema, or blood vessels.

Table 11.1 AJCC TNM staging system for renal cancer [42]

Category	Definition
Tx	Primary tumor cannot be assessed
T0	No evidence of primary tumor
T1a	≤4 cm in greatest diameter and limited to the kidney
T1b	>4 but ≤7 cm and limited to the kidney
T2a	>7 but ≤10 cm and limited to the kidney
T2b	>10 cm and limited to the kidney
T3a	Extension into renal vein or its branches or invading perirenal or renal sinus fat
T3b	Extension into IVC below diaphragm
T3c	Extension into IVC above the diaphragm or invading the IVC wall
T4	Invasion beyond perinephric (Gerota) fascia or into ipsilateral adrenal gland
Nx	Lymph nodes cannot be assessed
N0	No regional (retroperitoneal) lymph node involvement
N1	Regional (retroperitoneal) lymph node involvement
Mx	Distant metastatic status cannot be determined
M0	No distant metastasis
M1	Distant lymph node or other metastasis, including non-continuous adrenal involvement

> **Key Point**
>
> It is recommended that T3 disease is diagnosed on CT or MRI only when nodular tissue is identified in the perinephric space. Non-continuous adrenal gland invasion is regarded as M1 stage.

Figure 11.5 gives an overview about the diagnostic workup for renal cancer staging:

11.11.2 RENAL Nephrometry Score

Many urologists prefer that RENAL nephrometry scoring of suspected or known renal cancers also be obtained prior to surgery. According to the AUA and EAU guidelines, small T1a renal lesions should be treated with partial nephrectomy (PN) whenever technically feasible [3, 44]. Renal nephrometry scoring provides standard metrics to assess the tumor complexity, allowing the urologist to predict the likelihood that partial nephrectomy can be performed effectively and safely with a reduced risk of complications (39). For RENAL nephrometry scoring, a renal mass receives a score of 1–3 points for each of the five features: **R**enal mass size, **E**xophyticity, **N**earness to the renal collecting system or sinus, **A**nterior or posterior location, and **L**ocation with respect to the upper and lower polar lines (Table 11.2) [45]. Tumors that have composite nephrometry scores of 4–6 are very amenable to PN, while those that have scores of 10–12 are poor candidates for PN. Radical nephrectomy should be considered in the latter group.

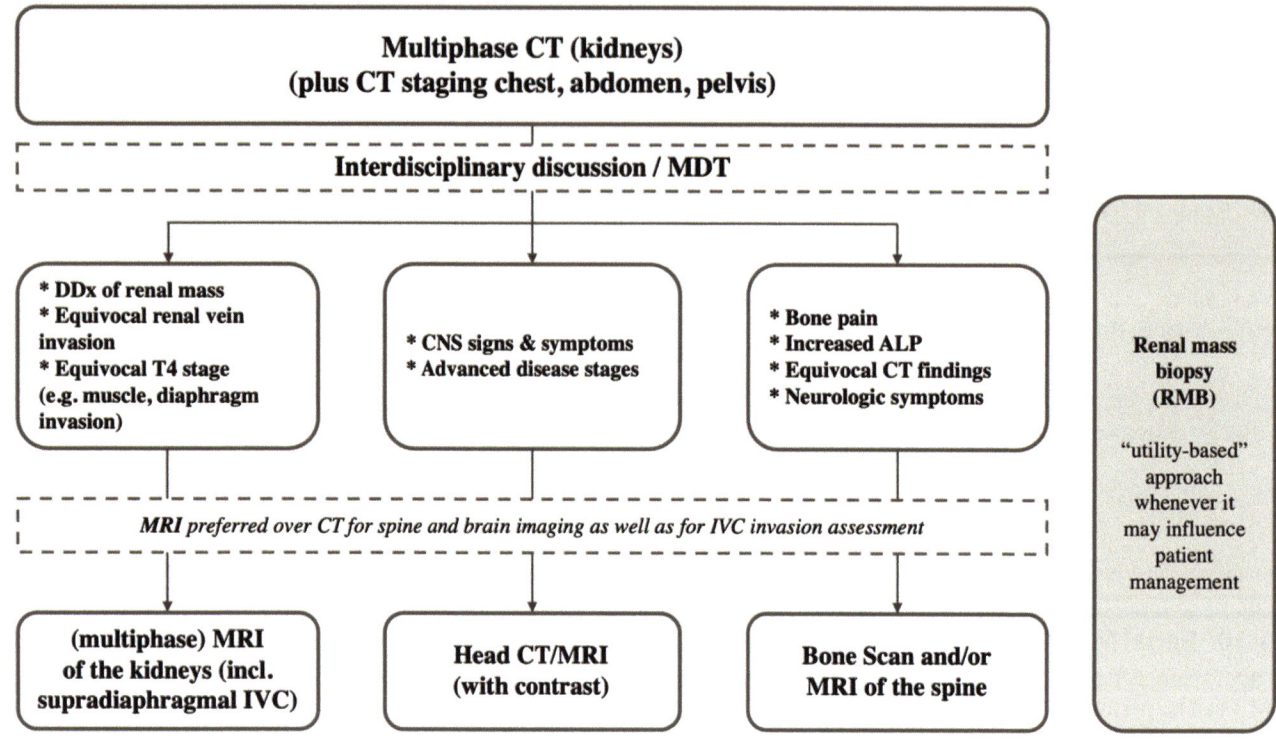

Fig. 11.5 Diagnostic workup for renal cancer staging [43]

Table 11.2 RENAL nephrometry score [45]

Feature	1 point	2 points	3 points
R = renal mass size	≤4 cm	>4–<7 cm	≥7 cm
E = Exophyticity/Endophyticity	≥50%	<50%	Entirely endophytic
N = nearness to collecting system or renal sinus	≥7 mm	>4–<7 mm	≤4 mm
A = anterior or posterior location	No points given. Mass is listed as a, p, or neither (x)		
L = location relative to upper and lower polar lines Add "**h**" if it touches renal artery or vein	Above upper or lower pole line	Crosses polar line	>50% of mass crosses polar line or crosses midline, or entirely interlobar

11.12 Management of Local or Locoregional Renal Cancer

Management of renal cancers that have not metastasized regionally or distantly now ranges from AS (for small (<4 cm) indolent (low Fuhrman grade) tumors in elderly patients with significant comorbidities) to local and/or thermal ablation (TA), partial nephrectomy (PN), or radical nephrectomy (RN) (32, 37). Over the last decades, there has been an increasing paradigm shift toward nephron-sparing treatments for small renal lesions (<4 cm) as well as an increasing role of AS as a management alternative to immediate treatment options. For patients with a solid renal mass <3 cm, or masses that are complex but predominantly cystic, not infiltrating on imaging, and a tumor growth of less than 5 mm per year, AS may be selected [4]. For patients with solid renal masses or complex Bosniak 3 (or 4) cystic renal masses who prefer AS, clinicians should consider RMB for oncologic risk stratification (if the risk-benefit analysis for AS vs. treatment is inconclusive). Patients on AS should undergo subsequent imaging every 3–6 months for a year to assess interval growth, followed by annual imaging for at least 5 years. Intervention in these patients is only considered when masses exceed 4 cm in size or grow by >5 mm per year [46, 47]. For small cT1a solid renal masses, there is growing evidence for the effectiveness of TA and/or local ablation as an alternative to PN, especially in patients who elect ablation [4]. The EAU guideline recommends performing an RMB before (ideally not concomitantly with) ablative therapy [44]. AS and/or TA is especially relevant for frail or comorbid patients with small renal masses who are not eligible for surgery. For advanced locoregional disease, the need for adjuvant therapy after surgery has been recently addressed [4, 48]. Furthermore, adjuvant pembrolizumab (a type of immunotherapy) can be considered as an alternative surgical MDT consideration for patients with locally advanced ccRCC following surgery with curative intent. Adjuvant pembrolizumab has been shown to be beneficial for intermediate- and high-risk ccRCC patients with a risk of recurrence (shown for pT2 G4 OR pT3 any G OR pT4 any G OR pN+ any G cancers) [48].

11.13 Management of (Oligo-)Metastatic Renal Cancer

For synchronous or early oligometastatic disease, the ESMO guideline 2019 does not usually recommend metastasectomy as an alternative to systemic therapy in patients with synchronous or early oligometastatic disease [35]. Oligometastatic disease may be observed without immediate treatment for up to 16 months before systemic therapy is required due to progression [44]. Furthermore, the role of stereotactic ablative radiotherapy (SABR) was recently investigated within the SABR-COMET trial for oligometastatic renal cancer disease in patients with one to five metastatic lesions, in comparison to standard-of-care palliative treatment [49]. Within the SABR-COMET trial, SABR was associated with an overall survival benefit and increased progression-free survival in oligometastatic patients in comparison to patients undergoing standard-of-care treatment. Overall, there is emerging evidence that SABR can be considered as a novel treatment reserved for patients with T1-T3a tumors (as well as for oligometastatic lesions) who are not medically or surgically operable [50].

11.14 Imaging after Renal Cancer Treatment

11.14.1 After Renal Mass Ablation

After successful renal mass radiofrequency ablation or cryoablation, there is an initial expansion of the ablation site. Initially, some enhancement may be detected normally in the ablation bed, particularly on MRI exams. This normal enhancement resolves over time. In the months following ablation, the ablation bed typically decreases, but rarely disappears completely. Other normal post-ablation findings include fat invagination between the ablation bed and normal renal parenchyma and a perilesional halo, changes that create an appearance that can be confused with an AML. Ablation bed expansion is not typically seen after microwave ablation.

> **Key Point**
> Frequent imaging should be performed after ablation (e.g., at 1, 3, 6, and 12 months). This is because residual or recurrent tumor is usually detectable within the first few months of ablation [51].

Persistent or recurrent tumors should be suspected after ablation if the ablation bed progressively increases (rather than decreases) in size, when there is increased perinephric nodularity, or when persistent or new areas of nodular or crescentic enhancement are detected, with these areas usually located at the interface of the ablation bed with adjacent renal parenchyma [51].

11.14.2 Imaging after Partial or Total Nephrectomy

After PN or RN, it is common to see post-operative inflammatory or fibrotic changes in the surgical bed, along with deformity of the renal contour at the site of partial nephrectomy. Post-ablation surgical findings may also include fat invagination between the surgical bed and normal renal parenchyma. Ablation bed expansion is not typically seen after microwave ablation. Gore-Tex mesh along the nephrectomy site appears as a linear area of high attenuation along the renal margin.

> **Key Point**
> Frequently used hemostatic material can be mistaken for infection or tumor, since it contains occasional gas within the material and its low attenuation components can persist for months after surgery.

Complication rates after partial nephrectomy are typically higher than after total nephrectomy, with complications including renal artery pseudoaneurysm (RAP), arteriovenous (AV) fistula, urinoma, or abscess. If urinoma is a concern, delayed imaging >1–2 h after contrast administration might prove useful to document the urinary leak. Although RAPs or AV fistulas after PN are rare conditions (in 1–5% of the cases after PN [52]) both represent a potentially life-threatening complication. Patients typically present 7–12 days after PN with hematuria and/or clinical signs of blood loss. Emergency treatment of choice is selective transarterial embolization as an effective minimally invasive treatment option for the management of hemodynamically unstable patients with RAP (or AV fistula) with minimal impact on renal function [52].

After PN or RN, recurrent tumor recurrence may develop in the surgical bed, regionally within the retroperitoneum or distantly. Surgical bed recurrences may initially be difficult to differentiate from post-operative scarring or fibrosis, although tumor recurrence often demonstrates detectable (hyper-)enhancement and enlarges over time (Fig. 11.6).

Renal cancer usually metastasizes to regional lymph nodes, liver, adrenal glands, lungs, and bones. Adrenal cancer metastases from ccRCC can be problematic, since they may contain large amounts of intracellular fat. As a result,

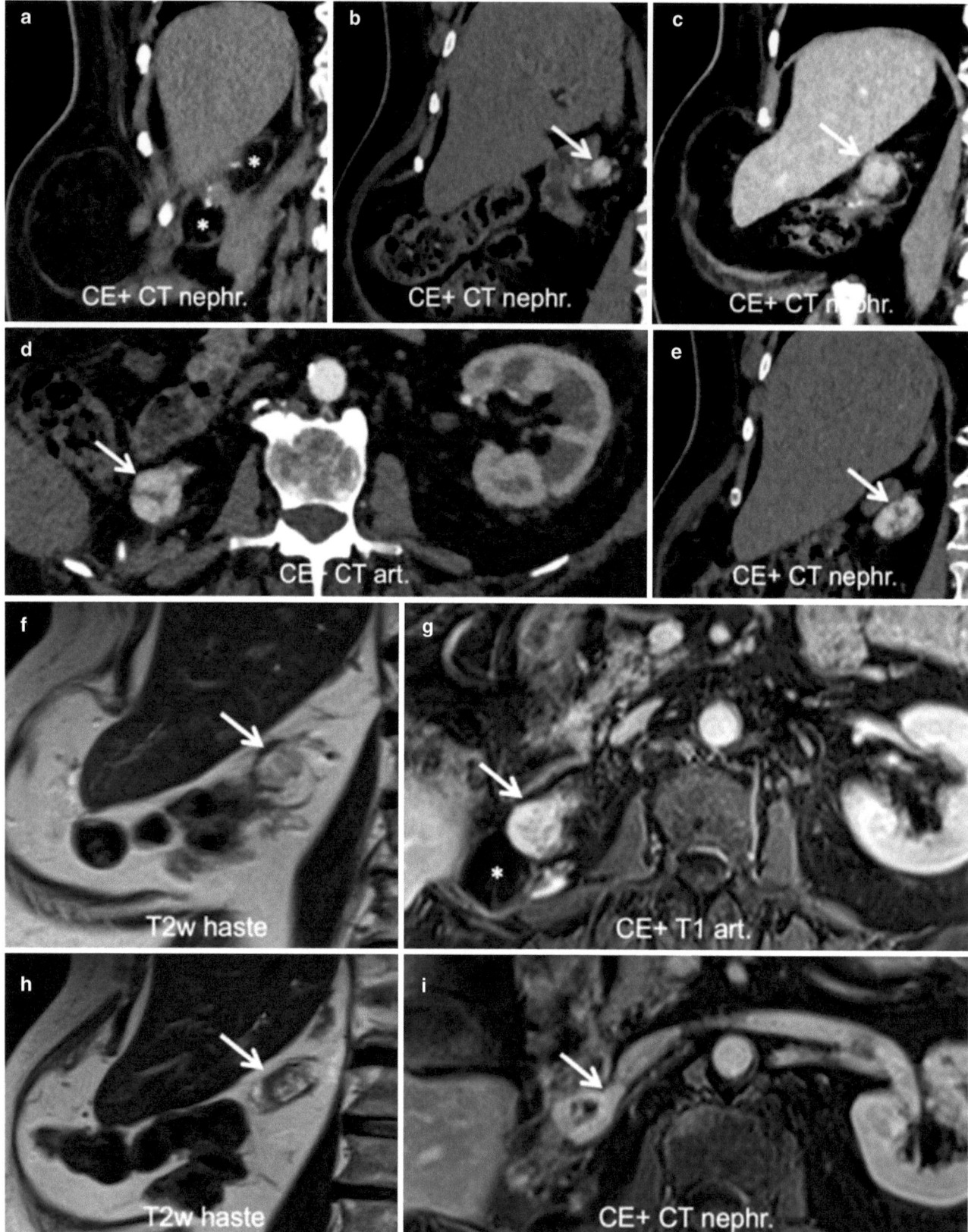

Fig. 11.6 Post-surgical appearance of the tumor bed on CT- (**a–e**) and MR-imaging (**f–i**) >3 years after PN of a ccRCC in the upper pole of the right kidney. (**a, g**) appearance of the post-surgical tumor bed (*) with fat invagination between the surgical bed and normal renal parenchyma on coronal CT (**a**) and coronal T2w haste images (**f**). (**b–i**) Surgical bed cancer recurrence (arrows) on CT- and MR imaging with a hypervascular soft tissue mass including renal vein invasion (**b, e, h, i**). Of note, tumor recurrence/tumor thrombus demonstrates T2 hyperintensity on MR imaging (**f, h**) as well as hypervascularity (**d, e, g**) consistent with ccRCC recurrence and venous invasion

like adenomas, adrenal metastases can demonstrate low signal intensity on opposed-phase MR images and can also demonstrate pronounced (>60%) washout on delayed enhanced CT. Renal cancer metastasizes to the pancreas more commonly than do other neoplasms [53].

11.14.3 Imaging After Treatment of Metastatic Disease

11.14.3.1 RECIST

Metastatic disease occurs approximately in 17% of patients at diagnosis of RCC. Patients who present with or develop metastatic disease must receive systemic treatment. Follow-up imaging is then performed regularly to determine whether (or not) patients are responding to adjuvant chemotherapy. The most commonly used measurement system for assessing tumor response to chemotherapy has been the Response Evaluation Criteria In Solid Tumors (RECIST) system according to the newest version 1.1 [54]. RECIST 1.1 involves measurements of up to five metastatic lesions (no more than two reference lesions per organ, with each measured lesion being at least 10 mm in length). Most metastases are measured in maximal dimensions; however, lymph nodes are measured in short-axis diameter. Complete response is diagnosed when all metastases resolve on follow-up imaging. A partial response is diagnosed when the sum of all target lesions decreases by ≥30% from one study to the next. Progressive disease is diagnosed when the sum of all target lesions increases by ≥20% or more. Any change between a 30% decrease and a 20% increase is considered a stable disease.

11.14.3.2 Multikinase Inhibitors

> **Key Point**
> While RECIST 1.1 has worked well for following metastatic disease treated by prior standard chemotherapy, there are problems with its use in patients treated with anti-angiogenesis drugs, including multi-kinase inhibitors. This is because multi-kinase inhibitors may produce necrosis (and resulting diminished attenuation on contrast-enhanced CT) in responding to metastatic lesions without these lesions decreasing significantly in size. As a result, a patient who is a partial responder can be misidentified as not having responded to treatment, if only RECIST 1.1 is used.

Several alternative measuring systems have been devised, which consider changes in lesion attenuation in addition to changes in size. This includes the Choi, modified Choi, and the "Morphology, Attenuation, Size, and Structure" (MASS)

systems [55, 56]. With the Choi criteria, a decrease in target lesion size of only 10% or more OR a decrease in target attenuation of 15% or more indicates a partial response. With the modified Choi criteria, both features must be present at the same time.

11.14.3.3 Immunotherapy

Recently, patients with metastatic RCC have been increasingly treated with immunotherapy. These agents are antibodies targeted to attack receptors on lymphocytes or surface ligands on tumor cells. They work by interfering with a tumor's ability to inhibit an immune response. At the present time, the immune checkpoints which are being inhibited include those related to cytotoxic T-lymphocyte-associated antigen 4 (CTLA4) and the program cell death protein 1 receptor on T-cells (PD-1) or its related ligands on tumor cells (PDL1, PDL2) (47).

> **Key Point**
> A unique feature of RCC metastases treated by immunotherapy is that some responding lesions may initially appear stable or even enlarge to such an extent that progressive disease would be diagnosed if RECIST 1.1 were to be used. An apparent initial increase in size should be considered as unconfirmed progressive disease (UPD). UPD must be confirmed by another follow-up imaging study in no less than 4 weeks [57]. If metastases continue to enlarge, then progressive disease can be diagnosed. In some instances, however, a subsequent study will indicate tumor response (consisting of decreased size and/or attenuation), confirming that the initial change in size was merely "pseudoprogression." The system for assessing metastatic tumor in immunotherapy patients has been modified to take these issues into account (iRECIST criteria) [57]. Initial studies on the efficacy of immunotherapy in treating patients with metastatic renal cancer have been promising. Many patients have had sustained responses, which have even persisted after therapy was discontinued.

11.14.3.4 Complications of Multikinase Inhibitor Treatment and Immunotherapy

Complications encountered in patients undergoing new systemic treatments include hepatic steatosis, cholecystitis, pancreatitis, bowel perforation, arterial thrombosis (after multikinase therapy) and segmental or diffuse colitis, pneumonitis, dermatitis, and, less commonly, thyroiditis, hypophysitis, pancreatitis, and adrenal dysfunction [57].

11.15 Concluding Remarks

Over the last years, there have been several exciting developments with respect to imaging, diagnosis, treatment, and management of cystic and solid renal masses. This has included the identification of imaging features that can differentiate among some of the many cystic and solid renal masses. In 2019, an updated Bosniak classification has been introduced also incorporating MR-based assessment of cystic renal masses and clear terms for radiology reporting. Unfortunately, in many patients, overlapping features still prevent the distinction of renal cancers from benign renal lesions or non-neoplastic cancer mimics. Therefore, RMB, which can be performed safely and without concern for tumor tract seeding, has an emerging role for definitive diagnosis and risk stratification. Imaging remains crucial for differential diagnosis, staging, and management of renal masses, as it is very accurate. In patients with organ-confined disease, imaging can be used to determine which patients are candidates for PN versus RN. It has become increasingly clear that some patients with small malignant renal masses may not undergo immediate treatment and that AS should be increasingly considered for selected patients. Novel chemotherapeutic agents have greatly prolonged the survival of patients with regional or distant oligometastatic disease and immunotherapy is increasingly implemented in adjuvant settings.

Take Home Messages
- Most renal masses are incidentally detected.
- Most solid renal masses are malignant.
- CT is the most frequent imaging technique to detect renal masses.
- CT is the main imaging modality for RCC staging.
- MRI can be helpful to characterize solid renal masses and serves as problem solver.
- Renal mass biopsy is an integral part of clinical staging.
- Multidisciplinary approach is key, and treatment should be tailored to each patient.

References

1. Herms E, Weirich G, Maurer T, Wagenpfeil S, Preuss S, Sauter A, et al. Ultrasound-based "CEUS-Bosniak"classification for cystic renal lesions: an 8-year clinical experience. World J Urol. 2022; https://doi.org/10.1007/s00345-022-04094-0.
2. Expert Panel on Urologic Imaging, Wang ZJ, Nikolaidis P, Khatri G, Dogra VS, Ganeshan D, et al. ACR appropriateness criteria(R) indeterminate renal mass. J Am Coll Radiol. 2020;17(11S):S415–S28. https://doi.org/10.1016/j.jacr.2020.09.010.
3. Campbell SC, Clark PE, Chang SS, Karam JA, Souter L, Uzzo RG. Renal mass and localized renal cancer: evaluation, management, and follow-up: AUA guideline: part I. J Urol. 2021;206(2):199–208. https://doi.org/10.1097/JU.0000000000001911.
4. Campbell SC, Uzzo RG, Karam JA, Chang SS, Clark PE, Souter L. Renal mass and localized renal cancer: evaluation, management, and follow-up: AUA guideline: part II. J Urol. 2021;206(2):209–18. https://doi.org/10.1097/JU.0000000000001912.
5. Znaor A, Lortet-Tieulent J, Laversanne M, Jemal A, Bray F. International variations and trends in renal cell carcinoma incidence and mortality. Eur Urol. 2015;67(3):519–30. https://doi.org/10.1016/j.eururo.2014.10.002.
6. Corwin MT, Altinmakas E, Asch D, Bishop KA, Boge M, Curci NE, et al. Clinical importance of incidental homogeneous renal masses that measure 10-40 mm and 21-39 HU at portal venous phase CT: a 12-institution retrospective cohort study. AJR Am J Roentgenol. 2021;217(1):135–40. https://doi.org/10.2214/AJR.20.24245.
7. Hindman NM. Approach to very small (<1.5 cm) cystic renal lesions: ignore, observe, or treat? AJR Am J Roentgenol. 2015;204(6):1182–9. https://doi.org/10.2214/AJR.15.14357.
8. Silverman SG, Pedrosa I, Ellis JH, Hindman NM, Schieda N, Smith AD, et al. Bosniak classification of cystic renal masses, version 2019: an update proposal and needs assessment. Radiology. 2019;292(2):475–88. https://doi.org/10.1148/radiol.2019182646.
9. Herts BR, Silverman SG, Hindman NM, Uzzo RG, Hartman RP, Israel GM, et al. Management of the Incidental Renal Mass on CT: a white paper of the ACR incidental findings committee. J Am Coll Radiol. 2018;15(2):264–73. https://doi.org/10.1016/j.jacr.2017.04.028.
10. Walker SM, Gautam R, Turkbey B, Malayeri A, Choyke PL. Update on hereditary renal cancer and imaging implications. Radiol Clin N Am. 2020;58(5):951–63. https://doi.org/10.1016/j.rcl.2020.04.003.
11. Bosniak MA, Birnbaum BA, Krinsky GA, Waisman J. Small renal parenchymal neoplasms: further observations on growth. Radiology. 1995;197(3):589–97. https://doi.org/10.1148/radiology.197.3.7480724.
12. Bosniak MA. The current radiological approach to renal cysts. Radiology. 1986;158(1):1–10. https://doi.org/10.1148/radiology.158.1.3510019.
13. Jinzaki M, Silverman SG, Akita H, Mikami S, Oya M. Diagnosis of renal Angiomyolipomas: classic, fat-poor, and epithelioid types. Semin Ultrasound CT MR. 2017;38(1):37–46. https://doi.org/10.1053/j.sult.2016.11.001.
14. Davenport MS, Neville AM, Ellis JH, Cohan RH, Chaudhry HS, Leder RA. Diagnosis of renal angiomyolipoma with hounsfield unit thresholds: effect of size of region of interest and nephrographic phase imaging. Radiology. 2011;260(1):158–65. https://doi.org/10.1148/radiol.11102476.
15. Catalano OA, Samir AE, Sahani DV, Hahn PF. Pixel distribution analysis: can it be used to distinguish clear cell carcinomas from angiomyolipomas with minimal fat? Radiology. 2008;247(3):738–46. https://doi.org/10.1148/radiol.2473070785.
16. Zhang YY, Luo S, Liu Y, Xu RT. Angiomyolipoma with minimal fat: differentiation from papillary renal cell carcinoma by helical CT. Clin Radiol. 2013;68(4):365–70. https://doi.org/10.1016/j.crad.2012.08.028.
17. Krishna S, Murray CA, McInnes MD, Chatelain R, Siddaiah M, Al-Dandan O, et al. CT imaging of solid renal masses: pitfalls and solutions. Clin Radiol. 2017;72(9):708–21. https://doi.org/10.1016/j.crad.2017.05.003.
18. Woo S, Cho JY, Kim SH, Kim SY, Lee HJ, Hwang SI, et al. Segmental enhancement inversion of small renal oncocytoma: differences in prevalence according to tumor size. AJR Am J Roentgenol. 2013;200(5):1054–9. https://doi.org/10.2214/AJR.12.9300.

19. O'Malley ME, Tran P, Hanbidge A, Rogalla P. Small renal oncocytomas: is segmental enhancement inversion a characteristic finding at biphasic MDCT? AJR Am J Roentgenol. 2012;199(6):1312–5. https://doi.org/10.2214/AJR.12.8616.

20. Low G, Huang G, Fu W, Moloo Z, Girgis S. Review of renal cell carcinoma and its common subtypes in radiology. World J Radiol. 2016;8(5):484–500. https://doi.org/10.4329/wjr.v8.i5.484.

21. Moch H, Cubilla AL, Humphrey PA, Reuter VE, Ulbright TM. The 2016 WHO classification of tumours of the urinary system and male genital organs-part a: renal, penile, and testicular tumours. Eur Urol. 2016;70(1):93–105. https://doi.org/10.1016/j.eururo.2016.02.029.

22. Zhu QQ, Wang ZQ, Zhu WR, Chen WX, Wu JT. The multislice CT findings of renal carcinoma associated with XP11.2 translocation/TFE gene fusion and collecting duct carcinoma. Acta Radiol. 2013;54(3):355–62. https://doi.org/10.1258/ar.2012.120255.

23. Roberts JL, Ghali F, Aganovic L, Bechis S, Healy K, Rivera-Sanfeliz G, et al. Diagnosis, management, and follow-up of upper tract urothelial carcinoma: an interdisciplinary collaboration between urology and radiology. Abdom Radiol (NY). 2019;44(12):3893–905. https://doi.org/10.1007/s00261-019-02293-9.

24. Osako Y, Tatarano S, Nishiyama K, Yamada Y, Yamagata T, Uchida Y, et al. Unusual presentation of intraparenchymal renal artery aneurysm mimicking cystic renal cell carcinoma: a case report. Int J Urol. 2011;18(7):533–5. https://doi.org/10.1111/j.1442-2042.2011.02775.x.

25. Dwivedi US, Goyal NK, Saxena V, Acharya RL, Trivedi S, Singh PB, et al. Xanthogranulomatous pyelonephritis: our experience with review of published reports. ANZ J Surg. 2006;76(11):1007–9. https://doi.org/10.1111/j.1445-2197.2006.03919.x.

26. Katabathina V, Menias CO, Pickhardt P, Lubner M, Prasad SR. Complications of immunosuppressive therapy in solid organ transplantation. Radiol Clin N Am. 2016;54(2):303–19. https://doi.org/10.1016/j.rcl.2015.09.009.

27. Pierorazio PM, Hyams ES, Mullins JK, Allaf ME. Active surveillance for small renal masses. Rev Urol. 2012;14(1–2):13–9.

28. Miskin N, Qin L, Matalon SA, Tirumani SH, Alessandrino F, Silverman SG, et al. Stratification of cystic renal masses into benign and potentially malignant: applying machine learning to the bosniak classification. Abdom Radiol (NY). 2021;46(1):311–8. https://doi.org/10.1007/s00261-020-02629-w.

29. Diaz de Leon A, Davenport MS, Silverman SG, Schieda N, Cadeddu JA, Pedrosa I. Role of virtual biopsy in the management of renal masses. AJR Am J Roentgenol. 2019:1–10. https://doi.org/10.2214/AJR.19.21172.

30. Kim NY, Lubner MG, Nystrom JT, Swietlik JF, Abel EJ, Havighurst TC, et al. Utility of CT texture analysis in differentiating Low-attenuation renal cell carcinoma from cysts: a bi-institutional retrospective study. AJR Am J Roentgenol. 2019;213(6):1259–66. https://doi.org/10.2214/AJR.19.21182.

31. Leng S, Takahashi N, Gomez Cardona D, Kitajima K, McCollough B, Li Z, et al. Subjective and objective heterogeneity scores for differentiating small renal masses using contrast-enhanced CT. Abdom Radiol (NY). 2017;42(5):1485–92. https://doi.org/10.1007/s00261-016-1014-2.

32. Coy H, Young JR, Douek ML, Brown MS, Sayre J, Raman SS. Quantitative computer-aided diagnostic algorithm for automated detection of peak lesion attenuation in differentiating clear cell from papillary and chromophobe renal cell carcinoma, oncocytoma, and fat-poor angiomyolipoma on multiphasic multidetector computed tomography. Abdom Radiol (NY). 2017;42(7):1919–28. https://doi.org/10.1007/s00261-017-1095-6.

33. Chen C, Kang Q, Wei Q, Xu B, Ye H, Wang T, et al. Correlation between CT perfusion parameters and Fuhrman grade in pT1b renal cell carcinoma. Abdom Radiol (NY). 2017;42(5):1464–71. https://doi.org/10.1007/s00261-016-1009-z.

34. Bindayi A, Hamilton ZA, McDonald ML, Yim K, Millard F, McKay RR, et al. Neoadjuvant therapy for localized and locally advanced renal cell carcinoma. Urol Oncol. 2018;36(1):31–7. https://doi.org/10.1016/j.urolonc.2017.07.015.

35. Escudier B, Porta C, Schmidinger M, Rioux-Leclercq N, Bex A, Khoo V, et al. Renal cell carcinoma: ESMO clinical practice guidelines for diagnosis, treatment and follow-up dagger. Ann Oncol. 2019;30(5):706–20. https://doi.org/10.1093/annonc/mdz056.

36. Delahunt B, Cheville JC, Martignoni G, Humphrey PA, Magi-Galluzzi C, McKenney J, et al. The International Society of Urological Pathology (ISUP) grading system for renal cell carcinoma and other prognostic parameters. Am J Surg Pathol. 2013;37(10):1490–504. https://doi.org/10.1097/PAS.0b013e318299f0fb.

37. Pedrosa I, Cadeddu JA. How we do it: managing the indeterminate renal mass with the MRI clear cell likelihood score. Radiology. 2022;302(2):256–69. https://doi.org/10.1148/radiol.210034.

38. Rasmussen RG, Xi Y, Sibley RC 3rd, Lee CJ, Cadeddu JA, Pedrosa I. Association of clear cell likelihood score on MRI and growth kinetics of small solid renal masses on active surveillance. AJR Am J Roentgenol. 2022;218(1):101–10. https://doi.org/10.2214/AJR.21.25979.

39. Halverson SJ, Kunju LP, Bhalla R, Gadzinski AJ, Alderman M, Miller DC, et al. Accuracy of determining small renal mass management with risk stratified biopsies: confirmation by final pathology. J Urol. 2013;189(2):441–6. https://doi.org/10.1016/j.juro.2012.09.032.

40. Park SH, Oh YT, Jung DC, Cho NH, Choi YD, Park SY. Abdominal seeding of renal cell carcinoma: radiologic, pathologic, and prognostic features. Abdom Radiol (NY). 2017;42(5):1510–6. https://doi.org/10.1007/s00261-016-1029-8.

41. Ozambela M Jr, Wang Y, Leow JJ, Silverman SG, Chung BI, Chang SL. Contemporary trends in percutaneous renal mass biopsy utilization in the United States. Urol Oncol. 2020;38(11):835–43. https://doi.org/10.1016/j.urolonc.2020.07.022.

42. Amin MB, Greene FL, Edge SB, Compton CC, Gershenwald JE, Brookland RK, et al. The eighth edition AJCC cancer staging manual: continuing to build a bridge from a population-based to a more "personalized" approach to cancer staging. CA Cancer J Clin. 2017;67(2):93–9. https://doi.org/10.3322/caac.21388.

43. Motzer RJ, Jonasch E, Boyle S, Carlo MI, Manley B, Agarwal N, et al. NCCN guidelines insights: kidney cancer, version 1.2021. J Natl Compr Cancer Netw. 2020;18(9):1160–70. https://doi.org/10.6004/jnccn.2020.0043.

44. Ljungberg B, Bensalah K, Canfield S, Dabestani S, Hofmann F, Hora M, et al. EAU guidelines on renal cell carcinoma: 2014 update. Eur Urol. 2015;67(5):913–24. https://doi.org/10.1016/j.eururo.2015.01.005.

45. Kutikov A, Uzzo RG. The R.E.N.a.L. nephrometry score: a comprehensive standardized system for quantitating renal tumor size, location and depth. J Urol. 2009;182(3):844–53. https://doi.org/10.1016/j.juro.2009.05.035.

46. Sury K, Pierorazio PM. Definitive treatment vs. active surveillance for small renal masses: closing the preference gap. Can Urol Assoc J. 2022;16(4):102–3. https://doi.org/10.5489/cuaj.7841.

47. Schieda N, Krishna S, Pedrosa I, Kaffenberger SD, Davenport MS, Silverman SG. Active surveillance of renal masses: the role of radiology. Radiology. 2022;302(1):11–24. https://doi.org/10.1148/radiol.2021204227.

48. Choueiri TK, Tomczak P, Park SH, Venugopal B, Ferguson T, Chang YH, et al. Adjuvant Pembrolizumab after nephrectomy in renal-cell carcinoma. N Engl J Med. 2021;385(8):683–94. https://doi.org/10.1056/NEJMoa2106391.

49. Palma DA, Olson R, Harrow S, Gaede S, Louie AV, Haasbeek C, et al. Stereotactic ablative radiotherapy versus standard of care palliative treatment in patients with oligometastatic can-

cers (SABR-COMET): a randomised, phase 2, open-label trial. Lancet. 2019;393(10185):2051–8. https://doi.org/10.1016/S0140-6736(18)32487-5.

50. Motzer RJ, Jonasch E, Agarwal N, Alva A, Baine M, Beckermann K, et al. Kidney cancer, version 3.2022, NCCN clinical practice guidelines in oncology. J Natl Compr Cancer Netw. 2022;20(1):71–90. https://doi.org/10.6004/jnccn.2022.0001.

51. Kawamoto S, Solomon SB, Bluemke DA, Fishman EK. Computed tomography and magnetic resonance imaging appearance of renal neoplasms after radiofrequency ablation and cryoablation. Semin Ultrasound CT MR. 2009;30(2):67–77. https://doi.org/10.1053/j.sult.2008.12.005.

52. Chen J, Yang M, Wu P, Li T, Ning X, Peng S, et al. Renal arterial Pseudoaneurysm and renal arteriovenous fistula following partial nephrectomy. Urol Int. 2018;100(3):368–74. https://doi.org/10.1159/000443700.

53. Corwin MT, Lamba R, Wilson M, McGahan JP. Renal cell carcinoma metastases to the pancreas: value of arterial phase imaging at MDCT. Acta Radiol. 2013;54(3):349–54. https://doi.org/10.1258/ar.2012.120693.

54. Nishino M, Jagannathan JP, Ramaiya NH, Van den Abbeele AD. Revised RECIST guideline version 1.1: what oncologists want to know and what radiologists need to know. AJR Am J Roentgenol. 2010;195(2):281–9. https://doi.org/10.2214/AJR.09.4110.

55. Smith AD, Shah SN, Rini BI, Lieber ML, Remer EM. Morphology, attenuation, size, and structure (MASS) criteria: assessing response and predicting clinical outcome in metastatic renal cell carcinoma on antiangiogenic targeted therapy. AJR Am J Roentgenol. 2010;194(6):1470–8. https://doi.org/10.2214/AJR.09.3456.

56. Thian Y, Gutzeit A, Koh DM, Fisher R, Lote H, Larkin J, et al. Revised Choi imaging criteria correlate with clinical outcomes in patients with metastatic renal cell carcinoma treated with sunitinib. Radiology. 2014;273(2):452–61. https://doi.org/10.1148/radiol.14132702.

57. Seymour L, Bogaerts J, Perrone A, Ford R, Schwartz LH, Mandrekar S, et al. iRECIST: guidelines for response criteria for use in trials testing immunotherapeutics. Lancet Oncol. 2017;18(3):e143–e52. https://doi.org/10.1016/S1470-2045(17)30074-8.

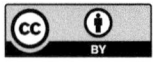

Imaging Features of Immunotherapy

12

Atul B. Shinagare and Ghaneh Fananapazir

Learning Objectives
- Understand the mechanisms of action of immunotherapy agents
- Recognize typical and atypical patterns of response to immunotherapy agents
- Recognize the complications of immunotherapy agents

12.1 Introduction

Immunotherapy has emerged as a major advance in the treatment of cancer. Immunotherapy utilizes the body's own immune system to target cancer cells and has proven effective against a variety of cancer subtypes, including melanoma, renal cell carcinoma, lung cancer, breast cancer, and lymphomas, to name a few. In this chapter, we will discuss the mechanism of action of common immunotherapy drugs, their response assessment, and adverse events.

12.2 Mechanism of Action

12.2.1 Cancer Immunity Cycle

Genetic alterations in cancer cells should, in theory, make them susceptible to attack by immune cells; however, cancer cells evade immune attack by producing certain surface pro-

teins (such as PD-1) that inhibit T cells [1]. The creation of immune response against cancer cells requires a series of events, called the cancer immunity cycle. The major steps involved in this process include the release of antigens from dying cancer cells and their capture by the dendritic cells (antigen-presenting cell), presentation of the cancer antigens by the dendritic cells to T cells resulting in activation of effector T cells against cancer, infiltration of the tumor by activated effector T cells, recognition of the cancer antigen by the T cells and T cell binding, and finally killing the target cancer cell. Dying cancer cells release additional tumor-associated antigens leading to wider immune activation against cancer. However, the cancer immunity cycle may not be effective due to failure of any of the above steps, most importantly because tumor microenvironment may suppress effector T cells.

12.2.2 Goal of Immunotherapy

The goal of cancer immunotherapy is to create a robust and self-sustaining cancer immunity cycle without creating an unchecked autoimmune inflammatory response against the host cells. This is achieved by selectively targeting certain steps of the cycle without amplifying the entire cycle.

12.2.3 Anti-CTLA-4 Antibodies

Anti-CTLA-4 (Cytotoxic T-Lymphocyte Antigen-4) antibodies, such as Ipilimumab, target the T cell activation step within lymph nodes. CTLA-4 on the T cell surface is a major negative regulator of T cells. If unchecked, it binds with B7 on the antigen-presenting cell and leads to inhibition of T cell response. Anti-CTLA-4 antibodies block this interaction of CTLA-4 and lead to T cell activation (Fig. 12.1). This also

A. B. Shinagare
Department of Radiology, Brigham and Women's Hospital, Boston, MA, USA
e-mail: ashinagare@bwh.harvard.edu

G. Fananapazir (✉)
Department of Radiology, UC Davis Medical Center, Sacramento, CA, USA
e-mail: fananapazir@ucdavis.edu

© The Author(s) 2023
J. Hodler et al. (eds.), *Diseases of the Abdomen and Pelvis 2023-2026*, IDKD Springer Series, https://doi.org/10.1007/978-3-031-27355-1_12

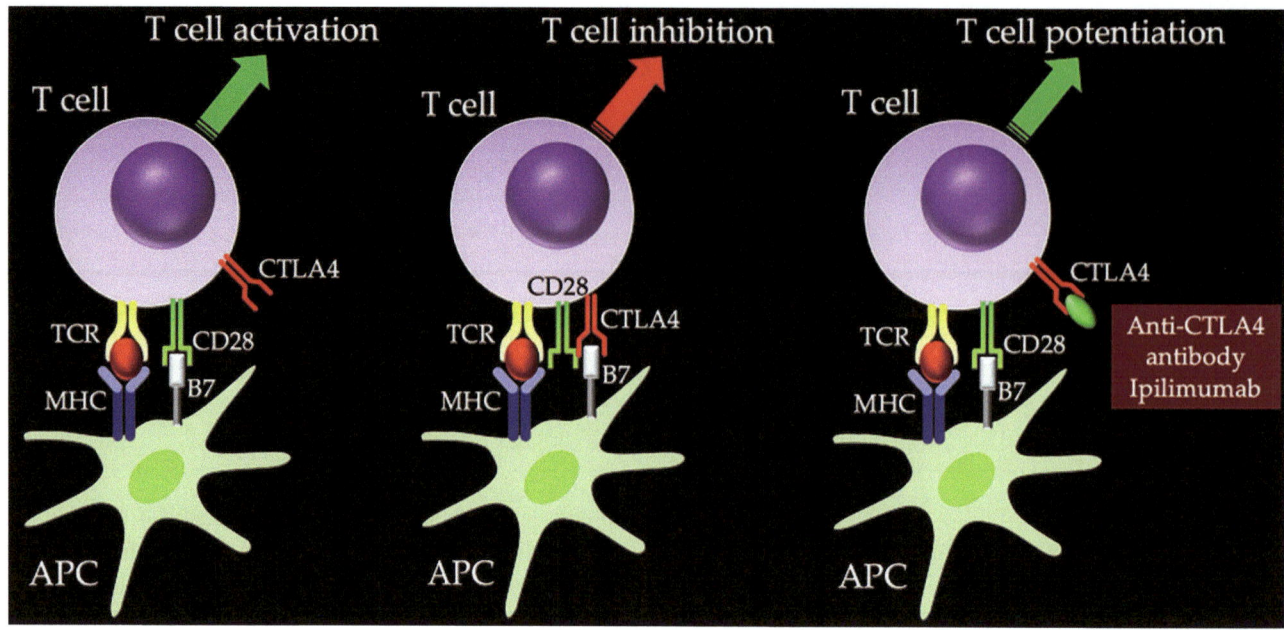

Fig. 12.1 Schematic showing the interaction between B7 on the antigen-presenting cell and CD28 on T cell leading to T cell activation (left), CTLA-4 on the T cell inhibiting this interaction leading to T cell inhibition (middle), and anti-CTLA-4 antibody (such as ipilimumab) blocking CTLA-4 leading to T cell activation (right)

helps explain the higher incidence of immune-related toxicities with anti-CTLA-4 antibodies. The activation of T cells is not necessarily limited against tumor-specific antigens. Lack of selectivity in T cell activation, combined with the fundamental importance of CTLA-4 as an immune checkpoint, leads to significant immune-related toxicities with agents such as ipilimumab [2].

12.2.4 PD-L1 and PD-1 Inhibitors

PD-L1 (Programmed death-ligand 1) is an immune modulator expressed in 20%–50% of human cancers, which binds to PD-1(Programmed cell death protein 1) on effector T cells, leading to blockade of cytotoxic mediators needed to kill the cancer cells. This is one of the most important mechanisms the cancer cells use to evade immune response. Agents that block PD-L1 on cancer cells (such as Atezolizumab, Avelumab, and Durvalumab) or PD-1 on T cells (such as Nivolumab and Pembrolizumab) restore antitumor immune response of effector T cells and result in excellent immune response (Fig. 12.2). Furthermore, acting within the tumor microenvironment, the PD-L1 and PD-1 inhibitors are more specific to cancer cells, and are thus associated with fewer and milder immune-related toxicities.

> **Key Point**
> Differences in the mechanism of action of anti-CTLA-4 antibodies and PD-L1/PD-1 inhibitors explain their different toxicity profiles. Anti-CTLA-4 antibodies lead to a more global activation of the immune system, leading to more frequent and severe toxicities, whereas PD-L1/PD-1 inhibitors are more specific to the tumor and therefore have fewer and milder toxicities.

12.2.5 Combination Immunotherapy

The approaches mentioned above, namely anti-CTLA-4 antibodies and PD-L1/PD-1 inhibitors are just two of many possible strategies to create immune response. Combining different agents acting at different steps of the cancer immunity cycle can create a more robust anticancer immune response, leading to potentially higher efficacy and frequency of response; however, such combination therapies may also be associated with a higher rate of toxicities.

> **Key Point**
> Once the immune system is activated, the response of immunotherapy agents is often durable, lasting even after the treatment is discontinued.

Fig. 12.2 Schematic showing the interaction between PD-1 on T cell and PD-L1 on the tumor cell. PD-1 and PD-L1 inhibitors act by blocking this interaction, thereby activating the effector T cell response against tumor cells

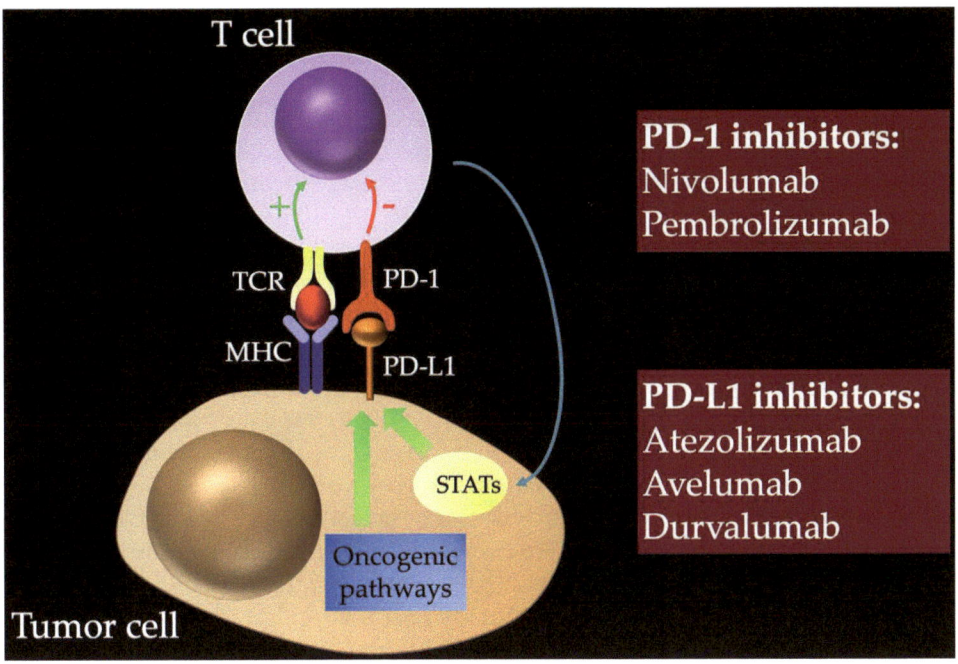

12.2.6 CAR T-Cell Therapy

Chimeric antigen receptor–engineered (CAR) T cell therapy is a novel form of immunotherapy predominantly used for hematologic malignancies. To date, there are four FDA-approved CAR T cell therapies. CAR T cell therapy involves harvesting of patient's own T cells. These T cells are modified using viral vectors to express artificial chimeric antigen receptors that can recognize tumor-associated antigens. Patient is given chemotherapy to temporarily deplete the patient's native lymphocytes, followed by infusion of CAR T cells. These cells then bind to the tumor-associated antigens thus activating an immune response [3].

12.3 Tumor Response to Immunotherapy

12.3.1 Development of Standards for Assessing Cancer Treatment Response

Imaging is important in assessing tumor response to treatment, of which contrast-enhanced CT plays a dominant role. The change in tumor burden with treatment, when compared to a baseline scan, is used as a surrogate for survival and quality of life [4]. Efforts in the 1980s by the World Health Organization (WHO) sought to standardize the process for assessing treatment response with bidimensional measurement of target lesions [5]. This was an important step since it allowed for data from multiple institutions to be compared in a reproducible and uniform fashion.

Around 2000, an international group called the Response Evaluation Criteria in Solid Tumors (RECIST), looking at 4500 patients from 14 clinical trials, simplified the process of standardized measurements and advocated for the use of unidimensional measurements of target lesions [6]. In 2009, RECIST 1.1 was developed which relies on the sum of unidimensional measurements of up to five target lesions (with a maximum of two per organ) [7]. Baseline CTs are performed less than 4 weeks prior to treatment. Target lesions are measured in longest dimension and have to be ≥10 mm. However, for lymph nodes as target lesions these need to be ≥15 mm in short-axis dimension. The sum of diameters of the target lesions is compared to a subsequent exam that is generally not less than 6–8 weeks after treatment. If all target lesions have disappeared and all measured lymph nodes are <10 mm in short-axis dimension, the treatment is designated as "complete response." If there is at least a 30% reduction in the sum of diameters, the therapy elicited a "partial response." "Progressive disease" occurs when there is at least a 20% increase in the size of the sum of diameters or the appearance of one or more lesions. Finally, if there is neither sufficient shrinkage or enlargement to meet partial response or progressive disease criteria, it is designated as a "stable disease."

12.3.2 Limitations of RECIST 1.1 in Assessing Immunotherapy Response

The WHO, RECIST 1.0, and RECIST 1.1 were all developed to assess the response to cytotoxic therapy, in which tumor shrinkage correlates with increased survival. Immunotherapy poses a challenge to current tumor assessment criteria since its mechanism of action results in different imaging characteristics. Tumors treated with immunotherapy can show an initial increase in size and can take longer to shrink compared with cytotoxic drugs.

> **Key Point**
> Additionally, infiltration by immune cells with robust response to immunotherapy can lead to increased size of the lesions (termed pseudoprogression) despite a robust response.

Cases that were classified by RECIST 1.1 as "progressive disease" have been shown to be "stable disease," "partial response," or "complete response" when carried out more longitudinally [8]. Designating response as "progressive disease" when it is actually responding can lead to inappropriate, premature cessation of treatment.

12.3.3 Development of Immunotherapy-Specific Response Standards

In 2009, in response to these concerns, a revised version of the WHO criteria (using bi-dimensional measurements) was proposed, termed the immune-related response criteria (irRC). This system allowed for new lesions to be included in the sum of diameters calculation as well as the need for a confirmatory scan for patients with "progressive disease" to performed ≥4 weeks later. In 2013, subsequent recommendations incorporated elements of RECIST 1.1 into immune therapy (number of target lesions and use of unidimensional measurements) and termed irRE-CIST. However, these were inconsistently applied, and the lack of standardization led the RECIST working group to create iRECIST in 2017, which is a modified version of RECIST 1.1 [9].

> **Key Point**
> iRECIST follows RECIST 1.1 with a new category termed "unconfirmed progressive disease" (iUPD) in cases where the subsequent examination seems to meet RECIST 1.1 criteria for "progressive disease." In such cases, a repeat scan is performed at 4–8 weeks, and if the sum of the dimensions continues to be 20% or greater from baseline or if there are new metastases, "confirmed progressive disease" (iCPD) is assessed [9].

12.4 Immune-Related Adverse Events (irAEs)

12.4.1 Overview

Immune-related adverse events (irAEs) are immunologic "flare" phenomenon. Clinically, irAEs have been reported in up to 72% of patients with high-grade toxicities in 24% of patients. On imaging, irAEs may be seen in up to 31% of patients with ipilimumab (anti-CTLA-4 antibody) and 14% of patients with nivolumab (anti-PD-1 agent); however, the actual frequency may vary based on the cancer population and the exact drugs used [10, 11]. The most common toxicities seen on imaging are colitis, pneumonitis, and sarcoid-like reaction (Table 12.1). irAEs are often mild and treatment can be continued if the patient tolerates it; however, when severe, they are treated with steroids and may necessitate treatment discontinuation.

12.4.2 Colitis

Immune-mediated colitis is the most common irAE, often seen within 2–3 months of starting treatment. It is often subtle on imaging, seen as fluid-filled bowel, mild bowel wall thickening, with or without surrounding fat stranding. Marked wall thickening, bowel perforation, and ascites are uncommon. Two distinct patterns of colitis are seen, namely diffuse and segmental [12]. Diffuse colitis involves the entire colon or a long segment and seen as fluid-filled colon and surrounding vascular engorgement with or without mild colonic wall thickening (Fig. 12.3). Segmental colitis often involves segments of preexisting diverticulosis, presumably secondary to inflammatory immune response, and seen as moderate degree of wall thickening and surrounding stranding (Fig. 12.4).

> **Key Point**
> It is important to communicate the pattern of colitis in the radiology report, because if treatment is needed, diffuse colitis is treated with steroids while segmental colitis may require treatment with steroids and antibiotics.

Table 12.1 Common toxicities of immunotherapy seen on imaging

Organ	Findings
Bowel	Colitis, enterocolitis
Liver	Hepatitis, cholangitis
Lungs	Pneumonitis
Lymph nodes	Sarcoid-like reaction
Pancreas	Pancreatitis
Endocrine	Hypophysitis, thyroiditis, adrenalitis

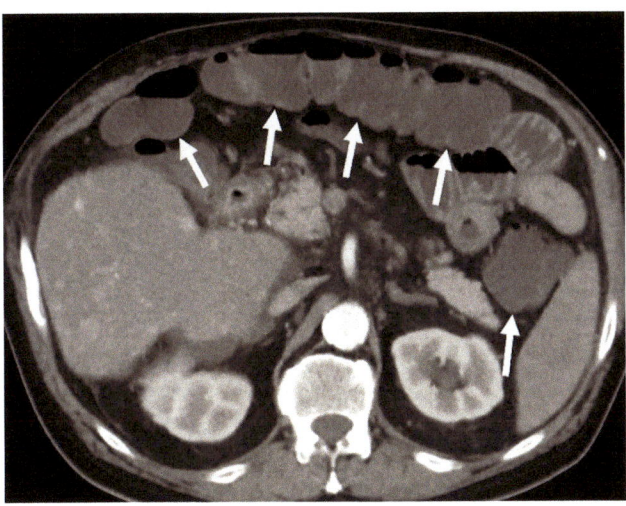

Fig. 12.3 Diffuse pattern of immune-mediated colitis. Axial contrast-enhanced CT showing fluid-filled transverse colon and splenic flexure (arrows) with very minimal vascular engorgement and without colonic wall thickening

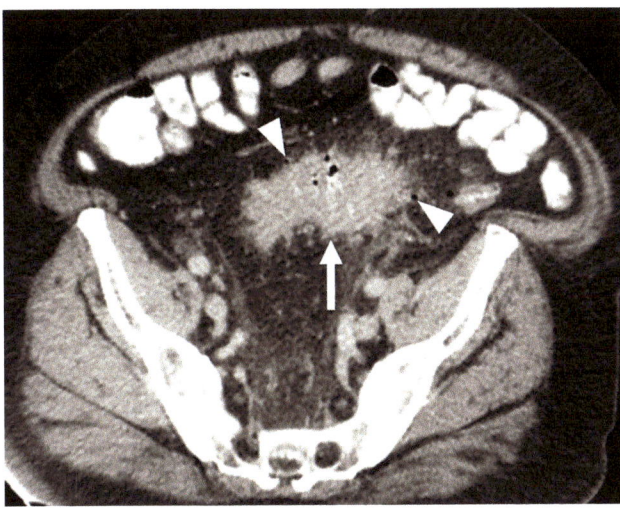

Fig. 12.4 Segmental pattern of immune-mediated colitis. Axial contrast-enhanced CT shows prominent wall thickening of the sigmoid colon (arrow) with surrounding fat stranding. A few small diverticula are seen (arrowheads)

12.4.3 Pneumonitis

Immune-mediated pneumonitis is reported in approximately 5% of patients; however, subtle imaging findings of inflammation may be seen more frequently. It usually presents within 2–6 months of starting therapy and is more common with combination immunotherapy, and more common with anti-PD-1 agents than anti-PD-L1 drugs [13]. Most commonly imaged with CT, pneumonitis usually presents as areas of groundglass or consolidative opacities with lower lobe predominance and often peripheral (Fig. 12.5). Reticular

changes may also be seen, especially when in the subacute phase. The findings are more commonly bilateral; however, may be unilateral. When presenting as a consolidation confined to a single lobe, it may mimic lobar pneumonia and may require treatment with both steroids and antibiotics if there is persistent confusion about the diagnosis. Some patients eventually develop a cryptogenic organizing pneumonia-like picture.

> **Key Point**
> Knowledge of immune-related pneumonitis is important even for abdominal radiologists as it is often seen in the lung bases on abdominal CT. Prompt communication of the toxicity is important as pneumonitis can quickly worsen and can be fatal.

12.4.4 Sarcoid-Like Reaction

Sarcoid-like reaction is best known with ipilimumab, often presenting with mediastinal lymphadenopathy, pulmonary nodules, and splenic involvement (Fig. 12.6) [14]. It may also involve other nodal stations.

> **Key Point**
> Sarcoid-like reactions may mimic disease progression. Mild increase or fluctuations in the size of previously uninvolved nodes upon starting immunotherapy should not be assumed to be metastatic disease. Progressive increase in nodal size on two or more scans is worrisome for metastatic involvement.

12.4.5 Hepatitis and Cholangitis

Immune-mediated hepatitis is an uncommon toxicity with often subtle and non-specific imaging findings. Imaging may be normal in mild cases. When severe, it may present with hepatomegaly, periportal edema, diffuse low attenuation or heterogeneous appearance of the liver and periportal lymphadenopathy (Fig. 12.7) [15]. On ultrasound, there is often prominent periportal echogenicity and gallbladder wall edema.

Immune-mediated cholangitis is uncommon and often difficult to diagnose. The imaging features are non-specific, appearing as biliary wall thickening and narrowing, mild biliary dilation, ill-defined peribiliary enhancement, and patchy diffusion restriction on MRI (Fig. 12.8). It is impor-

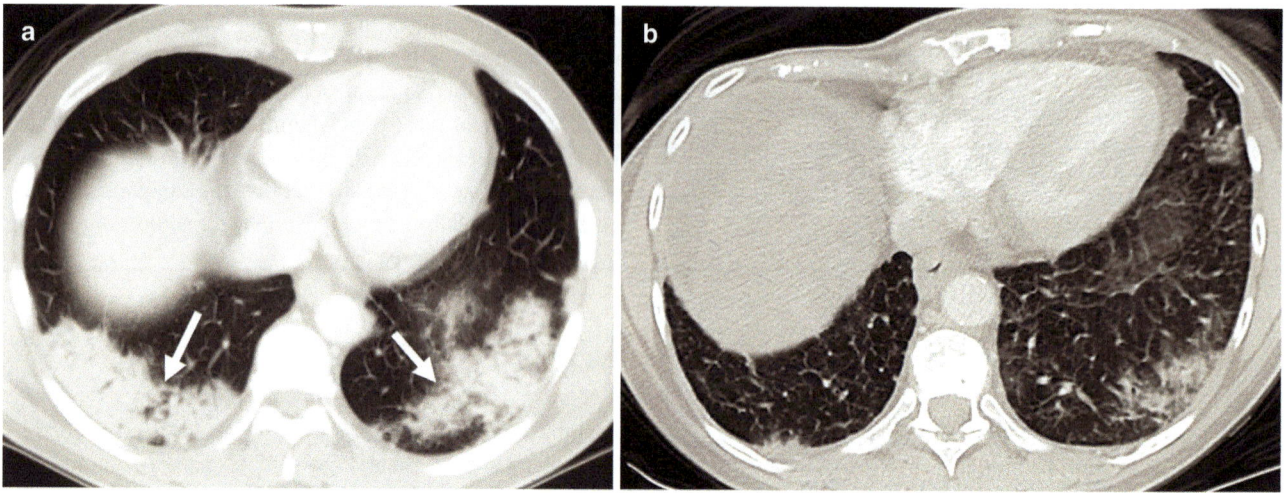

Fig. 12.5 Immune-mediated pneumonitis. (**a**) Axial CT of the chest through the lung bases shows bilateral lung base peripheral consolidative opacities (arrows). (**b**) The findings improved after treatment discontinuation and treatment with steroids

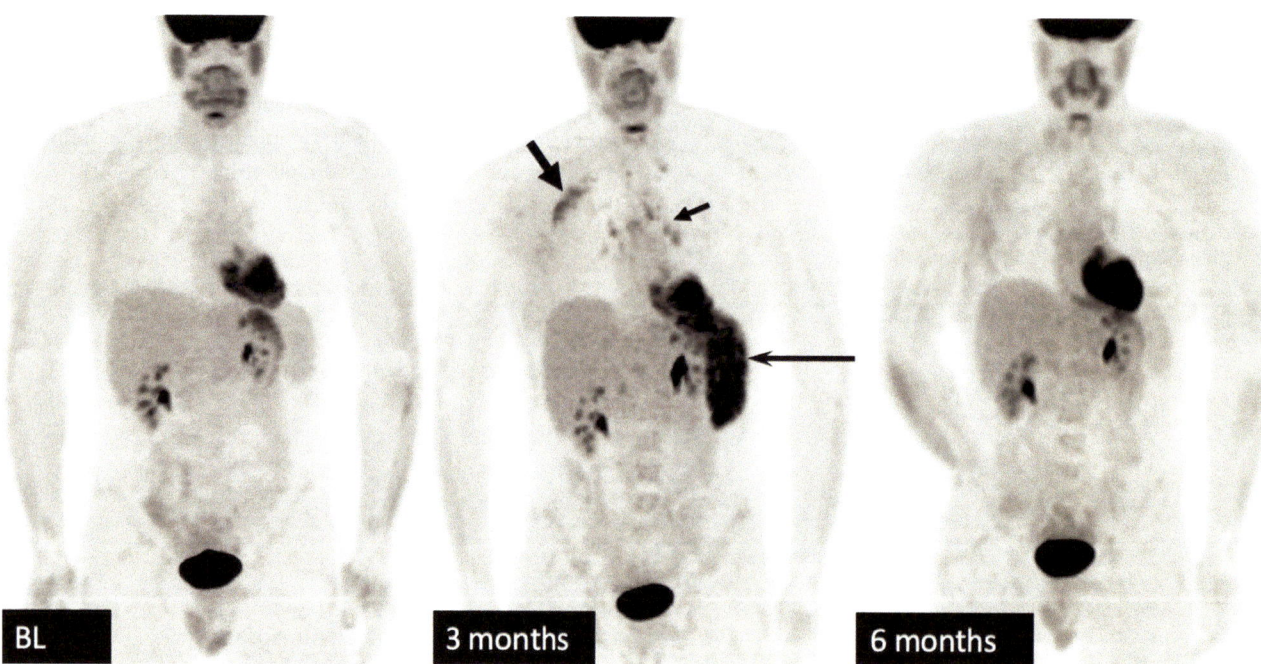

Fig. 12.6 Sarcoid-like reaction on ipilimumab. FDG-PET/CT performed 3 months after the first dose of ipilimumab showed new mediastinal lymphadenopathy (short thin arrow), lung nodules (short thick arrow), and splenic uptake (long thin arrow). The report raised a possibility of metastatic disease; however, the findings resolved on the follow-up FDG-PET/CT at 6 months

tant to rule out other autoimmune disorders including PSC or IgG4-related disease.

12.4.6 Pancreatitis

Immune-mediated pancreatitis is an uncommon but important toxicity of immunotherapy, often requiring treatment discontinuation. It is often focal but may be diffuse and presents with edematous appearance of the pancreas with mild surrounding stranding (Fig. 12.9). Occasionally the appearance may resemble autoimmune pancreatitis with a sausage-shaped pancreas. Severe pancreatitis with necrotic changes and peripancreatic collections is almost never seen.

> **Key Point**
> Imaging findings of immune-mediated pancreatitis are often mild and inconclusive. Correlation with serum lipase and/or amylase levels may be needed.

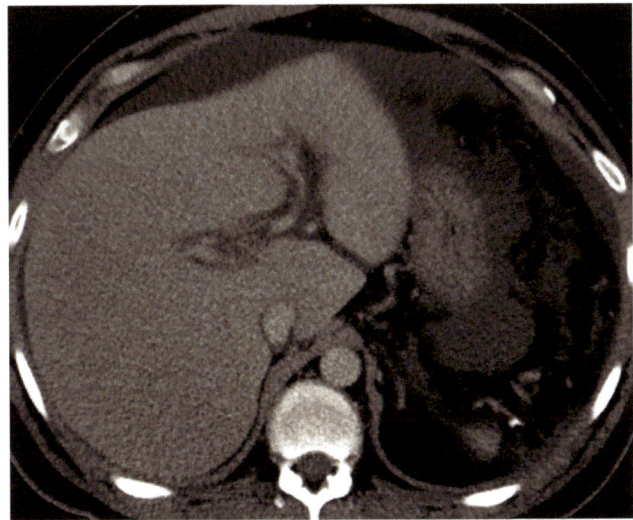

Fig. 12.7 Immune-mediated hepatitis. Axial contrast-enhanced CT shows periportal edema and diffuse mildly heterogeneous appearance of the liver

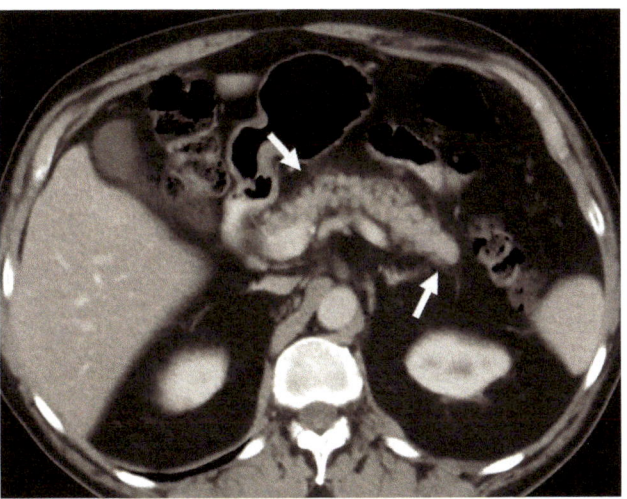

Fig. 12.9 Immune-mediated pancreatitis. Axial contrast-enhanced CT image shows edematous appearance of the pancreas with mild peripancreatic fat stranding (arrows)

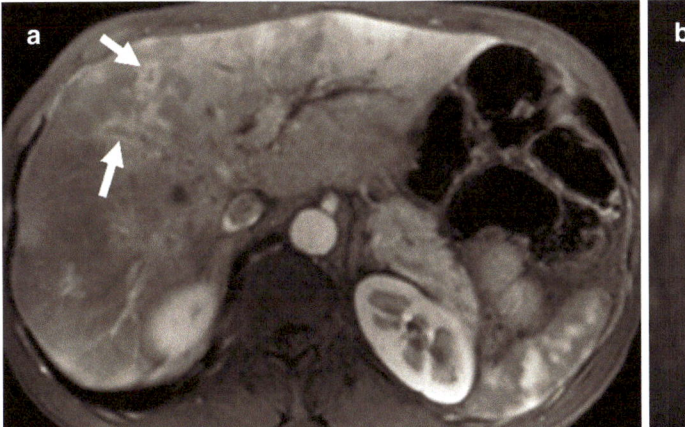
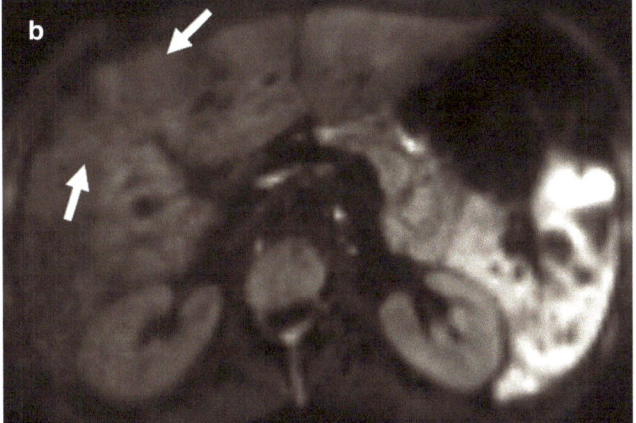

Fig. 12.8 Immune-mediated cholangitis. (**a**) Axial contrast-enhanced axial T1-weighted image shows mild thickening and enhancement of biliary ducts (arrows) with mild peribiliary enhancement. (**b**) Axial diffusion-weighted image shows patchy areas of diffusion restriction (arrows)

12.4.7 Endocrine Adverse Events

Endocrine adverse events are more commonly seen with combination immunotherapy and can be seen in the form of adrenalitis, hypophysitis, or thyroiditis. With adrenalitis, depending on the timing of imaging, the adrenals may be mildly thickened with surrounding stranding or may be atrophic.

> **Key Point**
> Immune-related toxicity can be a biomarker of response. Patients with severe adverse events are also more likely to have a robust response.

12.4.8 Toxicities of CAR T-Cell Therapy

The major toxicities of CAR T cell therapy include cytokine release syndrome (CRS) and neurotoxicity. While not specific to CAR T cell therapy, CRS occurs in 58–93% of patients receiving this treatment, typically 2–3 days after the infusion. Mild CRS presents as fatigue, fever, and malaise while severe cases present with hemodynamic instability, altered liver function tests, respiratory failure, consumptive coagulopathy, and can lead to death [3]. Imaging findings are nonspecific and may demonstrate pulmonary edema and pleural effusions.

12.5 Conclusion

Immunotherapy has been shown to be effective in treating many common cancers and is increasingly used in clinical practice. However, the imaging features of immunotherapy in determining response are different than those seen after chemotherapy and radiation therapy. Additionally, there is a range of adverse effects of immunotherapy that can be seen on imaging. Therefore, the radiologist should be aware of the history of immunotherapy use in determining response to treatment as well as being aware of immune-response adverse events.

> **Take Home Messages**
> - Immunotherapy activates the body's own immune system to elicit a response against tumor cells.
> - Inflammation from a robust immune response can lead to pseudoprogression of the target lesions.
> - iRECIST category "unconfirmed progressive disease" (iUPD) may indicate pseudoprogression or true progression, requiring a repeat scan to be performed at 4–8 weeks.
> - Toxicities related to immunotherapy can lead to colitis, hepatitis, cholangitis, pancreatitis, sarcomatoid-like reactions, pancreatitis pneumonitis, hypophysitis, thyroiditis, and adrenalitis.

References

1. Chen DS, Mellman I. Oncology meets immunology: the cancer-immunity cycle. Immunity. 2013;39(1):1–10.
2. Hodi FS, O'Day SJ, McDermott DF, Weber RW, Sosman JA, Haanen JB, et al. Improved survival with ipilimumab in patients with metastatic melanoma. N Engl J Med. 2010;363(8):711–23.
3. Yoon JG, Smith DA, Tirumani SH, Caimi PF, Ramaiya NH. CAR T-cell therapy: an update for radiologists. AJR Am J Roentgenol. 2021;217(6):1461–74.
4. Kim C, Prasad V. Cancer drugs approved on the basis of a surrogate end point and subsequent overall survival: an analysis of 5 years of US Food and Drug Administration approvals. JAMA Intern Med. 2015;175(12):1992–4.
5. Miller AB, Hoogstraten BF, Staquet MF, Winkler A. Reporting results of cancer treatment. Cancer. 1981;47(1):207–14.
6. Therasse P, Arbuck SG, Eisenhauer EA, Wanders J, Kaplan RS, Rubinstein L, Verweij J, Van Glabbeke M, van Oosterom AT, Christian MC, Gwyther SG. New guidelines to evaluate the response to treatment in solid tumors. J Natl Cancer Inst. 2000;92(3):205–16.
7. Eisenhauer EA, Therasse P, Bogaerts J, Schwartz LH, Sargent D, Ford R, Dancey J, Arbuck S, Gwyther S, Mooney M, Rubinstein L. New response evaluation criteria in solid tumours: revised RECIST guideline (version 1.1). Eur J Cancer. 2009;45(2):228–47.
8. Wolchok JD, Hoos A, O'Day S, Weber JS, Hamid O, Lebbé C, Maio M, Binder M, Bohnsack O, Nichol G, Humphrey R. Guidelines for the evaluation of immune therapy activity in solid tumors: immune-related response criteria. Clin Cancer Res. 2009;15(23):7412–20.
9. Tang YZ, Szabados B, Leung C, Sahdev A. Adverse effects and radiological manifestations of new immunotherapy agents. Br J Radiol. 2018;92:20180164.
10. Tirumani SH, Ramaiya NH, Keraliya A, Bailey ND, Ott PA, Hodi FS, et al. Radiographic profiling of immune-related adverse events in advanced melanoma patients treated with Ipilimumab. Cancer Immunol Res. 2015;3(10):1185–92.
11. Alessandrino F, Sahu S, Nishino M, Adeni AE, Tirumani SH, Shinagare AB, et al. Frequency and imaging features of abdominal immune-related adverse events in metastatic lung cancer patients treated with PD-1 inhibitor. Abdom Radiol (NY). 2019;44(5):1917–27.
12. Kim KW, Ramaiya NH, Krajewski KM, Shinagare AB, Howard SA, Jagannathan JP, et al. Ipilimumab-associated colitis: CT findings. AJR Am J Roentgenol. 2013;200(5):W468–74.
13. Khunger M, Rakshit S, Pasupuleti V, Hernandez AV, Mazzone P, Stevenson J, et al. Incidence of pneumonitis with use of programmed death 1 and programmed death-ligand 1 inhibitors in non-small cell lung cancer: a systematic review and meta-analysis of trials. Chest. 2017;152(2):271–81.
14. Vogel WV, Guislain A, Kvistborg P, Schumacher TNM, Haanen JBAG, Blank CU. Ipilimumab-induced sarcoidosis in a patient with metastatic melanoma undergoing complete remission. J Clin Oncol Off J Am Soc Clin Oncol. 2012;30(2):e7–10.
15. Kim KW, Ramaiya NH, Krajewski KM, Jagannathan JP, Tirumani SH, Srivastava A, et al. Ipilimumab associated hepatitis: imaging and clinicopathologic findings. Investig New Drugs. 2013;31(4):1071–7.

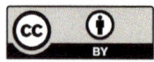

Benign Disease of the Uterus

13

Helen Addley and Fiona Fennessy

Learning Objectives
- Recognize the normal appearances of the uterus and avoid benign pitfall appearances, e.g., myometrial contractions.
- Diagnose common benign disease processes of the uterus, e.g., fibroids, adenomyosis, endometriosis, and endometrial pathology.
- Understand how congenital anomalies of the uterus are classified.

Key Points
- The diagnosis of DIE requires the presence of both morphological and signal intensity anomalies.
- Uterine leiomyomas use the FIGO classification system and are classified according to their location, to provide a uniform description to facilitate clinical care and research. It subdivides fibroids into submucosal, other (intramural and subserosal), and hybrid types.
- The Mullerian duct abnormality classification system is clinically orientated, based on anatomy. The external uterine contour and the uterine wall thickness—defined as the distance between the interostial line and a parallel line on the top of the fundus-are important considerations to appreciate.

13.1 Introduction

Benign diseases of the uterus are common and can be debilitating for patients with severe symptoms. Imaging is instrumental in diagnosing these conditions, ultrasound being the first-line investigation of choice. Correctly identifying congenital abnormalities of the uterus leads to optimal management, which in some cases can lead to a successful pregnancy outcome. Correct high-quality imaging performed optimally is therefore fundamental to patient management.

13.2 Modalities for Imaging the Uterus

13.2.1 Ultrasound

Pelvic ultrasound is the first-line examination in the investigation for gynecological symptoms both in pre- and post-menopausal patients [1]. Pelvic ultrasound is therefore the initial diagnostic test of choice for the investigation of symptoms that are due to benign diseases of the uterus. The most common of these are dysmenorrhea and menorrhagia. Ultrasound examination of the pelvis should include transvaginal examination (TVUS) which clearly demonstrates the uterus and its components, i.e., the myometrium, endometrium, and the myometrial/endometrial interface. The position of the uterus (anteverted, axial, or retroverted) should be assessed as well as uterine size (in longitudinal and transverse sections). The myometrium should be assessed for focal fibroids and diffuse heterogeneity. Heterogeneity of the myometrium and difficulty visualizing the myometrial and endometrial interface should raise the possibility of adenomyosis. The endometrial thickness should be measured as standard on the longitudinal section and the correlation with the pre-menopausal date in the cycle or post-menopausal status be made as routine.

H. Addley (✉)
Department of Radiology, Cambridge University Hospitals NHS Foundation Trust, Cambridge, Cambridgeshire, UK
e-mail: helenclare.addley@nhs.net

F. Fennessy
Department of Radiology, Brigham and Women's Hospital, Harvard Medical School, Boston, MA, USA
e-mail: ffennessy@bwh.harvard.edu

© The Author(s) 2023
J. Hodler et al. (eds.), *Diseases of the Abdomen and Pelvis 2023-2026*, IDKD Springer Series,
https://doi.org/10.1007/978-3-031-27355-1_13

13.2.2 MR/CT

MR imaging is utilized as second-line imaging following pelvic ultrasound with a focused question. When determining optimal fibroid treatment options, such as uterine artery embolization or MR-guided focused ultrasound surgery, MR imaging provides necessary pre-procedure anatomical and vascular supply detail. Similarly, MR imaging helps to plan the optimal surgical technique, such as open myomectomy versus hysteroscopic resection. In addition, MR imaging depicts the many different types of degeneration clearly, e.g., cystic, hyaline, or hemorrhagic, and may raise suspicious features for leiomyosarcoma which cannot be appreciated on pelvic ultrasound imaging.

MR imaging for endometriosis is required for surgical mapping of endometriosis patients prior to surgical resection. Subtle features of endometriosis, not apparent on US imaging, are often seen with MR imaging, such as thin endometriotic plaques and distortion.

The MR imaging protocol depends upon the study indication. Planning for uterine artery embolization or MR-guided focused ultrasound ablation, intravenous contrast administration is required. Most of the remaining indications for benign diseases of the uterus do not typically require intravenous contrast medium administration but require good preparation and technique for high-quality imaging interpretation. Patients should ideally be asked to empty their bladder at arrival for their appointment so that when their examination is started the bladder is not full or completely empty. This will help to decrease difficulty with movement artifact during the examination. An antiperistaltic agent, e.g., buscopan may be used, subject to contraindications, to also decrease movement artifact. The key sequences are multiplanar T2-weighted sequences in both sagittal and axial planes and then also T1-weighted sequences for the assessment of blood products. Dual-phase T1-weighted imaging (in-phase/out-of-phase) fat-saturated images allow for greater conspicuity of small areas of blood products in the assessment of endometriotic deposits and adenomyosis. A small field of view (FOV) axial oblique sequence perpendicular to the long axis of the uterus is required for optimal assessment of the endometrium and is also helpful for true assessment of the thickness of the junctional zone. This plane is also used to assess the fundal contour when suspicious of uterine anomaly sequence, which also requires evaluation of the upper abdominal in either a coronal or axial plane to visualize the kidneys fully to diagnose associated renal anomalies and agenesis.

There is no role for CT in the investigation of benign diseases of the uterus. However, benign diseases of the uterus are often incidentally identifiable on CT e.g. calcification of uterine fibroids. In addition, given the nature of the presentation of endometriosis with pelvic pain, it is important that the radiologist remains vigilant in the assessment of possible pathology during CT examinations for other requests.

13.3   Normal Anatomy

The flexion (angle between the longitudinal axis of the uterine fundus and cervix) and version (angle between the longitudinal axis of the cervix and vagina) are most commonly anteverted and anteflexed, but any of the four variants (anteverted and anteflexed, anteverted and retroflexed, retroverted and anteflexed, and retroverted and retroflexed) are considered normal. The size of the uterus is variable but typically between 6 and 9 cm in length. The pre-menopausal uterus demonstrates zonal anatomy (Fig. 13.1) from the central endometrial cavity (high signal intensity on T2-weighted MR imaging), inner myometrium junctional zone (low signal intensity on T2-weighted MR imaging) and the outer myometrium (higher signal intensity than the junctional zone on T2-weighted imaging). The outer serosal surface of the uterus is thin and of low signal intensity on T2-weighted imaging. On ultrasound examination, the endometrial cavity and myometrium are well demonstrated, and a thickened junctional zone can be seen as heterogeneity and difficulty in delineating the crisp endometrial margin with the myometrium. On MR imaging the zonal anatomy is best depicted on

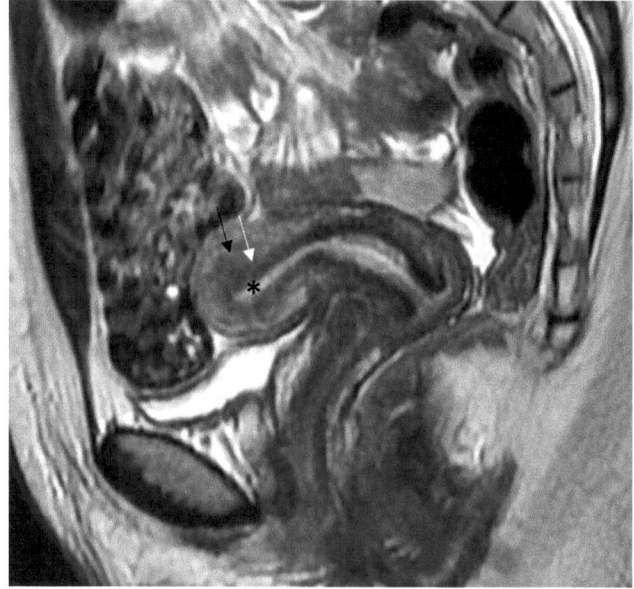

Fig. 13.1 Sagittal T2 weighted image demonstrating normal zonal anatomy of the anteverted and anteflexed uterus. Endometrium (*), inner myometrium (junctional zone white arrow), and outer myometrium (black arrow)

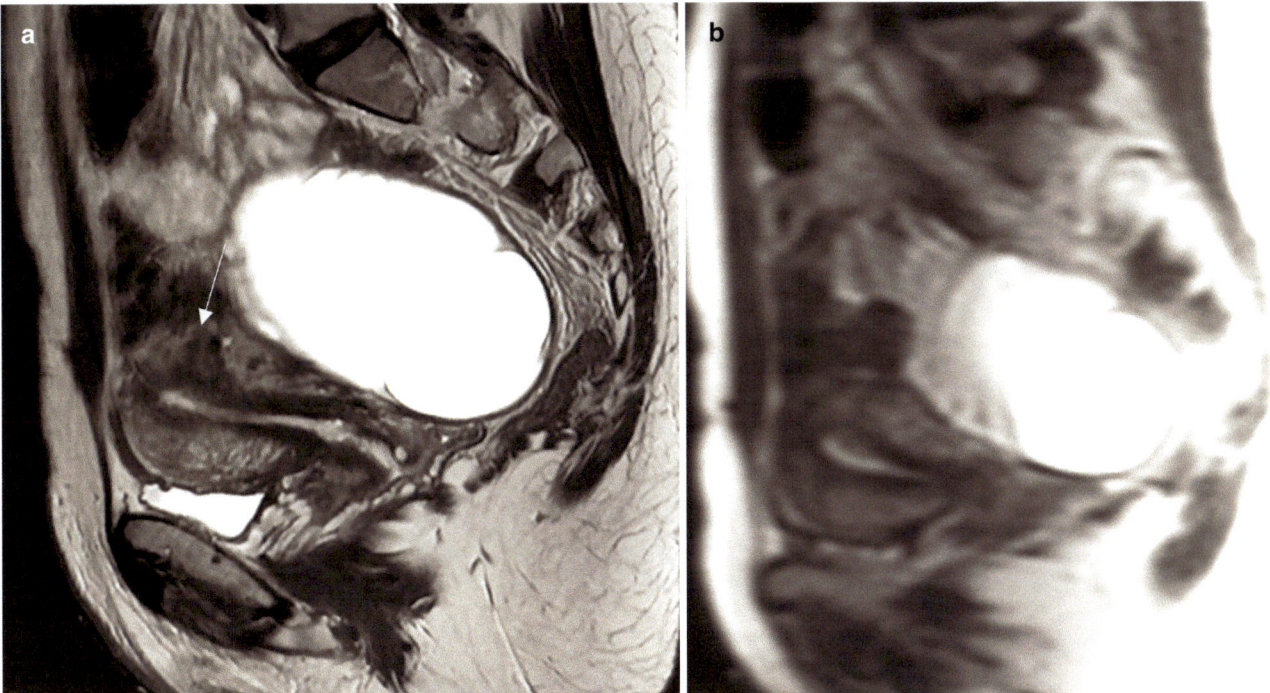

Fig. 13.2 Sagittal T2 weighted image (**a**) and localizer image (**b**) The low signal "band-like" area (white arrow) extending from the endometrial and myometrial interface into the myometrium may be mistaken for adenomyosis but correlation to the localizer images demonstrates a transient appearance in keeping with myometrial contraction. MR imaging in this case was performed for the ovarian cyst

sagittal T2-weighted imaging. The normal thickness of the junctional zone on MR imaging is approximately 8 mm with >12 mm in keeping with adenomyosis. A pitfall is when there is uterine contraction which can cause "band-like" artifact and subjective increases in thickness of the junctional zone. It is helpful to review the localizer sequences which in transient uterine contraction will demonstrate a normal junctional zone thickness on another sequence in the same examination (Fig. 13.2).

The endometrial thickness varies depending upon the menstrual cycle in the pre-menopausal uterus. During the proliferative phase, the endometrial thickness increases to become trilaminar in the mid-cycle which is seen clearly on ultrasound examination. The thickness in this phase is typically between 3 and 8 mm. In the latter secretory phase, the endometrium becomes more echogenic on ultrasound and increased in thickness to 8–12 mm. In the post-menopausal uterus, an endometrial thickness of >4 mm is used to guide further direct assessment of the endometrial cavity with hysteroscopy and sampling. The increased usage of hormone replacement therapy (HRT) tamoxifen has increased the referral of post-menopausal patients with endometrial thickness >4 mm, but this threshold remains for consideration of endometrial sampling to exclude a malignant cause. In addition to a decrease in endometrial thickness, the uterus decreases in size following menopause.

13.4 Benign Disease Processes

13.4.1 Endometriosis

Endometriosis is defined as ectopic functional endometrial glands and stroma outside of the uterus. The repeated bleeding of these areas causes fibrosis and anatomical distortion.

In recent years there has been increased awareness and support regarding the importance of earlier detection of endometriosis to avoid the delayed diagnoses of these patients who are typically in pain for many years prior to their ultimate diagnosis. This has led to increased imaging for pelvic pain and abnormal uterine bleeding at an earlier stage. First-line examination with ultrasound should ideally address four components as described from the IDEA (International Deep Endometriosis Analysis) group [2], namely: (1) routine examination of the uterus and adnexae (features for position of uterus, adenomyosis, and endometriomas); (2) evaluation of TVUS "soft-markers," e.g., site-specific tenderness; (3) assessment of status of pouch of Douglas using real-time ultrasound-based "sliding sign" and; (4) assessment for deep infiltrating endometriosis (DIE). Involvement of the torus uterinus from endometriosis with plaque formation is an example of deep infiltrating endometriosis and can extend to involve the adjacent rectosigmoid colon (Fig. 13.3a, b). Similarly, involvement of the retrocer-

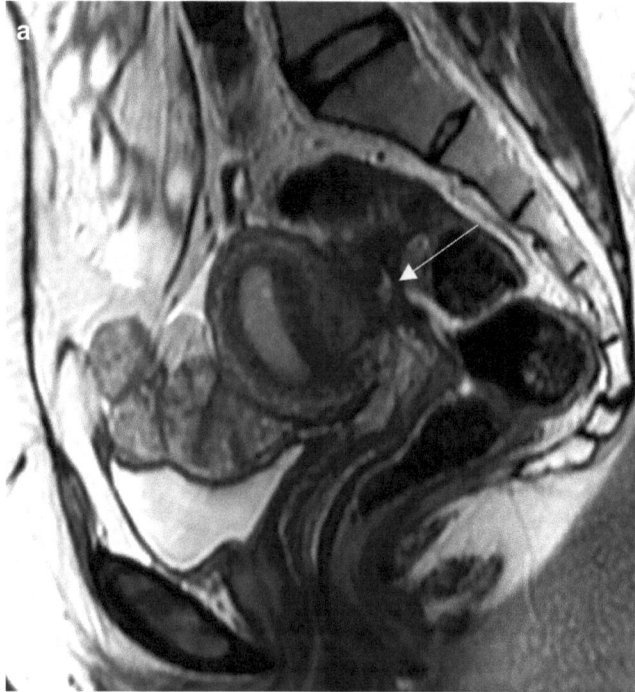

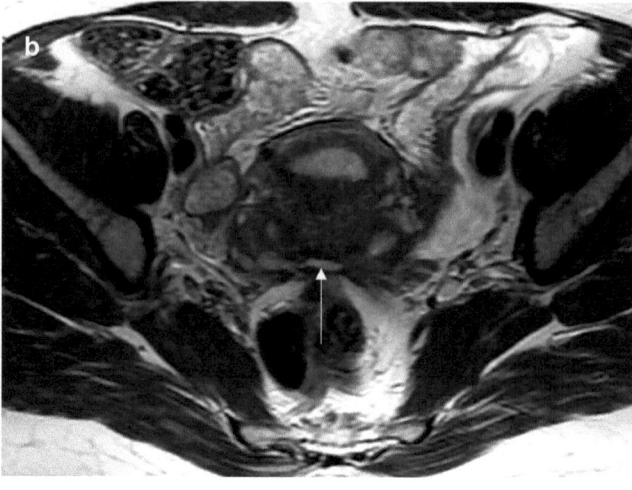

Fig. 13.3 Sagittal T2 weighted image (**a**) and axial T2 weighted image (**b**) demonstrating low signal intensity stellate plaque extending from posterior aspect of torus uterinus (**a** white arrow) in keeping with deep infiltrating endometriosis with anatomical distortion and tethering of both ovaries and rectosigmoid colon (**b** white arrow)

vical region into the pouch of Douglas can cause immobility and therefore restricted sliding sign. The features of these deposits on ultrasound and restricted movement can be subtle and therefore proactive examination and assessment is required by an experienced practitioner. DIE nodules can be seen most typically at the torus uterinus, retrocervical area, uterovesical area, and uterosacral ligaments. DIE nodules on ultrasound are seen as hypoechoic areas and should be measured in three orthogonal planes.

MR imaging for endometriosis has also been optimized by clear guidelines from the ESUR [3]. MR imaging for endometriosis mapping of disease sites prior to surgical resection has improved surgical morbidity and led to improved patient outcomes. The importance of a multidisciplinary approach with the involvement of radiology, gynecology and colorectal or urological surgery when required helps to ensure optimal discussion of treatment options for these patients. The ESUR guidelines agreed that the diagnosis of DIE required the presence of both morphological and signal intensity anomalies. The signal intensity depends upon the age of the hemorrhage and therefore can have varying appearances [4]. The typical appearance involving the uterus is adhesions and DIE nodules. Adhesions are seen as low signal intensity plaques (similar to fibrosis) on the posterior aspect of the uterus at the torus uterinus or retrocervical region extending to the posterior compartment. Associated features of anatomical distortion and tethering are common.

DIE nodules contain endometrial glands and stroma and in contradistinction to the adhesions which are low signal intensity on T1 and T2-weighted imaging these endometriotic deposits will typically demonstrate areas of focal high T1 signal intensity foci. Due to the multifocal nature of the disease, it is important to assess all pelvic compartments for endometriosis which is out of the scope for this chapter.

13.4.2 Adenomyosis

Adenomyosis is the presence of ectopic endometrial glandular cells within the myometrium. Adenomyosis may also be present in patients with leiomyomas or with endometriosis. In a recent study looking at the coexistence of leiomyomas, adenomyosis, and endometriosis and their risk for endometrial malignancy, >50% of patients with leiomyomas also had adenomyosis and half of the patients with endometriosis also had adenomyosis [5]. Differentiation of adenomyosis from leiomyomas is easier when adenomyosis is diffuse rather than focal but is very accurate on MR imaging. In focal adenomyosis there is less surrounding mass effect of the lesion relative to its size, e.g., distortion of the endometrial cavity for the size of the adenomyoma compared to leiomyomas, their outline is more indistinct, they appear more elliptical in shape compared to spherical leiomyomas and the adenomyoma contains typical key signal intensity characteristic with hyperintense foci on T2-weighted imaging and often striations out from the endometrial and myometrial junction (Fig. 13.4a). In diffuse adenomyosis, the thickness of the junctional zone >12 mm representing smooth muscle hyperplasia predicts diffuse adenomyosis with high accuracy (85%) [6]. In addition to the hyperintense foci on T2 weighted imaging, adenomyosis may also demonstrate high T1 signal intensity foci (in approximately 20% of cases) which represent small punctate hemorrhagic foci within ectopic endometrial tissue and has a 95% positive predictive value for adenomyosis. Cystic adenomyosis is less common and needs to be differentiated from cystic degeneration of a leiomyoma.

In comparison to MR imaging, which is highly accurate for diagnosis of adenomyosis, ultrasound appearances can be challenging in subtle cases such as mild diffuse adenomyosis. Given ultrasound is the first-line test it is important to be familiar with the appearances that raise suspicion for adenomyosis. The consensus statement from the morphological uterus assessment (MUSA) group [7] describes the key features on TVUS examination for adenomyosis as asymmetrical thickening of the myometrium (globular shaped uterus), presence of cystic areas within the myometrium, hyperechoic islands, fan-shaped shadowing, echogenic subendometrial lines and buds, translesional vascularity, irregular junctional zone and interrupted junctional zone (Fig. 13.4b).

13.4.3 Uterine Fibroids

Uterine fibroids (leiomyomas, myomas) are benign monoclonal tumors of uterine smooth muscle and are the single important indication for hysterectomy. Approximately 25%

of women of reproductive age and over 70% of women by the time they reach menopause are symptomatic with uterine fibroids. Their growth is dependent on estrogen and progesterone, and they may enlarge with pregnancy and oral contraceptive use, and usually request during menopause. They are commonly multiple, and their size can vary greatly.

Ultrasound is usually the initial imaging test of choice for symptomatic patients. However, MRI provides a more accurate assessment of the location, number, and type of uterine fibroids and is often used for complex cases or to help decide optimal therapy [8, 9]. MRI is also helpful as a problem-solving tool to distinguish uterine fibroids from adenomyosis, myometrial contractions, and malignant disease entities such as leiomyosarcoma [10].

13.4.3.1 Imaging Features on Ultrasound

Both transabdominal and transvaginal ultrasounds are often needed to adequately evaluate the uterus. Large or subserosal pedunculated fibroids may be missed by transvaginal imaging alone, whereas transvaginal ultrasound is often best to adequately evaluate submucosal fibroids. On ultrasound, fibroids typically appear as solid masses which are hypoechoic compared to the normal myometrium. They are occasionally hyperechoic and may have some foci of calcification. When there are many fibroids, or the fibroids are large and extend out of the pelvis, accurate assessment and measurement by ultrasound may be difficult.

13.4.3.2 Imaging Features on MRI

MRI is the most accurate modality for determining the size, number, location, and cellular characteristics of fibroids. Most commonly, uterine fibroids are well-circumscribed and

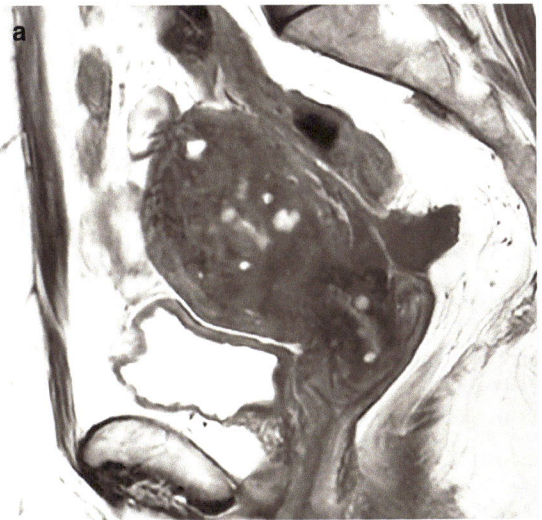
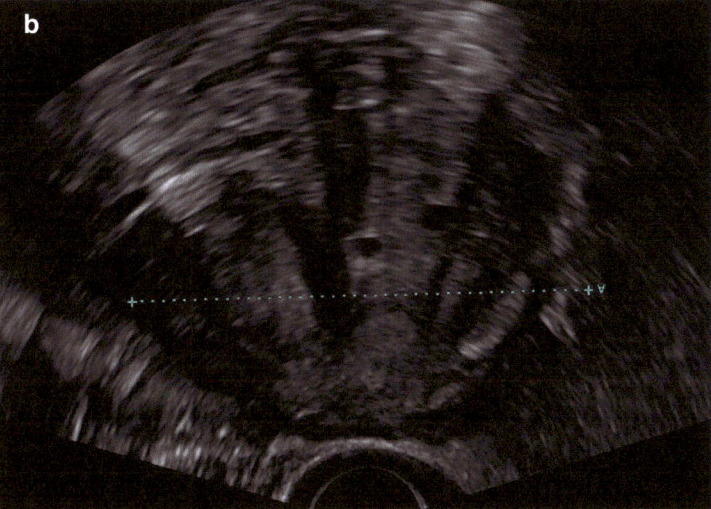

Fig. 13.4 Sagittal T2 weighted image (**a**) demonstrating thickening of the junctional zone and hyperintense focal punctate areas in keeping with extensive diffuse adenomyosis. Corresponding TVUS transverse section (**b**) of the uterus demonstrates the heterogeneity of the myometrium, indistinct endometrial and myometrial interface and focal small cystic areas

of low signal intensity on T2-weighted imaging compared to the surrounding myometrium. They are usually isointense on T1-weighted imaging and commonly enhance to the same or slightly less extent than the myometrium post-contrast administration.

Uterine leiomyomas are classified according to their location. The FIGO classification system (Fig. 13.5 and Table 13.1) was developed to provide a uniform description of location to "facilitate communication, clinical care and research" [11], and allows clinicians to determine the best treatment plan. Submucosal fibroids (FIGO 0, 1, and 2) are located beneath the mucosal lining: FIGO 0 are pedunculated intracavitary and attached to the endometrium by a stalk; FIGO 1 (Fig. 13.6) are ≥50% submucosal and <50%

intramural, whereas FIGO 2 leiomyomas are <50% submucosal and ≥50% intramural. Differentiating FIGO 1 from FIGO 2 can be helpful to gynecologists during hysteroscopic resection as it provides a better understanding of the intramural extent. FIGO classifies all remaining leiomyomas that do not have a submucosal component as "other." FIGO 3 leiomyomas (Fig. 13.6) are 100% intramural but may contact the endometrium with mass effect, but do not extend into the endometrial cavity. FIGO 4 leiomyomas (Fig. 13.6) are also 100% intramural but without any endometrial or serosal contact. Distinguishing FIGO 2 from FIGO 3 and 4 is important as the surgical approach is different, with FIGO 3 and 4

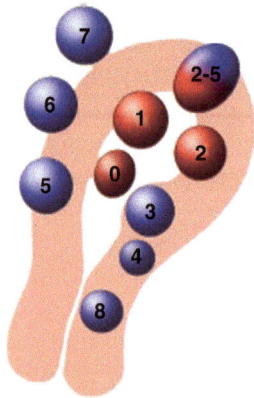

Fig. 13.5 FIGO fibroid subtypes. Submucosal fibroids (shown in red) include Type 0 (pedunculated intracavitary), Type 1 (≥ 50% submucosal), Type 2 (< 50% submucosal), and hybrid fibroids (here depicted as a Type 2–5 fibroid). Fibroids without submucosal components (shown in blue) include Type 3 (100% intramural fibroid with endometrial contact), Type 4 (100% intramural fibroid with no endometrial contact), Type 5 (≥ 50% intramural fibroid with subserosal component), Type 6 (< 50% intramural fibroid with subserosal component), Type 7 (pedunculated subserosal), and Type 8 (non-myometrial location, such as cervical, broad ligament, or parasitic fibroids) (*Permission requested from Springer journals. Original* Fig. 13.1 *from Abdominal Radiology (2021) 46: 2146–2155.* https://doi.org/10.1007/s00261-020-02882-z)

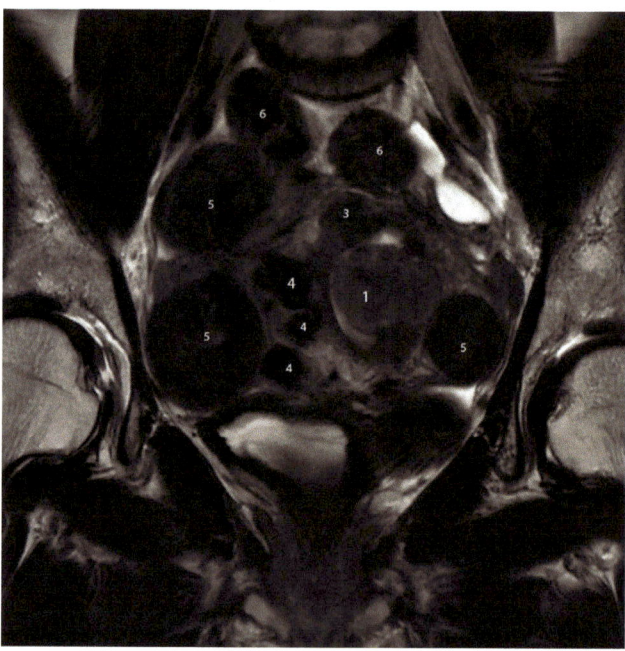

Fig. 13.6 Coronal T2-weighted image depicting numerable uterine leiomyomas. They are classified as FIGO 1 (#1): ≥50% submucosal and < 50% intramural; FIGO 4 (#4): intramural without any serosal or endometrial contact; FIGO 5 (#5): ≥50% intramural and < 50% subserosal; FIGO 6 (#6): <50% intramural and ≥ 50% subserosal

Table 13.1 FIGO fibroid classification system. *Permission requested from Springer journals. Original Table 1 from Abdominal Radiology (2021) 46: 2146–2155.* https://doi.org/10.1007/s00261-020-02882-z

Group	Type	Description
Submucosal	0	Pedunculated intracavitary
	1	< 50% intramural (≥ 50% submucosal)
	2	≥ 50% intramural (< 50% submucosal)
Other	3	100% intramural, contacting endometrium
	4	100% intramural, no endometrial or subserosal contact
	5	Subserosal, ≥ 50% intramural
	6	Subserosal, < 50% intramural
	7	Pedunculated subserosal
	8	Non-myometrial location: e.g., cervical, broad ligament, parasitic
Hybrid	X-X	Both submucosal and subserosal components. First number designates the submucosal component and second number designates the subserosal component

being removed via laparoscopy or laparotomy. Subserosal leiomyomas are divided into FIGO 5, 6, or 7 depending on the extent of subserosal involvement: FIGO 5 leiomyomas (Fig. 13.6) are ≥50% intramural and <50% subserosal, whereas FIGO 6 (Fig. 13.6) are <50% intramural and ≥50% subserosal. FIGO 7 leiomyomas are pedunculated without any intramural component. As they enlarge, they are at risk of torsion. Treatment options for subserosal fibroids usually include uterine artery embolization or myomectomy. Any extrauterine leiomyomas are classified as FIGO 8, including those arising from the cervix, broad ligament, or those parasitized in the pelvis. When a leiomyoma extends from the submucosal to the subserosal surface they are considered "hybrid" and denoted by two numbers (X-X), the first representing the submucosal component and the second representing the subserosal component. These are usually large and treatment options may include MR-guided focused ultrasound surgery, uterine artery embolization or hysterectomy. MRI is the preferred modality to assess for response post MR-guided focused ultrasound surgery or uterine artery embolization.

There are many different forms of degeneration that can occur in uterine fibroids and are usually well depicted on MRI. The most common form is that of hyaline degeneration which occurs when the smooth muscle is replaced by fibrous connective tissue. Areas of very low signal intensity, sometimes speckled, are identified within the fibroid on T2-weighted imaging and there is usually less enhancement after administration of gadolinium compared to the remainder of the uterine fibroid.

The clinical presentation and symptoms of leiomyomas may overlap with those of a rare though aggressive malignant smooth muscle tumor, leiomyosarcoma [12]. The rate of tumor growth cannot differentiate benignity from malignancy, nor can specific serum markers such as lactate dehydrogenase [13] or CA-125 [14]. However, more recent studies have suggested that specific MR features such as intra-tumoral hemorrhage, ill-defined border with the myometrium and enhancing finger-like projections post-contrast are associated with leiomyosarcoma [10]. It is also suggested that diffusion weighted imaging (with a b value of 1000 s/mm^2) and apparent diffusion coefficient mapping should also be used for the detection of leiomyosarcoma [15]. This differentiation is important, as although rare, leiomyosarcoma can have a devastating outcome.

13.4.4 Endometrial Pathology

Endometrial pathology is readily assessed with TVUS. The correlation with thickness of the expected appearance during the menstrual cycle is vital and if there is debate between normal appearances and pathology then further TVUS just shortly following menstruation when the endometrium should be at its thinnest can be helpful. Most endometrial polyps are seen in the postmenopausal patient group, and following ultrasound will undergo hysteroscopy and endometrial sampling.

Endometrial polyps are common causes of abnormal uterine bleeding. On ultrasound, these appear as a well-defined area within the endometrium and are typically homogeneous and isoechoic to the background endometrium. The ability to demonstrate a central feeding vessel on color doppler increases accuracy to >90% [16] (Fig. 13.7a). On MR imaging polyps are typically of intermediate T1 signal intensity but can be of heterogenous signal intensity on T2-weighted imaging as their size increases (Fig. 13.7b, c, d). The central fibrous core demonstrates low T2 signal intensity. Resection of the polyp is required to exclude malignancy or foci of atypical hyperplasia.

Endometrial hyperplasia is characterized by the proliferation of endometrial glands and is commonly seen in unopposed estrogen stimulation or in tamoxifen therapy. In postmenopausal patients, the TVUS appearances of a thickened endometrium >4 mm require further assessment with hysteroscopy and endometrial sampling. There are no definitive features on imaging currently which can differentiate benign endometrial hyperplasia from complex atypical hyperplasia or endometrial carcinoma and therefore a thickened endometrium should prompt cellular sampling.

Asherman's syndrome is an inflammatory response causing adhesions within the endometrial cavity typically following previous intervention or from previous repeated inflammatory events. In severe cases, fibrous adhesions within the cavity can cause cavity obliteration. This can be a cause of infertility or pregnancy loss. On TVUS, adhesions are identified as echogenic bands extending transversely across the endometrium. MR imaging is more accurate for this diagnosis and demonstrates obliteration of the endometrial cavity and fibrous signal intensity. Hysterosalpingogram or sonohysterography, which distends the endometrial cavity, can be helpful in demonstrating the extent of involvement.

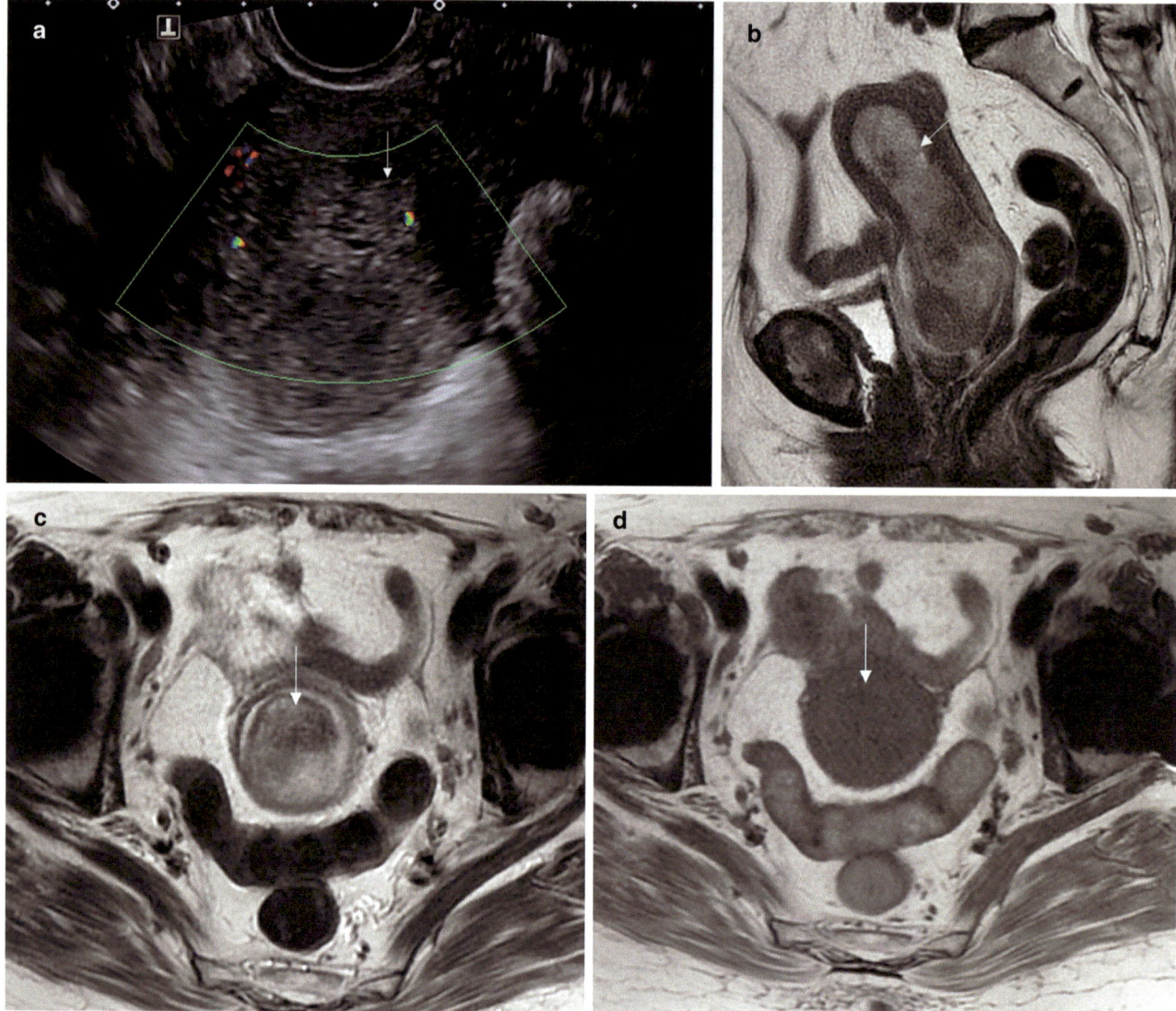

Fig. 13.7 TVUS transverse section (**a**) of the uterus demonstrates increased endometrial thickness (white arrow) with central vascularity. Hysteroscopy and subsequent pathology confirmed benign endometrial polyp. Corresponding MR examination sagittal T2 weighted image (**b**) and axial T2 weighted image (**c**) and T1 weighted image (**d**) demonstrate large central endometrial polyp (white arrow)

13.5 Mullerian Duct Anomalies of the Uterus

Mullerian duct anomalies (MDAs) are congenital disorders that arise from arrested development, incomplete fusion, or incomplete resorption of the mesonephric ducts. The Müllerian ducts undergo descent, fusion, and septum resorption to form the uterus, fallopian tubes, cervix, and upper two-third of the vagina. The ovaries and external genitalia/distal one-third of the vagina are spared because they originate from the primitive yolk sac and sinovaginal bud, respectively. MDAs are usually identified incidentally, and less commonly are identified as causes of infertility, endometriosis, recurrent miscarriages, or an obstructed reproductive tract. The prevalence of Mullerian duct anomalies in the general fertile population is 6.7%, versus 7.3% in the infertile population, and 13–17% in women with miscarriages [17].

The European Society of Human Reproduction and Embryology (ESHRE) and the European Society for Gynecological Endoscopy (ESGE) developed a clinically orientated classification system, based on anatomy [18]. US is commonly performed and may be diagnostic, especially when 3D US is used. MRI can be reserved for those cases in which the US is non-diagnostic or for complex cases. This system sorts the anomalies into classes based on increasing deviation from anatomical deviations (Fig. 13.8). Anomalies are classified into the following main classes, expressing uterine anatomical deviations deriving from the same embryological origin: U0, normal uterus; U1, dysmorphic uterus;

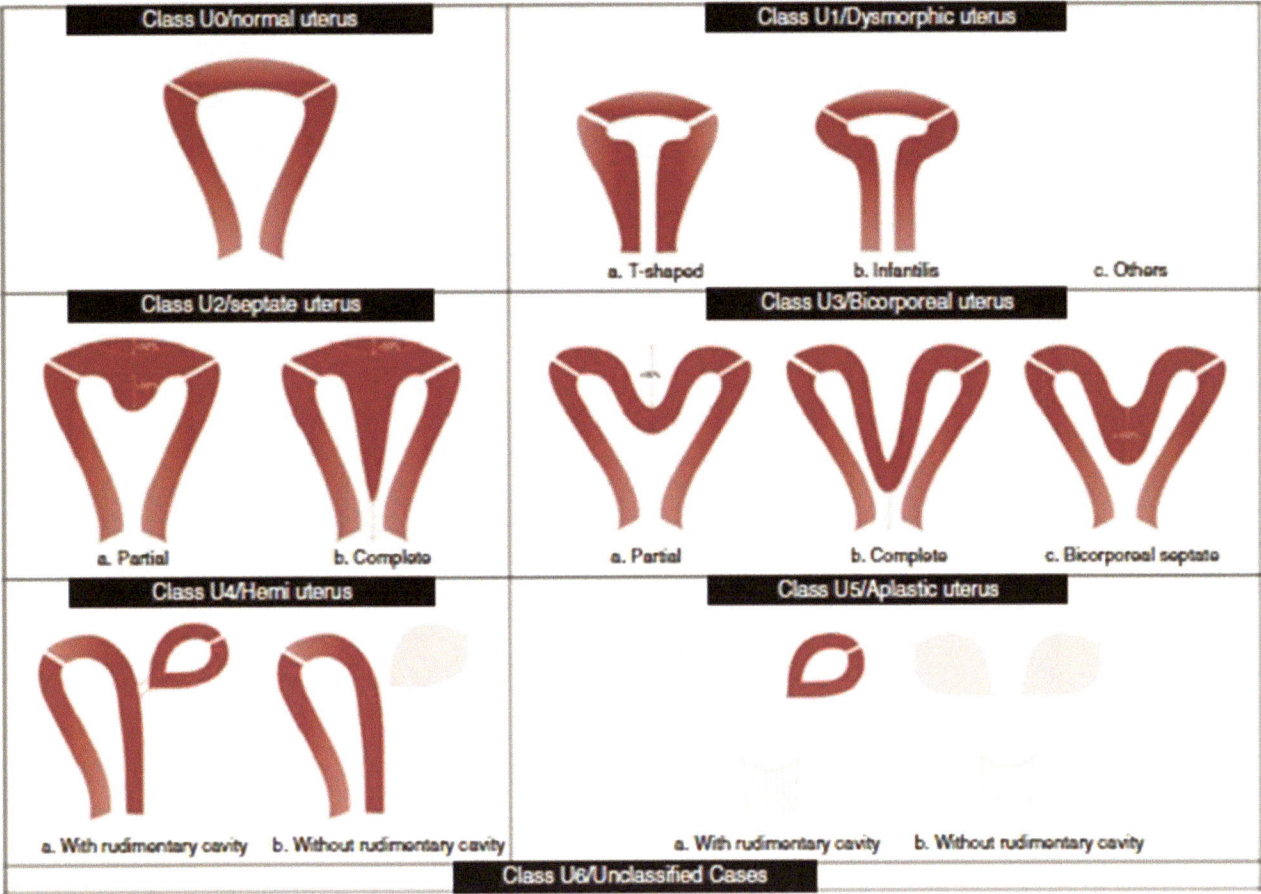

Fig. 13.8 Schematic drawing of the ESHRE/ESGE classification system of uterine congenital anomalies from Ref. [18], dividing uterine anomalies into six classes

U2, septate uterus; U3, bicorporeal/bicornuate uterus; U4, hemi-uterus; U5, aplastic uterus; U6, for unclassified cases. Uterine wall thickness (UWT) is an important parameter and a reference point for the definitions of dysmorphic T-shaped, septate, and bicorporeal uteri, and is defined as the distance between the tubal ostia (interostial line) and a parallel line on the top of the fundus [19] (Fig. 13.9).

13.5.1 Class U0

The normal uterus (U0) has either a straight or curved interostial line with an internal indentation ≤50% of the UWT at the fundal midline.

13.5.2 Class U1

Class U1 (dysmorphic uterus) has a normal uterine outline, but an abnormally shaped cavity (excluding septal abnormalities). An example is a T-shaped U1 which has thickened lateral walls. As with U0, the midline, fundal, inner indentation is <50% UWT.

13.5.3 Class U2

Class U2 uteri also have a normal outer contour, but there is abnormal resorption of the midline septum (either partial or complete) following normal Mullerian duct fusion. As such, for U2 cases there is midline, fundal, inner indentation is >50% of the UWT.

13.5.4 Class U3

Class U3 (bicorporeal) is due to abnormal fusion of the Mullerian ducts and has an abnormal outer contour with external indentation at the fundal midline >50% of the UWT. The extent to which the external fundal indentation divides the uterus above or to the level of the internal os defines partial or complete U3a vs U3b.

13.5.5 Class U

Class U4 category is unilateral uterine horn development, with associated incomplete (U4a) or absent (U4b) contralateral uterine horn remnant.

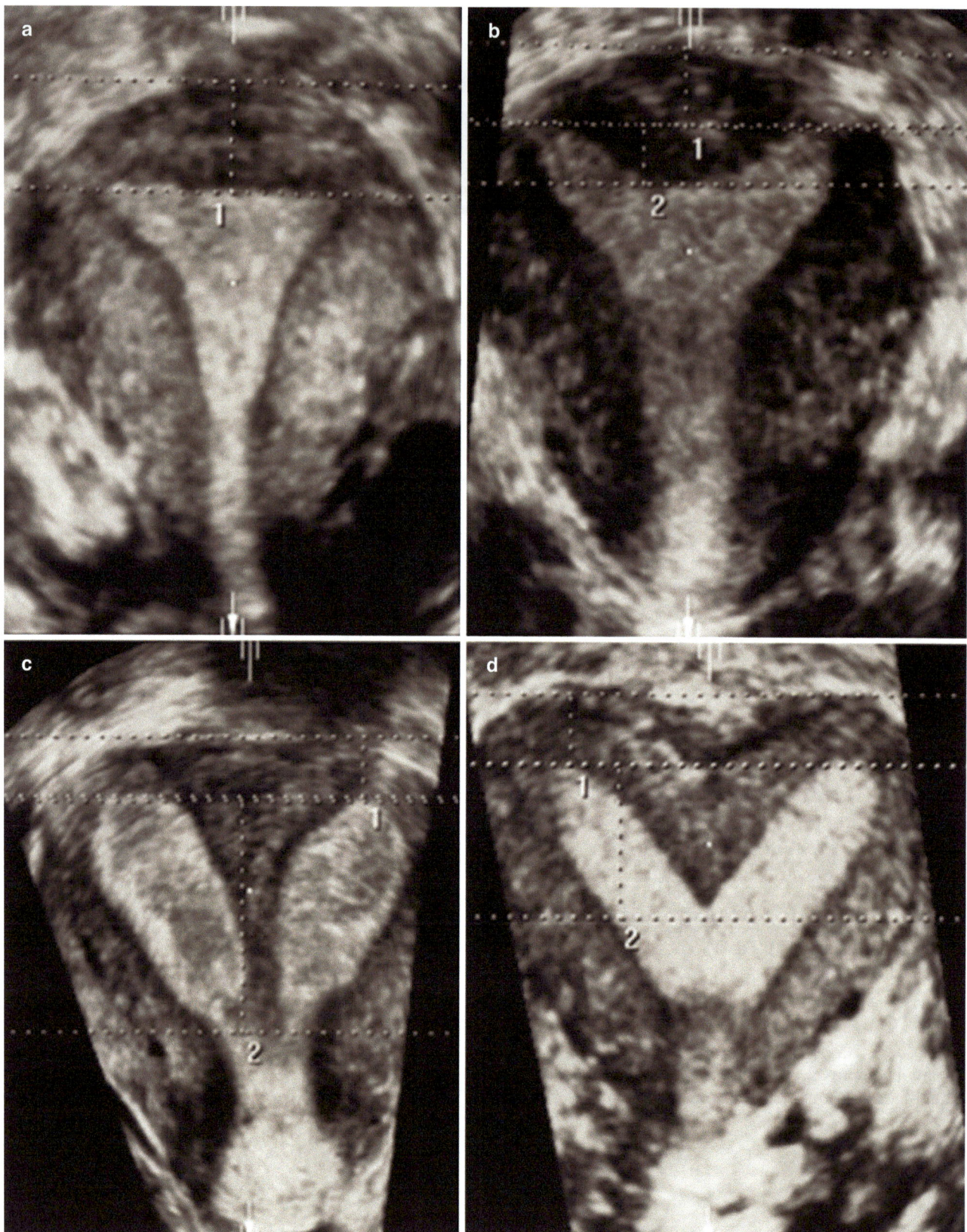

Fig. 13.9 Coronal 3D ultrasound views of the uterus depicting a normal uterus (**a**), a partial septate uterus (**b**), a complete septate uterus (**c**) and a bicornual uterus (**d**). Measurement 1 = uterine wall thickness: distance between tubal ostia and a parallel line on the top of the uterine fundus. Measurement 2 = internal midline indentation: distance between the tubal ostia and a parallel line on top of the indentation

13.5.6 Class U5

In Class U5 there is uterine aplasia, with no fully developed or unilaterally developed uterus. There may be a functional rudimentary horn or horns (U5a) or no functioning rudimentary horns (U5b).

13.5.7 Class U6

This class is reserved for subtle or combined abnormalities that do not fit into classes 0-5.

13.6 Concluding Remarks

Ultrasound is usually the first imaging modality in the assessment of benign diseases of the uterus. MRI is an important adjunct, especially for patients with complicated congenital anatomy, for the detection of deep infiltrating endometriosis or pre-operative intervention.

> **Take-Home Message**
> Ultrasound examination is the first-line investigation for benign disease of the uterus. MR imaging is focused on a particular question, often for complex diagnoses or for surgical planning, and may require specific protocol as a result.

References

1. Benacerraf BR, et al. Consider ultrasound first for imaging the female pelvis. Am J Obstet Gynecol. 2015;212:450–5.
2. Guerriero S, et al. Systematic approach to sonographic evaluation of the pelvis in women with suspected endometriosis, including terms, definitions and measurements: a consensus opinion from the International Deep Endometriosis Analysis (IDEA) group. Ultrasound Obstet Gynecol. 2016;48:318–32.
3. Bazot M, et al. European society of urogenital radiology (ESUR) guidelines: MR imaging of pelvic endometriosis. Eur Radiol. 2017;27:2765–75.
4. Foti PV, et al. Endometriosis: clinical features, MR imaging findings and pathologic correlation. Insights Imaging. 2018;9:149–72.
5. Johnatty SE, et al. Co-existence of leiomyomas, adenomyosis and endometriosis in women with endometrial cancer. Sci Rep. 2020;10:3621.
6. Novellas S, et al. MRI characteristics of the uterine junctional zone: from normal to the diagnosis of adenomyosis. AJR Am J Roentgenol. 2011;196:1206–13.
7. Van den Bosch T, et al. Terms, definitions and measurements to describe sonographic features of myometrium and uterine masses: a consensus opinion from the Morphological Uterus Sonographic Assessment (MUSA) group. Ultrasound Obstet Gynecol. 2015;46:284–98. https://doi.org/10.1002/uog.14806.
8. Hossain MZ, et al. A Comparative study of magnetic resonance imaging and transabdominal ultrasonography for the diagnosis and evaluation of uterine fibroids. Mymensingh Med J. 2017;26:821–7.
9. Dueholm M, Lundorf E, Hansen ES, Ledertoug S, Olesen F. Accuracy of magnetic resonance imaging and transvaginal ultrasonography in the diagnosis, mapping, and measurement of uterine myomas. Am J Obstet Gynecol. 2002;186:409–15.
10. Jagannathan JP, et al. Differentiating leiomyosarcoma from leiomyoma: in support of an MR imaging predictive scoring system. Abdom Radiol. 2021;46:4927–35.
11. Munro MG, Critchley HOD, Broder MS, Fraser IS, FIGO Working Group on Menstrual Disorders. FIGO classification system (PALM-COEIN) for causes of abnormal uterine bleeding in nongravid women of reproductive age. Int J Gynaecol Obstet. 2011;113:3–13.
12. Skorstad M, Kent A, Lieng M. Preoperative evaluation in women with uterine leiomyosarcoma. A nationwide cohort study. Acta Obstet Gynecol Scand. 2016;95:1228–34.
13. Goto A, Takeuchi S, Sugimura K, Maruo T. Usefulness of Gd-DTPA contrast-enhanced dynamic MRI and serum determination of LDH and its isozymes in the differential diagnosis of leiomyosarcoma from degenerated leiomyoma of the uterus. Int J Gynecol Cancer. 2002;12:354.
14. Juang CM, et al. Potential role of preoperative serum CA125 for the differential diagnosis between uterine leiomyoma and uterine leiomyosarcoma. Eur J Gynaecol Oncol. 2006;27:370–4.
15. Hindman N, et al. MRI evaluation of uterine masses for risk of leiomyosarcoma: a consensus statement. Radiology. 2022;306:e211658. https://doi.org/10.1148/radiol.211658.
16. Jakab A, et al. Detection of feeding artery improves the ultrasound diagnosis of endometrial polyps in asymptomatic patients. Eur J Obstet Gynecol Reprod Biol. 2005;119:103–7.
17. Saravelos SH, Cocksedge KA, Li TC. Prevalence and diagnosis of congenital uterine anomalies in women with reproductive failure: a critical appraisal. Hum Reprod Update. 2008;14:415–29.
18. Grimbizis GF, et al. The ESHRE/ESGE consensus on the classification of female genital tract congenital anomalies. Hum Reprod. 2013;28:2032–44.
19. Grimbizis GF, et al. The Thessaloniki ESHRE/ESGE consensus on diagnosis of female genital anomalies. Hum Reprod. 2016;31:2–7.

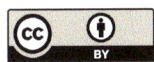

Malignant Diseases of the Uterus

14

Yulia Lakhman and Evis Sala

Learning Objectives
- Describe the role of MRI and FDG-PET to guide the management of patients with CC and EC.
- Highlight Tailored MRI Protocols for Staging of CC and EC
- Emphasize the advantages and limitations of MRI and FDG-PET in the evaluation of patients with CC and EC.
- Explain the role of imaging to confirm eligibility for fertility-sparing management.

14.1 Part I: Cervical Cancer

14.1.1 Epidemiology

Cervical cancer (CC) is the fourth most frequent malignancy in women worldwide with majority of new cases and deaths occurring in low-to-middle-income countries [1]. Persistent human papillomavirus (HPV) infection causes most CC. Infection with human immunodeficiency virus also increases the risk of CC [2]. CC can be prevented with HPV vaccination, HPV DNA testing, and timely treatment of precancerous lesions [1, 3].

14.1.2 Presentation and Diagnosis

Patients may have no symptoms or present with vaginal bleeding, discharge, pelvic pain, and dyspareunia. Squamous cell carcinoma accounts for 70–80% and adenocarcinoma for 20–25% of CC [4].

14.1.3 Staging

The International Federation of Gynecology and Obstetrics (FIGO) classification is used to stage CC [5]. The latest 2018 revision contains several key updates [5]. Pathologic and imaging findings can be used to supplement clinical findings, allowing the inclusion of lymph node (LN) status into the staging system. A notation (*r* for imaging, *p* for pathology) is added to indicate the method that was used to assign the stage. Pathologic findings take precedence over clinical exams and imaging. Stage IB is now divided into three subgroups (instead of two), IB1 ≤ 2 cm, IB2 > 2 cm to ≤4 cm, and IB3 > 4 cm, better capturing superior oncologic outcomes and potential for fertility-sparing treatment in patients with tumors ≤2 cm [6]. Stage III now includes Stage IIIC with IIIC1 indicating pelvic and IIIC2 para-aortic LN metastases.

Key Point
- The 2018 FIGO staging system allows pathologic and imaging findings to supplement clinical findings to assign the stage.

14.1.4 Management

Surgery (simple or radical hysterectomy) is advised for patients with cervix/upper vagina-confined tumors ≤4 cm [4, 7]. Fertility-sparing approach (conization, simple or radi-

Y. Lakhman (✉)
Department of Radiology, Memorial Sloan Kettering Cancer Center, New York, NY, USA
e-mail: lakhmany@mskcc.org

E. Sala
Department of Radiology, Fondazione Policlinico Universitario Agostino Gemelli IRCCS, Rome, Italy
e-mail: es220@medschl.cam.ac.uk

© The Author(s) 2023
J. Hodler et al. (eds.), *Diseases of the Abdomen and Pelvis 2023-2026*, IDKD Springer Series,
https://doi.org/10.1007/978-3-031-27355-1_14

cal trachelectomy) is an option for women who desire fertility and have cervix-confined tumors ≤2 cm. Parametrial resection differentiates radical from simple hysterectomy or trachelectomy. Pelvic LN assessment is added to the above procedures, with sentinel LN mapping favored over traditional lymphadenectomy [4, 7].

Chemoradiotherapy is preferred to surgery for cervix/upper vagina-confined tumors >4 cm [4, 7]. Chemoradiotherapy is also recommended for locally advanced disease, i.e., parametrial invasion and beyond (regardless of tumor size) but no distant metastases. External beam radiation is delivered concurrently with platinum-based chemotherapy followed by image-guided brachytherapy. Patients presenting with distant metastases are managed with systemic chemotherapy and, if needed, targeted radiation.

14.1.5 Role of Imaging in Initial Staging

Magnetic resonance imaging (MRI) allows to optimally assess loco-regional tumor extent and, if applicable, confirm eligibility for fertility-sparing surgery [8, 9]. MRI protocol should be tailored as described in Table 14.1 [8]. Patients are asked to empty their bladder and bowel before the exam to optimally position the uterus and minimize rectal gas. Anti-peristaltic agents can reduce bowel motion.

High-resolution small field-of-view T2-weighted images (T2WI) in sagittal and oblique axial planes (Table 14.1 and Fig. 14.1) are essential to local staging [8]. CC has intermediate-SI compared to low-SI cervical stroma on T2WI (Fig. 14.2). Diffusion-weighted images (DWI) [typical b values of 0–50 and 800–1000 s/mm^2] are acquired using the same

Table 14.1 Suggested tailored MRI protocols for staging of cervical cancer and endometrial cancer

Imaging sequences	Anatomic coverage	Imaging planes	Rationale in cervical cancer	Rationale in endometrial cancer
T2WI	Abdomen	Coronal or axial	• Presence of hydronephrosis • Para-aortic LN metastases	
T1WI	Pelvis	Axial	• Bone lesions • Pelvic LN metastases	

T2WI (non-fat saturated)	Pelvis	Sagittal & oblique axial	• Tumor size
			• If fertility is desired,
			  – Tumor-to-internal os distance
			• Locoregional extent
			  – Parametrial invasion
			  – Upper vs. lower vaginal involvement
			  – Pelvic wall invasion
			  – Pelvic LN enlargement
			  – Bladder or rectal mucosal involvement
				• Tumor size
				• If fertility is desired
				  – Exclusion of MI
				• Locoregional extent
				  – Depth of MI
				  – Cervical stromal invasion
				  – Uterine serosal invasion
				  – Ovarian involvement
				  – Vaginal or parametrial invasion
				  – Bladder or rectal mucosal involvement
				  – Peritoneal implants

DWI b = 0–50, 800–1000 mm²/s	Pelvis	Sagittal & Oblique axial	• Important adjunct to T2WI • Same FOV, plane(s), slice thickness as T2WI to facilitate side-by-side interpretation	• Same FOV, plane(s), slice thickness as T2WI to facilitate side-by-side interpretation

DCE	Pelvis	Sagittal & Oblique axial	• Primarily a research tool	• Early phase
				  – 30–60 s, sagittal plane
				• Equilibrium phase
				  – 120 s and at 180 s, sagittal and oblique axial planes, respectively
				• Delayed phase
				  – 4–5 min, oblique axial plane

Optional:
• Vaginal gel; may facilitate the detection of vaginal wall involvement
• Additional imaging planes may be obtained based on local preferences
• 3-dimensional T2WI; allows retrospective reconstruction in any plane

Abbreviations: DWI diffusion-weighted imaging, DCE dynamic contrast-enhanced, FOV field of view, LN lymph node, MI myometrial invasion

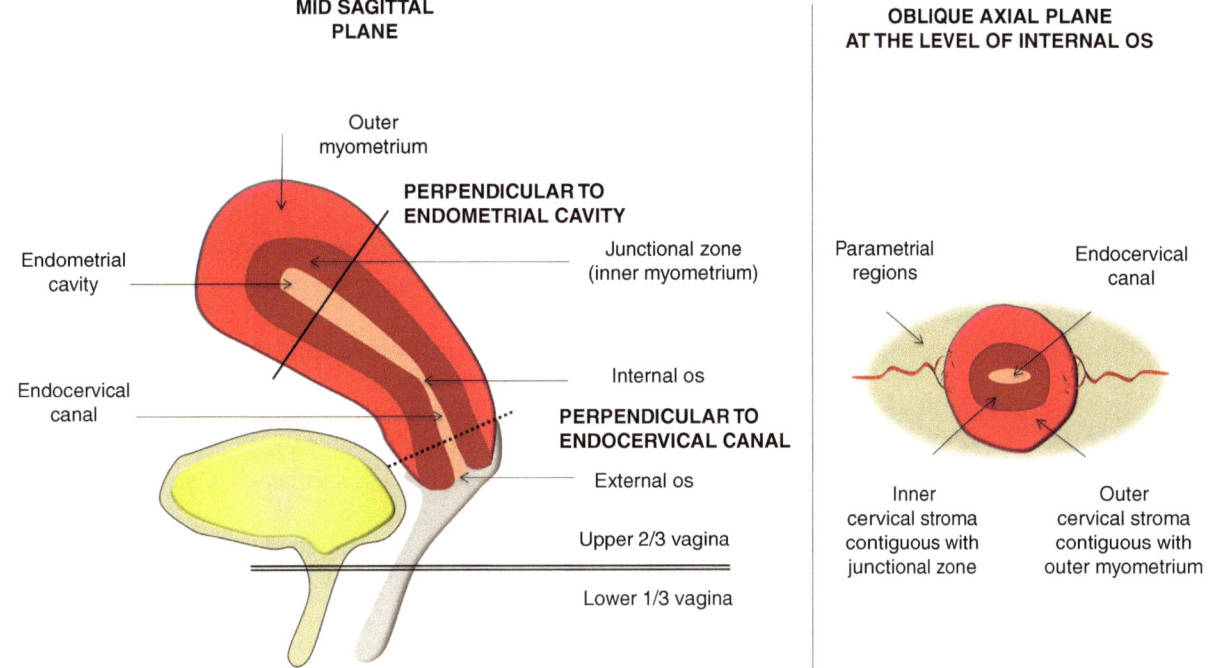

Fig. 14.1 A diagram illustrating relevant anatomy of the uterine corpus and cervix. Parametrial regions are comprised of connective tissues suited lateral to the cervix. On sagittal images, the location of internal os is identified as the narrowing of the endocervical canal superiorly before it widens again as endometrial cavity. On oblique axial images, the location of internal os is indicated by the entrance of uterine vessels

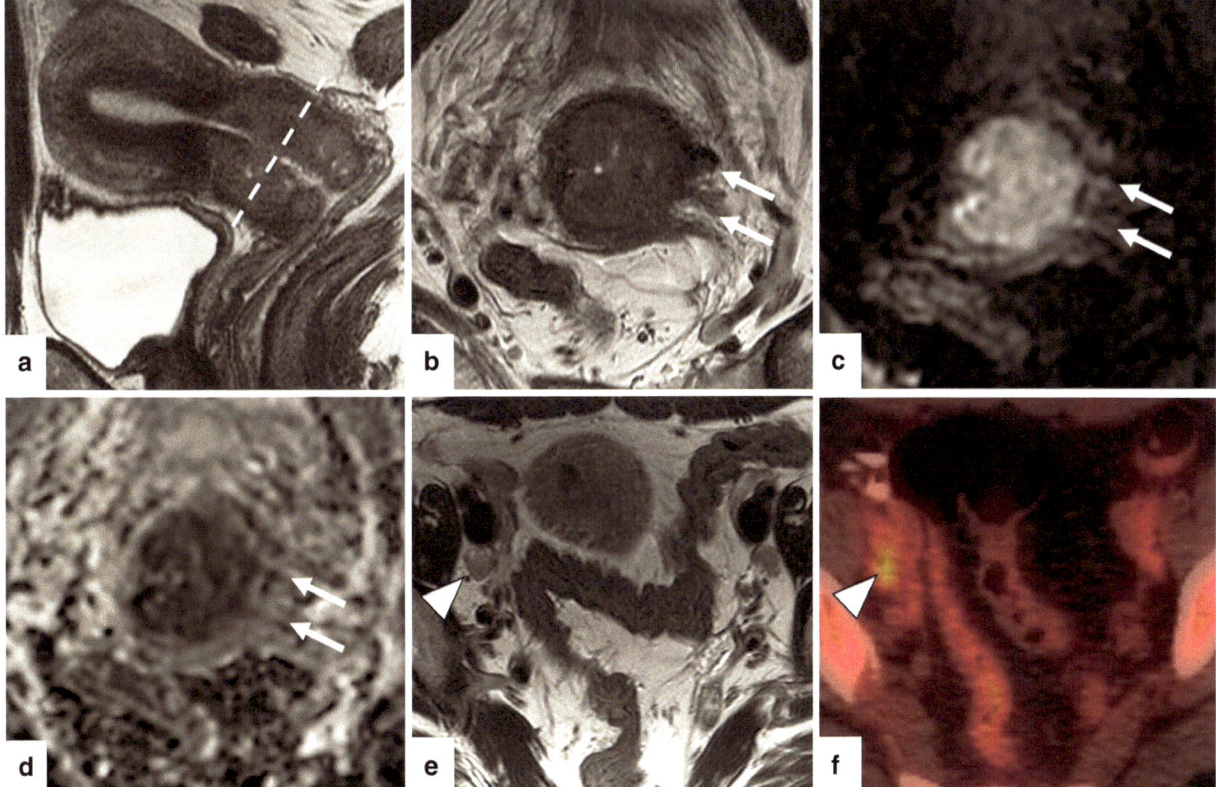

Fig. 14.2 39-year-old patient with squamous carcinoma of the cervix. (**a**) Sagittal T2-weighted image shows a 4.5 cm intermediate-SI tumor infiltrating entire cervical stroma. A dashed line indicates the orientation of oblique axial plane. B, C, and D. Oblique axial T2WI (**b**), DWI (**c**), and ADC map (**d**) demonstrate intermediate-SI tumor on T2WI with diffusion restriction (high-SI on high b-value DWI and low-SI on ADC map), full-thickness cervical stromal invasion and spiculated tumor-parametrial interface (arrows). (**e**) Axial T2WI image shows an enlarged (12 mm in short axis) right external iliac lymph node (arrowhead) and non-enlarged left external iliac lymph node. (**f**) Axial FDG-PET/CT image shows FDG avid right external iliac lymph node consistent with metastatic adenopathy

plane, field-of-view, and slice thickness as T2WI. Tumor demonstrates high-SI on high b-value DWI and low-SI on the apparent diffusion coefficient (ADC) map (Fig. 14.2). Side-by-side review of T2WI and DWI is useful to determine tumor margins and assign FIGO stage [8]. Dynamic contrast-enhanced imaging (DCE) is primarily a research tool and is not essential in routine clinical practice [8].

Fluorodeoxyglucose Positron Emission Tomography (FDG-PET) is advised for patients with cervix-confined tumors >4 cm and higher stage disease [7]. FDG-PET can be fused to either CT or MRI.

> **Key Point**
> - MRI is essential to determine loco-regional tumor extent and confirm eligibility for fertility-sparing surgery.
> - FDG-PET facilitates the detection of LN and distant metastases.

Stage I: *Cervix-confined disease [extension to the uterine corpus is disregarded].*

Stage IA is microscopic in size and, thus, below the imaging resolution. Stage IB includes IB1 ≤ 2 cm, IB2 > 2 cm to ≤4 cm, and IB3 > 4 cm based on the greatest tumor diameter [5]. The tumor can be measured in any plane that best demonstrates its maximum size. Intact rim of low-SI cervical stroma around intermediate-SI tumor on oblique axial T2WI excludes parametrial invasion [8, 9]. Combined review of T2WI and DWI may help to better delineate tumor margins and to distinguish tumor from post-procedural edema/inflammation. The latter has inter-mediate-SI on T2WI mimicking tumor but should not show diffusion restriction [8].

Women of childbearing age may be eligible for fertility-sparing management if they have cervix-confined tumors ≤2 cm of squamous cell carcinoma, adenocarcinoma, or adenosquamous carcinoma histology that are located ≥1 cm inferior to the internal os (Fig. 14.1) [4, 7].

Stage II: *Tumor is limited to the upper vagina (IIA) or parametrial regions (IIB).*

The involvement of upper two-thirds of the vagina (Stage IIA) is divided into IIA1 (≤4 cm) and IIA2 (>4 cm) disease [5]. If a horizonal line is placed at the bladder neck, the upper vagina is located above and the lower vagina is situated below this line (Fig. 14.1) [8, 9]. Vaginal involvement is suspected when intermediate-SI tumor interrupts low-SI vaginal wall.

Full-thickness cervical stromal invasion (replacement of low-SI cervical stroma by intermediate-SI tumor) on T2WI does not indicate parametrial invasion (Fig. 14.3). The diagnosis of parametrial invasion (Stage IIB) requires a nodular or spiculated tumor-parametrial interface in addition to full-thickness cervical stromal invasion (Fig. 14.2) [8, 9]. Tumor may also encase parametrial vessels. Adding DWI to T2WI does not change sensitivity for parametrial invasion (68–89%) but improves specificity from 85–89% to 97–99% [10].

Stage III: *Tumor involves lower third of vagina (IIIA), extends to pelvic wall and/or causes hydronephrosis or non-functioning kidney (IIIB), or involves pelvic and/or para-aortic LNs (IIIC) [including micro-metastases].*

Pelvic wall invasion is present when the tumor extends within 3 mm or directly abuts pelvic wall muscles or iliac vessels [8, 9]. Stage IIIC has been added in 2018 with IIIC1 denoting pelvic and IIIC2 para-aortic LN metastases [5].

PARAMETRIAL INVASION IS ABSENT
(Stage IB)

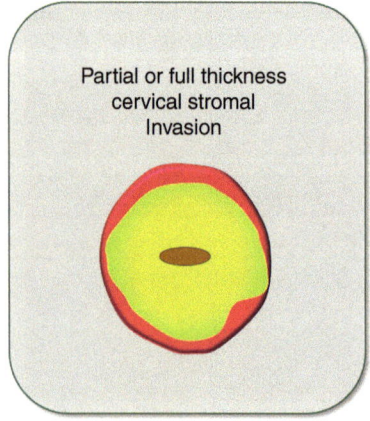

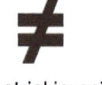

PARAMETRIAL INVASION IS PRESENT
(Stage IIB)

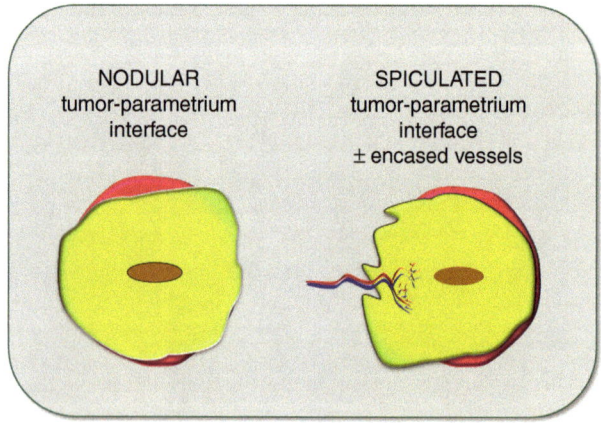

Fig. 14.3 A schematic of oblique axial images through the cervix. Full-thickness cervical stromal invasion does not indicate parametrial invasion. The diagnosis of parametrial invasion requires a nodular or spiculated tumor--parametrium interface in addition to full-thickness cervical stromal invasion. Tumor with parametrial regions may also encase parametrial vessels

LN metastases impact prognosis and, thus, treatment choice. MRI has moderate sensitivity (51–57%) and high specificity (90–93%) for LN metastases [11–13]. Short axis diameter ≥1 cm is the main criterion, although ancillary features like round shape, heterogenous-SI, same SI as primary tumor, LN clustering, and necrosis may help to identify small LN metastases (Fig. 14.2). Both benign and malignant LNs have high-SI on high b-value DWI making them easy to see. The ADC cut-off values are not used to identify LN metastases because mean ADCs of benign and malignant LNs overlap [8].

FDG-PET has both high sensitivity (88%) and specificity (93%) for pelvic LN metastases (Fig. 14.2) [14]. Detection of para-aortic LN metastases is less robust (sensitivity 40%, specificity 93%) due to low prevalence and small size [14].

Stage IV: *Tumor invades bladder/rectal mucosa [biopsy-proven] (IVA) or shows distant metastases (IVB).*

Bladder/rectal mucosal invasion (stage IVA) is present when intermediate-SI tumor disrupts low-SI bladder/rectal wall and extends into the edematous (bullous) mucosa or the lumen on T2WI [15]. Bullous edema alone is insufficient to assign stage IVA.

Stage IVB indicates distant metastases including LN metastases beyond pelvic and para-aortic regions. FDG-PET is the optimal approach to detect distant spread [16]. A biopsy confirmation is required due to the potential for false positives.

> **Key Point**
> - The diagnosis of parametrial invasion requires a nodular or spiculated tumor-parametrial interface in addition to full-thickness cervical stromal invasion.
> - Bullous edema alone is insufficient to assign Stage IVA.

14.1.6 Assessment of Treatment Response During and After Treatment

Pre-treatment MRI and FDG-PET facilitate chemoradiotherapy planning. Mid-treatment pre-brachytherapy MRI allows dose adjustment based on residual tumor volume to maximize local control and minimize adjacent organ dose [17]. Pretreatment mean ADC does not predict response to chemoradiotherapy, but tumor regression rate and the change in mean ADC values during treatment may inform response [18, 19].

Post-treatment MRI and FDG-PET are usually obtained 6 months after chemoradiotherapy. Reconstitution of low-SI cervical stroma on T2WI suggests tumor-free cervix, but edema/inflammation can persist 6–9 months post treat-

ment [8, 9]. Post-treatment FDG-PET informs prognosis with partial response (FDG avidity reduced from baseline) indicating moderate recurrence risk and progressive disease (unchanged, increased, or new foci of FDG avidity) suggesting persistent tumor [20].

14.1.7 Evaluation of CC Recurrence

Most patients recur within 2 years of initial treatment [8, 9]. Imaging characteristics of the recurrent disease are the same as primary tumor. MRI and FDG-PET allow a comprehensive assessment of tumor extent [21]. Chemotherapy is advised for localized recurrence after surgery. Radical surgery (pelvic exenteration) is the potential salvage option post chemoradiotherapy.

14.1.8 Future Directions

PET/MRI may offer a "one-stop shop" approach by providing anatomic, functional, and metabolic information in one exam [8]. Studies are needed to validate the added value of PET/MRI beyond the convivence of a single imaging session.

14.2 Part II: Endometrial Cancer

14.2.1 Epidemiology and Diagnosis

Endometrial cancer (EC) is the third most common malignancy in women worldwide and the most common gynecological cancer in developed countries [1]. The majority of cases are diagnosed at an early stage (70% stage I) with a 5-year survival rate of more than 95% [22]. While postmenopausal women are predominantly affected (75% are >50 years), 4% of the women diagnosed with EC are younger than 40 years, and therefore preservation of fertility is an important consideration [23].

Patients with abnormal vaginal bleeding are initially evaluated by transvaginal ultrasound. In postmenopausal patients, a focal or diffuse endometrial thickening of >4–5 mm is considered suspicious and should be followed by an endometrial pipelle or hysteroscopy and biopsy [24].

14.2.2 Histopathological Subtypes

There are two main histological subtypes. Type I (80–85%) is estrogen-dependent, affects younger patients, and has a good prognosis. Type II (10–15%) is not estrogen driven, affects older women, behaves more aggressively, and has a poorer prognosis (5-year survival rate of 40%) [24]. Most cases of

EC are sporadic, although 5% have a hereditary component linked to hereditary non-polyposis colon cancer (HNPCC or Lynch syndrome) [25]. Histologically, type I is a grade 1 or 2 endometrioid adenocarcinoma; type II includes grade 3 endometrioid adenocarcinoma, clear-cell carcinoma, undifferentiated, serous carcinoma, and carcinosarcoma. More recently, the Cancer Genome Atlas (TCGA) Research working group, introduced four molecular subtypes that relate to prognosis: (1) *POLE* (ultra-mutated tumors), (2) microsatellite unstable tumors, (3) copy-number high tumors with mostly TP53 mutations, and (4) copy-number low tumors without any of the above alterations, reflecting the profound genomic heterogeneity of EC [26].

14.2.3 Role of Imaging

Magnetic resonance imaging (MRI) is the best imaging modality to evaluate patients with newly diagnosed EC [27]. MRI findings facilitate risk assessment and ultimately guide treatment choice and surgical planning. The combination of T2WI, DWI, and DCE provides the "one-stop shop" approach [27]. The high-resolution T2WI is angled perpendicularly to the endometrium to obtain oblique axial images (Fig. 14.1). These are essential for accurate assessment of the depth of myometrial invasion (MI). A slice thickness of 4 mm and the use of non-fat suppressed sequences is advised [27]. DWI are obtained with a minimum of two b values of 0–50 and 800–1000 s/mm^2 in the same orientation as the sagittal and oblique axial T2WI (Table 14.1). MRI protocol for EC patients should also include a large-field-of-view axial T1WI and/or T2WI images of the pelvis and abdomen to identify enlarged lymph nodes, hydronephrosis, and bone marrow changes [27]. CT and PET/CT improve the evaluation of LN and distant metastases; PET/CT is currently not part of the standard-of-care for the initial staging of EC. However, it plays a crucial role in treatment selection and planning of pelvic exenteration in patients with tumor recurrence [21].

> **Key Points**
> - The combination of T2WI, DWI, and DCE provides the "one-stop shop" approach to the staging of EC.

14.2.4 MRI Indications

MRI has an essential role in treatment planning by (1) establishing the origin of the tumor and (2) assessing the local extent of the disease [9, 28]. The origin of the tumor is routinely established through clinical examination and histologic evaluation of biopsy specimens. However, in a limited number of cases, it is difficult to determine the tumor's origin due to, for example, unusual morphologic patterns, mixed-type histologic findings, or inadequate samples. Differentiating between endometrial and cervical origin is critical as it has major implications for patient management [29]. Most ECs are treated with simple hysterectomy and bilateral salpingo-oophorectomy, while CC patients undergo simple or radical hysterectomy in early stage and chemoradiotherapy in advanced disease [4, 7]. MRI has been proved useful in this clinical scenario, with an accuracy of 85–88% in correctly attributing the cancer origin to the corpus or cervix [9].

MRI has a reported accuracy of 85–93% in delineating the extent of the EC and is the imaging modality of choice to determine the depth of myometrial invasion preoperatively [9, 27, 28]. The latter is the most important morphologic prognostic factor, correlating with tumor grade, presence of LN metastases and overall survival [9, 27, 28]. Special attention should be given to the eligibility criteria prior to the fertility-sparing treatment for patients with grade 1 EC who desire fertility preservation. In these patients, MRI is crucial for confirming the absence of myometrial invasion, cervical stroma invasion, ovarian metastases, and lymphadenopathy.

> **Key Point**
> - MRI is crucial to confirm endometrium-confined disease prior to fertility-sparing management.

14.2.5 MRI Features of EC

On T2WI, EC appears as a thickened endometrium or a mass, occupying the endometrial cavity. It shows hyperintense SI when compared to hypointense myometrium, and intermediate-low SI relative to hyperintense normal endometrium (Fig. 14.4). Small tumors may not be associated with endometrial thickening or can have a similar SI to that of normal endometrium. In these cases, DWI and DCE are particularly helpful. On DWI, the tumor is hyperintense on high b-value images (800–1000 s/mm^2), with a corresponding hypointense SI on the ADC map (Fig. 14.4). On DCE images, the tumor shows an early enhancement compared to normal endometrium and on later phases it appears hypointense relative to the myometrium.

14.2.6 EC Staging with MRI

Endometrial cancer staging is usually performed using FIGO classification [30].

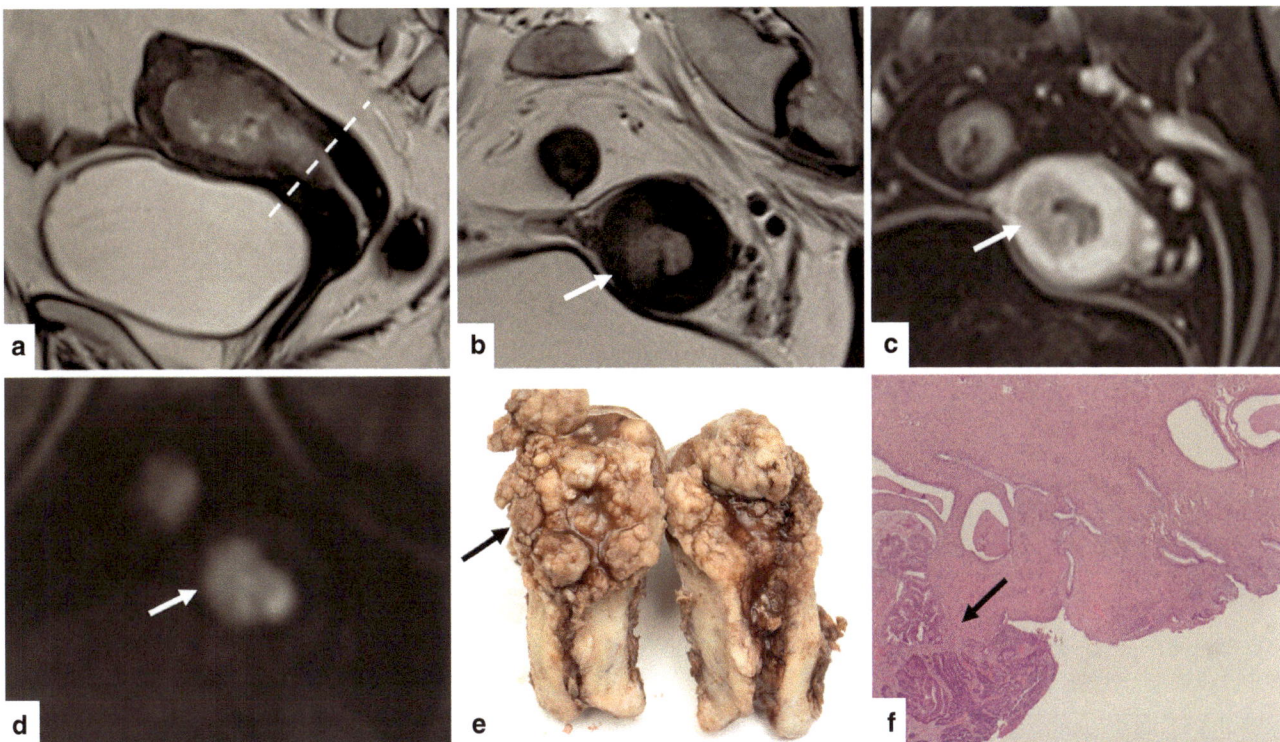

Fig. 14.4 "One-stop shop" approach, FIGO stage II endometrial cancer. A 66-year-old patient with vaginal bleeding. On T2WI there is an intermediate-SI endometrial tumor (**a**), which interrupts the low-SI of cervical stroma (**b**, arrow). On DCE (**c**) the normal enhancement of cervical stroma is disrupted by the hypo-enhancing tumor (arrow) which has restricted diffusion on DWI (**d**, arrow). The gross examination of the surgery specimen shows the solid tumor (**e**, arrow). The pathology revealed endometrioid adenocarcinoma involving the cervical stroma (**f**), consistent with FIGO stage II. These images were originally published in Pintican R, Bura V, Zerunian M, Smith J, Addley H, Freeman S, Caruso D, Laghi A, Sala E, Jimenez-Linan M. MRI of the endometrium—from normal appearances to rare pathology. Br J Radiol. 2021 Sep 1; 94 (1125): 20201347. doi: 10.1259/bjr.20201347. Epub 2021 Jul 8. PMID: 34233457; PMCID: PMC9327760

Fig. 14.5 A schematic of the oblique axial plane through the endometrium illustrating how the depth of myometrium invasion is measured

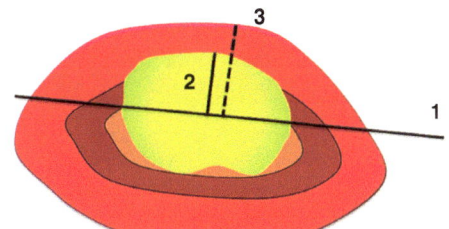

1. Place a line parallel to the inner myometrium
2. Measure tumor extent into the myometrium
3. Measure myometrial thickness
   Depth of myometrial invasion is the ratio between tumor extension into the myometrium (2) and myometrial thickness (3)

Stage I: Tumor invasion of <50% of the myometrial thickness indicates a stage IA tumor, while the invasion of ≥50% of the myometrial thickness indicates a stage IB tumor (Fig. 14.5). There are several pitfalls such as tumor extension into cornua, presence of adenomyosis and leiomyomas (Table 14.2) [9, 27, 28]. In such cases, DWI and DCE help better delineate the tumor margins and lead to improved accuracy.

Stage II: Tumor invades the cervical stroma. The hyperintense SI inflammation (edema) within cervical stroma on T2WI may lead to up-staging. The presence of intermediate T2 SI tumor with diffusion restriction and hypo-enhancement on delayed phase DCE suggests cervical stroma invasion (Fig. 14.4) [9, 27, 28].

Stage III: Tumor invades the uterine serosa or ovaries (Fig. 14.6). A concomitant primary ovarian tumor may be interpreted as a local-regional spread of EC. A primary tumor is suspected when a complex solid-cystic mass with enhancement and restricted diffusion is noted. Stage IIIB includes vaginal or parametrial involvement and IIIC indicates the presence of pelvic and/or para-aortic LN metastases.

Stage IV: In stage IVA disease tumor invades the bladder or rectal mucosa. A common pitfall is bullous edema of the bladder caused by tumor invasion of the subserosal or muscular layer. In stage IVB distant metastases are present, including lymphadenopathy above renal hilum or inguinal region, malignant ascites, peritoneal deposits, or distant

Table 14.2 Pearls and pitfalls of EC staging with MRI

FIGO stage	Pitfalls	Pearls
I: Depth of MI • IA < 50% • IB ≥ 50%	Over/underestimation of depth of MI: – Poor tumor-myometrium contrast on T2WI – Thin myometrium due to compression by a large tumor – Tumor extension into cornua where myometrium is thin physiologically – Leiomyomas, adenomyosis	– Use DWI and DCE for better delineation of tumor margins – Early phase DCE (30–60 s) is helpful exclude any myometrial invasion prior to fertility-sparing management – Equilibrium phase DCE (120–180 s) offers best tumor-myometrium contrast
II: Cervical stromal invasion	– Cervical stromal inflammation/edema – Tumor extension into endocervical canal – Poor tumor-cervical stroma contrast	– Correlate with DWI and DCE as T2WI can overestimate – Tumor extension into endocervical canal should be assigned stage I – DWI and delayed phase DCE (4–5 min) improve delineation of tumor margins and tumor-cervical stroma contrast
III: Loco-regional spread • IIIA-serosal or ovarian involvement • IIIB: vaginal invasion • IIIC: pelvic/para-aortic LN metastases	– Concomitant benign ovarian pathology – Questionable serosa deposits – Concomitant primary ovarian tumor – Inflammatory lymphadenopathy	– Dark SI on T2WI and DWI –> benign ovarian lesion – Check DWI for small serosa deposits – Complex solid-cystic mass –> suggest primary ovarian tumor – Report if ≥1 cm, round, spiculated, or clustered LNs – If uncertain recommend FDG-PET/CT
IV: Extrauterine spread • IVA: Bladder/rectum, mucosal invasion • IVB: Peritoneal deposits	– Bullous edema of the bladde – Questionable peritoneal implants	– Check for mucosal invasion; not just "lifting" of the mucosal line—best seen on T2WI – DWI helps identification of small peritoneal deposit

Abbreviations: DWI diffusion-weighted imaging, DCE dynamic contrast enhanced, LN lymph node, MI myometrial invasion

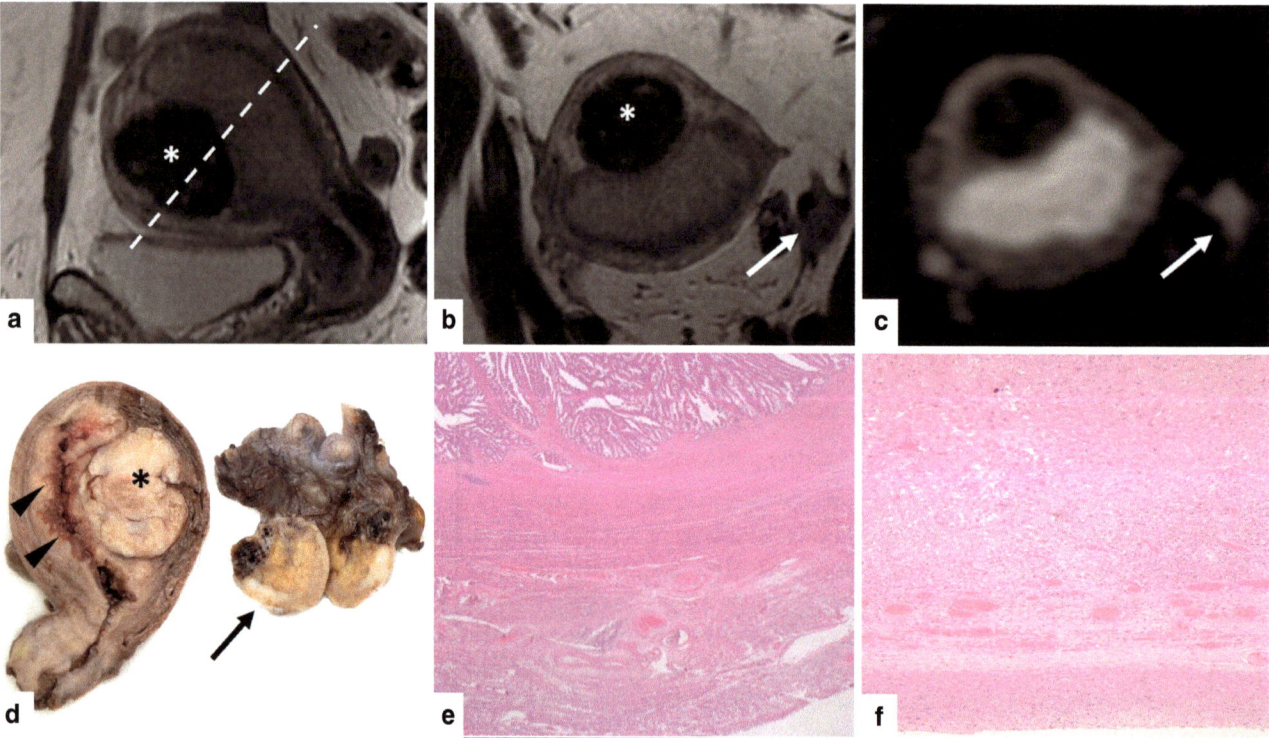

Fig. 14.6 Endometrial serous carcinoma: FIGO IIIA. A 78-year-old patient with vaginal bleeding. On T2WI there is a polypoid mass within the endometrial cavity (**a**, **b**) with restricted diffusion on DWI (**c**). Note the adjacent leiomyoma (*) with characteristic low-T2WI SI. The left ovary has intermediate-T2WI SI associated with high-DWI SI (C, arrow); the appearance is suspicious for the involvement of the left ovary. The gross examination of the surgery specimen (**d**) shows the endometrial tumor (arrowheads), the leiomyoma (*) and the left adnexa (arrow). The pathology revealed endometrial serous carcinoma (**e**) with spread to the left ovary (**f**), corresponding to Stage IIIA disease. These images were originally published in Pintican R, Bura V, Zerunian M, Smith J, Addley H, Freeman S, Caruso D, Laghi A, Sala E, Jimenez-Linan M. MRI of the endometrium - from normal appearances to rare pathology. Br J Radiol. 2021 Sep 1; 94 (1125): 20201347. doi: 10.1259/bjr.20201347. Epub 2021 Jul 8. PMID: 34233457; PMCID: PMC9327760

organ metastasis (e.g., lung, liver). CT and/or PET/CT are useful to detect LN and distant metastatic disease.

14.2.7 Evaluation of EC Recurrence

Recurrent endometrial cancer has a similar imaging appearance to the primary tumor. Risk factors for recurrence include advanced stage at presentation, high-grade disease, Type II tumor, and lymphovascular invasion. More than 80% of recurrences occur within 3 years of initial treatment with the vaginal vault (42%) and LNs (46%) as the most common sites. Recurrence in the peritoneum is uncommon but when present suggests Type II EC. MRI is useful for the evaluation of surgical resectability and for surgical planning by confirming that a disease is confined to the pelvis. PET/CT is helpful to exclude the presence of LN and distant metastases [21].

14.3 Concluding Remarks

Imaging evaluation of patients with CC and EC, particularly with MRI and FDG-PET, facilitates optimal treatment selection including confirming eligibility for conservative fertility-sparing management. Imaging is also central to the evaluation of treatment responses, detection of recurrent disease, and optimal selection of potential salvage treatment options.

> **Take Home Messages**
> - MRI excels at loco-regional staging of CC and EC.
> - PET improves N and M staging in uterine malignancies.
> - MRI facilitates patient selection for fertility-sparing management.

References

1. Sung H, Ferlay J, Siegel RL, Laversanne M, Soerjomataram I, Jemal A, Bray F. Global Cancer statistics 2020: GLOBOCAN estimates of incidence and mortality worldwide for 36 cancers in 185 countries. CA Cancer J Clin. 2021;71(3):209–49.
2. Stelzle D, Tanaka LF, Lee KK, Ibrahim Khalil A, Baussano I, Shah ASV, McAllister DA, Gottlieb SL, Klug SJ, Winkler AS, et al. Estimates of the global burden of cervical cancer associated with HIV. Lancet Glob Health. 2021;9(2):e161–9.
3. Lei J, Ploner A, Elfström KM, Wang J, Roth A, Fang F, Sundström K, Dillner J, Sparén P. HPV vaccination and the risk of invasive cervical Cancer. N Engl J Med. 2020;383(14):1340–8.
4. Marth C, Landoni F, Mahner S, McCormack M, Gonzalez-Martin A, Colombo N. Cervical cancer: ESMO clinical practice guidelines for diagnosis, treatment and follow-up. Ann Oncol. 2017;28(suppl_4):iv72–83.
5. Bhatla N, Berek JS, Cuello Fredes M, Denny LA, Grenman S, Karunaratne K, Kehoe ST, Konishi I, Olawaiye AB, Prat J, et al. Revised FIGO staging for carcinoma of the cervix uteri. Int J Gynaecol Obstet. 2019;145(1):129–35.
6. Bentivegna E, Gouy S, Maulard A, Chargari C, Leary A, Morice P. Oncological outcomes after fertility-sparing surgery for cervical cancer: a systematic review. Lancet Oncol. 2016;17(6):e240–53.
7. NCCN Clinical practice guidelines in oncology (NCCN guidelines®). Cervical Cancer. www.nccn.org/professionals/physician_gls/pdf/cervical.pdf.
8. Manganaro L, Lakhman Y, Bharwani N, Gui B, Gigli S, Vinci V, Rizzo S, Kido A, Cunha TM, Sala E, et al. Staging, recurrence and follow-up of uterine cervical cancer using MRI: updated guidelines of the European Society of Urogenital Radiology after revised FIGO staging 2018. Eur Radiol. 2021;31(10):7802–16.
9. Sala E, Rockall AG, Freeman SJ, Mitchell DG, Reinhold C. The added role of MR imaging in treatment stratification of patients with gynecologic malignancies: what the radiologist needs to know. Radiology. 2013;266(3):717–40.
10. Park JJ, Kim CK, Park SY, Park BK. Parametrial invasion in cervical cancer: fused T2-weighted imaging and high-b-value diffusion-weighted imaging with background body signal suppression at 3 T. Radiology. 2015;274(3):734–41.
11. Woo S, Atun R, Ward ZJ, Scott AM, Hricak H, Vargas HA. Diagnostic performance of conventional and advanced imaging modalities for assessing newly diagnosed cervical cancer: systematic review and meta-analysis. Eur Radiol. 2020;30(10):5560–77.
12. Xiao M, Yan B, Li Y, Lu J, Qiang J. Diagnostic performance of MR imaging in evaluating prognostic factors in patients with cervical cancer: a meta-analysis. Eur Radiol. 2020;30(3):1405–18.
13. Choi HJ, Ju W, Myung SK, Kim Y. Diagnostic performance of computer tomography, magnetic resonance imaging, and positron emission tomography or positron emission tomography/computer tomography for detection of metastatic lymph nodes in patients with cervical cancer: meta-analysis. Cancer Sci. 2010;101(6):1471–9.
14. Adam JA, van Diepen PR, Mom CH, Stoker J, van Eck-Smit BLF, Bipat S. [(18)F]FDG-PET or PET/CT in the evaluation of pelvic and Para-aortic lymph nodes in patients with locally advanced cervical cancer: a systematic review of the literature. Gynecol Oncol. 2020;159(2):588–96.
15. Rockall AG, Ghosh S, Alexander-Sefre F, Babar S, Younis MT, Naz S, Jacobs IJ, Reznek RH. Can MRI rule out bladder and rectal invasion in cervical cancer to help select patients for limited EUA? Gynecol Oncol. 2006;101(2):244–9.
16. Gee MS, Atri M, Bandos AI, Mannel RS, Gold MA, Lee SI. Identification of distant metastatic disease in uterine cervical and endometrial cancers with FDG PET/CT: analysis from the ACRIN 6671/GOG 0233 multicenter trial. Radiology. 2018;287(1):176–84.
17. Pötter R, Tanderup K, Schmid MP, Jürgenliemk-Schulz I, Haie-Meder C, Fokdal LU, Sturdza AE, Hoskin P, Mahantshetty U, Segedin B, et al. MRI-guided adaptive brachytherapy in locally advanced cervical cancer (EMBRACE-I): a multicentre prospective cohort study. Lancet Oncol. 2021;22(4):538–47.
18. Meyer HJ, Wienke A, Surov A. Pre-treatment apparent diffusion coefficient does not predict therapy response to Radiochemotherapy in cervical Cancer: a systematic review and meta-analysis. Anticancer Res. 2021;41(3):1163–70.
19. Harry VN, Persad S, Bassaw B, Parkin D. Diffusion-weighted MRI to detect early response to chemoradiation in cervical cancer: a systematic review and meta-analysis. Gynecol Oncol Rep. 2021;38:100883.
20. Schwarz JK, Siegel BA, Dehdashti F, Grigsby PW. Association of posttherapy positron emission tomography with tumor response and survival in cervical carcinoma. JAMA. 2007;298(19):2289–95.

21. Lakhman Y, Nougaret S, Micco M, Scelzo C, Vargas HA, Sosa RE, Sutton EJ, Chi DS, Hricak H, Sala E. Role of MR imaging and FDG PET/CT in selection and follow-up of patients treated with pelvic exenteration for gynecologic malignancies. Radiographics. 2015;35(4):1295–313.

22. Cancer Research UK. Uterine cancer incidence statistics. https://www.cancerresearchuk.org/health-professional/cancer-statistics/statistics-by-cancer-type/uterine-cancer/incidence#heading-Three. Accessed 17 Sept 2022.

23. Lee NK, Cheung MK, Shin JY, Husain A, Teng NN, Berek JS, Kapp DS, Osann K, Chan JK. Prognostic factors for uterine cancer in reproductive-aged women. Obstet Gynecol. 2007;109(3):655–62.

24. Timmermans A, Opmeer BC, Khan KS, Bachmann LM, Epstein E, Clark TJ, Gupta JK, Bakour SH, van den Bosch T, van Doorn HC, et al. Endometrial thickness measurement for detecting endometrial cancer in women with postmenopausal bleeding: a systematic review and meta-analysis. Obstet Gynecol. 2010;116(1):160–7.

25. Lynch HT, Snyder CL, Shaw TG, Heinen CD, Hitchins MP. Milestones of Lynch syndrome: 1895-2015. Nat Rev Cancer. 2015;15(3):181–94.

26. Kandoth C, Schultz N, Cherniack AD, Akbani R, Liu Y, Shen H, Robertson AG, Pashtan I, Shen R, Benz CC, et al. Integrated genomic characterization of endometrial carcinoma. Nature. 2013;497(7447):67–73.

27. Nougaret S, Horta M, Sala E, Lakhman Y, Thomassin-Naggara I, Kido A, Masselli G, Bharwani N, Sadowski E, Ertmer A, et al. Endometrial Cancer MRI staging: updated guidelines of the European Society of Urogenital Radiology. Eur Radiol. 2019;29(2):792–805.

28. Otero-García MM, Mesa-Álvarez A, Nikolic O, Blanco-Lobato P, Basta-Nikolic M, de Llano-Ortega RM, Paredes-Velázquez L, Nikolic N, Szewczyk-Bieda M. Role of MRI in staging and follow-up of endometrial and cervical cancer: pitfalls and mimickers. Insights Imaging. 2019;10(1):19.

29. Colombo N, Creutzberg C, Amant F, Bosse T, Gonzalez-Martin A, Ledermann J, Marth C, Nout R, Querleu D, Mirza MR, et al. ESMO-ESGO-ESTRO consensus conference on endometrial cancer: diagnosis, treatment and follow-up. Int J Gynecol Cancer. 2016;26(1):2–30.

30. Creasman W. Revised FIGO staging for carcinoma of the endometrium. Int J Gynaecol Obstet. 2009;105(2):109.

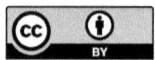

Adnexal Diseases

15

Sarah Swift and Sungmin Woo

Learning Points
1. To recognise common benign adnexal pathologies
2. To appreciate the limitations of US and CT for the assessment of adnexal masses
3. To understand when MRI is indicated and how it is performed
4. To become familiar with the O-RADS MRI scoring system
5. To be aware of and recognise non-gynaecological adnexal pathologies

15.1 Introduction

Adnexal lesions are common. In premenopausal women the majority of these are detected by Ultrasound and are benign lesions such as physiological cysts, endometriomas, mature ovarian teratomas (dermoid cysts), cyst adenomas or lesions of the fibroma lineage. In postmenopausal women adnexal masses are also likely to be benign.

The rapid expansion in the use of computed tomography (CT) for first-line assessment of the urinary and gastrointestinal tracts, investigation of patients presenting with non-specific symptoms, with an acute abdomen or following trauma has resulted in many adnexal masses being diagnosed but not characterised. Incidental adnexal masses are reported in approximately 5% of CT studies [1]. Of incidentally detected adnexal cysts at CT, the ovarian cancer rate is approximately 0.7% [2].

Whilst ultrasound is the initial imaging modality of choice in young women and those of any age presenting with pelvic symptoms and is excellent for characterisation of many lesions, benign diseases such as endometriosis, teratomas and adenofibromas can look complex with mixed cystic and solid components. The clinical presentation of the patient and ancillary information such as inflammatory indices and tumour markers are crucial in aiding interpretation of radiological findings and when there is a mismatch between the clinical picture and the level of radiological concern, additional imaging is then needed. This is also crucial for incidental CT findings. The role of additional imaging is to confirm benign diagnoses and to detect those lesions that are borderline or malignant in nature in order to ensure the patients are managed by the appropriate gynaecological oncology teams.

15.2 Imaging Modalities for Assessment of Adnexal Masses

15.2.1 Ultrasound

Ultrasound is considered the first-line imaging modality to characterise adnexal masses as benign or malignant. By using transvaginal and transabdominal approaches, in many cases not only determining the likelihood of malignancy but also predicting specific differential diagnoses is possible, with examples including simple or haemorrhagic cysts, endometriomas and mature cystic teratomas. In such cases management recommendations can often be made solely by ultrasound findings without the need for further imaging. However, when the adnexal mass remains indeterminate by ultrasound owing to factors of lesion complexity or limitations of the study due to patient characteristics, MRI can be helpful for further characterisation [3].

S. Swift (✉)
Department of Clinical Radiology, St James's University Hospital, Leeds, England, UK
e-mail: sarah.swift1@nhs.net

S. Woo
Department of Radiology, Memorial Sloan Kettering Cancer Centre, New York, NY, USA
e-mail: woos@mskcc.org

© The Author(s) 2023
J. Hodler et al. (eds.), *Diseases of the Abdomen and Pelvis 2023-2026*, IDKD Springer Series,
https://doi.org/10.1007/978-3-031-27355-1_15

15.2.2 Magnetic Resonance Imaging (MRI)

The usage of MRI is widely adopted by many national guidelines for characterisation of sonographically indeterminate adnexal masses [4]. Advantages of MRI include exquisite soft tissue resolution and lack of ionising radiation, in comparison with CT. Numerous studies have shown that MRI has the highest diagnostic accuracy among imaging modalities with pooled sensitivity of 0.94 (95% CI 0.91–0.95) and specificity of 0.91 (95% CI, 0.90–0.93) for differentiating malignant from benign adnexal tumours [5].

In order to achieve such high diagnostic accuracies as shown in the literature, guidelines recommend that certain protocols be followed when performing pelvic MRI for assessing adnexal lesions [6]. For preparation, fasting (e.g., 4 h), intravenous smooth muscle relaxants (e.g., glucagon), and partially filling the urinary bladder are recommended. MRI sequences should include (**a**) T2-weighted imaging (T2WI) in at least 2 planes—most commonly sagittal for orientation of the uterus and axial in high-resolution for analyzing the ovaries and (**b**) axial T1-weighted imaging (T1WI). Additional sequences for problem solving include (**a**) T2-weighted imaging in the plane along the long axis of the uterus (i.e., oblique axial) when ovaries are not seen well or when needing to evaluate for the presence of 'bridging vessels' to the uterus to determine organ of origin (i.e., adnexal vs. uterine); (**b**) fat-saturated T1-weighted imaging to differentiate fat vs. haemorrhagic cystic contents; (**c**) diffusion-weighted imaging (DWI) with b-values of 0–50 and ≥ 1000 s/mm^2 and (**d**) dynamic contrast-enhanced (DCE) MRI up to 4 min post-gadolinium-based contrast agent injection with temporal resolution of ≤ 15 s with derived subtraction images (especially for haemorrhagic lesions).

15.2.3 O-RADS MRI Scoring System for Risk Stratification of Adnexal Masses

It is recommended that risk stratification of sonographically indeterminate adnexal masses be done using an algorithmic approach. Recently the Ovarian-Adnexal Reporting and Data System (O-RADS) MRI scoring system was established by an international committee of multidisciplinary experts [7]. This was developed based on the ADNEX MR scoring system that incorporates assessment of fluid and solid components using anatomical and functional MRI which had been validated prospectively in multiple centres with a sensitivity and specificity of 0.93 and 0.91, respectively [8, 9]. O-RADS MRI risk stratification system allows assignment of 6 scores as follows:

1. O-RADS MRI score 0 (incomplete exam). Sometimes, adnexal lesions cannot fully be characterised due to incomplete coverage or technical issues (e.g., artifacts).
2. O-RADS MRI score 1 (normal ovaries). This score is given when there are only normal or physiological findings in the ovaries. This includes follicles, haemorrhagic cysts and corpus luteal cysts that are ≤ 3 cm in size in premenopausal women and small residua of follicles in postmenopausal women at the radiologist's discretion. A key tip to identifying the ovary (and in turn assessing whether the finding is adnexal or not) is to trace the gonadal veins. Of note, if the findings are not ovarian or adnexal origin, O-RADS MRI risk score is not applicable.
3. O-RADS MRI score 2 (almost certainly benign; positive predictive value [PPV] of cancer <0.5%). This category includes findings that are almost certainly benign. Examples are unilocular cyst with either simple or endometriotic fluid regardless of wall enhancement, proteinaceous haemorrhagic cysts without wall enhancement, simple hydrosalpinx, peritoneal inclusion cyst. Mature teratoma can have small amount of solid tissue, commonly in the form of a Rokitansky nodule [10]. Only solid masses that demonstrate very low signal on both T2-weighted imaging and DWI, known as the "dark/dark" pattern are also included.
4. O-RADS MRI score 3 (low risk for malignancy [PPV around 5%]). Unilocular cysts containing proteinaceous, haemorrhagic, or mucinous fluid with a smooth enhancing wall, or multilocular cysts with any type of fluid with smooth enhancing wall/septa. In the presence of solid tissue not showing 'dark/dark' pattern, the tissue should enhance slower than the uterine myometrium without a shoulder or plateau (low risk time intensity curve [TIC]). Dilated fallopian tubes showing thick/smooth walls/folds or containing non-simple fluid are also included here.
5. O-RADS MRI score 4 (intermediate risk for malignancy [PPV around 50%]). This category includes lesions with solid tissue that are not 'dark/dark' and demonstrate moderate enhancement less than or equal to myometrium, with a shoulder and plateau (intermediate risk TIC). Additionally, lesions with fat-containing large volume of enhancing solid tissue are considered O-RADS MRI score or 4.
6. O-RADS MRI score 5 (high risk for malignancy [PPV around 90%]). This category is assigned to adnexal lesions with non- 'dark/dark' solid tissue showing brisk enhancement greater than myometrium (high-risk TIC) or when definite signs of malignancy such as peritoneal or omental deposits are present.

Although using TIC pattern analysis has been recommended, it is acceptable to base the degree of enhancement at 30–40 s if DCE MRI is not available [11].

15.2.4 Computed Tomography (CT)

CT has become the first-line imaging modality for assessment of the urinary tract for calculi and other causes of haematuria, for assessing the colon and in the investigation of patients who present with non-specific symptoms and those who prevent emergently to the Accident & Emergency Department with acute abdominal pain or following trauma. It is the modality of choice for staging of many cancers, and it is therefore not surprising, given the volume of CT performed, that a significant number of adnexal masses are discovered. CT is poor for characterisation of an isolated adnexal mass. On single-phase CT of the pelvis, it cannot differentiate between cystic lesions containing non-simple fluid and homogeneous poorly enhancing solid masses such as fibromas. Adenofibromas may appear cystic and solid, and masses of the fibroma lineage can be associated with ascites in the setting of Meigs syndrome. Foci of calcification may suggest fibroma or Brenner tumour but can also be seen in low-grade serous carcinoma and some borderline tumours. A pelvic mass on CT in the absence of secondary signs of malignancy such as peritoneal disease or adenopathy is often indeterminate. Low volume free fluid and streaky change in the peri-lesional fat may be due to an inflammatory process such as a tubo-ovarian abscess or torsion of a lesion, and knowledge of the presenting clinical symptoms is crucial for correct interpretation. CA 125 may be elevated by any process which causes peritoneal irritation and biochemical and imaging findings need to be interpreted in the relevant clinical setting to avoid over diagnosis of malignancy.

Once a diagnosis of ovarian cancer is made, however, CT is the modality of choice to stage disease and provide information needed in the MDT meeting to make decisions regarding the likelihood of successful primary surgery versus primary chemotherapy followed by interval debulking surgery [12].

15.2.5 Positron Emission Tomography/ Computed Tomography (PET/CT)

Fluorodeoxyglucose (FDG) activity can be seen in response to physiological change in the ovaries and in benign adnexal diseases such as endometriomas, teratomas and fibroids. Conversely malignant lesions such as necrotic, mucinous and low-grade tumours can be FDG negative or show only low level activity. Consequently, FDG PET/CT is not recommended for the characterisation of adnexal masses nor is it used routinely in the management of patients with ovarian cancer. It can have a role in the assessment of patients with an elevated CA 125 who have no visible disease or only equivocal findings on CT and MRI [13, 14].

15.3 Benign Adnexal Masses

15.3.1 Benign Adnexal Masses and Ultrasound

Most adnexal masses discovered incidentally in pre- and postmenopausal women will be benign. Characterisation of a lesion as benign allows the managing clinician to decide whether intervention is needed based upon the imaging findings, the mode of presentation and the patient's overall health status.

Simple cysts are one of the most common adnexal findings and often visualised using ultrasound. These mostly represent follicles or follicular cysts in premenopausal women and para-ovarian cysts in postmenopausal women. On ultrasound they are seen as round or oval anechoic fluid that is contained by smooth and thin walls without internal septations, solid areas, nor flow on colour Doppler studies. It has been well documented that simple cysts in asymptomatic women have no difference in cancer risk compared with women without such findings, regardless of menopausal status and size of the lesion [15]. Multidisciplinary consensus guidelines recommend that most simple cysts do not require follow-up, but this should be reserved for larger cysts of >3–5 cm in pre- and > 5–7 cm in postmenopausal women, or for less well-defined cysts where follow-up may be helpful to ensure that no suspicious findings were missed on initial imaging. Follow-up to 2 years could be done for simple cysts that have not decreased in size initially, to ensure stability and to identify development of suspicious areas such as papillary projections. Haemorrhagic cysts may have more variable appearance depending on the stage of the blood products and the presence of clot. These latter can also be typically characterised on ultrasound as showing reticular or fishnet pattern of internal echoes or having a retracting clot, which can be differentiated from a mural nodule by identifying sharp and concave margins and lack of flow on Doppler studies. In cases where ultrasound is indeterminate, MRI can be used to further determine its nature. On MRI, haemorrhagic cysts show T1 hyperintense fluid that remains high despite fat suppression and variable T2 signal with lack of enhancing solid tissue.

> **Key Point**
> - Adnexal masses are common in pre- and postmenopausal women and are most often benign. Ultrasound can characterise many benign lesions.

15.3.2 Benign Adnexal Masses and MRI

MRI can make confident benign diagnoses in simple and non-simple fluid-containing cystadenomas, ovarian teratomas, endometriomas, solid and mixed cystic and solid lesions of the fibroma/adenofibroma lineage.

The demonstration of gross fat using T1-weighted sequences with and without fat saturation, with attention to using the same plane of imaging, makes the diagnosis of a teratoma (Fig. 15.1).

Teratomas can show complex internal architecture depending on the content of the lesion, which may include enamel, glial and thyroid tissue in addition to fat, but it is scrutiny of the wall of the lesion that is crucial to identify rare but poor prognosis malignant teratomas. The malignant elements are usually squamous carcinomas that arise within skin elements. These are usually located in the wall of the lesion and can be seen as solid enhancing mural nodules that may demonstrate transmural extension (Fig. 15.2).

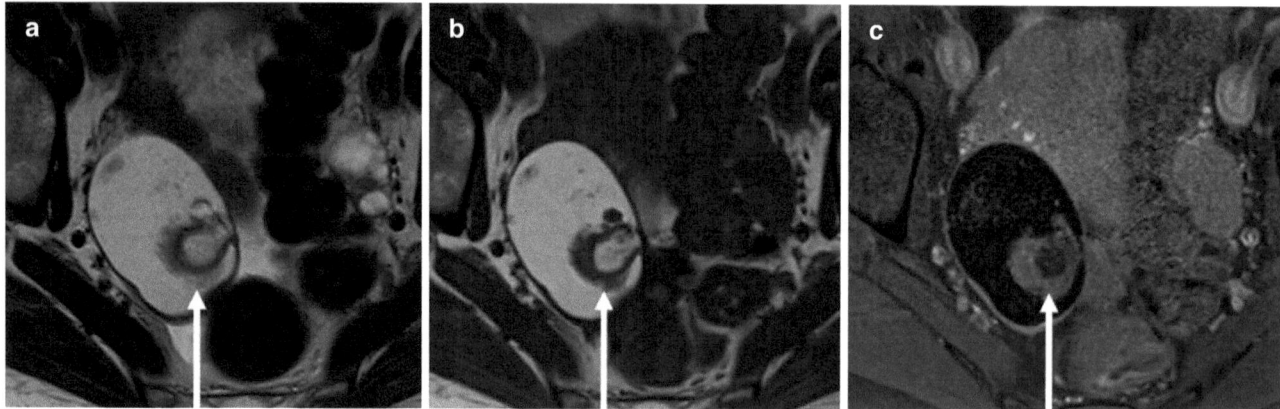

Fig. 15.1 Benign mature ovarian teratoma. The right ovarian lesion displays high signal intensity (SI) on the T2-weighted sequence (**a**), high SI on T1-weighted (**b**) and shows signal loss on the fat saturation sequence (**c**). A Rokitansky nodule is seen posteriorly on all sequences (arrow)

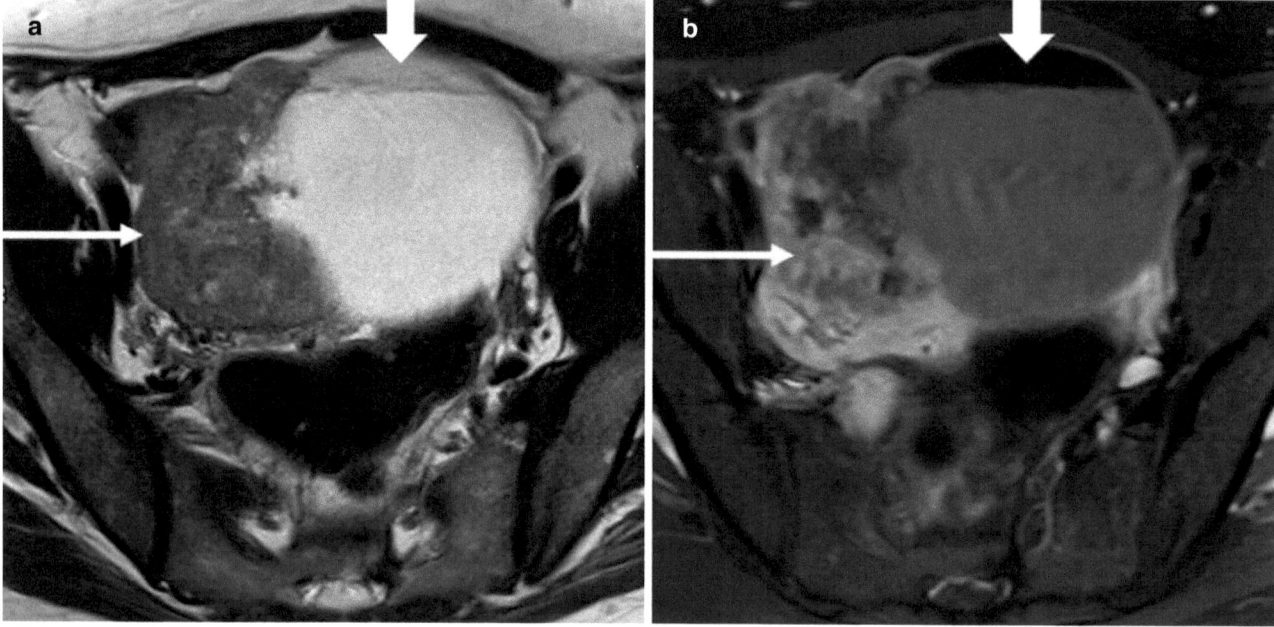

Fig. 15.2 Malignant change in a teratoma. The right ovarian lesion has an intermediate T2 SI solid, transmural component in its right lateral aspect (thin arrow—**a**) that demonstrates enhancement post Gadolinium (thin arrow—**b**). Note the fat-fluid level anteriorly—thick arrow

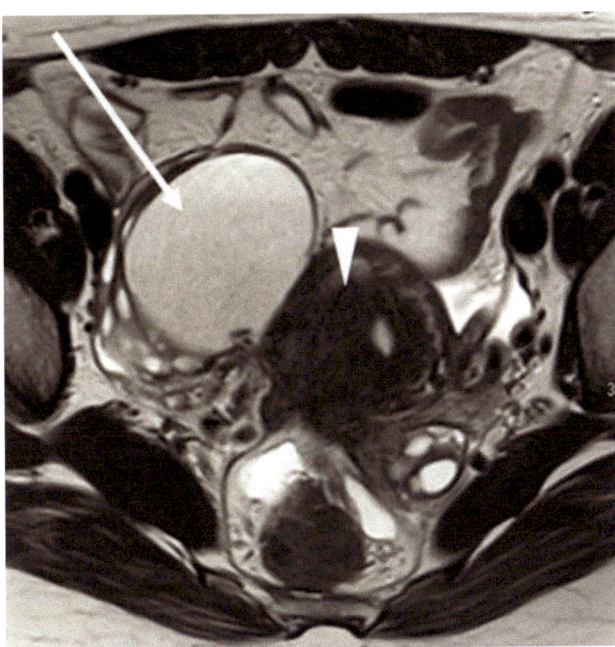

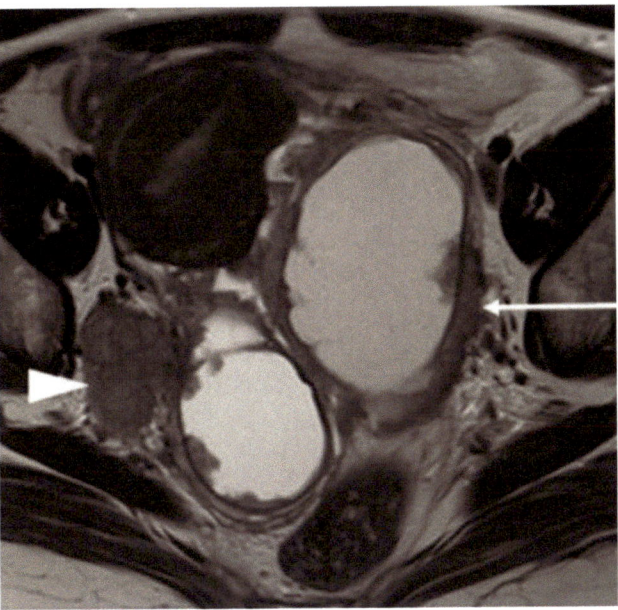

Fig. 15.3 Right ovarian endometrioma displaying shading of contents on T2-weighted imaging (arrow). Note thickening of the uterine junctional zone reflecting adenomyosis (arrowhead)

Fig. 15.4 Malignant change in endometriosis. Bilateral endometriomas with thick irregular walls (arrow) and evidence of nodal metastases (arrowhead)

Endometriomas reflect episodes of repeated haemorrhage due to endometrial tissue in an ectopic location, usually in the ovary or Fallopian tube. This pathophysiology results in a cystic mass containing blood of differing ages and gives the pathognomonic finding of 'shading' of contents on T2-weighted imaging and this is seen as the gradation of signal from high T2 signal intensity (SI) non-dependently to lower T2 signal in the dependent portion of a lesion (Fig. 15.3).

Small low T2 signal foci reflecting haemosiderin may also be apparent. Endometriomas are of high SI on T1 weighted sequences without signal loss post fat saturation and display restricted diffusion. Ancillary signs of endometriosis may be present elsewhere with thickening of the junctional zone of the uterine body due to ectopic endometrial glands within the myometrium reflecting adenomyosis, haematosalpinges and low T2 signal fibrotic endometriosis commonly seen between the posterior uterine serosa and the undersurface of the recto-sigmoid and related to the vaginal fornices in the Pouch of Douglas. The ovaries may lie medially in the pelvis, often tethered to the posterior uterine serosa—'kissing ovaries'—due to adhesions. Malignant

change can occur in endometriomas, most commonly to clear cell carcinoma and suspicious features are mural thickening and solid components (Fig. 15.4).

Solid adnexal masses cause significant diagnostic challenges on CT. The first question is where do they arise from? The excellent soft tissue contrast of T2-weighted MRI may allow identification of normal ovaries separate to the lesion and its relationship to the uterus. Tortuous vessels seen as signal void within a mass, within a vascularised pedicle or in the para-uterine region are a feature of fibroid disease and suggest the lesion may be uterine rather than adnexal in origin. This should prompt search for separate ovaries.

Ovarian fibromas are typically low signal intensity on T2-weighted imaging, do not show restricted diffusion and display minimal enhancement post-Gadolinium (Fig. 15.5).

Adenofibromas may show variable cystic change which accounts for diagnostic difficulty on US or CT, but the T2 dark solid areas which are low signal on high b value diffusion-weighted imaging (DWI) allow MRI to make the correct diagnosis [16].

Ascites is commonly seen when fibromas are present in the setting of Meigs syndrome (Fig. 15.6). This causes fur-

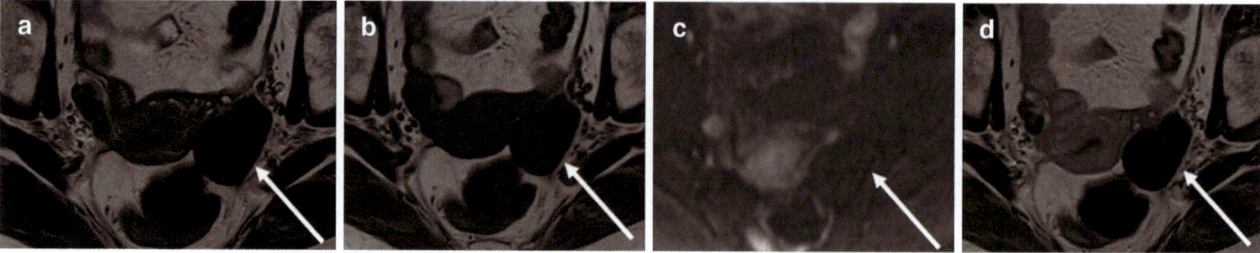

Fig. 15.5 Left ovarian fibroma (arrow) displaying low SI on T2-weighted and T1-weighted images (**a, b**), low SI on high b value DWI (**c**) and no enhancement post Gadolinium (**d**)

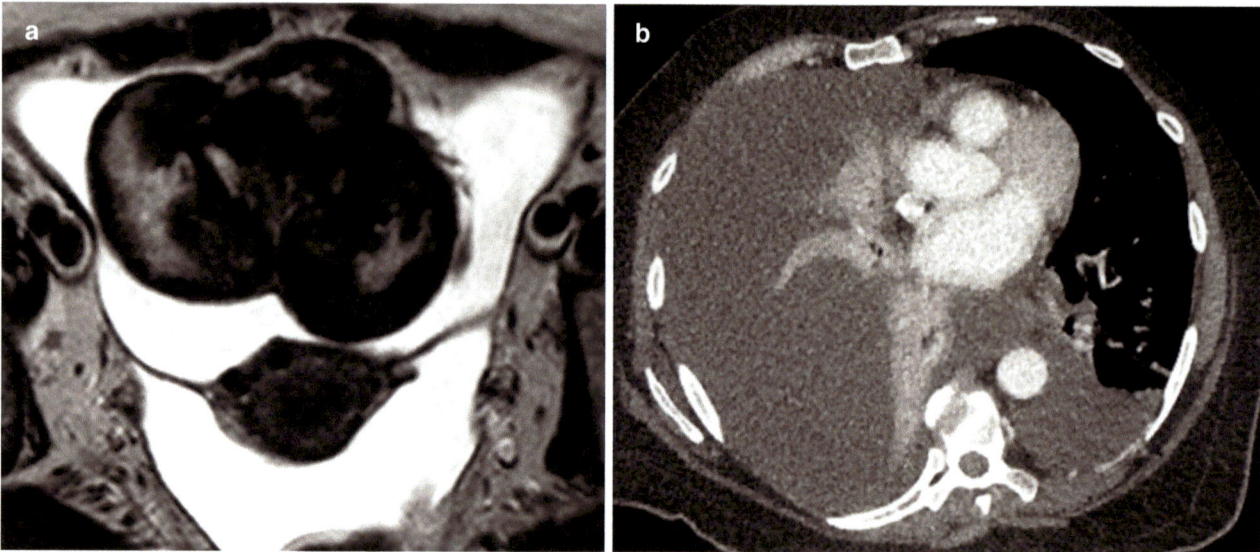

Fig. 15.6 Meigs Syndrome—T2 dark ovarian fibroma with ascites (**a**) and pleural effusions on CT (**b**)

ther diagnostic difficulty with US and CT and if the clinical picture is not one of malignancy and the CA 125 level is not particularly raised, this diagnosis should be considered, and MRI is again of use to characterise the lesion.

Granulosa cell tumours may display avid enhancement on both CT and MRI and give an intermediate to high risk of malignancy O-RADS score of 4 or 5, although clinically they are considered of low malignant potential. Due to their hormonal activity, they may present with vaginal bleeding and be associated with ancillary MRI signs such as preservation of zonal anatomy and uterine size in a postmeno-pausal woman and these findings should prompt consideration of such tumours as a differential diagnosis (Fig. 15.7).

> **Key Point**
> • MRI should be used to characterise lesions that are indeterminate on Ultrasound and CT, and where the clinical picture does not reflect the initial imaging findings.

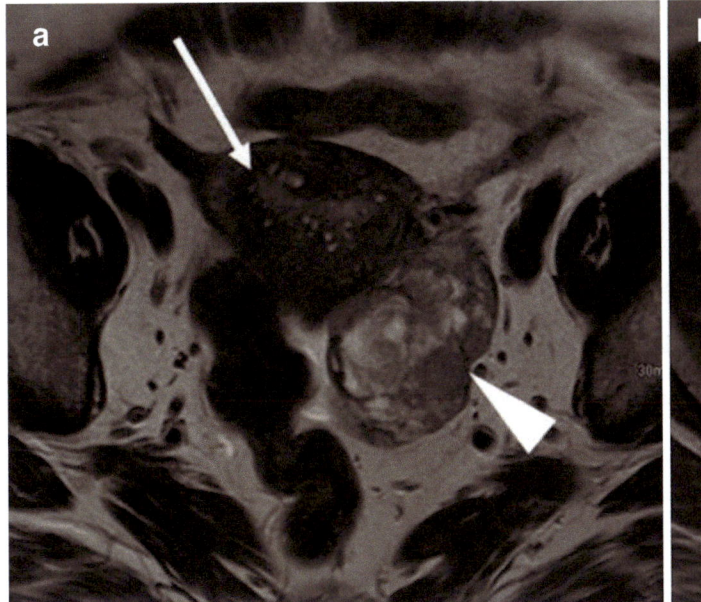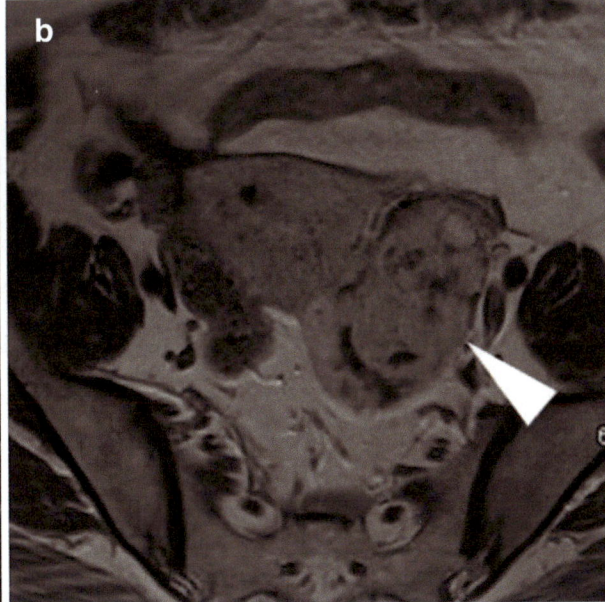

Fig. 15.7 Granulosa cell tumour. A predominantly solid left adnexal mass in a postmenopausal woman (arrowhead). The T2-weighted sequence shows preserved uterine zonal anatomy and cystic adenomyo- sis (arrow) which is abnormal in a patient of this age (**a**) and there is an avid enhancement of the lesion post-gadolinium (**b**)

15.4 Borderline Adnexal Masses

Borderline ovarian tumours occur in younger patients and have a better prognosis. This is an important diagnosis to make pre-operatively as fertility-sparing surgery is then considered as a treatment option. Serous borderline ovarian tumours have pathognomonic imaging features on MRI with papillary projections related to the internal aspect of the wall of the lesion in the cystic form or related exo- phytically to the lesion wall in the surface form (Fig. 15.8a) [17]. These distinctive findings are not readily apparent on CT or US.

Borderline ovarian tumours may also be mucinous in nature and appear as multiloculated cystic masses with loc- ules containing fluid of differing signal intensities on T1-weighted MRI sequences (Fig. 15.8b, c). The wall and internal septations are thin and no solid foci are apparent [18].

> **Key Point**
> - Adnexal lesions with mucinous features on MRI should prompt scrutiny of the GI tract including the appendix for a possible primary tumour site.

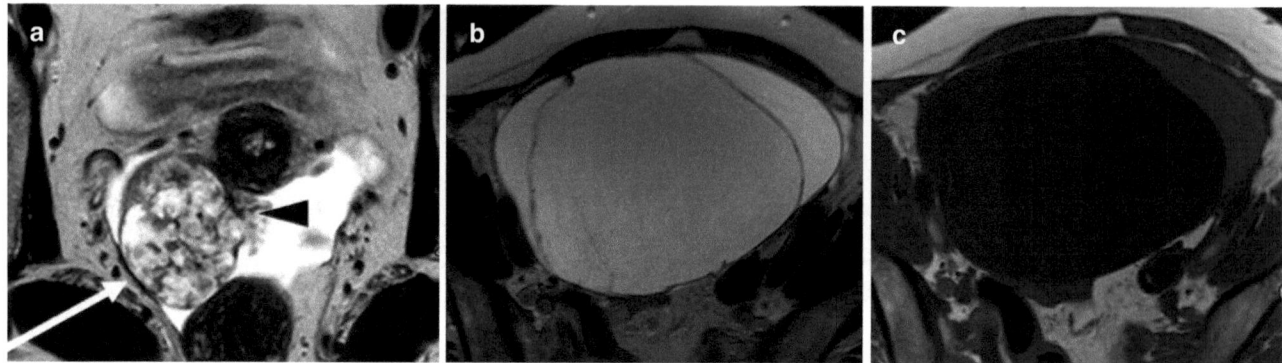

Fig. 15.8 Borderline ovarian tumours. Papillary projections both within the lumen (white arrow) and related to the surface (black arrowhead) of a serous borderline tumour on T2-weighted imaging (**a**). Borderline mucinous tumours typically display locules of differing signal intensities on T2 and T1-weighted sequences (**b, c**)

15.5 Malignant Adnexal Masses

A complex adnexal mass on ultrasound or CT which is then shown to have intermediate T2 signal intensity solid areas which display restricted diffusion and contrast enhancement on MRI, i.e. O-RADS score 4 or 5, is considered malignant and these patients need further management by specialist Gynaecology oncology teams (Fig. 15.9).

Additional imaging may be needed to determine the extent and spread of disease within the abdomen and pelvis. This can be performed with MRI at the time of the pelvic characterisation study or by CT (Fig. 15.10).

Primary ovarian cancer spreads primarily by peritoneal dissemination of disease causing ascites, omental disease, serosal disease often involving the undersurface of the diaphragm, the surface of the liver, spleen and bowel. Nodal disease may be present in the abdomen and pelvis, and the presence of anterior paracardiac and diaphragmatic nodes implies diaphragmatic involvement. Stage IV involvement of the thorax is often reflected by pleural disease with pleural fluid positive for malignant cells and adenopathy spreading through the mediastinum to the supraclavicular fossae. Multidisciplinary discussion is then needed to determine whether primary surgery will achieve optimal debulking or whether the extent of disease combined with the patients' clinical status suggests primary chemotherapy followed by interval debulking surgery (IDS) is more appropriate.

Knowledge of tumour markers in addition to the pattern of disease spread is crucial as the radiological features of metastatic ovarian cancer may be identical to those of metastatic non-ovarian cancer [19]. Metastatic disease to the ovaries is not always solid nor bilateral as originally described by Friedrich Ernst Krukenberg in 1896. The term Krukenberg tumour refers to metastatic mucin-rich signet-ring adenocarcinoma to the ovary from a gastrointestinal primary site. Gastric cancer accounts for approximately 70% of ovarian metastases, with a combination of gastric and colorectal metastases making up 90%. Other tumour sites may also metastasise to the ovaries and primary ovarian cancer may be associated with other non-ovarian malignancies such as breast cancer in those with BRCA gene mutations. The finding of abnormal tumour markers other than CA 125 should prompt detailed scrutiny of the GI tract, including the appendix, the solid upper abdominal organs and the breasts (Fig. 15.11).

Ovarian cancer is recognised as the 'silent killer', patients having advanced disease by the time they present with abdominal swelling or other non-specific symptoms. An acute presentation with abdominal pain is atypical for malignant disease and patients with such symptoms are usually assessed in the emergency department by general surgeons, unless they are known to have a pre-existing adnexal lesion, and initial investigation is invariably CT. The presence of an adnexal mass with low volume free fluid and streaky change within the pelvic fat could be interpreted as cancer with early peritoneal disease. CA 125 is non-specific and invariably elevated in acute abdominal conditions that cause peritoneal irritation, however, torsion of an adnexal mass must be considered and then a search made for relevant radiological signs including a thickened, twisted vascular pedicle and deviation of the uterus to the side of the lesion [20]. Masses may appear as low attenuation on CT due to lack of contrast enhancement if they are already infarcted or they may appear of high attenuation due to intralesional haemorrhage. If the

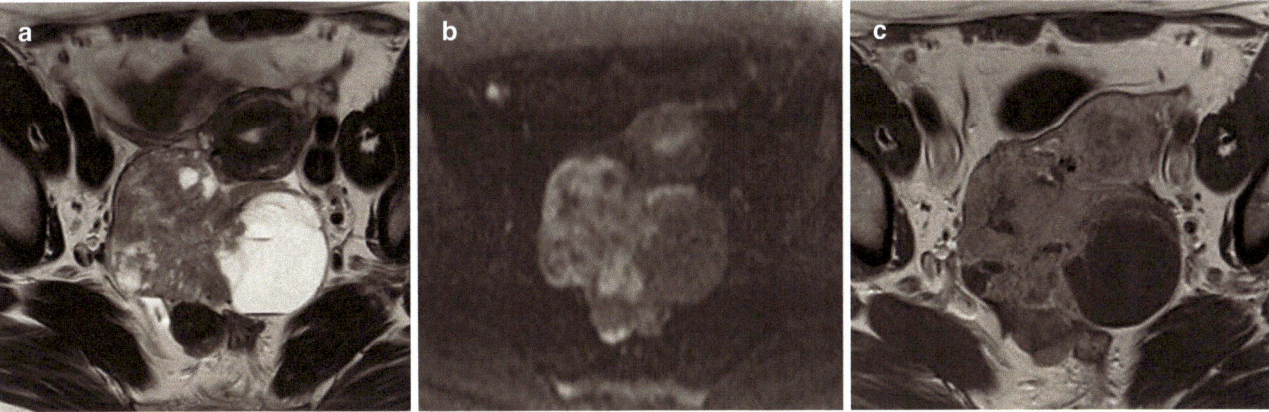

Fig. 15.9 Malignant ovarian mass. Complex adnexal mass with intermediate T2SI solid area (**a**), which shows restricted diffusion on the high b value DWI sequence (**b**) and enhancement post-Gadolinium (**c**)

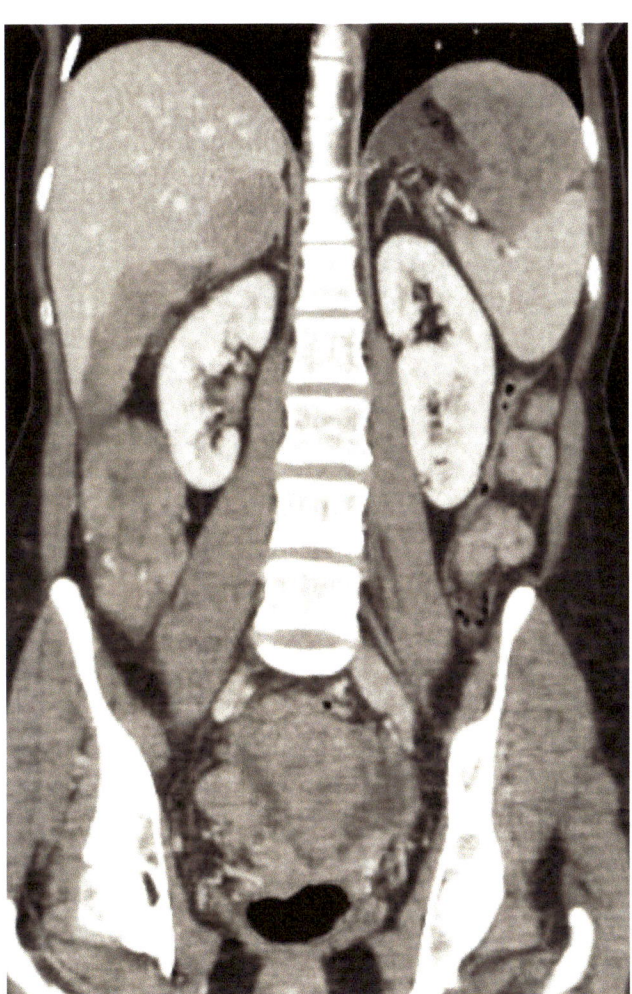

Fig. 15.10 CT scan in a patient presenting with advanced ovarian cancer displaying multifocal peritoneal disease

diagnosis of torsion is considered, assessment with MRI—if it can be performed in a timely fashion—can confirm the diagnosis. The twisted vascular pedicle is more readily apparent and intramural haemorrhage related to the lesion or the pedicle is a pathognomonic finding (Fig. 15.12) [21].

> **Key Point**
> - Clinical presentation with pain suggests an 'accident' to an adnexal mass, commonly torsion or haemorrhage. Most lesions that present acutely are benign.

Women with inflammatory adnexal disease may also present generally unwell and with non-specific symptoms. Ascending infection should be considered in sexually active women and uncommon infections such as actinomycosis remembered as a potential diagnosis if there is a long history of an IUD in situ.

It should be remembered that non-gynaecological structures can also present as an adnexal mass. Mucocoele of the appendix may appear as a tubular adnexal structure on all imaging modalities suggesting it is of tubal origin; however, its relationship to the caecal pole and identification of distant normal ovaries allow the correct diagnosis to be made. These lesions may display calcification on CT (Fig. 15.13).

Gastrointestinal Stromal Tumours (GISTs) are a rare type of sarcoma found in the wall of the digestive system and can occur anywhere from the oesophagus to the rectum [22]. Although most commonly located in the stomach, approxi-

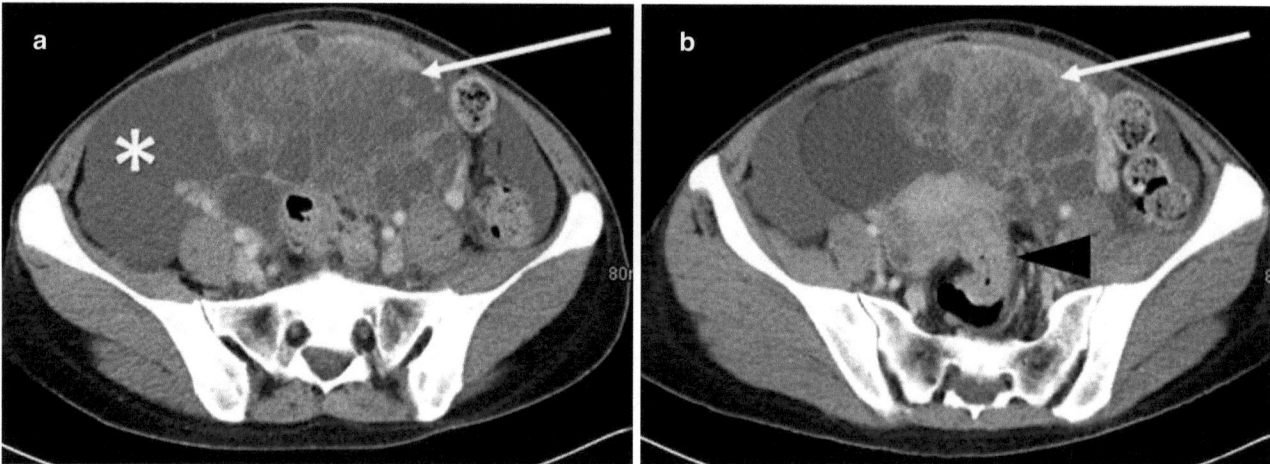

Fig. 15.11 Krukenberg tumour. CT scan in a patient presenting with a mucinous-looking ovarian mass (white arrow) and ascites (*) (**a**). Abnormal mural thickening is visible involving the sigmoid colon indicating the primary tumour site (black arrowhead) (**b**)

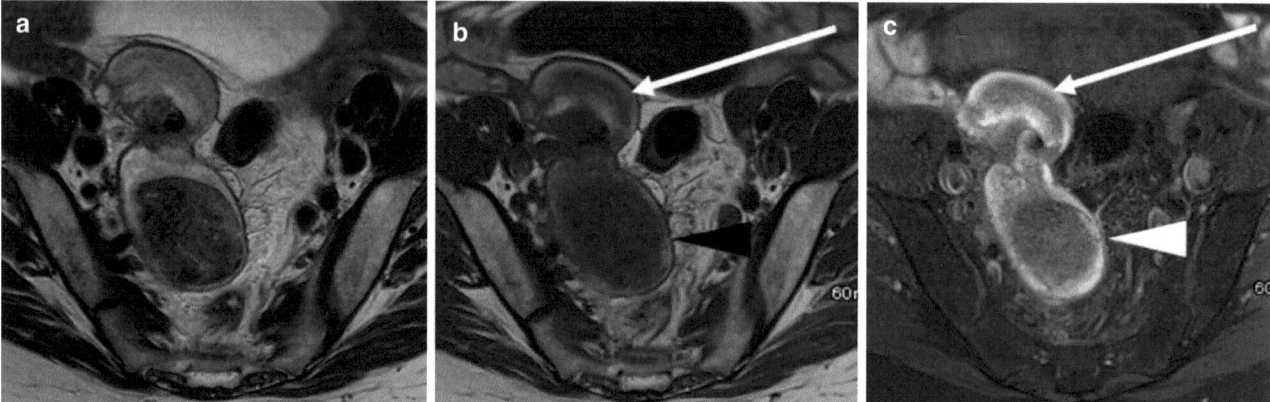

Fig. 15.12 Torsion of a benign fibroma in a patient presenting with abdominal pain. The lesion is seen to be oedematous with a thickened vascular pedicle on the T2-weighted image (**a**), intramural haemor-rhage which is high SI on T1 and high b value DWI (**b, c**) is seen related to the lesion (arrow head) and the pedicle (arrow)

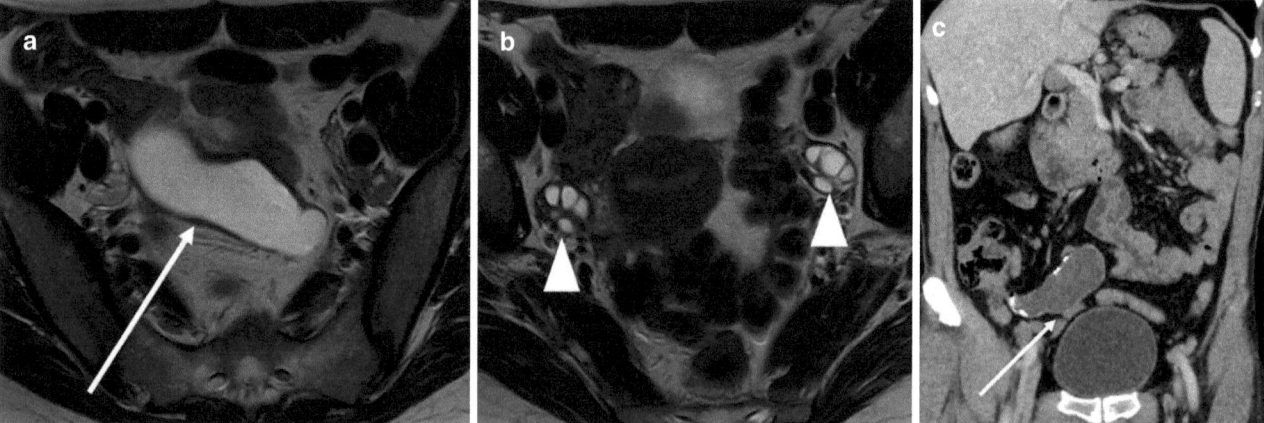

Fig. 15.13 Mucocoele of the appendix. A high T2 SI tubular lesion is seen within the pelvis (**a**). Both ovaries are visible separately and are normal (arrowheads) (**b**). Peripheral calcification may be apparent on CT (arrow) (**c**)

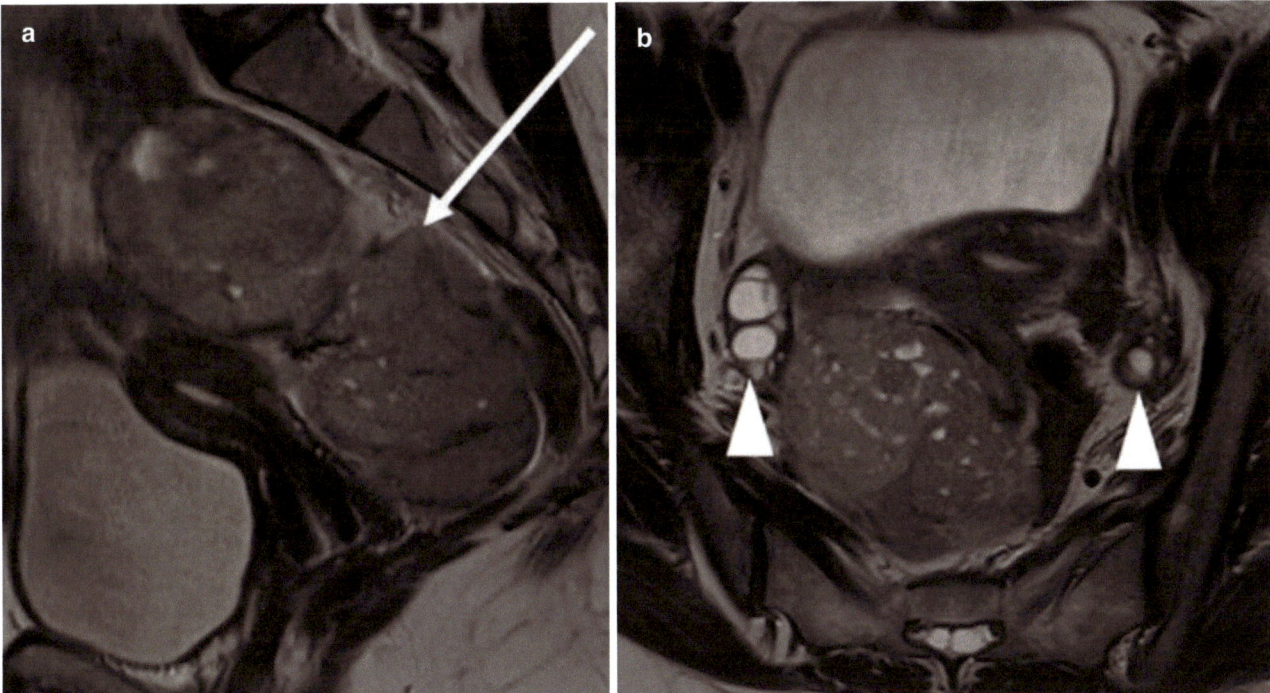

Fig. 15.14 Malignant looking mass filling the Pouch of Douglas (arrow) in a 36 year old woman (**a**). Both ovaries are identified separately (arrowheads) and are normal (**b**). Transrectal biopsy demonstrated a Gastrointestinal Stromal Tumour (GIST)

mately 55%, they can rarely occur in the colon or rectum 3%, and are an uncommon but important differential diagnosis for an adnexal mass with otherwise normal gynaecological structures (Fig. 15.14).

15.6 Concluding Remarks

Adnexal masses are common in pre- and postmenopausal women, and many are discovered as incidental findings, particularly on CT scans performed for a wide variety of indications. The role of imaging is to characterise the lesions and identify those with borderline or malignant features in order to ensure that patients are managed by appropriate specialist gynaecological oncology teams. Where initial imaging findings on US or CT are indeterminate, or their findings do not correlate with the clinical picture or presentation, MRI is an excellent problem-solving modality and allows confident benign and malignant diagnoses to be made and this has been supported by the developed MRI scoring systems, ADNEX MR and subsequently O-RADS MRI.

Take-Home Messages
1. Radiological findings of an adnexal mass need to be interpreted in the knowledge of the mode of presentation, the patient's clinical status and tumour markers.
2. Whilst Ultrasound is an excellent initial imaging modality and may make confident diagnoses, CT is poor for characterisation of adnexal masses particularly in the absence of secondary signs of malignancy.
3. MRI is an excellent problem-solving modality, allows correct benign and malignant diagnoses to be made and therefore ensure patients are managed by the appropriate specialist teams.
4. Radiologists should be aware of the range of differential diagnoses and the pathognomonic MRI findings of common benign lesions, which may be indeterminate on CT and Ultrasound.

References

1. Slanetz PJ, Hahn PF, Hall DA, Mueller PR. The frequency and significance of adnexal lesions incidentally revealed by CT. AJR Am J Roentgenol. 1997;168(3):647–50.
2. Boos J, Brook OR, Fang J, Brook A, Levine D. Ovarian cancer: prevalence in incidental simple adnexal cysts initially identified in CT examinations of the abdomen and pelvis. Radiology. 2018;286(1):196–204.
3. Spencer JA, Ghattamaneni S. MR imaging of the Sonographically indeterminate adnexal mass. Radiology. 2010;256(3):677–94.
4. Friedrich L, Meyer R, Levin G. Management of adnexal mass: a comparison of five national guidelines. Eur J Obstet Gynecol Reprod Biol. 2021;265:80–9.
5. Wang WH, Zheng CB, Gao JN, Ren SS, Nie GY, Li ZQ. Systematic review and meta-analysis of imaging differential diagnosis of benign and malignant ovarian tumors. Gland Surg. 2022;11(2):330–40.
6. Sadowski EA, Thomassin-Naggara I, Rockall A, Maturen KE, Forstner R, Jha P, et al. O-RADS MRI risk stratification system: guide for assessing adnexal lesions from the ACR O-RADS committee. Radiology. 2022;303(1):35–47.
7. O-RADS™ ACoRCo. O-RADS MRI Risk Stratification System. https://www.acr.org/-/media/ACR/Files/RADS/O-RADS/O--RADS-MR-Risk-Stratification-System-Table-September-2020.pdf. Accessed 4 Oct 2022.
8. Thomassin-Naggara I, Aubert E, Rockall A, Jalaguier-Coudray A, Rouzier R, Daraï E, et al. Adnexal masses: development and preliminary validation of an MR imaging scoring system. Radiology. 2013;267(2):432–43.
9. Thomassin-Naggara I, Poncelet E, Jalaguier-Coudray A, Guerra A, Fournier LS, Stojanovic S, et al. Ovarian-adnexal reporting data system magnetic resonance imaging (O-RADS MRI) score for risk stratification of Sonographically indeterminate adnexal masses. JAMA Netw Open. 2020;3(1):e1919896.
10. Cheng M, Causa Andrieu P, Kim TH, Gangai N, Sonoda Y, Hricak H, et al. Fat-containing adnexal masses on MRI: solid tissue volume and fat distribution as a guide for O-RADS score assignment. Abdom Radiol. 2022.
11. Vargas HA, Woo S. Quantitative versus subjective analysis of dynamic contrast-enhanced MRI for O-RADS? Radiology. 2022;303(3):576–7.
12. Forstner R, Sala E, Kinkel K, Spencer JA. ESUR guidelines: ovarian cancer staging and follow-up. Eur Radiol. 2010;20(12):2773–80.
13. The Royal College of Radiologists RCoP, British Nuclear Medicine Society, Administration of Radioactive Substances Advisory Committee. Evidence-based indications for the use of PET/CT in the United Kingdom. Clin Radiol. 2022;71(7):e171–88.
14. Dejanovic D, Hansen NL, Loft A. PET/CT variants and pitfalls in gynecological cancers. Semin Nucl Med. 2021;51(6):593–610.
15. Smith-Bindman R, Poder L, Johnson E, Miglioretti DL. Risk of malignant ovarian cancer based on ultrasonography findings in a large unselected population. JAMA Intern Med. 2019;179(1):71–7.
16. Montoriol PF, Mons A, Da Ines D, Bourdel N, Tixier L, Garcier JM. Fibrous tumours of the ovary: aetiologies and MRI features. Clin Radiol. 2013;68(12):1276–83.
17. Naqvi J, Nagaraju E, Ahmad S. MRI appearances of pure epithelial papillary serous borderline ovarian tumours. Clin Radiol. 2015;70(4):424–32.
18. Woo S, Kim SH, Kim MA, Park IA, Lee MS, Kim SY, et al. Magnetic resonance imaging findings of mucinous borderline ovarian tumors: comparison of intestinal and endocervical subtypes. Abdom Imaging. 2015;40(6):1753–60.
19. Chang WC, Meux MD, Yeh BM, Qayyum A, Joe BN, Chen LM, et al. CT and MRI of adnexal masses in patients with primary non-ovarian malignancy. AJR Am J Roentgenol. 2006;186(4):1039–45.
20. Buamah P. Benign conditions associated with raised serum CA-125 concentration. J Surg Oncol. 2000;75(4):264–5.
21. Duigenan S, Oliva E, Lee SI. Ovarian torsion: diagnostic features on CT and MRI with pathologic correlation. AJR Am J Roentgenol. 2012;198(2):W122–31.
22. Levy AD, Remotti HE, Thompson WM, Sobin LH, Miettinen M. Gastrointestinal stromal tumors: radiologic features with pathologic correlation. Radiographics. 2003;23(2):283–304. 456; quiz 532

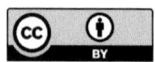

Magnetic Resonance Imaging of the Prostate in the PI-RADS Era

16

Alberto Vargas, Patrick Asbach, and Bernd Hamm

Learning Objectives
- To learn about the advancing role of MR imaging for the management of prostate cancer.
- To learn how to optimize multiparametric prostate MR imaging.
- To know common pitfalls in MR imaging of the prostate.
- To understand how the PI-RADS classification system is applied and interpreted.
- To know the relevance of structured reporting in prostate cancer.

16.1 Introduction

Ongoing technical innovation in combination with a broad research activity has resulted in increased adoption and widespread utilization of magnetic resonance imaging (MRI) of the prostate. The Prostate Imaging Reporting and Data System (PI-RADS), first introduced in 2012 and subsequently updated in 2015 and 2019, standardized image acquisition and reporting and facilitated the communication of imaging findings to referring physician teams and is now considered an obligatory key element in prostate MRI. This has had a tremendous impact on the diagnostic workup of patients with suspected prostate cancer. Indications for MRI have been incorporated in multiple prostate cancer guidelines (e.g., NICE, AUA, EAU, German S3-Guideline), and in

turn imaging-based targeted prostate biopsy has markedly increased. Referring physicians not only heavily rely on accurate interpretation of MRI of the prostate but actively seek high-quality MRI scans for their daily practice because prostate MRI has direct impact on their cancer detection rate. Furthermore, a paradigm shift is taking place in the prostate cancer community regarding the care of low-risk prostate cancer patients, where active surveillance (AS) is increasingly favored over definitive therapy. Prostate MRI plays an important role in AS not only during the initial assessment to determine eligibility but also over the course of follow-up of the disease.

All abdominal and genitourinary radiologists require training and skill in performing and interpreting prostate MRI, especially as prostate MRI has become an indispensable diagnostic tool for *all* patients with clinical suspicion of prostate cancer, during surveillance of low-risk disease and follow-up after prostate cancer treatment.

16.2 The Prostate Imaging Reporting and Data System (PI-RADS)

PI-RADS was introduced by the European Society of Uroradiology (ESUR) in 2012. An updated version (PI-RADS v2) was published in 2015 in collaboration with the American College of Radiology (ACR) and the AdMeTech Foundation. Further refinements through the same collaboration were conducted in 2019 and published as PI-RADS version 2.1. PI-RADS is not based on evidence from clinical research trials but rather on expert knowledge; however, several studies have confirmed that the PI-RADS system improves the diagnostic accuracy of multiparametric (mp) MRI. The overall rationale for implementation of PI-RADS was to ´improve detection, localization, characterization, and risk stratification in patients with suspected cancer in treatment naïve prostate glands´. PI-RADS is currently not applicable to post-treatment assessment in prostate can-

A. Vargas
Department of Radiology, Memorial Sloan Kettering Cancer Center, New York, NY, USA
e-mail: vargasah@mskcc.org

P. Asbach · B. Hamm (✉)
Department of Radiology, Charité Universitätsmedizin Berlin, Berlin, Germany
e-mail: patrick.asbach@charite.de; bernd.hamm@charite.de

© The Author(s) 2023
J. Hodler et al. (eds.), *Diseases of the Abdomen and Pelvis 2023-2026*, IDKD Springer Series,
https://doi.org/10.1007/978-3-031-27355-1_16

cer patients, although there are now other efforts proposed specifically for this purpose. The following specific definitions and aims regarding MR imaging and reporting are targeted by PI-RADS:

16.2.1 Clinical Considerations

Timing of mpMRI after prostate biopsy does not necessarily need to be postponed since clinically significant cancer is less likely affected by post biopsy changes when the biopsy was negative, a phenomenon referred to as the "hemorrhage exclusion sign." For local staging of prostate cancer a delay of a minimum of 6 weeks might be advantageous. No specific patient preparation is necessary; however, the administration of a spasmolytic drug may be beneficial. Bowel cleaning is not recommended, but the patient should evacuate the rectum if possible to reduce the occurrence of susceptibility-related imaging artifacts.

16.2.2 Technical Considerations

Magnetic field strengths of 1.5 or 3 Tesla can both be used (even without an endorectal coil at 1.5 Tesla) when the scan parameters are tailored to small field-of-view imaging of the prostate and contemporary scanner technology is used (specifically multi-channel phased-array surface coils and high=performance gradients). In general, latest generation 3 Tesla systems are preferred (higher signal-to-noise ratio, shorter scan time), although an optimized acquisition protocol is considered even more important than field strength.

mpMRI of the prostate should include the following sequences:

T2-weighted imaging: 2D turbo spin-echo sequence, slice thickness ≤ 3 mm (no interslice gap), in-plane spatial resolution ≤ 0.7 mm (phase-encoding direction) $x \leq 0.4$ mm (frequency-encoding direction). Images in the axial plane (either straight axial to the patient or oblique axial perpendicular to the long axis of the prostate) should be acquired as well as images in at least one additional orthogonal plane (sagittal and/or coronal).

Diffusion-weighted imaging (DWI): spin-echo EPI (echo planar imaging) sequence with fat saturation, slice thickness ≤ 4 mm (no interslice gap), in-plane spatial resolution ≤ 2.5 mm (phase- and frequency-encoding direction), at least two b-values (low b-value of 50–100 s/mm^2 and an intermediate b-value of 800–1000 s/mm^2). Additional b-values in the range of 100–1000 s/mm^2 are optional. A high b-value (≥ 1400 s/mm^2) image set is also mandatory (preferably should be obtained from a separate acquisition rather than from the abovementioned sequence (used for ADC map calculation), or calculated from the low and intermediate b-value images.

Dynamic contrast-enhanced (DCE) imaging: 2D or 3D (3D preferred) gradient-echo sequence with a temporal resolution below 15 s (preferably below 10 s) per acquisition, slice thickness ≤ 3 mm (no interslice gap), in-plane spatial resolution ≤ 2 mm (phase- and frequency-encoding direction).

Slice orientation and slice thickness should match for all mpMRI sequences to allow side-by-side comparison. Also, a large field-of-view sequence covering the pelvic lymph nodes and the skeleton should be acquired.

16.2.3 Assessment of Prostatic Lesions

One major key element of PI-RADS is scoring the likelihood of a prostatic lesion to be *clinically significant* prostate cancer on a 5-point Likert-type scale (Table 16.1).

Since several different definitions of clinically significant prostate cancer exist PI-RADS defines it as "Gleason score ≥ 7 (including 3 + 4 with prominent but not predominant Gleason 4 component), and/or tumor volume ≥ 0.5cc, and/or tumor extra prostatic extension (EPE)." The scoring system is based on typical imaging findings on the respective multiparametric MR sequence (exact definitions according to PI-RADS see Tables 16.2, 16.3, and 16.4, for examples see Figs. 16.1, 16.2, 16.3, 16.4, 16.5, 16.6, 16.7, 16.8, 16.9, 16.10, 16.11, 16.12, and 16.13). For this purpose, typical examples for each score and sequence are included in the PI-RADS publication. The goal is to increase the diagnostic accuracy for detection of prostate cancer and to reduce the variability in image interpretation. Most preliminary studies report good reader agreement, which is higher for peripheral zone (PZ) lesions than transition zone (TZ) lesions. Also, agreement is higher for PI-RADS scores 4 and 5 compared to lower scores.

Compared to PI-RADS version 1, PI-RADS version 2 introduced the diagnostic weighting of the multiparametric sequences to generate a combined score by introducing the concept of a dominant imaging sequence. The dominant sequence depends on the prostatic zone the lesion is located; therefore identification of the zonal anatomy is crucial. The area at the base of the prostate where the central zone borders

Table 16.1 (Reproduced from https://doi.org/10.1007/978-3-319-75019-4_11)

PI-RADS 1	Very low (clinically significant cancer is highly unlikely)
PI-RADS 2	Low (clinically significant cancer is unlikely)
PI-RADS 3	Intermediate (the presence of clinically significant cancer is equivocal)
PI-RADS 4	High (clinically significant cancer is likely)
PI-RADS 5	Very high (clinically significant cancer is highly likely)

Table 16.2 T2-weighted imaging (modified from https://doi.org/10.1007/978-3-319-75019-4_11)

Score	Peripheral zone (PZ)	Transition zone (TZ)
1	Uniform hyperintense signal intensity (normal)	Normal appearing TZ (rare) or a round, completely encapsulated nodule ("typical nodule")
2	Linear or wedge-shaped hypointensity or diffuse mild hypointensity, usually indistinct margin	A mostly encapsulated nodule OR a homogeneous circumscribed nodule without encapsulation. "Atypical nodule") OR a homogeneous mildly hypointense area between nodules
3	Heterogeneous signal intensity or non-circumscribed, rounded, moderate hypointensity includes others that do not qualify as 2, 4, or 5	Heterogeneous signal intensity with obscured margins includes others that do not qualify as 2, 4, or 5
4	Circumscribed, homogenous moderate hypointense focus/mass confined to prostate and < 1.5 cm in greatest dimension	Lenticular or non-circumscribed, homogeneous, moderately hypointense, and < 1.5 cm in greatest dimension
5	Same as 4 but ≥1.5 cm in greatest dimension or definite extraprostatic extension/invasive behavior	Same as 4, but ≥1.5 cm in greatest dimension or definite extraprostatic extension/invasive behavior

Table 16.3 Diffusion-weighted imaging (DWI) (modified from https://doi.org/10.1007/978-3-319-75019-4_11)

Score.	Peripheral zone (PZ) or transition zone (TZ)
1	No abnormality (i.e., normal) on ADC and high b-value DWI
2	Linear/wedge shaped hypointense on ADC and/or linear/wedge shaped hyperintense on high b-value DWI
3	Focal (discrete and different from the background) hypointense on ADC and/or focal hyperintense on high b-value DWI; may be markedly hypointense on ADC or markedly hyperintense on high b-value DWI, but not both.
4	Focal markedly hypointense on ADC and markedly hyperintense on high b-value DWI; <1.5 cm in greatest dimension
5	Same as 4 but ≥1.5 cm in greatest dimension or definite extraprostatic extension/invasive behavior

Table 16.4 Dynamic contrast-enhanced (DCE) imaging (reproduced from https://link.springer.com/chapter/10.1007/978-3-319-75019-4_11)

Score.	Peripheral zone (PZ) or transition zone (TZ)
Negative	No early or contemporaneous enhancement; or diffuse multifocal enhancement NOT corresponding to a focal finding on T2W and/or DWI or focal enhancement corresponding to a lesion demonstrating features of BPH on T2WI (including features of extruded BPH in the PZ)
Positive	Focal, and; earlier than or contemporaneously with enhancement of adjacent normal prostatic tissues, and; corresponds to suspicious finding on T2W and/or DWI

the peripheral zone and the anterior gland where the anterior horn of the peripheral zone borders the transition zone and the anterior fibromuscular stroma might be challenging in this respect. DWI is the dominant sequence for the peripheral zone, where most prostate cancers are located. T2W is the dominant sequence for the transition zone. The dominant sequence defines the final PI-RADS score with the exception of PI-RADS 3 lesions, where for the peripheral zone, the DCE sequence and for the transition zone, the DWI sequence defines the final PI-RADS score (see Tables 16.5 and 16.6). PI-RADS version 2.1 also included a subcategorization of PI-RADS score 2 TZ lesions on T2-weighted images, as reflected in Table 16.6.

There is growing interest and support for the use of bi-parametric (bp) MRI (T2W + DWI), eliminating the need for DCE-MRI. The current PI-RADS version 2.1 contains no specific recommendations for the use of bpMRI; however, it does address situations where a particular sequence cannot be acquired or is non-diagnostic due to artifacts (e.g., DWI when certain hip implants are present). In these situations, the following rules apply:

Assessment without DWI (applies to PZ and TZ): the T2-weighted sequence defines the final PI-RADS score with the exception of PI-RADS 3 - if the lesion is DCE negative the final score remains 3, if the lesion is DCE positive the final score is 4.

Assessment without DCE (only applies to the peripheral zone since DCE is not used for transition zone scoring): the DWI score represents the final PI-RADS score.

16.2.4 Structured Reporting

A very important task of PI-RADS is to simplify and standardize the terminology and content of radiology reports and to enhance interdisciplinary communications with referring clinicians. A comprehensive mpMRI report should therefore include the following contents:

The volume of prostate should be reported according to the ellipsoid formula: maximum AP diameter × maximum transverse diameter × maximum longitudinal diameter × 0.52. PI-RADS version 2.1 suggests that maximum AP and longitudinal diameters be measured on a mid-sagittal T2W image if obtained, and that maximum transverse diameter measurement is made on an axial T2W image. PI-RADS scores are assigned to up to 4 intraprostatic lesions with overall score ≥ 3. In case of multiple lesions, an index lesion should be defined. The index lesion is the one with the highest PI-RADS score. In case multiple lesions qualify for the highest PI-RADS score, extraprostatic extension (EPE) outweighs lesion size. For each lesion a PI-RADS score is

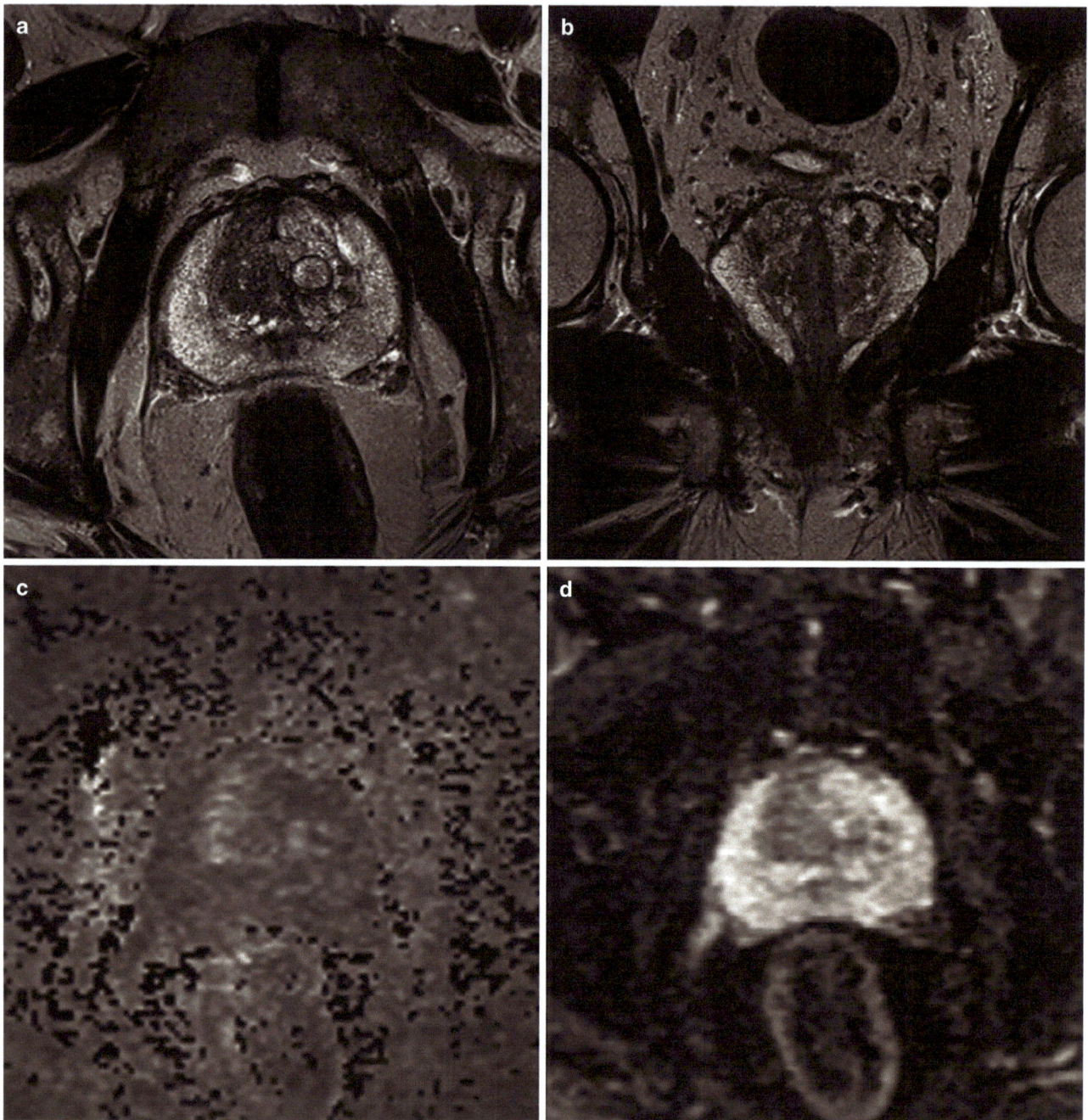

Fig. 16.1 (a–d) Normal peripheral zone. (a) Axial and (b) coronal T2-weighted sequence showing uniform hyperintense signal intensity of the peripheral zone (PI-RADS score 1). (c) Diffusion-weighted high b-value (calculated $b = 1400$ s/mm^2) image and (d) ADC map (domi-nant sequence for the peripheral zone) with no abnormality consistent with an overall PI-RADS score of 1. (Reproduced from. https://doi.org/10.1007/978-3-319-75019-4_11)

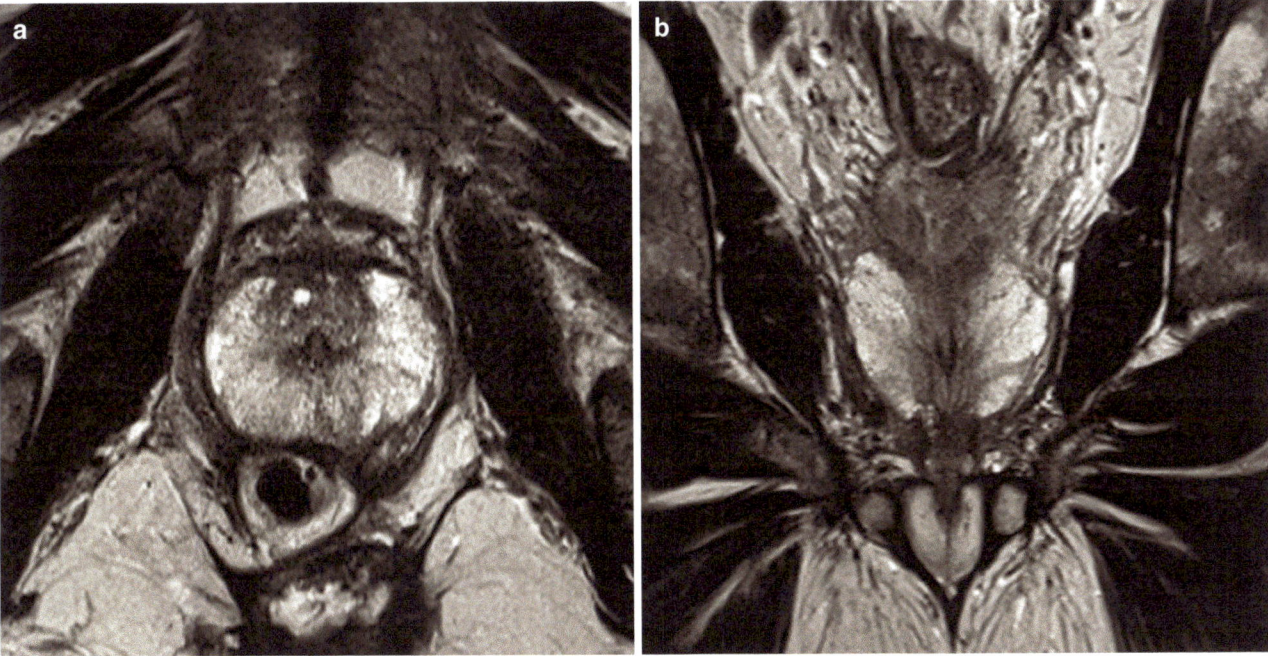

Fig. 16.2 (**a**, **b**) Normal transition zone. (**a**) Axial and (**b**) coronal T2-weighted sequence (dominant sequence for the transition zone) showing heterogeneous intermediate signal intensity of the non-

enlarged transition zone (PI-RADS score 1). (Reproduced from. https://doi.org/10.1007/978-3-319-75019-4_11)

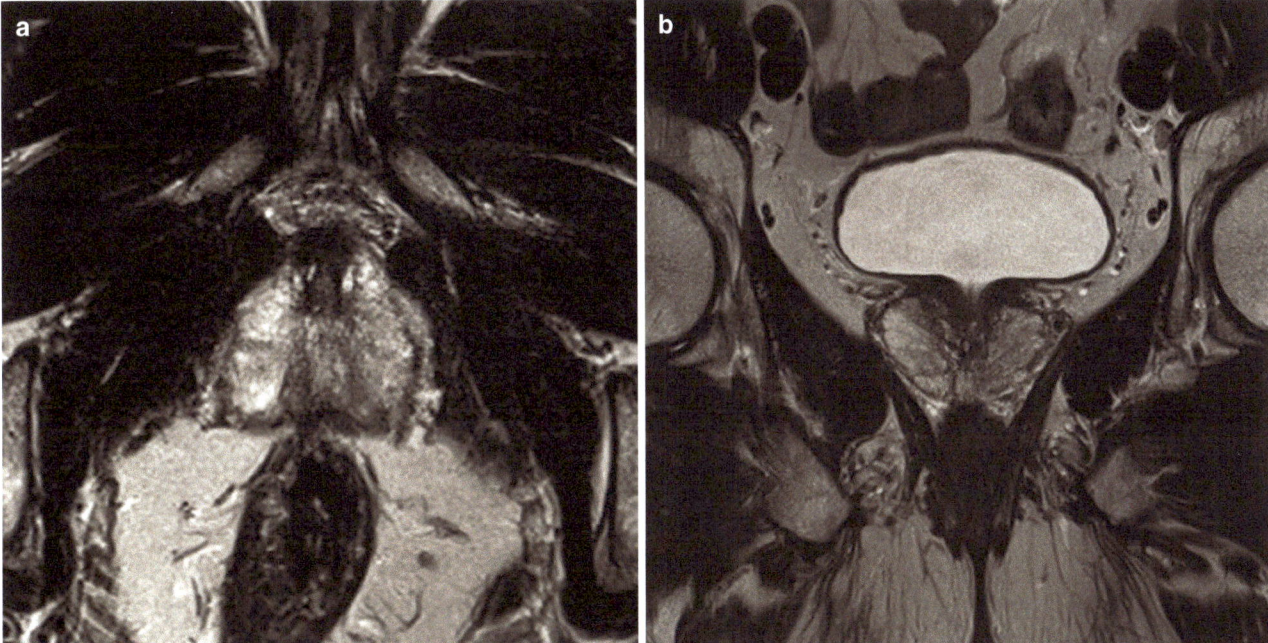

Fig. 16.3 (**a–e**) PI-RADS score 2 findings in the peripheral zone. (**a**) Axial and (**b**) coronal T2-weighted sequence showing linear hypointensities in the bilateral peripheral zone (PI-RADS score 2). (**c**) Diffusion weighted high b-value (calculated $b = 1400$ s/mm^2) image shows no areas of increased signal intensity. (**d**) ADC map shows no focal hypointense areas (dominant sequence for the peripheral zone) in the

peripheral zone (PI-RADS score 2). (**e**) DCE sequence shows no focal or early enhancement (DCE negative) consistent with an overall PI-RADS score of 2. Linear T2-hypointensities in the peripheral zone are a frequent finding and may represent changes related to chronic prostatitis or post biopsy scarring. (Reproduced from. https://doi.org/10.1007/978-3-319-75019-4_11)

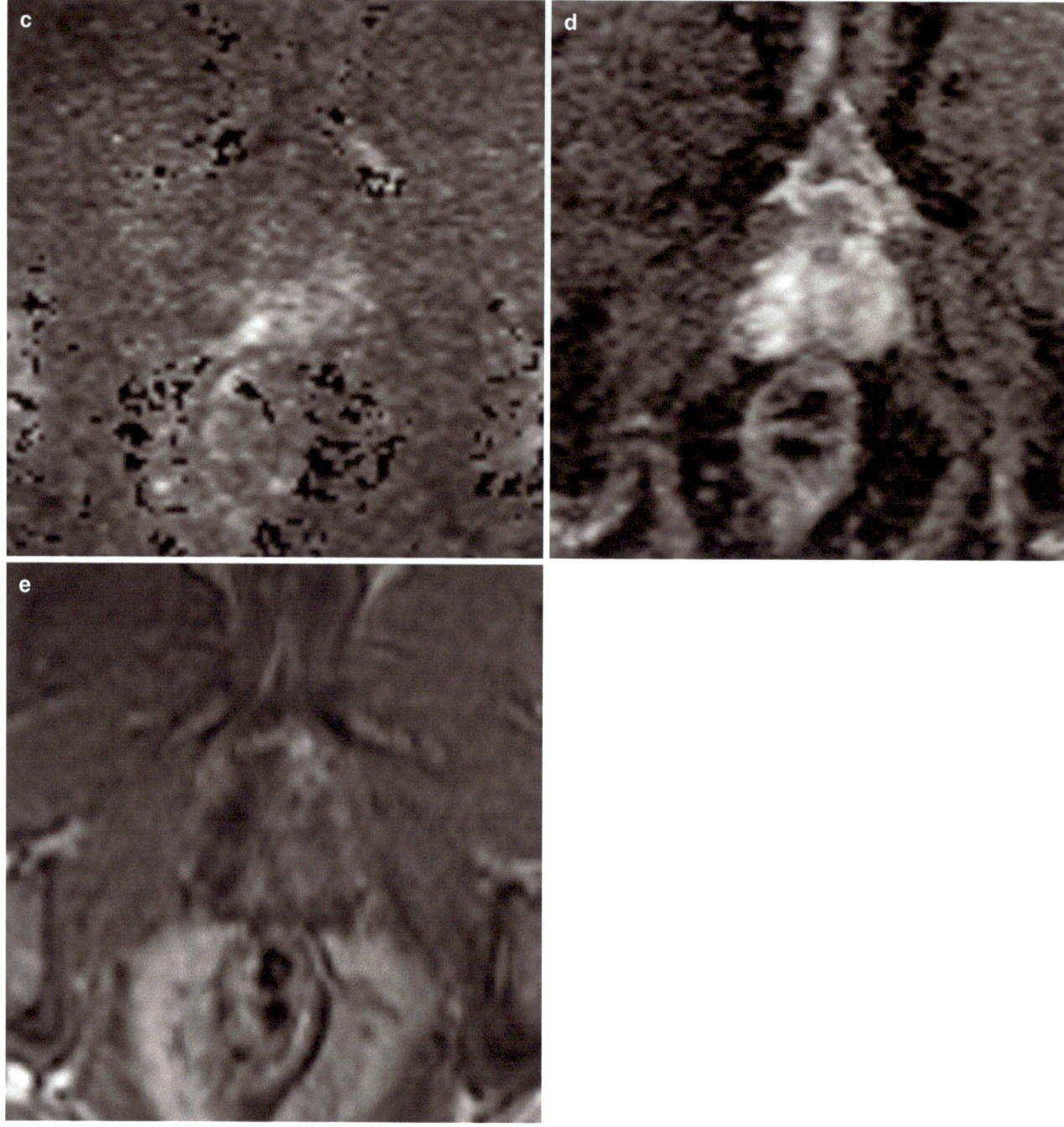

Fig. 16.3 (continued)

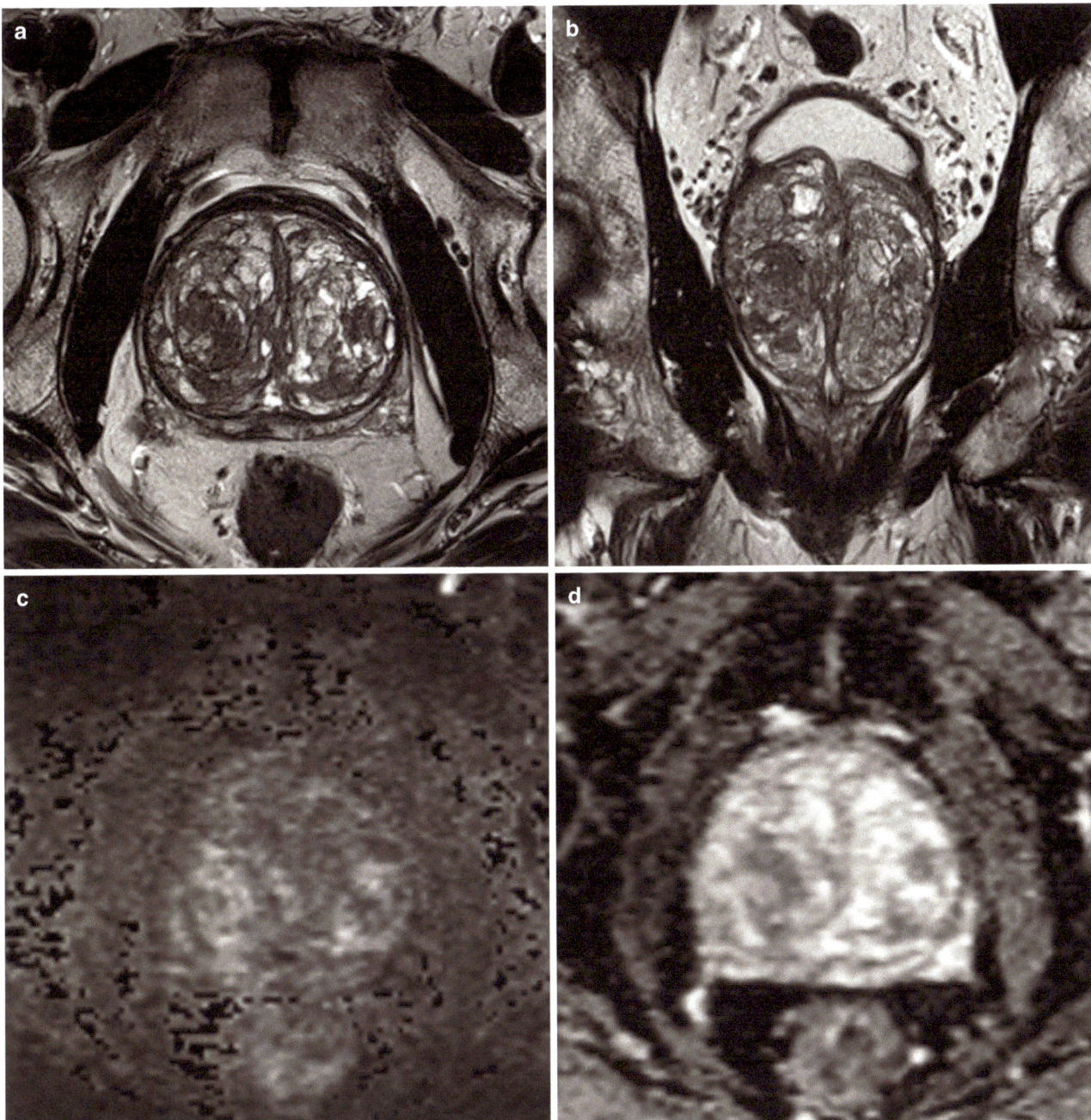

Fig. 16.4 (**a**–**d**) PI-RADS 1 findings of the transition zone in a patient with benign prostatic hyperplasia (BPH). (**a**) Axial and (**b**) coronal T2-weighted sequence (dominant sequence for the transition zone) showing multiple circumscribed heterogeneous encapsulated nodules (dark T2-rim) within the enlarged transition zone (PI-RADS score 1). (**c**) Diffusion-weighted high b-value (calculated $b = 1400$ s/mm^2) image shows no focal areas of moderately increased signal intensity. (**d**) ADC map shows no focal hypointense areas (PI-RADS score 1). (Reproduced from. https://doi.org/10.1007/978-3-319-75019-4_11)

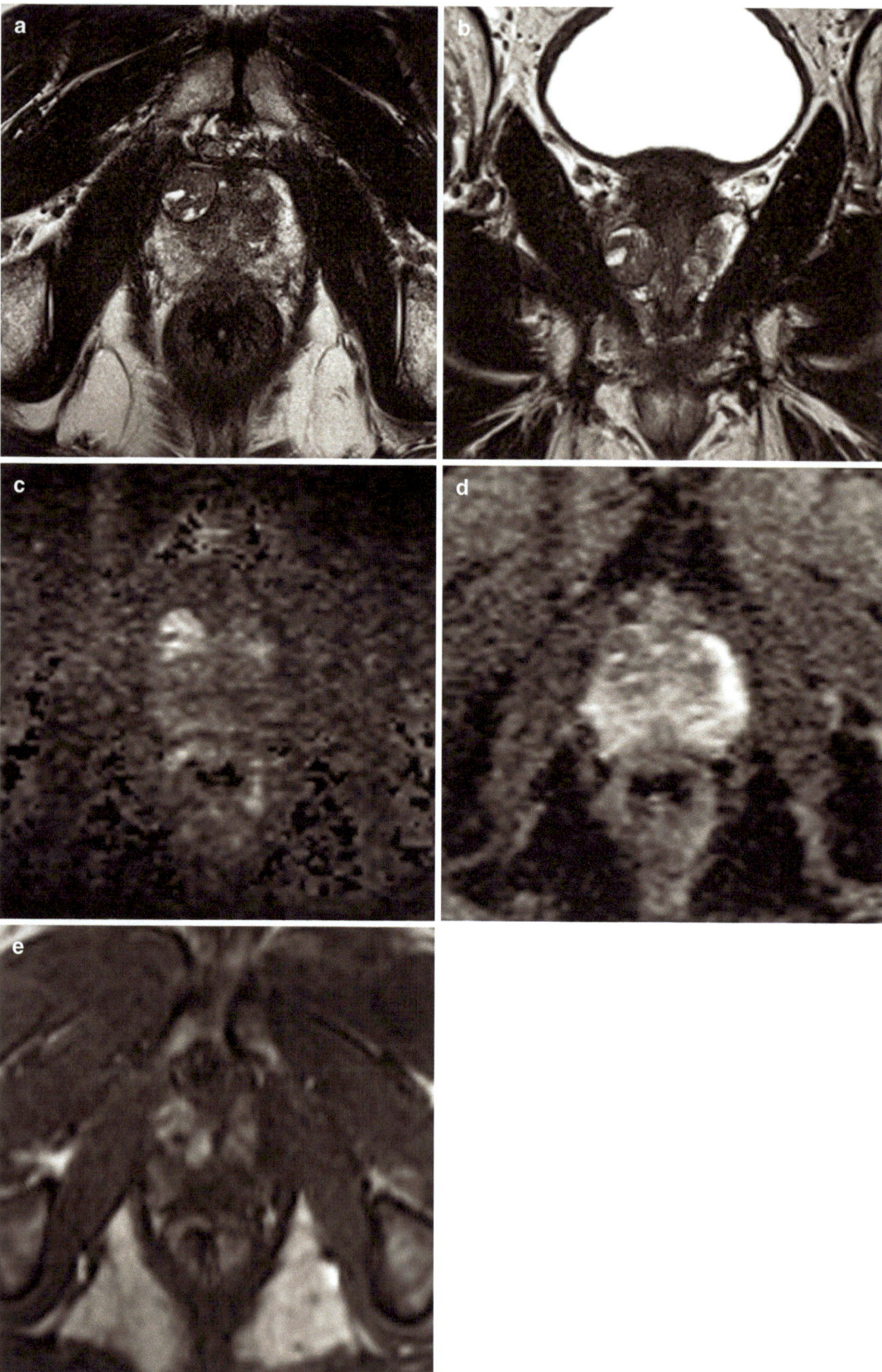

Fig. 16.5 (**a–e**) Protruded BPH node in the right anterior gland. (**a**) Axial and (**b**) coronal T2-weighted sequence (dominant sequence for the transition zone) showing a circumscribed heterogeneous completely encapsulated nodule (overall PI-RADS score 1). (**c**) Diffusion weighted high b-value (calculated $b = 1400$ s/mm^2) image shows increased signal intensity. (**d**) ADC map shows a focal hypointensity which is related to stromal BPH components which corresponds to the BPH nodule. (**e**) DCE sequence showing focal enhancement which corresponds to the lesion that demonstrates clear features of a BPH node (therefore DCE negative) consistent with an overall PI-RADS score of 1. (Reproduced from. https://doi.org/10.1007/978-3-319-75019-4_11)

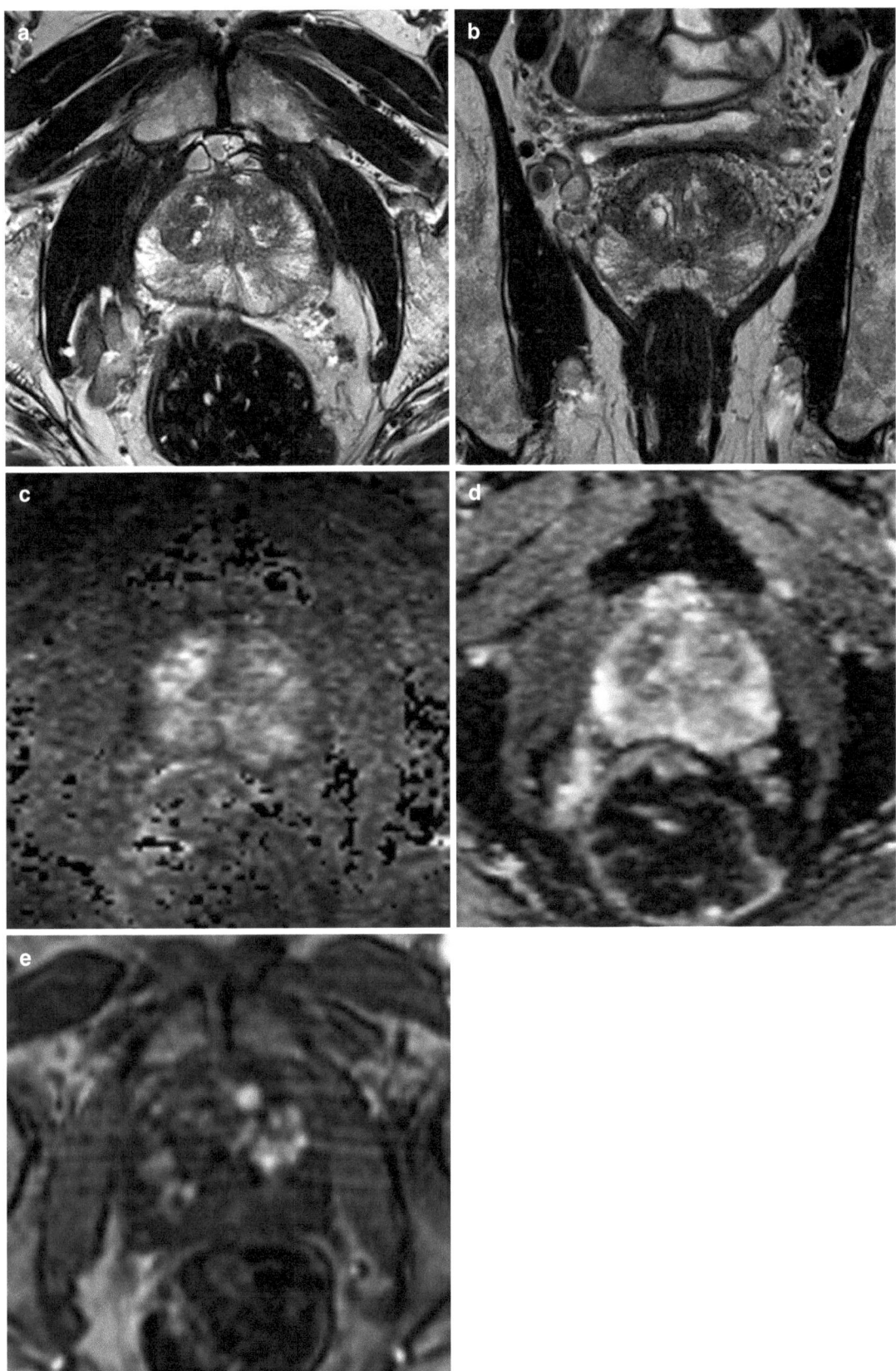

Fig. 16.6 (**a–e**) PI-RADS 3 findings of the peripheral zone. (**a**) Axial and (**b**) coronal T2-weighted sequence showing heterogeneous non-circumscribed changes of the peripheral zone bilaterally (PI-RADS score 3). (**c**) Diffusion weighted high b-value (calculated $b = 1400$ s/mm^2) image shows a mildly hyperintense signal intensity. (**d**) ADC map (dominant sequence for the peripheral zone) shows moderately hypoin-tense changes in the bilateral peripheral zone (PI-RADS score 3). (**e**) DCE sequence shows no focal early enhancement (DCE negative) consistent with an overall PI-RADS score of 3. TRUS-guided prostate biopsy revealed mild chronic prostatitis with no evidence of prostate cancer. (Reproduced from. https://doi.org/10.1007/978-3-319-75019-4_11)

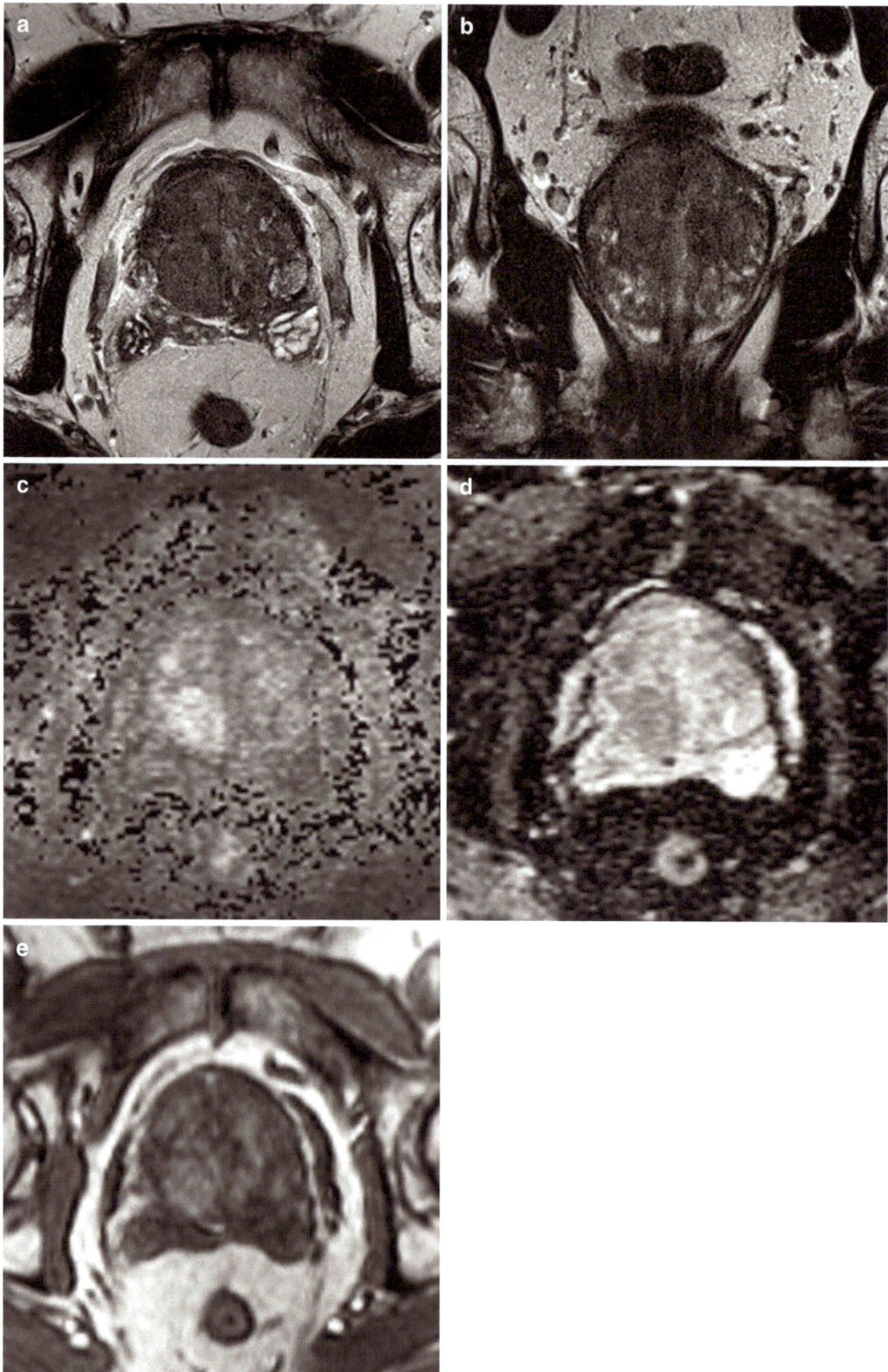

Fig. 16.7 (a–e) PI-RADS 3 changes of the transition zone in a patient with benign prostatic hyperplasia (BPH). (a) Axial and (b) coronal T2-weighted sequence (dominant sequence for the transition zone) showing heterogeneous signal intensity with obscured margins within the enlarged transition zone (overall PI-RADS score 3). (c) Diffusion weighted high b-value (calculated b = 1400 s/mm^2) image shows mildly hyperintense signal intensity. (d) ADC map shows moderately hypointense areas (PI-RADS score 3). (e) DCE sequence shows diffuse enhancement not corresponding to a focal finding on any other sequence (DCE negative). Random TRUS-guided biopsy revealed no cancer, the findings were clinically attributed to BPH with predominantly stromal (T2 hypointense) components. (Reproduced from. https://doi.org/10.1007/978-3-319-75019-4_11)

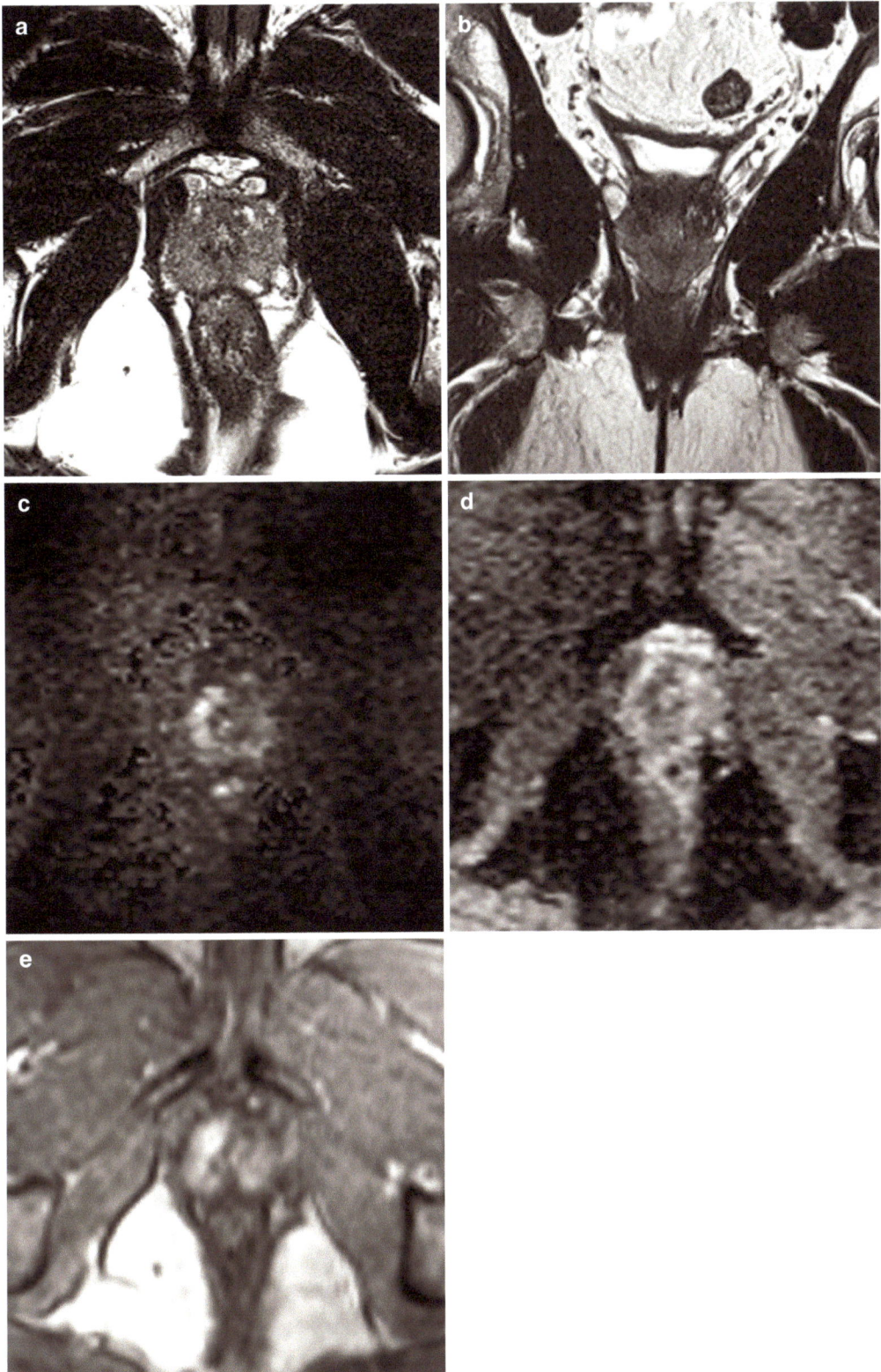

Fig. 16.8 (**a–e**) PI-RADS 4 lesion in the peripheral zone. (**a**) Axial and (**b**) coronal T2-weighted sequence showing moderate diffuse (non-circumscribed) hypointensity of the bilateral peripheral zone (PI-RADS score 3). (**c**) Diffusion weighted high b-value (calculated $b = 1400$ s/mm^2) image shows mildly hyperintense signal intensity in the right anterior and lateral peripheral zone (PI-RADS score 3). (**d**) ADC map correspondingly shows moderate hypointense signal intensity (domi-nant sequence for the peripheral zone) in the right anterior and lateral peripheral zone (PI-RADS score 3). (**e**) DCE sequence shows focal and contemporary enhancement (DCE positive) consistent with an upgrading to an overall PI-RADS score of 4. MRI/US fusion guided biopsy revealed a Gleason $3 + 4 = 7$ adenocarcinoma (PSA level 6.9 ng/mL). (Reproduced from. https://doi.org/10.1007/978-3-319-75019-4_11)

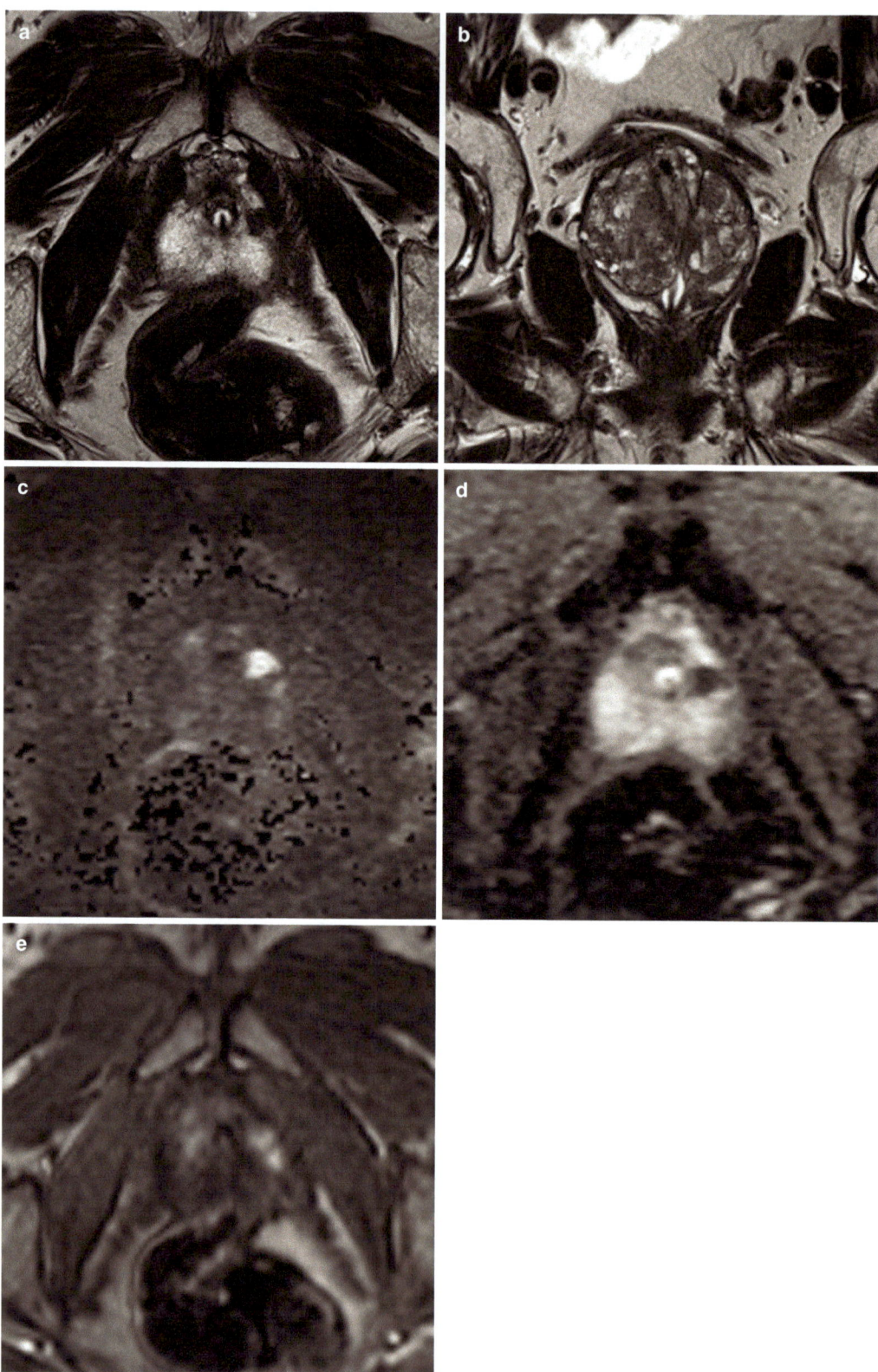

Fig. 16.9 (a–e) PI-RADS 4 lesion in the peripheral zone. (a) axial and (b) coronal T2-weighted sequence showing a circumscribed 11 mm hypointense lesion in the left lateral peripheral zone (PI-RADS score 4). (c) Diffusion weighted high b-value (calculated $b = 1400$ s/mm^2) image shows focal markedly hyperintense signal intensity. (d) ADC map (dominant sequence for the peripheral zone) correspondingly shows focal markedly hypointense signal intensity (PI-RADS score 4). (e)DCE sequence shows focal and early enhancement (DCE positive) corresponding to the lesion seen on T2w and DWI consistent with an overall PI-RADS score of 4. MRI/US fusion guided biopsy revealed a Gleason 4 + 3 = 7 adenocarcinoma (PSA level 8.1 ng/mL). (Reproduced from. https://doi.org/10.1007/978-3-319-75019-4_11)

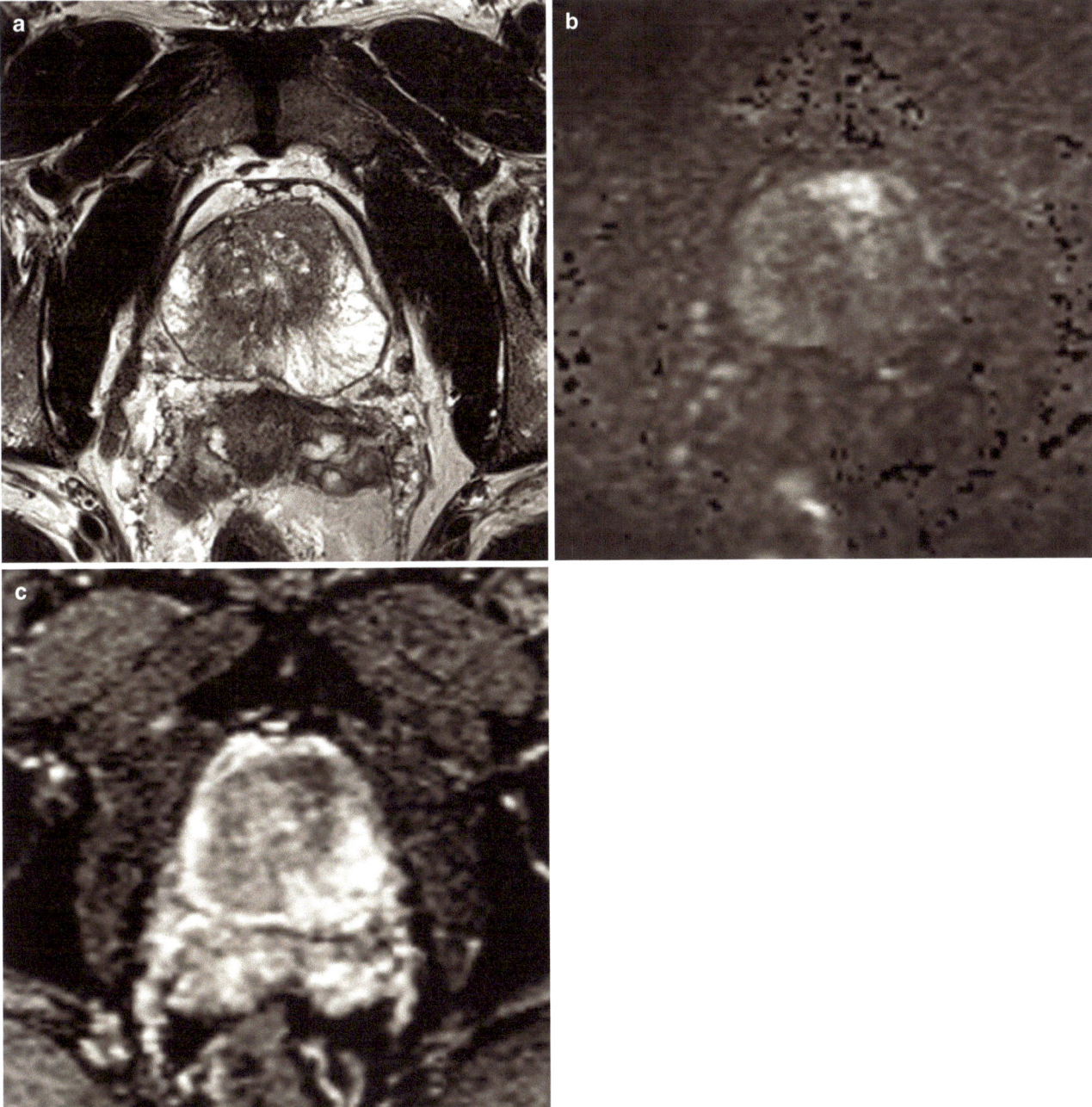

Fig. 16.10 (a–c) PI-RADS 4 lesion in the transition zone. (a) Axial T2-weighted sequence (dominant sequence for the transition zone) showing a circumscribed lenticular 14 mm hypointense lesion in the left anterior transition zone with bulging of the fibromuscular stroma (PI-RADS score 4). (b) Diffusion weighted high b-value (calculated $b = 1400$ s/mm^2) image shows focal markedly hyperintense signal intensity. (c) ADC map correspondingly shows focal markedly hypointense signal intensity (PI-RADS score 4). MRI/US fusion guided biopsy revealed a Gleason $4 + 4 = 8$ adenocarcinoma (PSA level 9.8 ng/mL). The patient had undergone a random TRUS-guided biopsy 3 months earlier with no evidence of malignancy. The anterior location is typical for adenocarcinoma missed by random prostate biopsies, thus MRI is particularly useful in patients with negative random biopsy and persisting clinical suspicion for prostate cancer. (Reproduced from. https://doi.org/10.1007/978-3-319-75019-4_11)

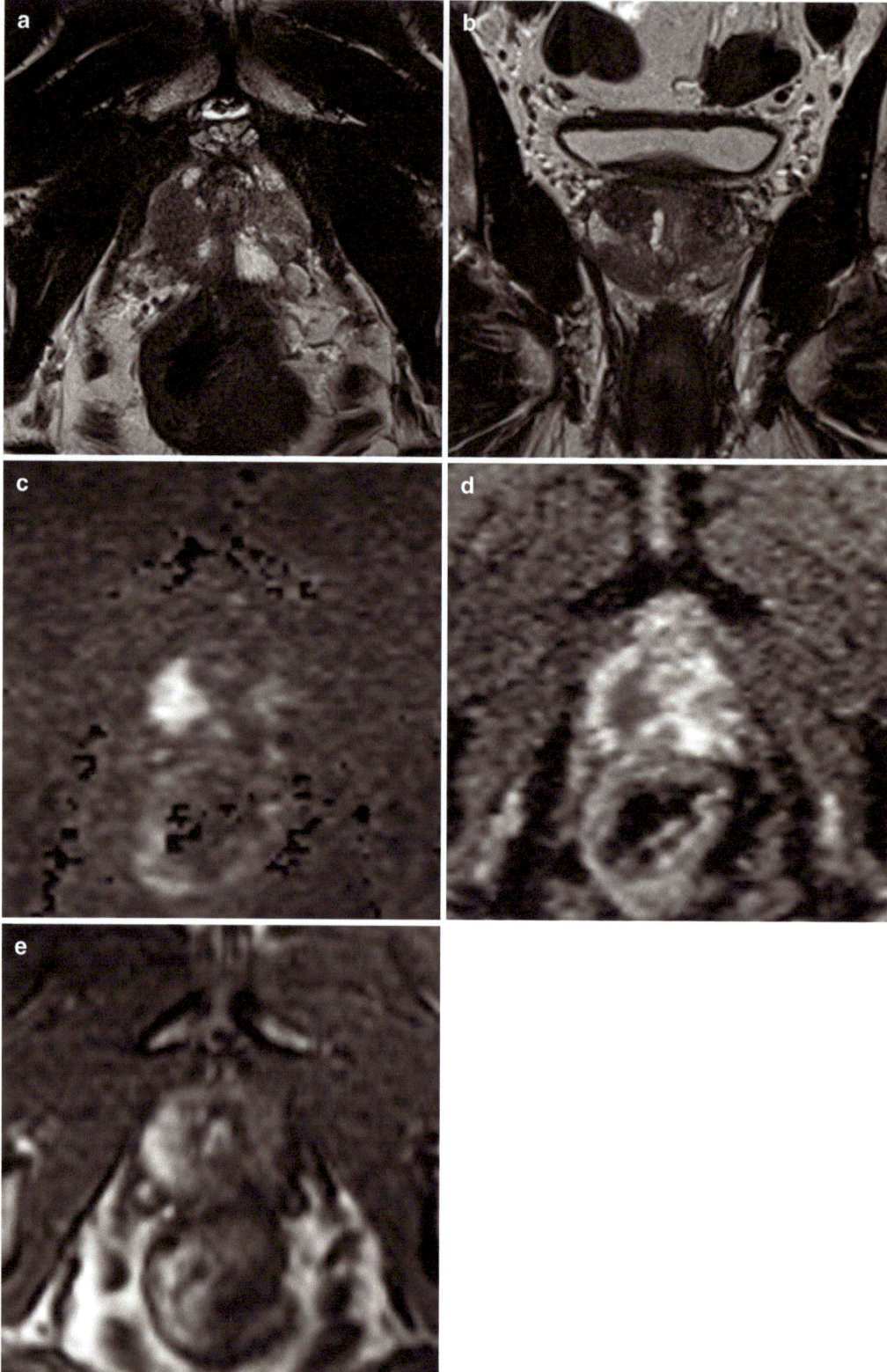

Fig. 16.11 (**a–e**) PI-RADS 5 lesion in the peripheral zone. (**a**) Axial and (**b**) coronal T2-weighted images showing a circumscribed 18 mm hypointense lesion in the right lateral peripheral zone (PI-RADS score 5). (**c**) Diffusion weighted high b-value (calculated $b = 1400$ s/mm²) image shows focal markedly hyperintense signal intensity. (**d**) ADC map (dominant sequence for the peripheral zone) correspondingly shows focal markedly hypointense signal intensity (PI-RADS score 5). (**e**) DCE sequence shows focal and early enhancement (DCE positive) corresponding to the lesion seen on T2w and DWI consistent with an overall PI-RADS score of 5. MRI/US fusion guided biopsy revealed a Gleason $4 + 3 = 7$ adenocarcinoma (PSA level 11.2 ng/mL). Also note the wedge-shaped T2-hypointensities in the left lateral peripheral zone which demonstrate moderately hypointense signal on the ADC map and no focal enhancement (PI-RADS 3). On biopsy multifocal prostate cancer was diagnosed with Gleason $3 + 3 = 6$ pattern in the left side of the prostate. (Reproduced from. https://doi.org/10.1007/978-3-319-75019-4_11)

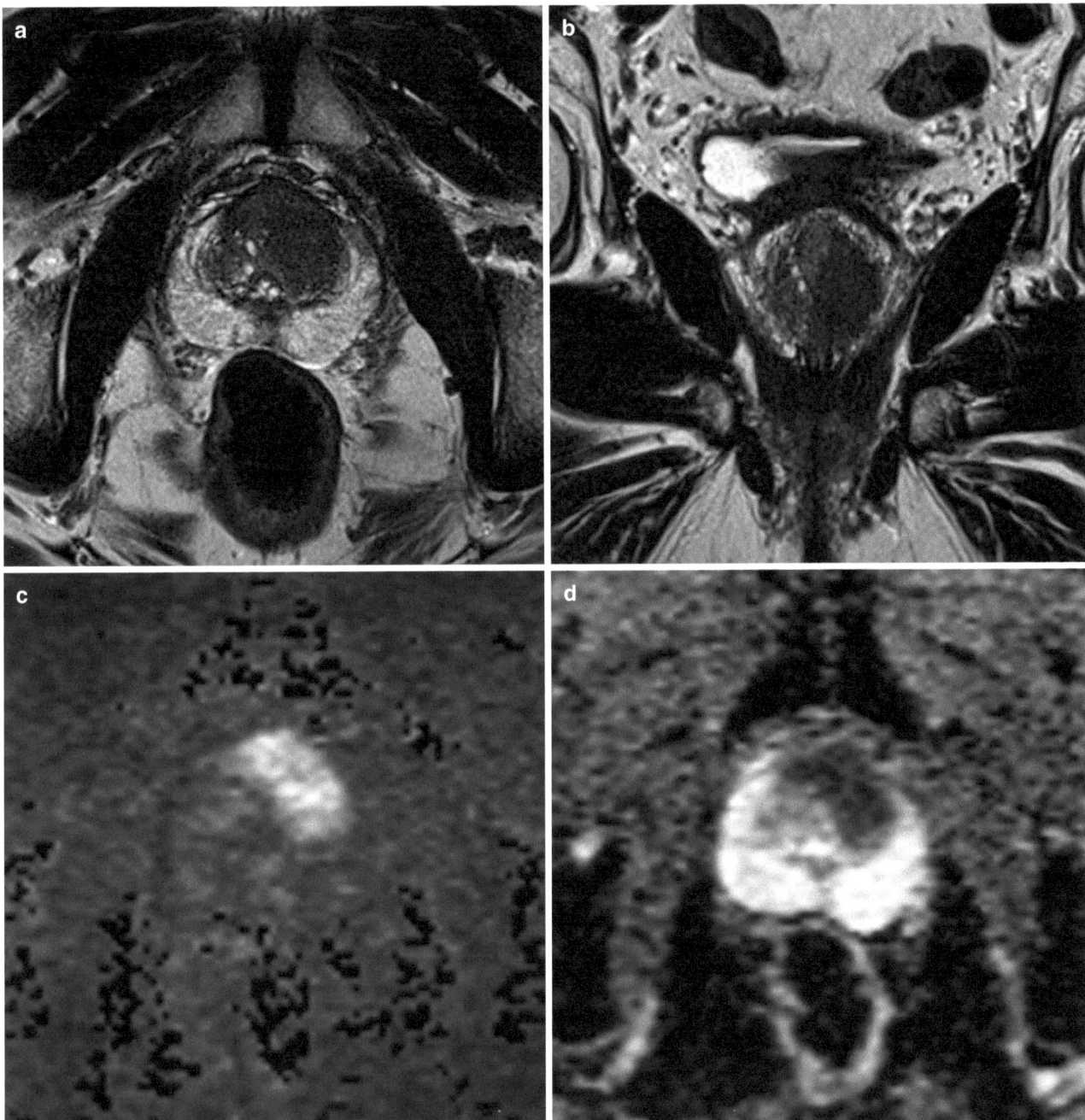

Fig. 16.12 (**a**–**d**) PI-RADS 5 lesion in the transition zone. (**a**) Axial and (**b**) coronal T2-weighted images (dominant sequence for the transition zone) showing a circumscribed lenticular 20 mm hypointense mass the anterior transition zone with bulging of the prostatic capsule (PI-RADS score 5). (**c**) Diffusion weighted high b-value (calculated $b = 1400$ s/mm^2) image shows focal markedly hyperintense signal intensity. (**d**) ADC map correspondingly shows focal markedly hypointense signal intensity (PI-RADS score 4). MRI/US fusion guided biopsy revealed a Gleason $4 + 3 = 7$ adenocarcinoma (PSA level 14.7 ng/mL). (Reproduced from. https://doi.org/10.1007/978-3-319-75019-4_11)

assigned to a visual snapshot, or *the series* and *the image number* where the lesion is best visualized should be reported to assist the selection of optimal images for MRI/US fusion-guided prostate biopsy. The lesion size also needs to be reported. Measurement of each lesion is preferred on the axial images, the DWI sequence should be used for peripheral zone lesions and the T2-weighted images for transition zone lesions. If a lesion is not well delineated on the axial sequences then another plane can be used.

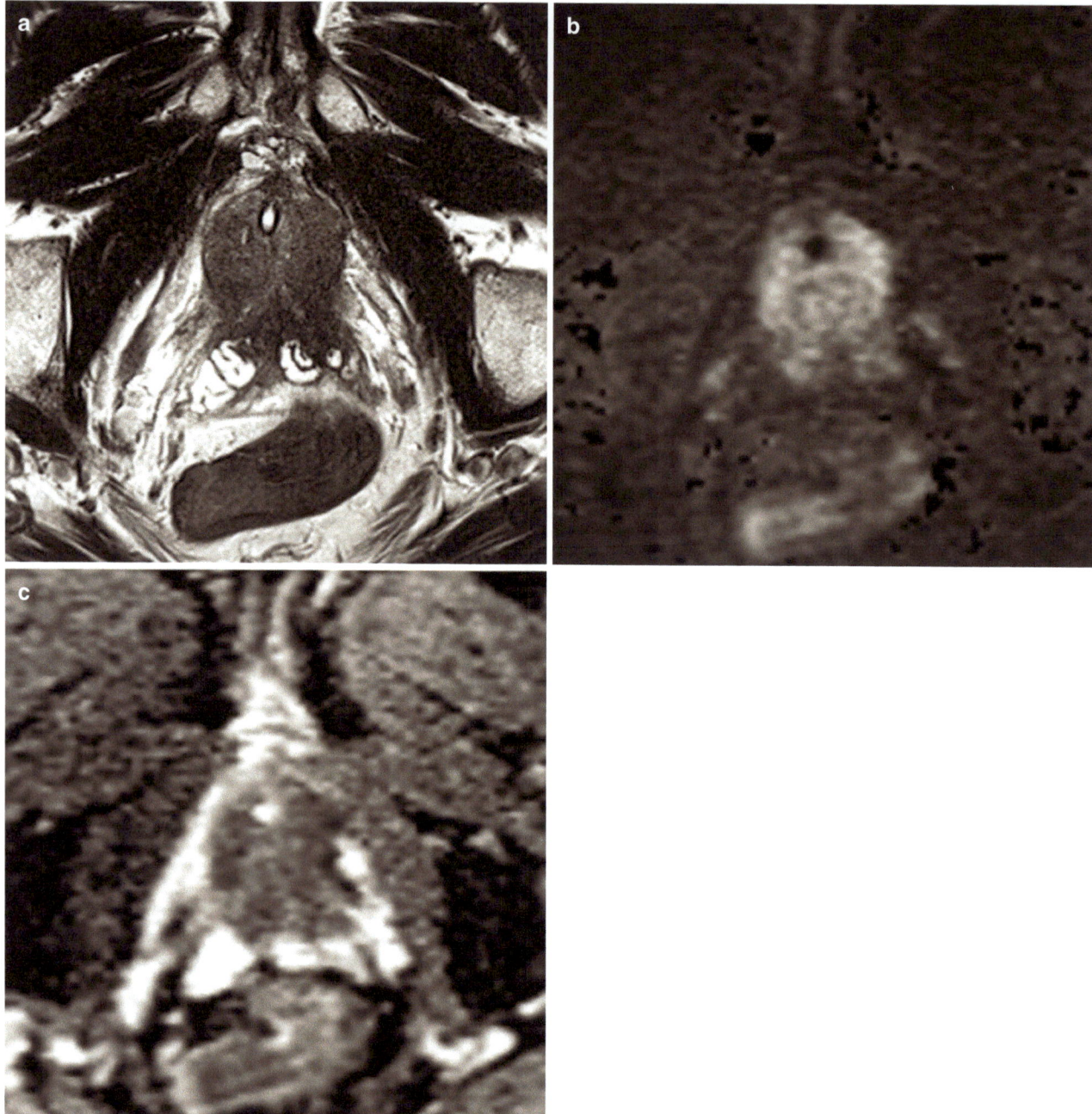

Fig. 16.13 (**a–c**) Locally advanced prostate cancer with seminal vesicle invasion. (**a**) Axial T2-weighted sequence showing diffuse hypointensity of the entire prostate (zonal anatomy not visible) with extension into the bilateral seminal vesicles (PI-RADS score 5). (**b**) Diffusion weighted high b-value (calculated $b = 1400$ s/mm²) image shows markedly hyperintense signal intensity of the entire prostate. (**c**) ADC map correspondingly shows markedly hypointense signal intensity of the prostate (PI-RADS score 5). Randomized TRUS guided biopsy revealed a Gleason 4 + 5 = 9 adenocarcinoma (PSA level 26.5 ng/mL). (Reproduced from. https://doi.org/10.1007/978-3-319-75019-4_11)

Table 16.6 Transition Zone (TZ) (reproduced from https://link.springer.com/chapter/10.1007/978-3-319-75019-4_11)

T2	DWI	DCE	PI-RADS score
1	Any	Any	1
2	≤ 3	Any	2
	≥ 4		3
3	≤ 4	Any	3
	5		4
4	Any	Any	4
5	Any	Any	5

Table 16.5 Peripheral zone (PZ) (reproduced from https://link.springer.com/chapter/10.1007/978-3-319-75019-4_11)

DWI	T2	DCE	PI-RADS score
1	Any	Any	1
2	Any	Any	2
3	Any	Negative	3
		Positive	4
4	Any	Any	4
5	Any	Any	5

Another crucial element of a full PI-RADS report is a sector map in which the lesions should be indicated, since this particularly enhances the communication with referring physician teams. For this matter, the prostate is subdivided into three axial regions craniocaudally, the base, the midgland and the prostatic apex. The seminal vesicles should also be included for cases of extraprostatic extension. The zonal anatomy (peripheral zone, transition zone, central zone and anterior fibromuscular stroma) and the urethra should also be incorporated into the sector map.

16.3 Conclusion

Comprehensive multiparametric MRI of the prostate should include lesion scoring and reporting according to the PI-RADS system. This will assist to achieve a high level of diagnostic accuracy and assure a thriving communication with the multidisciplinary care team.

Further Reading

Ahmed HU, El-Shater Bosaily A, Brown LC, et al. Diagnostic accuracy of multi-parametric MRI and TRUS biopsy in prostate cancer (PROMIS): a paired validating confirmatory study. Lancet. 2017;389:815–22.

Barentsz JO, Richenberg J, Clements R, et al. ESUR prostate MR guidelines 2012. Eur Radiol. 2012;22:746–57.

Barrett T, Vargas HA, Goldman D, Akin O, Hricak H. The value of the "Hemorrhage exclusion" sign on T1-weighted prostate MRI for the detection of prostate cancer. Radiology. 2012;263(3):751–7.

Barth BK, De Visschere PJ, Cornelius A, Nicolau C, Vargas HA, Eberli D, Donati OF. Detection of clinically significant prostate cancer: short dual-pulse sequence versus standard multiparametric MR Imaging-A multireader study. Radiology. 2017;284(3):725–36.

Cash H, Günzel K, Maxeiner A, et al. Men with a negative real-time MRI/ultrasound-fusion guided targeted biopsy but prostate cancer detection on TRUS-guided random biopsy – what are the reasons for targeted biopsy failure? BJU Int. 2016a;118:35–43.

Cash H, Maxeiner A, Stephan C, et al. The detection of significant prostate cancer is correlated with the Prostate Imaging Reporting and Data System (PI-RADS) in MRI/transrectal ultrasound fusion biopsy. Word J Urol. 2016b;34:525–32.

Greer MD, Shih JH, Lay N, et al. Validation of the dominant sequence paradigm and role of dynamic contrast-enhanced imaging in PI-RADS version 2. Radiology in press. 2017;285(3):859–69.

Haas M, Gnzel K, Penzkofer T, et al. Implications of PI-RADS version 1 and updated version 2 on the scoring of prostatic lesions on multiparametric MRI. Aktuelle Urol. 2016;47:383–7.

Panebianco V, Villeirs G, Weinreb J, et al. Prostate Magnetic Resonance Imaging for Local Recurrence Reporting (PI-RR): International consensus-based guidelines on multiparametric magnetic resonance imaging for prostate cancer recurrence after radiation therapy and radical prostatectomy. Eur Urol Oncol. 2021;4(6):868–76.

Polanec S, Helbich TH, Bickel H, et al. Head-to-head comparison of PI-RADS v2 and PI-RADS v1. Eur J Radiol. 2016;85:1125–31.

Purysko AS, Bittencourt LK, Bullen JA, et al. Accuracy and interobserver agreement for Prostate Imaging Reporting and Data System, Version 2, for the characterization of lesions identified on multiparametric MRI of the prostate. AJR Am J Roentgenol. 2017;209:339–49.

Rosenkrantz AB, Ginocchio LA, Cornfeld D, et al. Interobserver reproducibility of the PI-RADS version 2 lexicon: a multicenter study of six experienced prostate radiologists. Radiology. 2016;280:793–804.

Turkbey B, Rosenkrantz AB, Haider MA, et al. Prostate Imaging Reporting and Data System Version 2.1: 2019 Update of Prostate Imaging Reporting and Data System Version 2. Eur Urol. 2019;76(3):340–51.

Ullrich T, Quentin M, Oelers C, et al. Magnetic resonance imaging of the prostate at 1.5 versus 3.0 T: a prospective comparison study of image quality. Eur J Radiol. 2017;90:192–7.

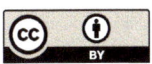

Pathways for the Spread of Disease in the Abdomen and Pelvis

17

James A. Brink and Brent J. Wagner

Learning Objectives
To understand the ligamentous anatomy of the upper abdomen and how it can inform the spread of disease by direct invasion and lymphatic extension.

To understand the anatomy of the peritoneal spaces and how it can inform the spread of disease by intraperitoneal seeding.

17.1 Introduction

Disease may spread through the abdomen and pelvis by a variety of mechanisms. For example, intraabdominal malignancies may metastasize through hematologic routes, and tumors may spread by directly invading adjacent tissues and organs or via the lymphatic system. When tumors break through the visceral peritoneum, they may also spread via intraperitoneal seeding. While hematologic spread of disease is beyond the scope of this chapter, direct invasion, lymphatic extension, and intraperitoneal seeding will be discussed relative to the anatomy that guides these pathways for the spread of disease in the abdomen and pelvis [1].

Direct invasion and lymphatic extension occur through peritoneal ligaments and mesenteries that interconnect the abdominal viscera with other organs in the abdomen and pelvis, the retroperitoneum, and the body wall. Moreover, these structures guide the flow of peritoneal fluid through the abdomen and pelvis, thereby dictating the routes of spread through intraperitoneal seeding. In short, understanding these pathways

for the spread of disease ties closely to a clear understanding of a ligamentous anatomy of the abdomen and pelvis.

17.2 Peritoneal Ligaments as Conduits for the Spread of Disease

The upper abdominal viscera are interconnected by three pairs of ligaments: the gastrohepatic and hepatoduodenal ligaments (that together comprise the lesser omentum), the gastrosplenic and splenorenal ligaments, and the gastrocolic ligament and transverse mesocolon. Each of these ligamentous pairs contains one ligament that bridges to the retroperitoneum: the hepatoduodenal ligament, the splenorenal ligament, and the transverse mesocolon. Thus, disease from the abdominal viscera may spread to the retroperitoneum and vice versa through these ligamentous pairs.

17.2.1 Gastrohepatic and Hepatoduodenal Ligaments

The gastrohepatic and hepatoduodenal ligaments form an important pathway of disease from the lesser curvature of the stomach to the porta hepatis and retroperitoneum. The gastrohepatic ligament extends from the lesser curvature of the stomach to the porta hepatis, inserting into the fissure for the ligamentum venosum. Containing the left gastric artery, the left gastric vein or coronary vein, and associated lymphatics, the gastrohepatic ligament may be recognized on cross sectional imaging as the fatty plane connecting the lesser curvature of the stomach to the left lobe of the liver and containing these vessels (Fig. 17.1). Nodes in the gastrohepatic ligament are typically 8 mm or less in diameter, somewhat smaller than elsewhere in the abdomen [2]. Care must be taken to avoid misidentifying unopacified loops of bowel, the pancreatic neck, or the papillary process of the caudate lobe as enlarged nodes in the gastrohepatic ligament [3, 4].

J. A. Brink (✉)
Departments of Radiology, Massachusetts General Hospital, Brigham and Women's Hospital, Boston, MA, USA
e-mail: jabrink@mgh.havard.edu

B. J. Wagner
American Board of Radiology, Tucson, AZ, USA
e-mail: bwagner@theabr.org

© The Author(s) 2023
J. Hodler et al. (eds.), *Diseases of the Abdomen and Pelvis 2023-2026*, IDKD Springer Series,
https://doi.org/10.1007/978-3-031-27355-1_17

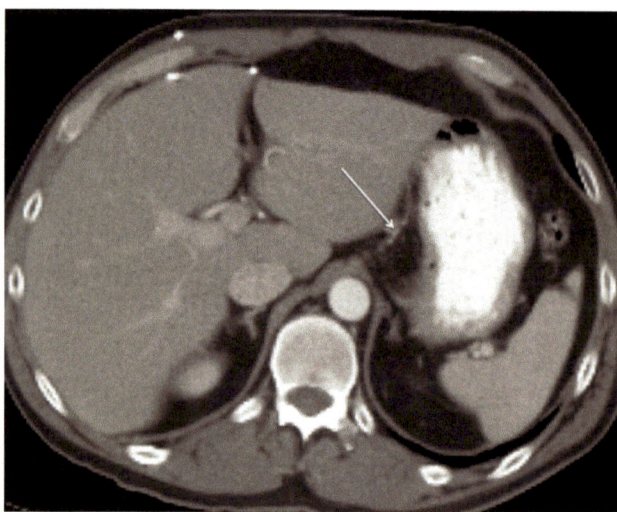

Fig. 17.1 Transaxial CT image demonstrates the gastrohepatic ligament (GHL), seen as a fatty plane interposed between lesser curvature of the stomach and the lobe of the liver. The GHL contains the left gastric artery (arrow), the left gastric vein (coronary vein) and associated lymphatics

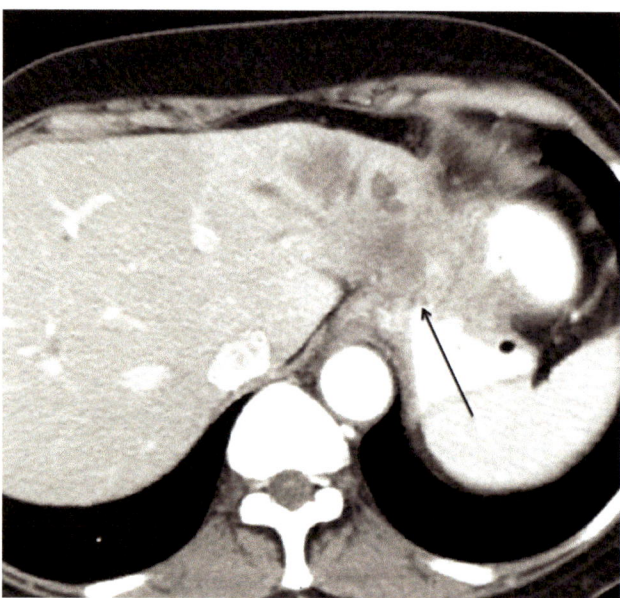

Fig. 17.2 Transaxial CT image demonstrates a heterogenous mass centered in the gastrohepatic ligament (GHL), with invasion of the left hepatic lobe and the stomach. Prospectively, it was unclear as to the organ of origin, but it proved to be a hepatoma extending through the GHL to involve the stomach

A unique feature of the gastrohepatic ligament is continuity of its subperitoneal areolar tissue with the perivascular fibrous capsule of the liver (Glisson capsule). This anatomic continuity provides a direct pathway for the spread of disease from the gastric lesser curvature into the left hepatic lobe via the gastrohepatic ligament and vice versa. Both neoplastic and inflammatory conditions can spread in this fashion (Fig. 17.2). Gastric and esophageal cancer commonly spread via lymphatic extension and direct invasion through the gastrohepatic ligament, allowing these tumors to spread to the

liver, and conversely hepatoma and cholangiocarcinoma may spread to the stomach through these pathways as well.

The free edge of the gastrohepatic ligament is the hepatoduodenal ligament, and together, the gastrohepatic and hepatoduodenal ligaments comprise the lesser omentum. The hepatoduodenal ligament is the thickest ligament in the upper abdomen owing to the portal structures that it contains: the portal vein, the hepatic artery, the common bile duct and associated lymphatics. The hepatoduodenal ligament extends from the porta hepatis to the flexure between the first and second duodenum, forming a tent-like structure that extends from superior to inferior as it courses from anterior to posterior. The foramen of Winslow or epiploic foramen lies immediately posterior to the ligament connecting the right posterior perihepatic space with the lesser sac [5]. Here, nodes at the base of the hepatoduodenal ligament at the epiploic foramen (in the portocaval space) can be quite prominent in size and still normal. These nodes can be up to 2.0 cm in transverse dimension and up to 1.5 cm in anteroposterior dimension and still be normal. Pathology within these nodes may be difficult to identify but may be suggested when the nodes assume a more spherical shape or have central necrosis [6, 7].

A host of neoplastic and inflammatory conditions spread commonly via the hepatoduodenal ligament from the porta hepatis to the retroperitoneum, following antegrade flow of lymphatic fluid from the liver and biliary tree to nodes surrounding the duodenum and pancreas. However, lymphatic extension can also occur in a retrograde fashion through these lymphatics, originating from disease in nodes surrounding the superior mesenteric artery, as may occur in pancreatic and colon cancer, and spreading up the lymphatic channels in the hepatoduodenal ligament to the liver.

Structures intimately related to the hepatoduodenal ligament may also spread via direct invasion through the ligament, as occurs commonly with gastric cancer arising in the lesser curvature and spreading to peripancreatic and periduodenal lymph nodes via the gastrohepatic and hepatoduodenal ligaments. Many inflammatory conditions also spread commonly through the hepatoduodenal ligament including inflammatory processes within the gall bladder and biliary tree. Pancreatitis may also spread via this pathway as well. Occasionally, vascular complications may be seen in the hepatoduodenal ligament related to both malignant and inflammatory conditions coursing through it. These include portal vein thrombosis as well as hepatic arterial pseudoaneurysms [1, 5] (Fig. 17.3).

17.2.2 Gastrosplenic and Splenorenal Ligaments

An important highway of disease is provided in the left upper abdomen by the gastrosplenic and splenorenal ligaments, connecting the gastric greater curvature to the splenic hilum and the retroperitoneum, respectively (Fig. 17.4). The gastrosplenic ligament is a rather thin delicate structure that connects the superior third of the greater curvature of the

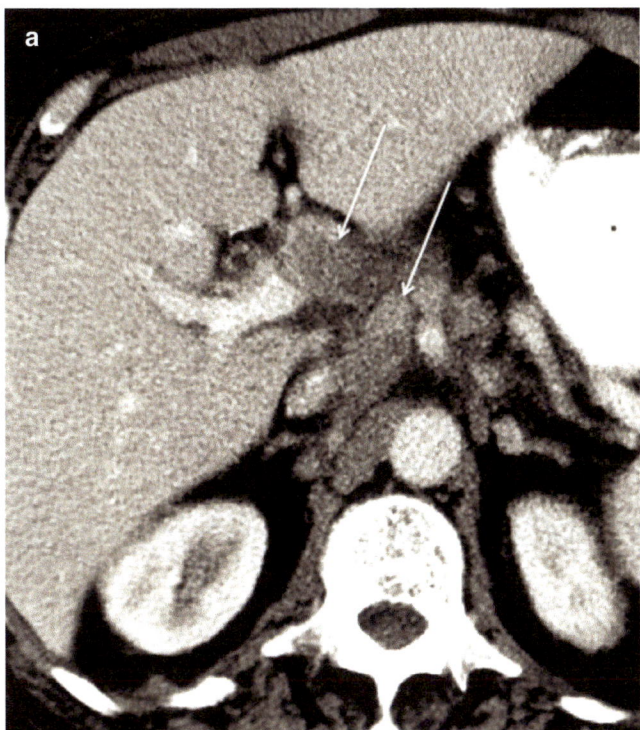
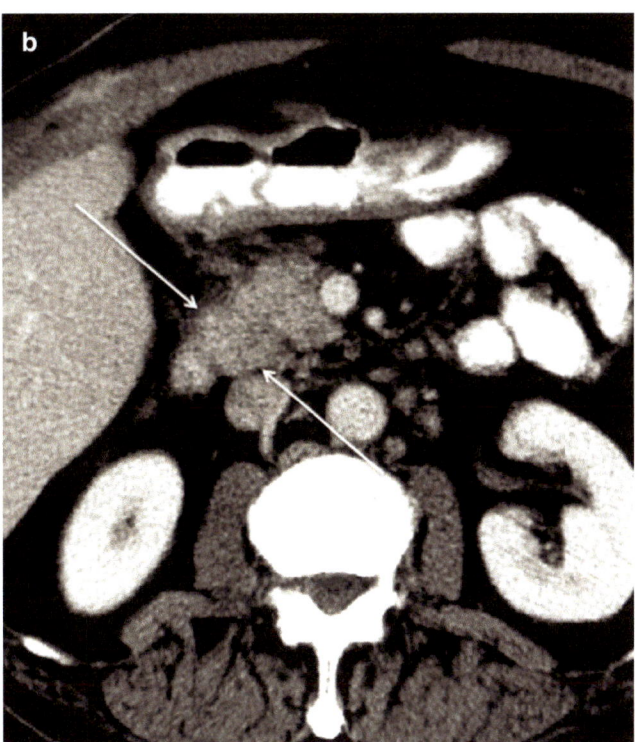

Fig. 17.3 Transaxial CT images through the porta hepatis (**a**) and the uncinate process (**b**) demonstrate bulky lymphadenopathy (arrows) in the hepatoduodenal ligament (HDL) in a patient with gallbladder carci-

noma. Tumor has spread bi-directionally within the HDL proximally (**a**), and distally to the insertion of the HDL on the second portion of the duodenum

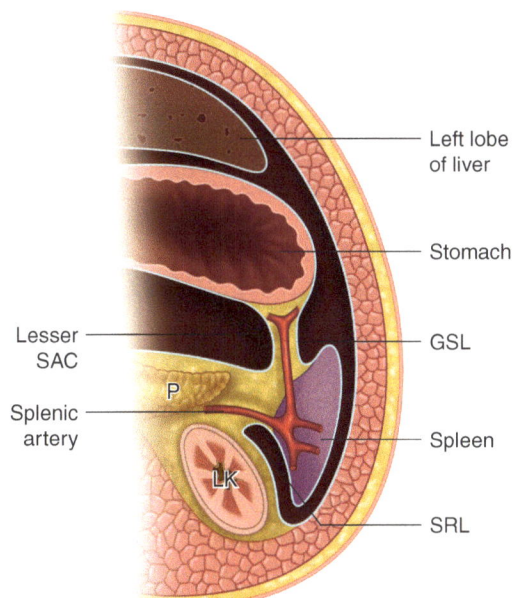

Fig. 17.4 The gastrosplenic ligament (GSL) and splenorenal ligament (SRL) comprise the left wall of the lesser sac and provide a conduit for the spread of metastatic disease from the greater curvature of the stomach to the retroperitonium and vice versa. (Adapted from Myers MA. Dynamic Radiology of the Abdomen: Normal and Pathologic Anatomy, New York: Springer, 1994)

stomach to the splenic hilum. This ligament contains the left gastroepiploic and short gastric vessels and their associated

lymphatics. The gastrosplenic ligament can direct diseases arising in the stomach to the splenic hilum, and both neoplastic and inflammatory diseases may invade the spleen via this pathway.

Posteriorly and medially, the gastrosplenic ligament is continuous with the splenorenal ligament. Once disease reaches the splenic hilum from the stomach via the gastrosplenic ligament, it may turn and extend to the retroperitoneum via the splenorenal ligament. Here, disease may surround and invade the pancreatic tail and compromise the splenic artery and splenic vein (Fig. 17.5) [8, 9]. Just as gastric disease can spread to the retroperitoneum via this ligamentous pair, both inflammatory and neoplastic disease of the pancreas may spread in the opposite direction to the splenic hilum and greater curvature via the splenorenal and gastrosplenic ligaments, respectively [1].

17.2.3 Gastrocolic Ligament and Transverse Mesocolon

As the gastrohepatic and hepatoduodenal ligaments in the right abdomen, and the gastrosplenic and splenorenal ligaments in the left abdomen form important pathways of disease from the upper abdominal viscera to the retroperitoneum, the gastrocolic ligament and transverse mesocolon form a similar pathway in the mid abdomen. The gastrocolic ligament (greater omentum) connects the inferior two-thirds

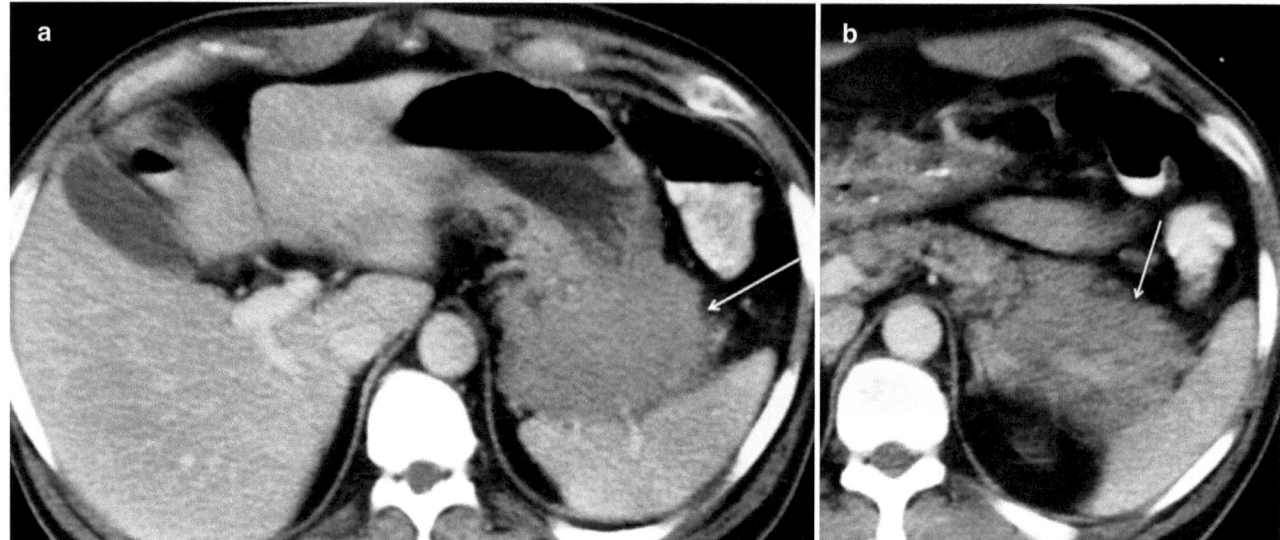

Fig. 17.5 Transaxial CT images through the gastrosplenic ligament (GSL) (**a**), and the splenorenal ligament (SRL) (**b**), in a patient with lymphoma. Tumor is seen within the GSL, interposed between the gas- tric greater curvature and the spleen (**a**), and within the SRL, encasing the splenic vasculature (**b**)

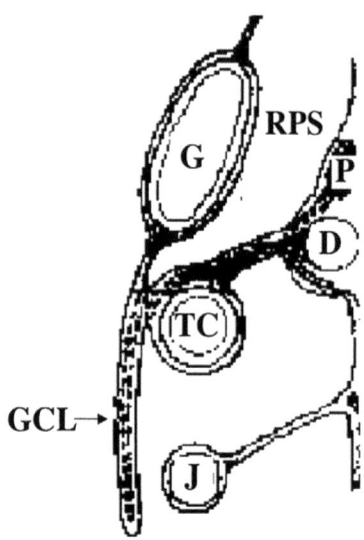

Fig. 17.6 The gastrocolic ligament (GCL) joins the greater curvature of the stomach (G) to the transverse colon (TC). In concert with the transverse mesocolon, a pathway of disease is formed between retro- peritoneal structures such as the pancreas (P) and the duodenum (D) to the anterior aspect of the intraperitoneal cavity (modified from Langman J., Medical Embriology, New York: Saunders, 1971)

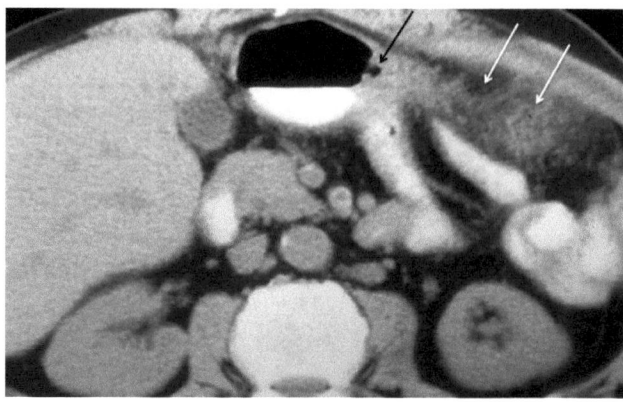

Fig. 17.7 Transaxial CT image through the gastrocolic ligament (GCL) demonstrates a gastric ulcer extending into the GCL (black arrow) with associated inflammation in the greater omentum (white arrows)

of the greater curvature of the stomach to the transverse colon (Fig. 17.6). On the left, the gastrocolic ligament is continu- ous with the gastrosplenic ligament, and on the right, it ends at the gastroduodenal junction near the hepatoduodenal liga- ment. Embryologically, the gastrosplenic ligament gives rise to the gastrocolic ligament and the transverse mesocolon in the adult, with fusion of the anterior and posterior leaves of the embryonic gastrosplenic ligament. In consequence, the gastrocolic ligament has a potential space within it that can fill with fluid when tense ascites in the lesser sac dissects open

this potential space. This can result in a cyst-like appearance within the gastrocolic ligament/greater omentum.

The gastrocolic ligament contains the gastroepiploic ves- sels and associated lymphatics which can help identify the ligament as the fatty plane connecting the stomach to the transverse colon. Both benign and malignant disease from the inferior two-thirds of the greater curvature of the stomach may spread to the transverse colon via this pathway and vice versa (Fig. 17.7). The transverse mesocolon completes the pathway from the stomach to the retroperitoneum in the mid abdomen; disease involving the stomach and transverse colon are connected via the gastrocolic ligament, and disease involving the transverse colon and pancreas/retroperitoneum are connected by the transverse mesocolon. In addition, the greater omentum continues inferior to the transverse colon as a fatty veil that forms an important nidus for carcinomatosis,

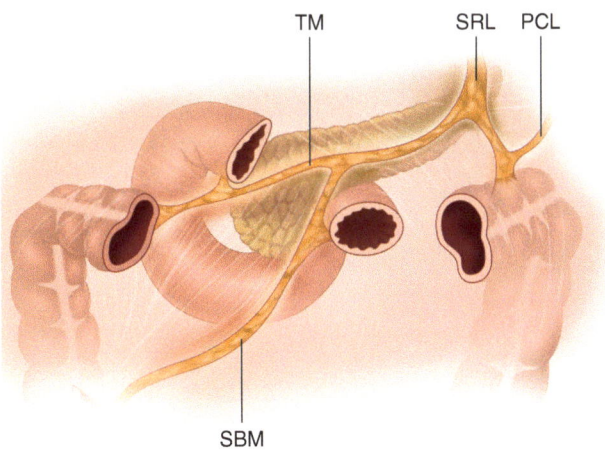

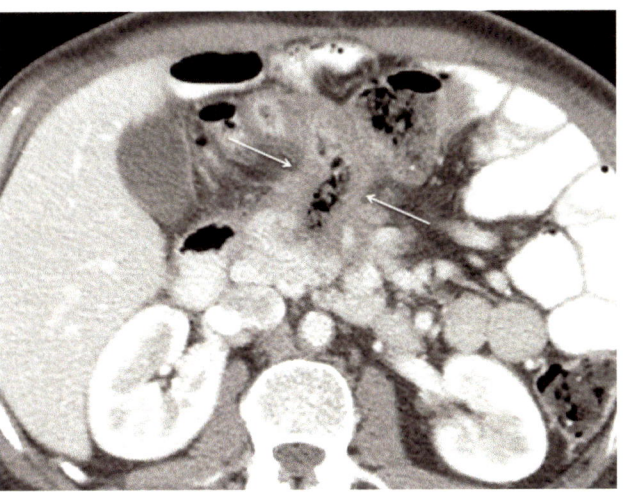

Fig. 17.8 The transverse mesocolon (TM) provides an important conduit for the spread of disease across the mid-abdomen. It is continuous with the splenorenal ligament (SRL) and phrenicocolic ligament (PCL) on the left and with the duodenocolic ligament on the right. In its mid-portion, it is continuous with the small bowel mesentery (SBM). (Adapted from Myers MA. Dynamic Radiology of the Abdomen: Normal and Pathologic Anatomy, New York: Springer, 1994)

Fig. 17.9 Transaxial CT image through the transverse mesocolon (TMC) in a patient with pancreatic adenocarcinoma demonstrates invasion of the TMC with necrotic tumor (arrows). The tumor in the TMC has fistulized with the transverse colon resulting in gas accumulating within the necrotic debris

as commonly occurs with ovarian, gastric, colon, and pancreatic cancer [10–12]. Sometimes, gastroepiploic collaterals may be recognized in the gastrocolic ligament which should raise concern about the possibility of splenic venous compromise as commonly occurs in pancreatic carcinoma.

The transverse mesocolon connects the transverse colon to the retroperitoneum but also forms a broad conduit for disease across the mid abdomen; bare areas link the pancreas to the transverse colon, spleen, and small bowel (Fig. 17.8). The transverse mesocolon is continuous with the phrenicocolic ligament and the splenorenal ligaments in the left abdomen, with the small bowel mesentery in the mid abdomen, and with the duodenocolic ligament in the right abdomen. The transverse mesocolon may be recognized as the fatty plane that connects the transverse colon to the retroperitoneum at the level of the uncinate process of the pancreas. As this structure lies commonly in a paracoronal orientation, recognition of the middle colic vessels and associated lymphatics within the mesocolon can aid in its identification. Pancreatic disease, both benign and malignant, often spreads ventrally into the transverse mesocolon and then on to the transverse colon (Fig. 17.9). Pancreatitis often results in adjacent fluid collections that can dissect open the potential space within the transverse mesocolon formed by fusion of the anterior and posterior leaves of the embryonic gastrosplenic ligament. Free fluid in the lesser sac is often confused with contained fluid collections within the transverse mesocolon.

The duodenocolic ligament, the right edge of the transverse mesocolon, forms an important pathway for the spread of right colon cancers via lymphatic drainage from the right colon passing through this ligament. Tumors of the right colon may spread via these lymphatics to deposit in nodes around the duodenum and pancreas [1]. Gastric outlet

obstruction may occur once this adenopathy becomes sufficiently severe to obstruct the second duodenum explaining how cancers of the right colon may result in upper gastrointestinal obstruction on rare occasion.

17.3 Peritoneal Spaces as Pathways for the Spread of Disease

Peritoneal fluid flows naturally through the peritoneal spaces that are defined by the peritoneal ligaments and mesenteries in the abdomen and pelvis. However, certain neoplastic and inflammatory conditions within the peritoneal cavity may leverage this natural flow of peritoneal fluid to spread throughout the peritoneal spaces. Tumors that arise from the peritoneal lining or break through the visceral peritoneum may shed their cells directly into the peritoneal fluid. Similarly, inflammatory processes within the peritoneal cavity may also leverage this natural flow of ascitic fluid and spread throughout the peritoneal spaces of the abdomen and pelvis. A thorough knowledge and understanding of this anatomy can help narrow the differential diagnosis for intraabdominal pathologies and may help radiologists better predict the organ of origin and likely route of spread for certain conditions (Fig. 17.10).

17.3.1 Left Peritoneal Space

The left peritoneal space is comprised of four compartments: the left anterior perihepatic space, the left posterior perihepatic space (gastrohepatic recess), the left anterior subphrenic space, and the left posterior subphrenic space (perisplenic space).

Fig. 17.10 Posterior peritoneal reflections and recesses. Intraperitoneal fluid flows naturally from the pelvis to the upper abdomen. Flow occurs preferentially through the right rather than left paracolic gutters owing to the broader diameter of the right gutter. In addition, flow in the left paracolic gutter is cut off from reaching the left subphrenic space by the phrenicocolic ligament. The transverse mesocolon divides the abdomen into supra- and inframesocolic spaces. In the right inframesocolic space, fluid is impeded from draining into the pelvis via the small bowel mesentery. Owing to natural holdup of fluid at the root of the small bowel mesentery and sigmoid mesocolon, these structures are naturally predisposed to involvement with serosal-based metastases in the setting of peritoneal carcinomatosis. (Adapted from Myers MA. Dynamic Radiology of the Abdomen: Normal and Pathologic Anatomy, New York: Springer, 1994).

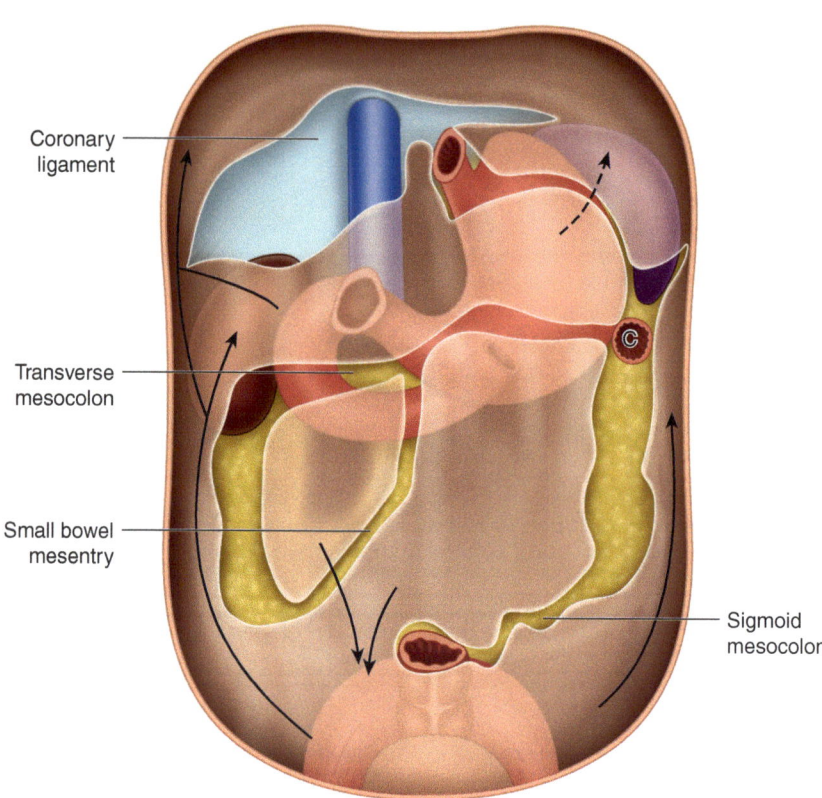

Anteriorly, the left peritoneal space extends to the right as the left anterior perihepatic space, ventral to the left lobe of the liver. It is bounded laterally on the right by the falciform ligament and on the left by the anterior wall of the stomach. Posteriorly, it extends along the diaphragm and is limited by the left coronary ligament, the left-superior extension of the bare area of the liver (Fig. 17.11a).

Along the medial margin of the left hepatic lobe, the left anterior perihepatic space turns to form the left posterior perihepatic space as it extends along the inferior margin of the left hepatic lobe posteriorly, deep into the fissure for the ligamentum venosum. Also known as the gastrohepatic recess, the left posterior perihepatic space is bounded on the left by the lateral wall of the stomach and is juxtaposed to the anterior wall of the duodenal bulb, the anterior wall of the gallbladder, and the porta hepatis [8]. Fluid in the gastrohepatic recess is separated from fluid in the superior recess of the lesser sac by the lesser omentum as it inserts into the fissure for the ligamentum venosum. Fluid collections in the gastrohepatic recess are relatively easy to drain owing to the lack of intervening structures between this space and the body wall, along the medial margin of the left hepatic lobe. Conversely, fluid collections in the lesser sac may be more difficult to approach percutaneously owing to the presence of intervening vasculature in the lesser omentum.

Laterally in the left abdomen, the left anterior subphrenic space connects with the left anterior perihepatic space across

the midabdomen. This space is cut off from the left paracolic gutter by the phrenicocolic ligament, unlike the right subphrenic space, which communicates freely with the right paracolic gutter. Thus, fluid can accumulate within the left anterior subphrenic space by passing ventral to the stomach, but once it enters this space, it is relatively static owing to the phrenicocolic ligament. Thus, fluid in the left anterior subphrenic space is a common site for peritoneal carcinomatosis and abscess formation consequent to peritonitis [13].

The posterior extension of the left anterior subphrenic space is the left posterior subphrenic space also known as the perisplenic space (Fig. 17.12). The bare areas of the spleen that result from the insertion of the gastrosplenic and splenorenal ligaments into the splenic hilum may be highlighted by fluid that surrounds the spleen within the perisplenic space [14–16]. Superiorly, the perisplenic space surrounds completely the upper margin of the spleen [17].

17.3.2 Right Peritoneal Space

The right peritoneal space is comprised of three compartments: the right subphrenic space/right anterior perihepatic space, the right posterior perihepatic space (hepatorenal recess/Morison's pouch), and the lesser sac.

The right subphrenic space surrounds the upper margin of the liver, separating it from the right hemidiaphragm

Fig. 17.11 Left (**a**) and right (**b**) perihepatic spaces. The left and right perihepatic spaces are bounded posteriorly by the coronary ligaments. The reflections of the coronary ligaments mark the site of the nonperitonealized "bare area" of the liver. (*LL* left lobe of the liver, *LK* left kidney, *S* stomach, *TC* transverse colon, *P* pancreas, *D* duodenum, *Lu* lung, *L* liver [right lobe], *A* adrenal, *K* kidney, *C* colon) (Adapted from Myers MA. Dynamic Radiology of the Abdomen: Normal and Pathologic Anatomy, New York: Springer, 1994)

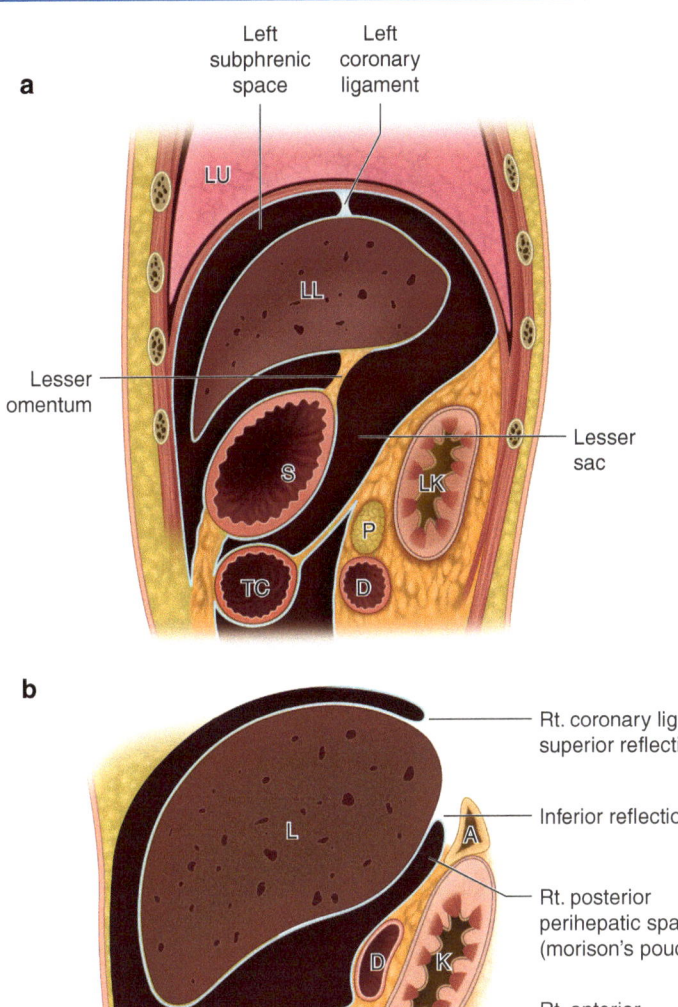

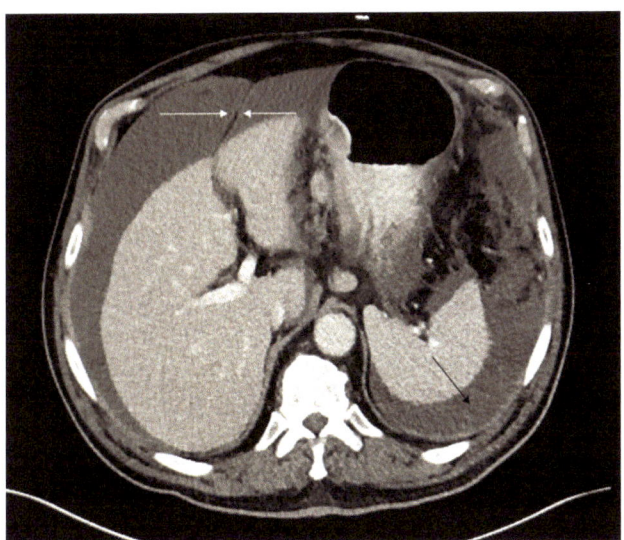

Fig. 17.12 Transaxial CT image from a patient with carcinomatosis secondary to gastric cancer demonstrates fluid in the left posterior subphrenic space (black arrow) and fluid in the right and left anterior perihepatic spaces, separated by the falciform ligament (white arrows)

(Figs. 17.11b and 17.12). Posteriorly and medially, the right coronary ligament (bare area of the liver) forms the posteromedial border of the right subphrenic space [18] (Fig. 17.13).

Inferior to the right coronary ligament, the hepatorenal recess (Morison's pouch) is the medial extension of the right subphrenic space, located between the right lobe of the liver and the anterior border of the kidney.

The lesser sac is the leftward extension of the right posterior perihepatic space/hepatorenal recess/Morison's pouch as it extends through the foramen of Winslow. The lesser sac is comprised of superior and inferior recesses [9, 19]. Fluid in the superior recess of the lesser sac surrounds the caudate lobe producing a reverse C-shaped configuration as it surrounds this structure (Figs. 17.14 and 17.15). A raised peritoneal reflection along the posterior aspect of the lesser sac serves as an anatomic boundary that separates the superior

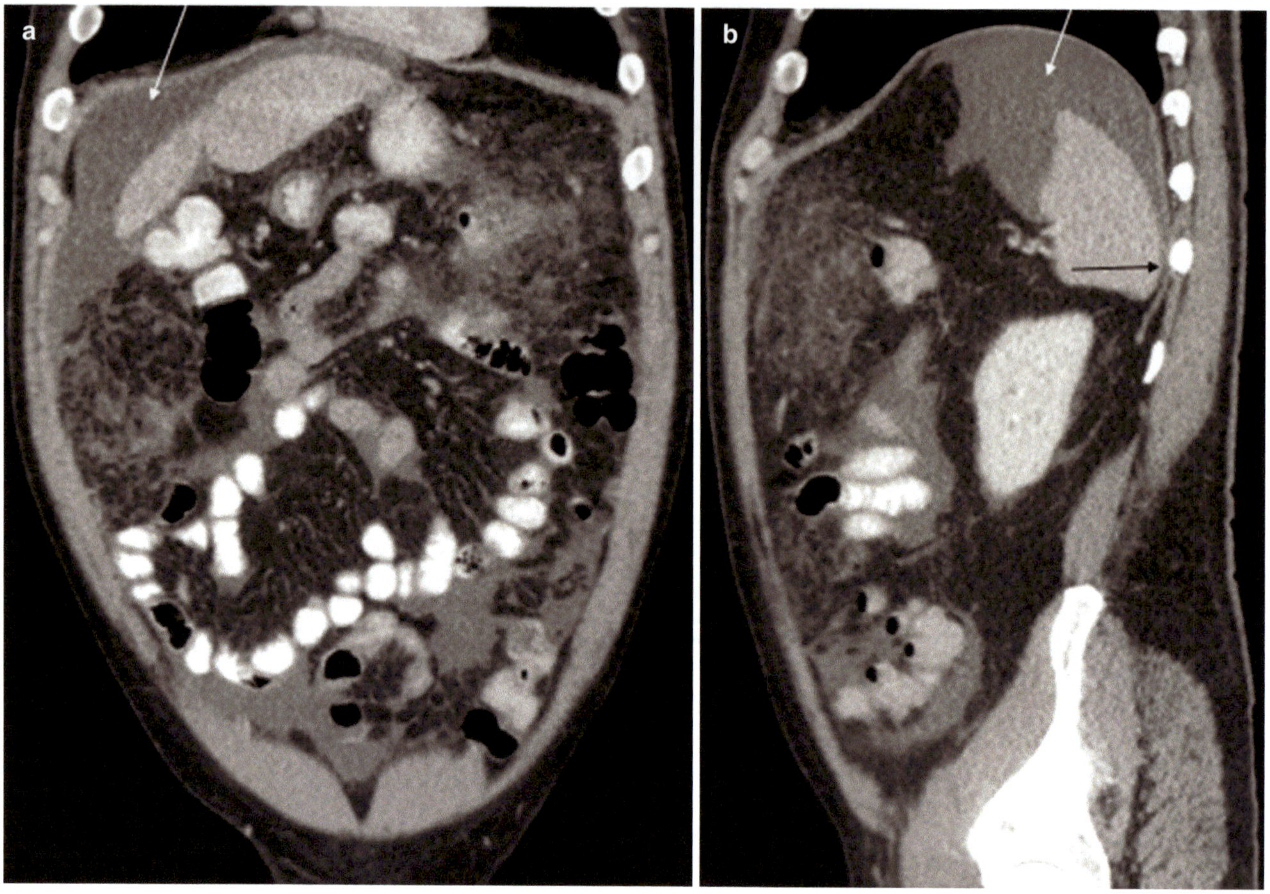

Fig. 17.13 Coronal (**a**) and sagittal (**b**) reformatted CT images from a patient with peritoneal mesothelioma demonstrates fluid in the right sub-phrenic space (white arrows) bounded posteriorly by the right coronary ligament (black arrow)

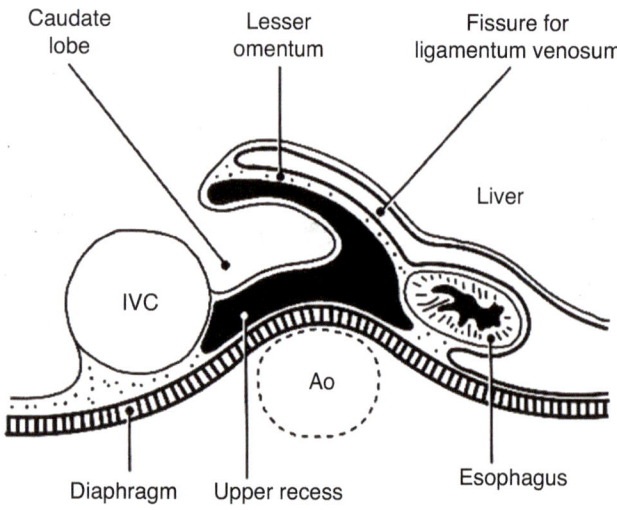

from the inferior recesses. This gastropancreatic plicae contains the proximal left gastric artery and may be recognized, particularly when surrounded by ascitic fluid in the superior and inferior recesses.

The inferior recess of the lesser sac is bounded laterally by the gastrosplenic and splenorenal ligaments, inferoposteriorly by the transverse mesocolon, and anteriorly by the stomach. Percutaneous drainage of fluid in lesser sac collections is problematic owing to the presence of abdominal organs, ligaments, and mesenteries that surround both superior and inferior recesses completely [20]. When evaluating lesser sac pathology for potential intervention, it is important to recognize variants. The most common variant involves the gastrosplenic ligament that can be pleated longitudinally and potentially confused with a soft tissue mass [21].

Fig. 17.14 The boundaries of the superior recess of the lesser sac may be recognized when fluid engulfs the caudate lobe. The lesser omentum separates this fluid from fluid in fissure for the ligamentum venosum which is in continuity with the left posterior periheptatic space (gastrohepatic recess). (*IVC* inferior vena cava, *Ao* aorta) (Reprinted with permission from Myers MA. Dynamic Radiology of the Abdomen: Normal and Pathologic Anatomy, New York: Springer, 1994)

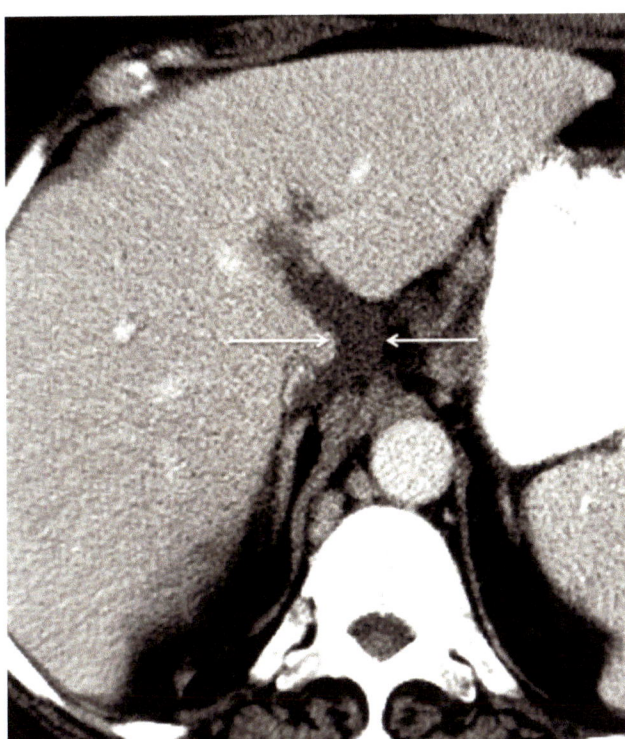

Fig. 17.15 Transaxial CT image through the superior recess of the lesser sac in a patient with gallbladder cancer (same patient as is illustrated in figure 3). Malignant ascites has accumulated in the superior recess of the lesser sac (arrows), seen with a characteristic reverse c-shaped configuration surrounding the caudate lobe

17.4 Concluding Remarks

Upper abdominal disease may spread from the upper abdominal organs to the retroperitoneum and vice versa via the gastrohepatic and hepatoduodenal ligaments in the right abdomen, the gastrosplenic and splenorenal ligaments in the left abdomen, and the gastrocolic ligament and transverse mesocolon in the mid abdomen. Disease in any of these ligamentous pairs can suggest the organ of origin, and in some cases, the location of the disease within the organ. Peritoneal ligaments and mesenteries also guide the flow of intraperitoneal fluid throughout the peritoneal spaces that they define. Neoplastic and inflammatory diseases that arise de novo or extend into the peritoneal cavity may spread through these spaces and deposit in predictable areas within the peritoneal cavity.

Key Points
- Disease may spread through the abdomen and pelvis by the following mechanisms:
  - Via the bloodstream
  - Via lymphatic extension
  - Via direct invasion
  - Via intraperitoneal seeding.
- Direct invasion and lymphatic extension occur commonly through the peritoneal ligaments and mesenteries that interconnect the abdominal viscera.
- Intraperitoneal spread occurs by seeding the peritoneal cavity with cells that spread via the natural flow of peritoneal fluid via the peritoneal spaces.

Take-Home Messages
A thorough understanding of the peritoneal ligaments and mesenteries as well as the peritoneal spaces that they define can inform the pathways by which inflammatory and neoplastic diseases may spread throughout the abdomen and pelvis.

1. Transaxial CT image demonstrates the gastrohepatic ligament (GHL), seen as a fatty plane interposed between lesser curvature of the stomach and the lobe of the liver. The GHL contains the left gastric artery (arrow), the left gastric vein (coronary vein) and associated lymphatics.
2. Transaxial CT image demonstrates a heterogenous mass centered in the gastrohepatic ligament (GHL), with the invasion of the left hepatic lobe and the stomach. Prospectively, it was unclear as to the organ of origin, but it proved to be a hepatoma extending through the GHL to involve the stomach.
3. Transaxial CT images through the porta hepatis (A) and the uncinate process (B) demonstrate bulky lymphadenopathy (arrows) in the hepatoduodenal ligament (HDL) in a patient with gallbladder carcinoma. Tumor has spread bi-directionally within the HDL proximally (A), and distally to the insertion of the HDL on the second portion of the duodenum.
4. The gastrosplenic ligament (GSL) and splenorenal ligament (SRL) comprise the left wall of the lesser sac and provide a conduit for the spread of metastatic disease from the greater curvature of the stomach to the retroperitonium and vice versa. (Reprinted with permission from Myers MA. Dynamic

Radiology of the Abdomen: Normal and Pathologic Anatomy, New York: Springer, 1994).

5. Transaxial CT images through the gastrosplenic ligament (GSL) (A) and the splenorenal ligament (SRL) (B) in a patient with lymphoma. Tumor is seen within the GSL, interposed between the gastric greater curvature and the spleen (A), and within the SRL, encasing the splenic vasculature (B).

6. The gastrocolic ligament (GCL) joins the greater curvature of the stomach (G) to the transverse colon (TC). In concert with the transverse mesocolon, a pathway of disease is formed between retroperitoneal structures such as the pancreas (P) and the duodenum (D) to the anterior aspect of the intraperitoneal cavity (modified from Langman J., Medical Embriology, New York: Saunders, 1971).

7. Transaxial CT image through the gastrocolic ligament (GCL) demonstrates a gastric ulcer extending into the GCL (black arrow) with associated inflammation in the greater omentum (white arrows).

8. The transverse mesocolon (TM) provides an important conduit for the spread of disease across the mid abdomen. It is continuous with the splenorenal ligament (SRL) and phrenicocolic ligament (PCL) on the left and with the duodenocolic ligament on the right. In its mid-portion, it is continuous with the small bowel mesentery (SBM). (Reprinted with permission from Myers MA. Dynamic Radiology of the Abdomen: Normal and Pathologic Anatomy, New York: Springer, 1994).

9. Transaxial CT image through the transverse mesocolon (TMC) in a patient with pancreatic adenocarcinoma demonstrates invasion of the TMC with necrotic tumor (arrows). The tumor in the TMC has fistulized with the transverse colon resulting in gas accumulating within the necrotic debris.

10. Posterior peritoneal reflections and recesses. Intraperitoneal fluid flows naturally from the pelvis to the upper abdomen. Flow occurs preferentially through the right rather than left paracolic gutters owing to the broader diameter of the right gutter. In addition, flow in the left paracolic gutter is cut off from reaching the left subphrenic space by the phrenicocolic ligament. The transverse mesocolon divides the abdomen into supra- and inframesocolic spaces. In the right inframesocolic space, fluid is impeded from draining into the pelvis via the small bowel mesentery. Owing to natu-

ral holdup of fluid at the root of the small bowel mesentery and sigmoid mesocolon, these structures are naturally predisposed to involvement with serosal-based metastases in the setting of peritoneal carcinomatosis. (Reprinted with permission from Myers MA. Dynamic Radiology of the Abdomen: Normal and Pathologic Anatomy, New York: Springer, 1994).

11. Left (A) and right (B) perihepatic spaces. The left and right perihepatic spaces are bounded posteriorly by the coronary ligaments. The reflections of the coronary ligaments mark the site of the non-peritonealized "bare area" of the liver. (LL = left lobe of the liver, LK = left kidney, S = stomach, TC = transverse colon, P = pancreas, D = duodenum, Lu = lung, L = liver [right lobe], A = adrenal, K = kidney, C = colon) (Reprinted with permission from Myers MA. Dynamic Radiology of the Abdomen: Normal and Pathologic Anatomy, New York: Springer, 1994).

12. Transaxial CT image from a patient with carcinomatosis secondary to gastric cancer demonstrates fluid in the left posterior subphrenic space (black arrow) and fluid in the right and left anterior perihepatic spaces, separated by the falciform ligament (white arrows).

13. Coronal (A) and sagittal (B) reformatted CT images from a patient with peritoneal mesothelioma demonstrates fluid in the right subphrenic space (white arrows) bounded posteriorly by the right coronary ligament (black arrow).

14. The boundaries of the superior recess of the lesser sac may be recognized when fluid engulfs the caudate lobe. The lesser omentum separates this fluid from fluid in fissure for the ligamentum venosum, which is in continuity with the left posterior periheptatic space (gastrohepatic recess). (IVC = inferior vena cava, Ao = aorta) (Reprinted with permission from Myers MA. Dynamic Radiology of the Abdomen: Normal and Pathologic Anatomy, New York: Springer, 1994).

15. Transaxial CT image through the superior recess of the lesser sac in a patient with gallbladder cancer (same patient as is illustrated in Fig. 17.15). Malignant ascites has accumulated in the superior recess of the lesser sac (arrows), seen with a characteristic reverse c-shaped configuration surrounding the caudate lobe.

References

1. Meyers MA, Oliphant M, Berne AS, Feldberg MAM. The perito-neal ligaments and mesenteries: pathways of intraabdominal spread of disease. Radiology. 1987;163:593–604.

2. Balfe DM, Mauro MA, Koehler RE, Lee JKT, Weyman PJ, Picus D, Peterson RR. Gastrohepatic ligament: normal and pathologic CT anatomy. Radiology. 1984;150:485–90.

3. Auh YH, Rosen A, Rubenstein WA, Engel IA, Whalen JP, Kazam E. CT of the papillary process of the caudate lobe of the liver. AJR. 1984;142:535–8.

4. Donoso L, Martinez-Noguera A, Zidan A, Lora F. Papillary process of the caudate lobe of the liver: sonographic appearance. Radiology. 1989;173:631–3.

5. Weinstein JB, Heiken JP, Lee JKT, DiSantis DJ, Balfe DM, Weyman PJ, Peterson RR. High resolution CT of the porta hepatis and hepatoduodenal ligament. Radiographics. 1986;6:55–74.

6. Zirinsky K, Auh YH, Rubenstein WA, Kneeland JB, Whalen JP, Kazam E. The portacaval space: CT with MR correlation. Radiology. 1985;156:453–60.

7. Ito K, Choji T, Fujita T, Kuramitsu T, Nakaki H, Kurokawa F, Fujita N, Nakanishi T. Imaging of the portacaval space. AJR. 1993;161:329–34.

8. Vincent LM, Mauro MA, Mittelstaedt CA. The lesser sac and gas-trohepatic recess: sonographic appearance and differentiation of fluid collections. Radiology. 1984;150:515–9.

9. Dodds WJ, Foley WD, Lawson TL, Stewart ET, Taylor A. Anatomy and imaging of the lesser peritoneal sac. AJR. 1985;144:567–75.

10. Cooper C, Jeffrey RB, Silverman PM, Federle MP, Chun GH. Computed tomography of omental pathology. J Comput Assist Tomogr. 1986;10(1):62–6.

11. Rubesin SE, Levine MS, Glick SN. Gastric involvement by omental cakes: radiographic findings. Gastrointest Radiol. 1986;11:223–8.

12. Nougaret S, Sadowski E, Lakhman Y, Rousset P, Lahaye M, Worley M, Sgarbura O, Shinagare AB. The BUMPy road of peritoneal metastases in ovarian cancer. Diagn Interv Imaging. 2022;103:448–59.

13. Halvorsen RA, Jones MA, Rice RP, Thompson WM. Anterior left subphrenic abscess: characteristic plain film and CT appearance. AJR. 1982;139:283–9.

14. Vibhakar SD, Bellon EM. The bare area of the spleen: a constant CT feature of the ascitic abdomen. AJR. 1984;141:953–5.

15. Rubenstein WA, Auh YH, Zirinsky K, Kneeland JB, Whalen JP, Kazam E. Posterior peritoneal recesses: assessment using CT. Radiology. 1985;156:461–8.

16. Love L, Demos TC, Posniak H. CT of retrorenal fluid collections. AJR. 1985;145:87–91.

17. Crass JR, Maile CW, Frick MP. Catheter drainage of the left posterior subphrenic space: a reliable percutaneous approach. Gastrointest Radiol. 1985;10:397–8.

18. Rubenstein WA, Auh TH, Whalen JP, Kazem E. The perihepatic spaces: computed tomographic and ultrasound imaging. Radiology. 1983;149:231–9.

19. Jeffrey RB, Federle MP, Goodman PC. Computed tomography of the lesser peritoneal sac. Radiology. 1981;141:117–22.

20. Meyers MA. Dynamic radiology of the abdomen: normal and pathologic anatomy. 4th ed. New York: Springer; 1994.

21. Elmohr MM, Blair KJ, Menias CO, Nada A, Shaaban AM, Sandrasegaran K, Elsayes KM. The lesser sac and foramen of Winslow: anatomy, embryology, and CT appearance of pathologic processes. AJR. 2020;215:843–51.

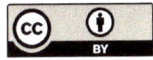

Small Bowel: The Last Stronghold of Gastrointestinal Radiology

18

Moriyah Naama and Pablo R. Ros

Learning Objectives
- To become familiar with small bowel key imaging modalities and the clinical considerations in choosing the appropriate study
- To identify imaging signs of small bowel inflammation for diagnosis and characterization of the main causative entities
- To recognize radiological characteristics of the various benign and malignant small bowel neoplasms
- To learn about signs of mesenteric ischemia imaging and resulting ischemic bowel damage

18.1 Imaging Techniques

As direct endoscopic visualization of most of the midgut proximal to the ileocecal valve is impossible, radiological imaging plays a vital role in assessing and diagnosing pathology of the small bowel. The optimal choice of imaging technique depends on the clinical setting, the presumptive differential diagnosis, whether the patient presents as an outpatient or in the acute setting, and individual patient characteristics, such as age and ability to cooperate.

The two major cross-sectional imaging techniques for small bowel evaluation are computed tomography (CT) and magnetic resonance imaging (MRI), each utilizing various acquisition protocols. The appropriate selection between these techniques has been a subject of interest in multiple studies, as each has characteristic advantages and disadvantages. For example, a main concern of CT imaging is repeated exposure of patients to ionizing radiation, which is particularly a concern in young patients, as frequently occurs in inflammatory bowel disease (IBD). Additionally, CT lacks visualization of superficial lesions and thus, may be inferior in detecting subtle mucosal disease [1]. Conversely, MRI may be more sensitive for identifying mild inflammation, in differentiating inflammation from fibrosis and additionally, may be used to assess motility with cine sequences. Disadvantages of MRI include a higher prevalence of motion artifacts than in CT, which affect image quality and thus, sensitivity, especially with uncooperative patients and in the acute setting. Other advantages of contrast-enhanced CT over MRI in the setting of an acute abdomen include availability, rapid acquisition, superiority in the assessment of certain complications such as perforation or bowel obstruction and the ability to rapidly screen for a wide range of pathologies in and outside the small bowel [2]. In addition, in clinical practice CT is the imaging workhorse for abdominal symptomatology and frequently the first diagnostic test performed. Thus, familiarity with small bowel CT findings is, in many cases, the initial key to diagnosis and in suggesting more specific tests such as CT-E, MR-E, CT Angiography (CT-A) and MR Angiography (MR-A).

Indeed, the widespread use of cross-sectional imaging has obviated the need for radiographic enteroclysis, in which contrast material is injected through a naso-jejunal tube to distend the small bowel, which is then imaged fluoroscopically. The disadvantages of this technique include indirect visualization of the bowel wall, inability to assess extramural pathology and the bowel loop overlapping, limiting the study. Thus, CT and MR-enteroclysis have largely replaced radiographic enteroclysis. Currently, the prevalent imaging technique to depict the small bowel is either CT or MR enterography (CT-E, MR-E), which utilizes orally

M. Naama
Department of Radiology, Stony Brook University, Stony Brook, NY, USA

Department of Radiology, Hadassah Hebrew University Medical Center, Jerusalem, Israel
e-mail: Moriyah.Naama@mail.huji.ac.il

P. R. Ros (✉)
Department of Radiology, Stony Brook University, Stony Brook, NY, USA
e-mail: Pablo.Ros@stonybrookmedicine.edu

© The Author(s) 2023
J. Hodler et al. (eds.), *Diseases of the Abdomen and Pelvis 2023-2026*, IDKD Springer Series,
https://doi.org/10.1007/978-3-031-27355-1_18

administered contrast rather than inserting a naso-jejunal tube to distend the bowel. Though enterography results in reduced luminal distention compared to enteroclysis, especially of the jejunum, this technique is less invasive than enteroclysis and thus, results in better patient acceptance [2]. Notwithstanding, the initial imaging study in the acute setting is often contrast-enhanced CT rather than CT-E, due to its rapid acquisition and reduced patient ability to ingest a large volume of contrast material. Unless contraindicated, intravenous contrast is always administered for characterization of mural and lesion enhancement patterns. Additionally, spasmolytic agents may be administered shortly before imaging to reduce motion artifact.

In some centers, intestinal ultrasound (IUS) is frequently used to image the small bowel in chronic and acute settings, with color Doppler being especially informative in assessing mural vascularity and inflammatory activity [3, 4]. Other available imaging modalities for the assessment of specific small bowel pathologies include capsule endoscopy, balloon-assisted enteroscopy, and elastography [5].

> **Key Point**
> The two major cross-sectional imaging modalities for the evaluation of the small bowel are MR-E and CT-E, with CT having a central role in the emergency setting.

18.2 Inflammatory and Infectious Diseases

18.2.1 Inflammatory Bowel Disease

Inflammatory bowel disease (IBD) consists of two entities: Crohn's disease (CD), which can involve any part of the gastrointestinal tract though most commonly the terminal ileum, and ulcerative colitis (UC), which is limited to the colon, along with various extraintestinal manifestations in both conditions. CD is characterized as a transmural, granulomatous inflammatory disease of uncertain etiology. The diagnosis of CD is made based on combined clinical, radiologic, endoscopic, and histologic findings demonstrating discontinuous transmural inflammation of the gastrointestinal tract. Complications of CD include inflammatory and/or fibrotic strictures, which may manifest as complete or partial bowel obstruction as well as abscesses, perforation, fistulae and, after long-standing disease, an increased risk for malignancy. In Europe and North America, the diagnosis, staging, and management of CD constitute the most common clinical scenarios necessitating imaging of the small bowel [5].

Determining the extent of disease and surveillance of disease activity in CD is heavily reliant on cross-sectional imaging. Importantly, radiological response to treatment is associated with better long-term outcomes in patients and may be used as a target for treatment [6]. Imaging findings indicative of active small bowel inflammation include segmental mural hyperenhancement, which may be homogenously transmural, asymmetric, or involving only the inner wall resulting in a "halo sign". Other findings are bowel wall thickening above a normal 3 mm, intramural edema seen on fat-saturated T2-weighted MRI, ulcerations which appear as focal discontinuity in the intraluminal surface, diminished motility on cine MRI sequences, and inflammatory strictures with upstream luminal dilatation >3 cm (Fig. 18.1). Diffusion-weighted MR imaging may also be helpful in identifying areas of active inflammation, though diffusion restriction should not be used as a sole indicator of active disease. Penetrating disease may manifest as fistulas, which are categorized as simple or complex depending on whether there are single or multiple extra-enteric tracts. Complex fistulas often appear as a "clover leaf" or "star sign" involving multiple bowel loops or adjacent organs. Fibrofatty proliferation or "creeping fat" is seen as increased fat along the mesenteric border of abnormal bowel. The characteristic "comb sign" denotes engorged vasa recta that supply inflamed bowel loops, though it may also reflect past inflammation (Fig. 18.2). Inflammatory masses, abscesses, perienteric edema, acute or chronic mesenteric vein thrombosis, and mesenteric adenopathy are additional imaging findings consistent with penetrating disease [7]. It is important to remember that signs of bowel inflammation are nonspecific to CD and careful clinical correlation is needed to exclude other causes, including infectious etiologies such as yersiniosis.

Accurately determining disease activity based on imaging and reporting findings in a clinically useful manner is highly challenging. Consensus recommendations for the use and interpretation of CT-E and MR-E studies in small bowel CD have been established by the American Gastroenterological Association [7].

> **Key Point**
> Major imaging findings in active small bowel inflammation include mural hyperenhancement, engorged vasa recta, bowel wall thickening above 3 mm, intramural edema, ulcerations, diminished motility and inflammatory strictures with upstream luminal dilatation >3 cm.

18.2.2 Celiac Disease

Celiac disease is a maldigestion syndrome due to the aberrant recognition of gliadin, a component of gluten, as an immunogenic agent in genetically predisposed individuals. This trig-

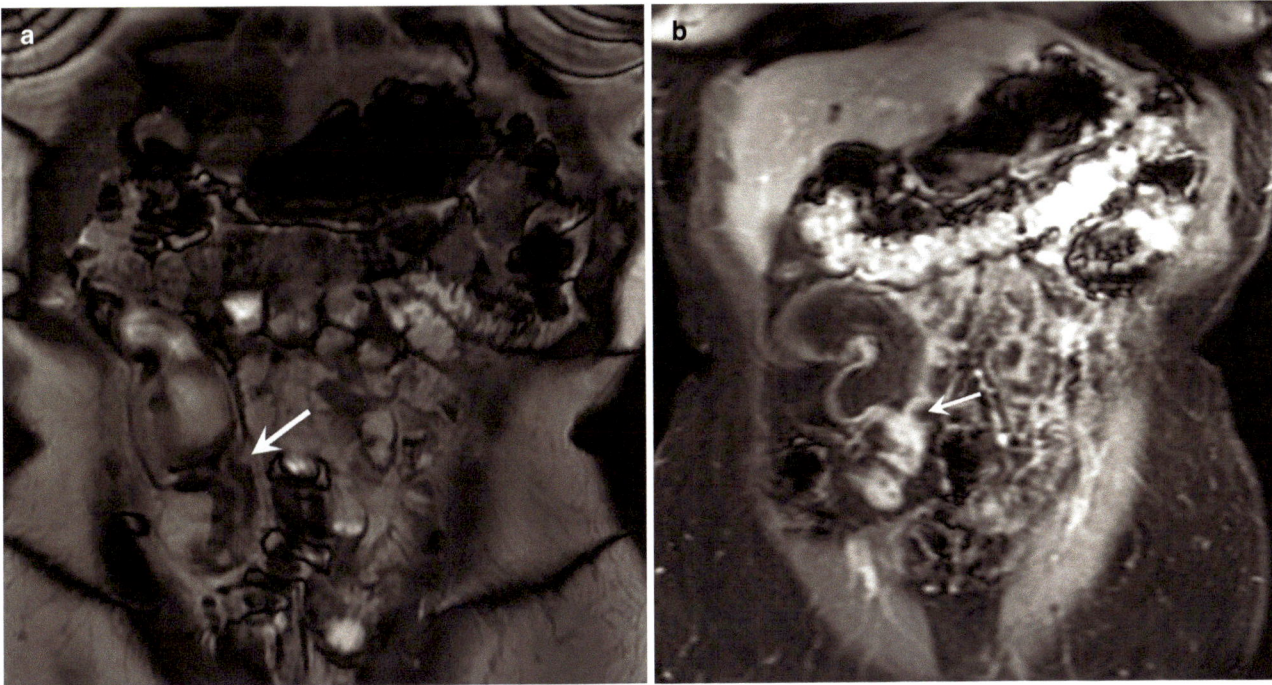

Fig. 18.1 MR-E in Crohn's disease. Coronal T1 pre- (**a**) and T1 post-contrast (**b**) MR-E images demonstrate an enhancing stricture (arrow) with upstream bowel dilatation in the terminal ileum

gers an antibody and cell-mediated response toward the villi and the intestinal mucosa, leading to severe mucosal deficit. Clinically, celiac disease is diverse, though typical symptoms include diarrhea, abdominal pain, steatorrhea, weight loss, vomiting, and manifestations of various nutritional deficits including iron-deficiency anemia. Hyposplenism, neuropsychiatric symptoms and dermatological manifestations, classically dermatitis herpetiformis, are also possible [5]. Symptoms usually abate with cessation of gluten ingestion. Long-standing, refractory disease may progress to enteropathy-associated T-cell lymphoma (EATL) or small bowel adenocarcinoma. Due to varying and atypical presentations, diagnosis may be challenging and is often delayed, as it primarily relies on obtaining biopsies of affected portions of the duodenum. These reveal characteristic histological findings of villous atrophy, crypt hyperplasia, and inflammatory cell infiltrate of the lamina propria. Medical imaging plays a supporting role in the timely diagnosis and management of this disease [5].

It is key to recognize radiological signs suspicious for celiac disease, so further diagnostic testing can be pursued. Fluoroscopic guided small bowel follow-through previously constituted the main imaging test for celiac disease by depicting small bowel malabsorption pattern (MABP) [8]. Features of MABP include excess fluid secretion resulting in multiple dilated, fluid-filled loops with reversal of the jejunal-ileal fold pattern ("moulage sign"), laminar flow of contrast due to decreased peristalsis, dilution, and flocculation of contrast

material, and telescoping of bowel loops with transient intussusception. Of these signs, small intestinal fold pattern alterations, reflective of underlying villous atrophy, are the most specific sign for celiac disease and its depiction necessitates adequate distention of the jejunum [9]. As the use of fluoroscopic barium examinations has declined, cross-sectional imaging often constitutes the initial radiological assessment of abdominal complaints. CT-E and MR-E are both capable of depicting MABP of the small bowel and additional findings of active inflammation in the bowel wall and mesentery. These include mesenteric lymphadenopathy, proximal bowel wall thickening with or without submucosal fat deposition, and a hypervascular, engorged mesentery. Splenic atrophy is present in 30–60% of patients [10]. Refractory celiac disease (RCD), which develops in 2–10% of patients, can result in life-threatening complications including cavitary mesenteric lymph node syndrome, ulcerative jejunoileitis, EATL, adenocarcinoma and an increased risk for other gastrointestinal malignancies [9].

18.2.3 Graft Versus Host Disease

Graft versus host disease (GVHD) is an immune dysfunction most commonly following allogenic bone marrow transplants, though it may occur following transplantations of any organ rich in lymphocytes or after blood transfusions. In this disorder, competent donor lymphocytes attack recipient tis-

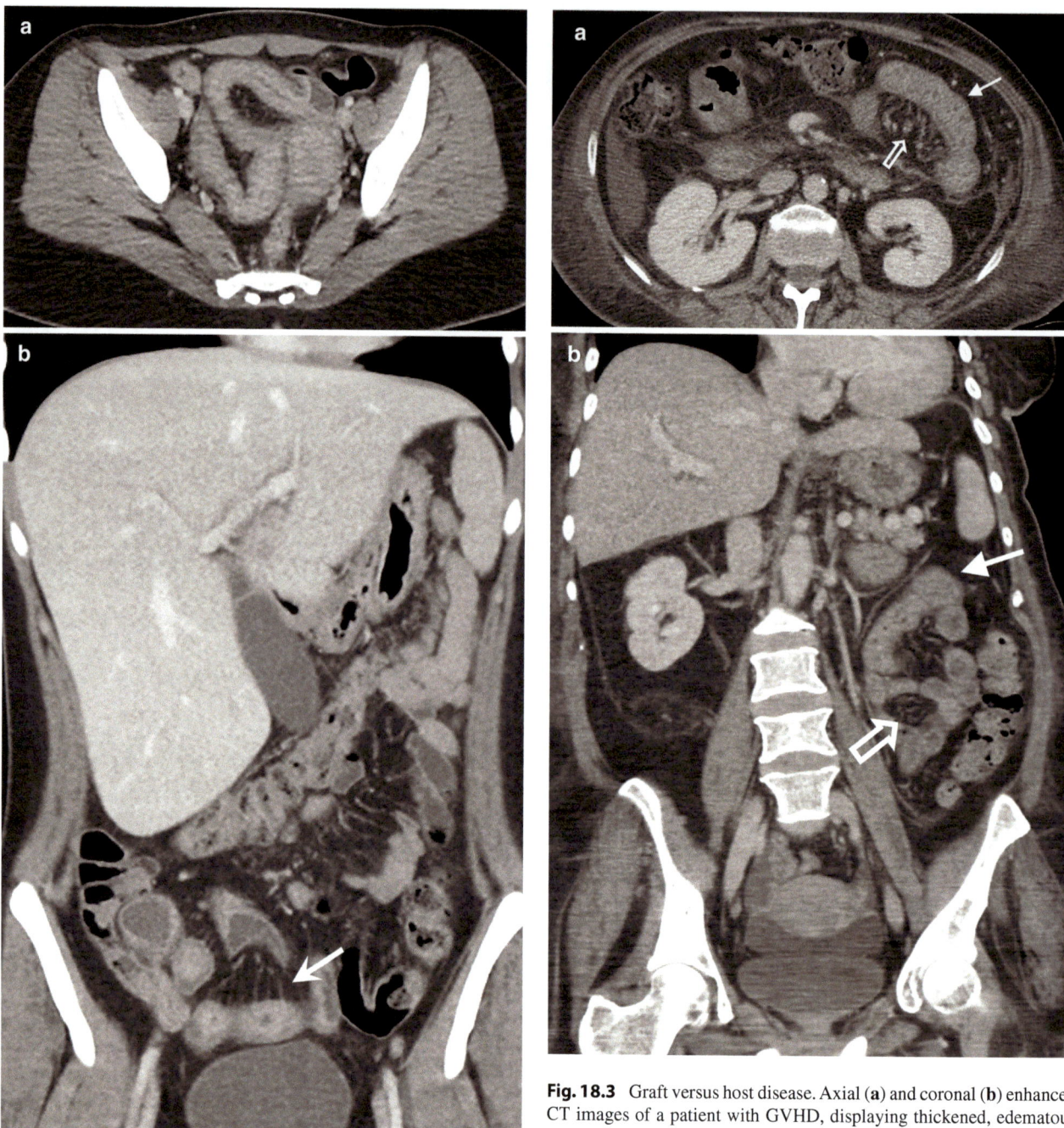

Fig. 18.3 Graft versus host disease. Axial (**a**) and coronal (**b**) enhanced CT images of a patient with GVHD, displaying thickened, edematous bowel wall (solid arrow) or normal caliber small bowel loops with engorged mesenteric vessels (hollow arrow)

Fig. 18.2 Enhanced CT in Crohn's disease. Axial (**a**) and coronal (**b**) enhanced CT images of a long segment of distal ileum with bowel wall thickening, mesenteric fat stranding, and engorged vasa recta ("comb sign," arrow) in keeping with active inflammation

sue, leading to inflammation and tissue destruction. Moderate to severe GVHD occurs in 30–50% of patients undergoing matched allogenic bone marrow transplants. Small bowel involvement is ubiquitous [11]. Symptoms include watery diarrhea, ileus, fever, and abdominal pain [5].

Typical imaging findings are nonspecific signs of bowel inflammation, including a thickened, enhancing bowel wall, engorged vasa recta, fluid-filled bowel loops, and mesenteric fat stranding (Fig. 18.3). The extent of involved bowel tends to be greater in GVHD than in IBD. It is critical to differentiate GVHD from infection, as treatment of GVHD involves immunosuppressive agents. As such, biopsies are often needed to confirm this diagnosis [5].

18.2.4 Infections

Infection remains an important etiology in the differential diagnosis in all cases of small bowel inflammation. Acute gastroenteritis, most frequently of viral etiology, is a common illness resulting in many emergency department visits [12]. While most cases are self-limiting, infectious enteritis occasionally requires targeted treatment and hospitalization. Moreover, it is often crucial to exclude infectious enteritis before treatment of other suspected inflammatory processes. Imaging findings are nonspecific and usually require additional testing, such as biopsy, to confirm the diagnosis (Fig. 18.4).

A variety of atypical pathogens can cause enteritis:

1. Tuberculous enteritis is found in Asia and Africa and most commonly involves distal ileal and ileocecal areas. Patients typically present with constitutional symptoms. Radiologically, it may appear as an ileocecal mass with deformity of the cecum and low attenuation mesenteric lymphadenopathy, though it cannot be reliably distinguished from CD or lymphoma.
2. Yersiniosis is an infectious disease presenting radiologically as a mild terminal ileitis with ulceration, lymphoid hyperplasia, wall thickening and increased, stratified enhancement. It is a cause of mesenteric adenitis in children and may mimic acute appendicitis. Yersiniosis may mimic radiologically mild CD.
3. Actinomycosis may cause clinical infection in predisposed individuals. This presents as a chronic, progressive, granulomatous infection with suppurative inflammation with sinus tracts and fistulation. The radiological appearance may mimic small bowel adenocarcinoma.
4. Whipple's disease is a rare bacterial infection caused by *Tropheryma whipplei*, which may infect any organ though always involves the small bowel. Imaging demonstrates thickening of the valvulae conniventes, nodularity of the duodenum and jejunum and possible bowel dilatation and characteristically low attenuation mesenteric lymphadenopathy (Fig. 18.5).
5. Infestations with helminths and other parasites are prevalent in tropical and subtropical areas. Strongyloidiasis and Giardiasis may demonstrate non-specific bowel wall thickening on imaging. Heavy infestations with Ascariasis lumbricoides may present with obstructive symptoms. Chagas' disease is a chronic condition caused by infection with *Trypanosoma cruzi* and can eventually damage the enteric nervous system resulting in dilatation and slow transit in any segment of the GI tract from the esophagus to the rectum. Small bowel involvement results in megaduodenum [5].
6. SARS-CoV-2, the causative virus of the COVID-19 pandemic, has been reported to cause gastrointestinal symptoms in a significant portion of patients [13]. Small bowel complications include ileus with persistent bowel dilatation, feeding intolerance and mesenteric ischemia dis-

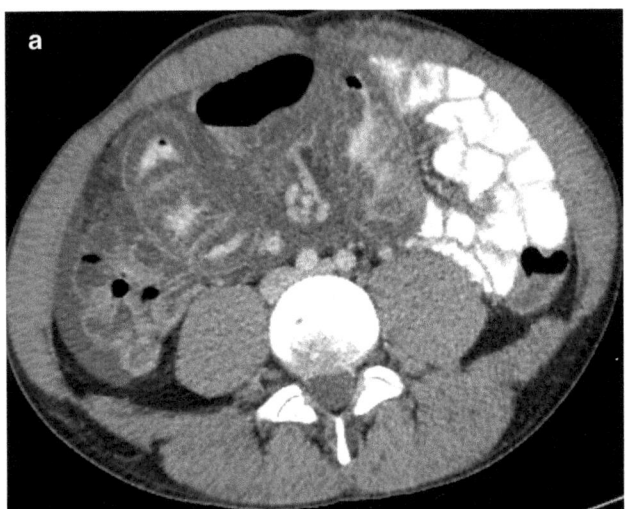

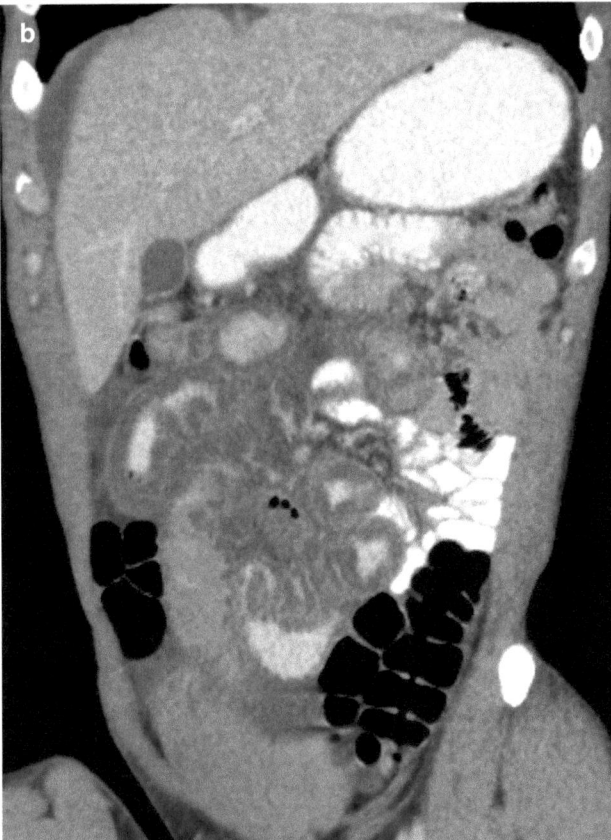

Fig. 18.4 Infectious gastroenteritis. Axial (**a**) and coronal (**b**) CT images of infectious gastroenteritis, with diffuse nonspecific markedly thickened, low attenuation small bowel loops with mesenteric fat inflammatory changes

playing bowel wall thickening, pneumatosis, and even portal venous air on CT imaging. It is unclear whether these complications are SARS-CoV-2-specific or are indirect sequalae common in critically ill patients. Interestingly, the ACE2 receptor, through which the virus infects host cells, is heavily expressed on the brush border of the intestinal epithelium [14].

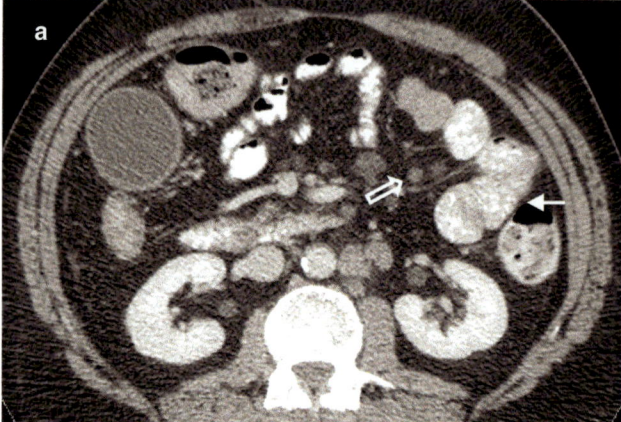

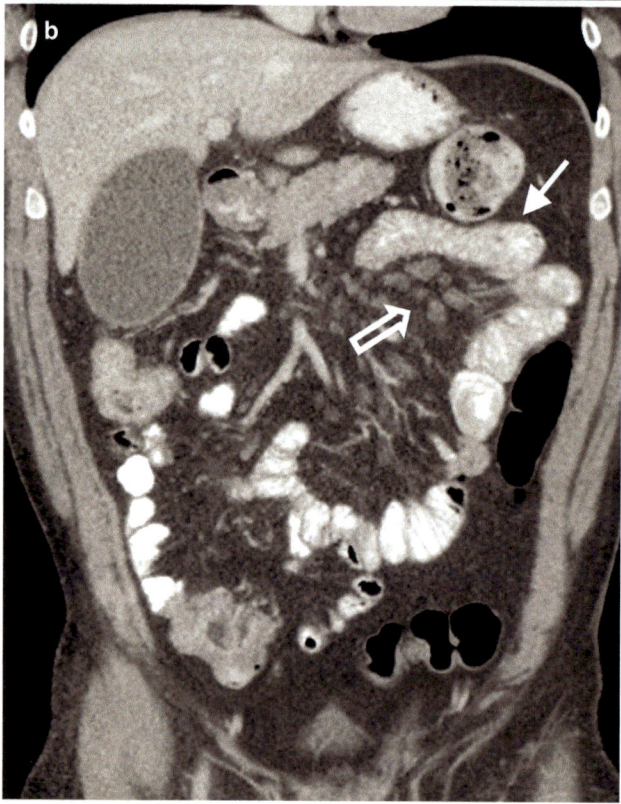

Fig. 18.5 Whipple's disease. Axial (**a**) and coronal (**b**) CT images in a patient with Whipple's disease, displaying characteristic nodularity of the duodenal and jejunal folds (solid arrows), along with multiple prominent low attenuation mesenteric lymph nodes (hollow arrows)

Key Point

It is critical to differentiate infection from other causes of bowel inflammation, as radiological signs may be similar and treatment as a non-infectious condition, for example with immunosuppressive agents, may result in exacerbation if the etiology is infectious.

18.3 Small Bowel Neoplasms

Despite constituting above 90% of the surface area of the gastrointestinal tract, small bowel neoplasms are relatively rare. Malignant tumors of the small intestine constitute only 3% of gastrointestinal cancers and 0.6% of all cancers in the USA [15]. For reasons unclear, the incidence of small bowel cancers is rising, particularly neuroendocrine tumors (NET) or carcinoid tumors.

Small bowel tumors are often clinically silent for long periods of time, and many are found incidentally during surgery or radiological exams performed for other reasons. Incidence is greatest in the proximal small bowel and decreases distally up to the terminal ileum. CT-E and MR-E have a central role in diagnosis and characterization of small bowel tumors [16].

18.3.1 Benign Neoplasms

Benign small bowel tumors are usually solitary, unless there is an underlying intestinal polyposis syndrome. Appearance on imaging is often that of a round and well-circumscribed intrinsic filling defect with smooth margins, single or multiple in polyposis. Adenomas and leiomyomas are the most common benign tumors of the small bowel and the only two with malignant predisposition. Rarer lesions include lipomas, vascular and neurogenic tumors, hamartomas, and heterotopias, which have no malignant predisposition [5].

Adenomas originate from glandular epithelium and may have a tubular, villous, or tubulovillous morphology, like in the colon. Tubular adenomas often appear on imaging as a solitary intrinsic filing defect with smooth margins, either sessile or pedunculated, while villous adenomas appear cauliflower-like and tend to be larger (>3 cm). Adenomas larger than 2 cm are routinely resected due to malignant potential. Adenomas are usually solitary unless there is an underlying polyposis syndrome. Multiple adenomas are typically of varying sizes and within a single bowel segment.

Lipomas are composed of mature adipose tissue arising from the submucosa and have no malignant potential. Less than 50% are symptomatic, and they may present with obstruction, bleeding, or manifest as the lead point for intussusception. Most small bowel lipomas arise in the ileum or in the duodenum. On imaging, they appear as a smooth, homogenous mass with fat attenuation on CT and no enhancement. On MRI they follow uniform macroscopic fat signals across all sequences. Symptomatic lesions may be resected.

Leiomyomas are the most common symptomatic benign small bowel neoplasm. These mesenchymal tumors, when in the small bowel, appear most frequently in the jejunum.

They are well circumscribed, homogenously enhancing soft tissue density masses on CT and MRI, which may calcify or ulcerate if large. Differentiation from GIST is not possible by imaging and requires histological analysis. Lesions larger than 6 cm, with irregular margins or associated lymphadenopathy, are suspicious for leiomyosarcoma. Symptomatic lesions, including those which present with obstruction, hemorrhage, and anemia, are surgically resected (Fig. 18.6).

Several non-neoplastic lesions present as mass-like on imaging, constituting a potential source of confusion. Small bowel diverticulitis, though rare, presents as a round, debris-filled mass-like structure with associated bowel wall thickening and mesenteric fat inflammatory changes. A Meckel diverticulum may appear as a mass-like blind-ended debris-filled pouch on the antimesenteric border of the distal ileum. An intramural hematoma appears as thickened, hyperattenuating bowel wall with possible luminal narrowing and obstruction and occurs in trauma or blood dyscrasias such as hemophilia.

18.3.2 Polyposis Syndromes

Polyposis syndromes include Familial Adenomatous Polyposis (FAP), and its variants Gardner and Turcot syndromes and Peutz-Jeghers syndrome, among others. Because many polypoid lesions are present, the risk of malignancy is greater. Patients may be symptomatic due to the polyps acting as lead points, causing intussusception. MR-E is the imaging exam of choice for the detection and characterization of multiple polyps.

FAP is an autosomal dominant condition manifesting with many premalignant colonic adenomas, with over 80% of patients also developing adenomas in the small bowel, most commonly in the periampullary region. Due to the near definite risk of developing colon cancer, patients undergo prophylactic proctocolectomy, though these patients are still at risk of developing small bowel malignancies. As it is not possible to remove all small intestine adenomas, only large ones are resected, and patients are monitored at regular intervals. Patients are also at risk of developing Gardner's syndrome, or mesenteric fibromatosis (locally aggressive desmoid tumors), which can infiltrate adjacent structures including the small bowel and cause obstruction.

Peutz-Jegher's syndrome is a rare, autosomal dominantly inherited condition with multiple hamartomatous polyps in the digestive tract, specifically the small bowel. In general, these lesions have much lower malignant potential than adenomas. Patients may suffer episodes of intermittent intussusception and bleeding. On CT or MRI, these lesions appear as smooth or lobulated, enhancing intrinsic

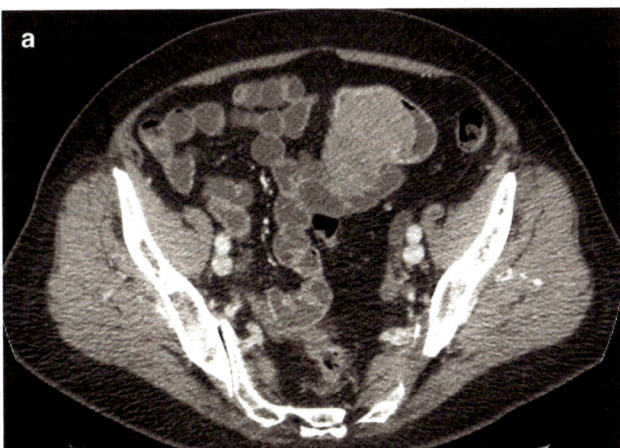

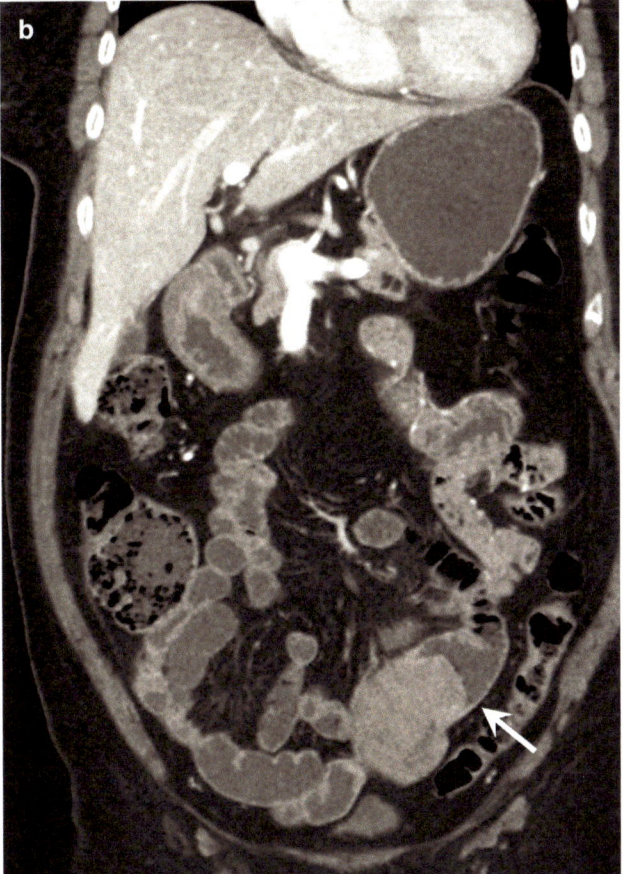

Fig. 18.6 Leiomyoma. Axial (**a**) and coronal (**b**) CT images of a patient with a well-marginated, homogenously enhancing small bowel mass causing partial obstruction with mild proximal bowel dilatation (arrow). This lesion was ultimately diagnosed as leiomyoma on histology. Based on this imaging, the main differential diagnosis is GIST

filling defects in the small bowel lumen. This syndrome is also characterized by mucocutaneous perioral and genital melanin pigmentation, known as pluriorificial ectodermosis. Patients are also at increased risk of developing gynecological malignancies [5, 16].

18.3.3 Malignant Neoplasms

Imaging characteristics suggestive of a malignant lesion include irregular margins with heterogeneous enhancement, and invasion of adjacent structures. Due to nonspecific symptoms and low clinical suspicion, small bowel malignancies are often diagnosed at advanced stages and thus carry a poor prognosis [16]. Risk factors for primary malignancies include chronic inflammation, HIV infection and inherited conditions including hereditary nonpolyposis colorectal cancer (HNPCC), familial adenomatous polyposis (FAP) and Peutz-Jeghers syndrome. Metastatic lesions, most commonly from breast and lung cancer and melanoma, are more frequent than primary small bowel malignancy (Fig. 18.7).

For many years, adenocarcinoma constituted the most common histologic type of primary small bowel malignancy, though in recent years, it has been surpassed by neuroendocrine (carcinoid) tumors (NETs) [17].

Small bowel adenocarcinomas arise most commonly in the distal duodenum and proximal jejunum. On CT and MRI, they appear as an enhancing soft tissue density/intensity mass with possible luminal narrowing, either with eccentric or circumferential growth ("apple core" sign, like adenocarcinomas in the colon). They may present with vascular invasion, lymphadenopathy, peritoneal masses and obstruction. Adenocarcinomas, like other small bowel malignancies, often metastasize to the liver due to rich mesenteric venous drainage.

Gastrointestinal stromal tumor (GIST) originates from the interstitial cells of Cajal and is defined by its expression of KIT (CD117), a tyrosine kinase growth factor receptor. GISTs usually behave non-aggressively, though a minority display overtly malignant clinical behavior. GISTs often extend exophytically into the bowel lumen and the mesentery and may variably contain calcifications. On MRI, they display low T1 and high T2 signal intensity. It may be difficult to differentiate aggressive from non-aggressive GIST based on imaging alone. Non-aggressive lesions tend to be smaller than 5 cm, well circumscribed, have poor contrast enhancement and a low mitotic index on histology [5]. Aggressive lesions tend to be large and have a lobulated margin and heterogeneous enhancement, often with areas of necrosis and cavitation which may communicate with the bowel lumen. GIST may metastasize to the omentum, peritoneum, liver, or even extra-abdominally. Associated bulky adenopathy is rare with GIST. Since all GISTs are potentially malignant, they are considered for resection even if relatively small [16].

Gastrointestinal NETs arise from intraepithelial endocrine cells. 90% of small bowel NETs arise in the distal ileum and many are multifocal. Often the primary lesion is not visible on initial imaging, or it presents as a small intraluminal filling defect. More commonly, NET presents as a spiculated

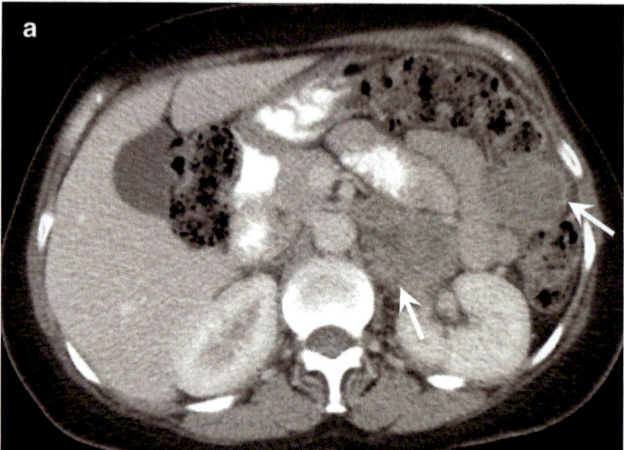

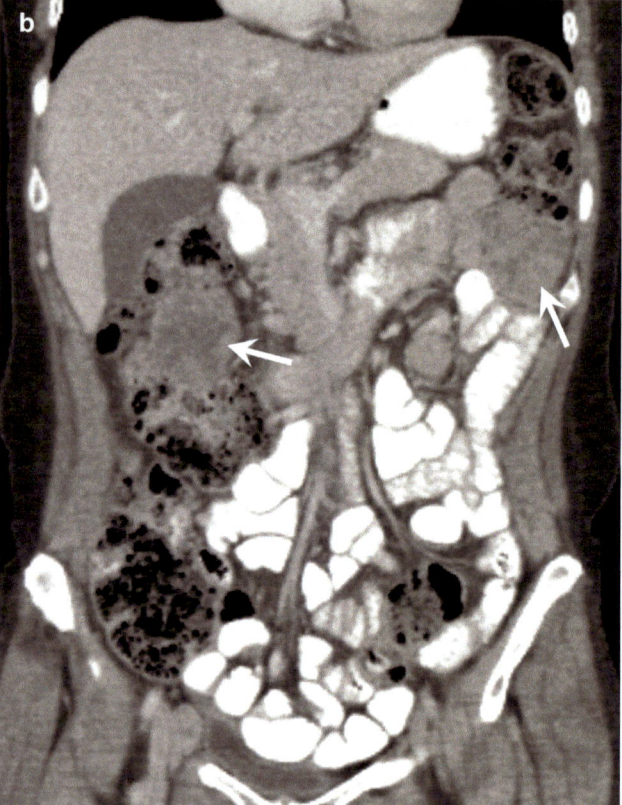

Fig. 18.7 Melanoma metastasis to small bowel. Axial (**a**) and coronal (**b**) CT images in a patient with metastatic melanoma, with multiple small bowel masses (arrows)

mesenteric mass eliciting a desmoplastic reaction, the result of regional metastasis. The tumor may have avid arterial contrast enhancement and contain calcifications. The tumor, along with the surrounding desmoplastic reaction, may cause small bowel obstruction or ischemia. Metastases to the liver may lead to carcinoid syndrome, manifesting with diarrhea, skin rash, sweating and, in severe cases, bronchospasm, flushing, and hypotension (Fig. 18.8).

Small bowel lymphoma may be primary (with no other lymphoma lesions) or part of systemic lymphoma at discov-

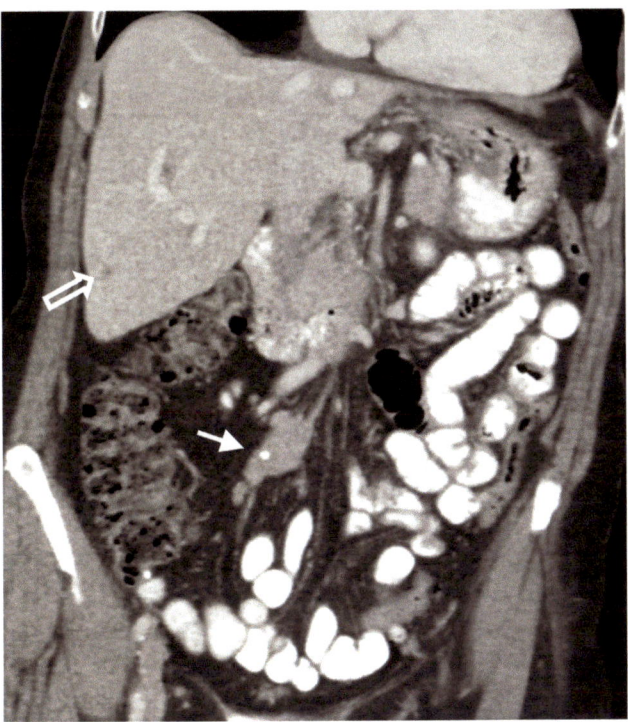

Fig. 18.8 NET. Coronal CT image of a patient with small bowel NET manifesting with a lobulated mesentery mass representing regional metastatic focus with internal calcifications (solid arrow). A liver metastasis at the inferior pole of the liver is partially visualized (hollow arrow)

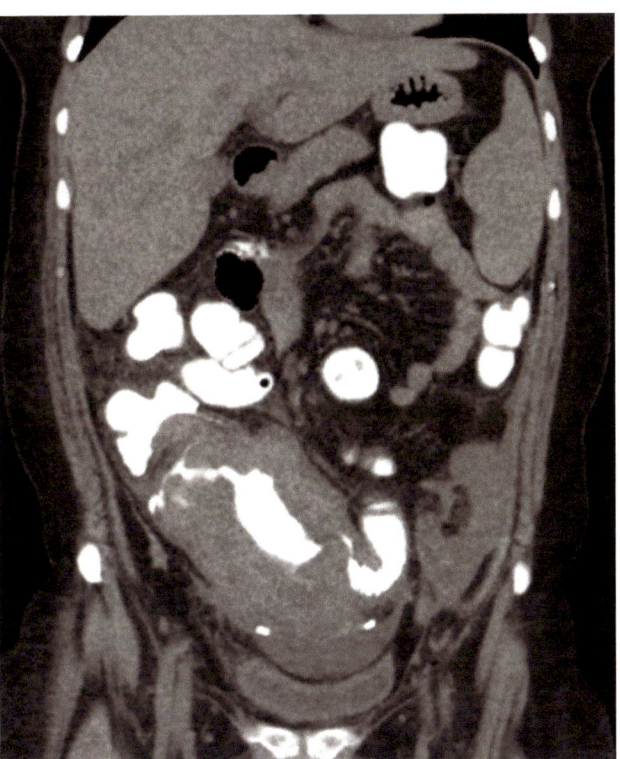

Fig. 18.9 Coronal CT image of a patient with small bowel lymphoma after undergoing a kidney transplant. Note mass-like concentric thickening of the bowel wall with luminal narrowing

ery. When primary, the most common location is in the ileum due to abundant lymphoid tissue. There is often associated bulky adenopathy and multifocal disease. Lymphoma has multiple possible radiologic appearances, including mass-like wall thickening and dilatation (pseudoaneurysmal), a polypoid mass projecting into the lumen, a cavitary soft tissue mass (endoexoenteric) or with extension into the surrounding mesentery (Fig. 18.9). The stenosing form is rare and is frequently a complication of long-standing celiac disease. The most common form is pseudoaneurysmal. Due to its various presentations, lymphoma may be difficult to distinguish from other small bowel malignancies on imaging. A more distal location and multifocal involvement may assist in differentiating lymphoma from adenocarcinoma, while bulky adenopathy associated with lymphoma is not common in GIST.

Sarcoma is a relatively rare primary malignancy in the small bowel, constituting about 10% of small bowel cancers. The most common type is leiomyosarcoma, most frequently appearing in the jejunum. On CT and MRI, leiomyosarcoma appears as a large heterogeneously enhancing mass with central necrosis. The mass may cavitate and communicate with the bowel lumen. Radiological characteristics may overlap those of GIST [16].

> **Key Point**
> Benign characteristics of a small bowel tumor include a round and well-circumscribed intrinsic filling defect with smooth margins. Benign lesions include adenoma, lipoma, and leiomyoma. Malignant characteristics include irregular margins with heterogeneous enhancement and invasion of adjacent structures. Malignant tumors include adenocarcinoma, NET, malignant GIST, lymphoma, and sarcoma.

18.4 Mesenteric Ischemia

The superior mesenteric artery (SMA), which supplies the jejunum and ileum, is a large caliber vessel with a narrow origin, rendering it susceptible to embolic phenomena and occlusion. When collateral vascular pathways cannot compensate for SMA occlusion and the perfusion of the small bowel is compromised, mesenteric ischemia occurs [5]. Mesenteric ischemia may be acute or chronic. Prompt diagnosis and intervention are critical, particularly when the ischemia is acute, as delayed intervention often results in catastrophic complications [18]. Since neither laboratory tests nor clinical examination is specific for mesenteric ischemia, imaging plays a critical role in its diagnosis. The gold standard imaging test for mesenteric ischemia is CT-A. Oral contrast material is usually not appropriate in acute cases, as it can interfere with detecting subtle changes in bowel wall enhancement, its administration can cause diagnostic delays and it is often not propagated well due to development of dynamic ileus and fluid-filled bowel loops.

Mesenteric ischemia manifests initially as mucosal injury, as the bowel mucosa is the most susceptible to vascular compromise, with progression in severity to transmural necrosis (bowel infarction), perforation, and peritonitis. Stricture formation and obstruction may occur with long-standing chronic ischemia [5].

The etiology of acute mesenteric ischemia is embolic occlusion in 40–50% of cases. Emboli may appear as high-attenuation findings in the SMA on non-contrast CT images or cause filling defects distally. In acute infarction, the diameter of the SMA is often enlarged with simultaneous reduction of the caliber of the SMV, causing reversal of the normal size relation between them. Contrast enhancement in the affected bowel wall is diminished or absent. As damage progresses, muscular tone is lost, and the bowel wall becomes progressively thinner as the bowel dilates as transmural infarction occurs ("paper thin wall"). If bowel thickening occurs, notably with a halo or target pattern on contrast images, it is usually due to reperfusion and is an encouraging sign. Conversely, intramural gas (pneumatosis intestinalis) and air in the mesenteric and portal venous system are highly suggestive of bowel infarction (Fig. 18.10). Visualization of extraintestinal gas is indicative of perforation, which also may be associated with mesenteric fat stranding and ascites. Hyperattenuation of bowel loops on non-contrast phases may be caused by hemorrhagic infarction.

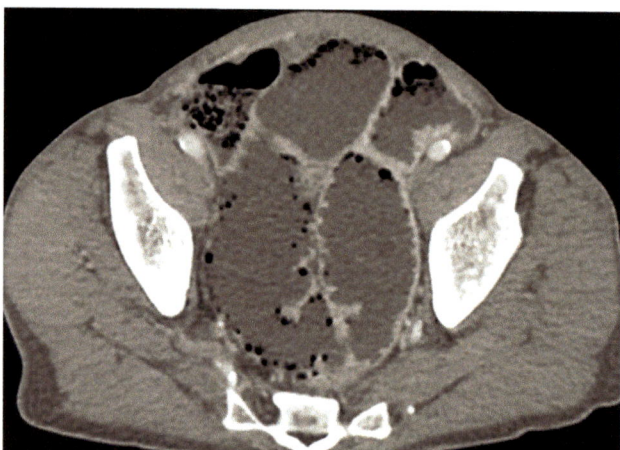

Fig. 18.10 Axial enhanced CT image of a patient with mesenteric ischemia displaying distended, fluid-filled bowel loops and thin bowel walls, with pneumatosis intestinalis

Other causes of acute infarction include thrombus formation in a previously stenotic vessel, dissection, or arterial inflammation. Some cases, notably in thrombus formation within chronically diseased vessels, may have a more indolent course due to the development of vascular collaterals [18, 19]. An additional form of this condition is non-obstructive mesenteric ischemia (NOMI), in which systemic hypotension leads to vascular spasm of the mesenteric vessels. It is associated with low-flow states, such as cardiac insufficiency, severe trauma or, classically, patients undergoing hemodialysis [18]. Unlike in obstructive forms of mesenteric ischemia, in NOMI a main finding is narrowing origins of mesenteric branches and alternate dilatation and narrowing of intestinal branches, with discontinuous and segmental bowel involvement. Because distal branches of the SMA are difficult to visualize on CT, angiography has an important role in the diagnosis of this entity [19].

The vast majority (>90%) of chronic mesenteric ischemia is related to progressive atherosclerosis at the origins of mesenteric vessels [18]. The diagnosis of chronic mesenteric ischemia is based on clinical symptoms, classically postprandial abdominal pain and weight loss, and anatomic findings, including atherosclerotic occlusion of at least two of the three main splanchnic arteries without evidence of other gastrointestinal pathologies [5]. Although significant atherosclerotic calcifications of mesenteric vessels can also often be visualized in SMA acute thrombus formation, in chronic ischemia without acute thrombosis the appearance of the bowel is usually normal [19].

A minority of cases (5–15%) are due to mesenteric venous thrombosis and resultant bowel edema and diminished perfusion, usually in the setting of hypercoagulable states. Unlike acute arterial mesenteric ischemia, these are not surgical emergencies and often respond to anticoagulation [18]. On imaging, thrombi may be visualized in the mesenteric and portal veins as filling defects surrounded by rim-enhanced venous walls, along with accompanying engorgement of mesenteric veins and prominent bowel wall thickening with halo or target pattern enhancement. Mesenteric fat stranding and ascites are common findings and do not correlate with severity of bowel damage as in acute arterial ischemia. However, bowel wall enhancement may be diminished or absent with severe ischemia [19].

Ischemia may also develop due to secondary causes, such as bowel obstruction. In these cases, treatment of the primary cause is essential.

Key Point

Acute mesenteric ischemia is a surgical emergency and diagnosis must be made rapidly. Signs of irreversible ischemic bowel damage include a "paper-thin" bowel wall, pneumatosis intestinalis and portal venous air, prolonged absence of bowel wall enhancement and signs of perforation including extraintestinal air.

18.5 Concluding Remarks

The small bowel encompasses most of the surface area of the gastrointestinal tract and much of it is inaccessible to endoscopic study. As such, cross-sectional radiological imaging is an imperative component of assessing pathology in the small bowel. Numerous important clinical entities arise in the small intestine, with varying degrees of clinical urgency. In all the above pathologies, imaging constitutes an essential role in establishing a timely diagnosis and directing management. To this end, special care must be taken to choose the appropriate imaging study in any given clinical setting. Comprehensive knowledge of normal and pathologic bowel appearance on various studies is a prerequisite in delivering good care for patients.

Take-Home Messages
- CT and MRI have largely replaced conventional fluoroscopic-based methods of small bowel imaging, with CT-E and MR-E constituting the most specific techniques of small bowel imaging. While MR-E holds a greater role in outpatient settings, CT is often used in acute clinical scenarios.
- MR-E plays a vital role in the assessment of disease activity, complications, and response to treatment for Crohn's disease. Because of radiation concerns in a population of largely young patients, CT is utilized sparingly and reserved for identification of surgical complications in the emergency setting.
- Due to varied and nonspecific symptomology, celiac disease is often left undiagnosed for years. It is important to recognize characteristic features of small bowel malabsorption pattern (MABP) on abdominal imaging, which can indicate the need for further diagnostic testing, in order to minimize complications.
- Though rare, it is critical to identify and characterize small bowel tumors, including on non-targeted abdominal imaging when possible, as often symptoms are nonspecific and diagnosis is delayed. Small bowel malignancies include adenocarcinoma and NETs, and more rarely malignant GIST, lymphoma and sarcoma. MR-E serves as a primary tool for follow-up of multiple small bowel polyps in polyposis syndromes.
- Imaging plays a critical role in the diagnosis of mesenteric ischemia, with CT angiography being the gold standard imaging modality. Acute embolic mesenteric ischemia is a surgical emergency with high mortality rates and prompt intervention is vital.

References

1. Horsthuis K, Stokkers PC, Stoker J. Detection of inflammatory bowel disease: diagnostic performance of cross-sectional imaging modalities. Abdom Imaging. 2008;33(4):407–16.
2. Masselli G, Gualdi G. CT and MR enterography in evaluating small bowel diseases: when to use which modality? Abdom Imaging. 2013;38:249–59.
3. Saevik F, Eriksen R, Eide GE, Gilja OH, Nylund K. Development and validation of a simple ultrasound activity score for crohn's disease. J Crohns Colitis. 2021;15(1):115–24.
4. Taylor SA, Avni F, Cronin CG, Hoeffel C, Kim SH, Laghi A, Napolitano M, Petit P, Rimola J, Tolan DJ, Torkzad MR, Zappa M, Bhatnagar G, Puylaert C, Stoker J. The first joint ESGAR/ESPR consensus statement on the technical performance of cross-sectional small bowel and colonic imaging. Eur Radiol. 2017;27(6):2570–82.
5. Hamm B, Ros PR. Abdominal imaging. Berlin, Heidelberg: Springer; 2013.
6. Deepak P, Fletcher JG, Fidler JL, Barlow JM, Sheedy SP, Kolbe AB, Harmsen WS, Loftus EV, Hansel SL, Becker BD, Bruining DH. Radiological response is associated with better long-term outcomes and is a potential treatment target in patients with small bowel Crohn's disease. Am J Gastroenterol. 2016;111(7):997–1006.
7. Bruining DH, Zimmermann EM, Loftus EV Jr, Sandborn WJ, Sauer CG, Strong SA, Society of Abdominal Radiology Crohn's Disease-Focused Panel. Consensus recommendations for evaluation, interpretation, and utilization of computed tomography and magnetic resonance enterography in patients with small bowel Crohn's disease. Gastroenterology. 2018;154(4):1172–94.
8. Scholz FJ, Afnan J, Behr SC. CT findings in adult celiac disease. Radiographics. 2008;31(4):977–92.
9. Sheedy SP, Barlow JM, Fletcher JG, Smyrk TC, Scholz FJ, Codipilly DC, Al Bawardy BF, Fidler JL. Beyond moulage sign and TTG levels: the role of cross-sectional imaging in celiac sprue. Abdom Radiol. 2017;42(2):361–88.
10. Soyer P, Boudiaf M, Dray X, Fargeaudou Y, Vahedi K, Aout M, Vicaut E, Hamzi L, Rymer R. CT enteroclysis features of uncomplicated celiac disease: retrospective analysis of 44 patients. Radiology. 2009;253(2):416–24.
11. Sarwani N, Tappouni R, Tice J. Pathophysiology of acute small bowel disease with CT correlation. Clin Radiol. 2011;66(1):73–82.
12. Bresee JS, Marcus R, Venezia RA, Keene WE, Morse D, Thanassi M, Brunett P, Bulens S, Beard RS, Dauphin LA, Slutsker L, Bopp C, Eberhard M, Hall A, Vinje J, Monroe SS, Glass RI, US Acute Gastroenteritis Etiology Study Team. The etiology of severe acute gastroenteritis among adults visiting emergency departments in the United States. J Infect Dis. 2012;205(9):1374–81.
13. Cheung KS, Hung IFN, Chan PPY, Lung KC, Tso E, Liu R, Ng YY, Chu MY, Chung TWH, Tam AR, Yip CCY, Leung KH, Fung AY, Zhang RR, Lin Y, Cheng HM, Zhang AJX, To KKW, Chan KH, Yuen KY, Leung WK. Gastrointestinal manifestations of SARS-CoV-2 infection and virus load in fecal samples from a Hong Kong cohort: systematic review and meta-analysis. Gastroenterology. 2020;159(1):81–95.
14. Lamers MM, Beumer J, van der Vaart J, Knoops K, Puschhof J, Breugem TI, Ravelli RBG, Paul van Schayck J, Mykytyn AZ, Duimel HQ, van Donselaar E, Riesebosch S, Kuijpers HJH, Schipper D, van de Wetering WJ, de Graaf M, Koopmans M, Cuppen E, Peters PJ, Haagmans BL, Clevers H. SARS-CoV-2 productively infects human gut enterocytes. Science. 2020;369(6499):50–4.
15. Siegel RL, Miller KD, Fuchs HE, Jemal A. cancer statistics, 2022. CA Cancer J Clin. 2022;72(1):7–33.
16. Jasti R, Carucci LR. Small bowel neoplasms: a pictorial review. Radiographics. 2020;40(4):1020–38.

17. Bilimoria KY, Bentrem DJ, Wayne JD, Ko CY, Bennett CL, Talamonti MS. Small bowel cancer in the United States: changes in epidemiology, treatment, and survival over the last 20 years. Ann Surg. 2009;249(1):63–71.

18. Clair DG, Beach JM. Mesenteric ischemia. N Engl J Med. 2016;374(10):959–68.

19. Kanasaki S, Furukawa A, Fumoto K, Hamanaka Y, Ota S, Hirose T, Inoue A, Shirakawa T, Hung Nguyen LD, Tulyeubai S. Acute mesenteric ischemia: multidetector CT findings and endovascular management. Radiographics. 2018;38(3):945–61.

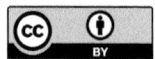

Small Bowel Disease: An Approach to Optimise Imaging Technique and Interpretation

Damian J. M. Tolan

Learning Objectives
- To understand the main clinical presentations of patients with small bowel disease.
- To know the place of radiological assessment for investigation compared with endoscopic techniques.
- To know how to select an appropriate CT protocol to evaluate patients from the clinical presentation.
- To know imaging features that warrant consideration of emergency surgery.

19.1 Introduction

The aim of this chapter is to provide an approach to deal with small bowel disease in routine clinical practice. It will provide advice on imaging protocols and the imaging signs to search for to produce a diagnosis, particularly those which indicate urgent clinical intervention. The focus is on common conditions and the usual management. Rare conditions are mentioned to illustrate that not everything is common or usual!

19.2 Setting the Scene: Case Presentation and Patient Factors

Small bowel diseases form a small contribution to the total workload of an abdominal radiologist but are challenging because of the length of small bowel being evaluated and the difficulty detecting abnormalities while trying to avoid false-positive diagnosis. Generally, patients present either as an emergency after acute admission or in a more indolent man-

ner as an outpatient. The chapter will be divided into those two distinct referral sources to reflect daily radiology practice.

Furthermore, the approach will focus on the main clinical presentations leading to a request for imaging to assist in diagnosis of small bowel disease. In the emergency setting, three main presenting scenarios are presented; overt or obscure GI bleeding; suspicion of bowel obstruction; and unexplained acute abdominal pain, with or without signs of sepsis. In outpatients the assessment focuses on two presentations; symptoms of weight loss, abdominal pain and altered bowel habit, where there is concern for malignancy or inflammatory bowel disease; and iron deficiency anaemia with occult obscure GI bleeding.

19.2.1 Emergency Small Bowel Conditions: Common Clinical Presentations

CT has an established critical role in the assessment of the acute abdomen. While some patient diagnoses are quite clear at the time of presentation, like acute GI haemorrhage, others are not, such as small bowel ischaemia or perforation and the radiologist may be the first to consider or confirm the diagnosis. This presents difficulties when deciding the optimal protocol as the clinical differential diagnosis can be quite wide and a compromise must be made to prevent routine excessive radiation exposure in all cases while providing an accurate diagnosis for a majority of patients.

19.2.1.1 CT Intravenous Contrast Considerations

A weight-based iso- or hypo-osmolar intravenous iodinated contrast should be preferred. Evaluation of renal function should not delay CT scans in a critical care setting where prompt accurate diagnosis is the greatest priority [1]. Estimated Glomerular Filtration Rate assessment may be helpful before CT for clinicians to understand potential

D. J. M. Tolan (✉)
Department of Radiology, St James's University Hospital, Leeds teaching Hospitals NHS Trust, Leeds, West Yorkshire, UK
e-mail: damian.tolan@nhs.net.uk

© The Author(s) 2023
J. Hodler et al. (eds.), *Diseases of the Abdomen and Pelvis 2023-2026*, IDKD Springer Series,
https://doi.org/10.1007/978-3-031-27355-1_19

impact of contrast on renal function and reduction in renal function can be supported with renal replacement therapy if necessary. Where possible a rapid contrast injection (3–5 mL/s) allows optimal identification of vessels, hypervascular lesions, and bleeding locations with 350 mg/mL Iodinated contrast dose at 1.2–1.5 mL/kg.

19.2.1.2   CT Scan Phase Choices for Acquisition

- **Non-contrast CT** for detection of free gas, dilated small bowel in the presence of obstruction, blood in the lumen of the bowel from bleeding and intramural haemorrhage which is associated with ischaemia and infarction.
- **Late arterial phase CT** (10 s post peak aortic enhancement) for acute gastrointestinal bleeding to optimise arterial enhancement to see occlusions and arterial jets of contrast at the site of brisk haemorrhage.
- **Enteric phase CT** (45–50 s post injection) for optimal evaluation of small bowel enhancement and detection of focal bowel lesions.
- **Portal venous phase CT** (65–75 s post injection) for delayed or slow contrast pooling from extravasation and global assessment of bowel and other viscera in the setting of ischaemia or obstruction.

Routine thin slice reconstructions (1 mm or less) are important for evaluation of vessels and detection of sites of bleeding and multiplanar reformation to appreciate global small bowel enhancement patterns and to detect focal abnormalities like strictures, transition points in obstruction and bleeding [2].

19.2.1.3   CT Luminal Contrast: What Role?

Luminal contrast has a very limited role emergency small bowel CT. Oral contrast delays scanning and it is not appropriate in patients with small bowel obstruction or perforation because of subsequent general anaesthesia and risk of aspiration, in addition to unpleasantness of drinking contrast when patients are unwell with an acute abdomen.

Positive oral contrast should be avoided as it obscures many signs being sought (such as intramural or intraluminal haemorrhage), and the contrast density makes it more difficult to appreciate reduced bowel enhancement.

Specific neutral contrast agents (like Mannitol or Polyethylene Glycol) are usually unnecessary in an acute setting since most of the diseases that might cause an acute hospital admission, such as enteritis from infection or Crohn's disease, are easily appreciated without it. Water may be given for pre-hydration to reduce the opportunity for contrast induced kidney injury in a sub-acute situation.

19.2.1.4   What Role for MR and Ultrasound?

MRI offers a global assessment of the small bowel without radiation. This may be advantageous in young patients and in pregnancy but relies on sufficient expertise in interpretation and access out of normal working hours (Fig. 19.1). The examinations are longer (20–30 min) and require greater patient cooperation with multiple breath holds and the enclosed environment may not be appropriate if patients are acutely unwell with risk of vomiting. MR enterography is particularly useful in reassessing patients with Crohn's disease with deterioration in symptoms requiring hospital admission and sub-acute reassessment for complications and evaluation of disease activity, as they may have multiple examinations and accumulate a high lifetime radiation dose from CT. However in the situation of possible perforation, it is inappropriate to wait for MRI and CT is an acceptable test to plan emergency patient management.

Ultrasound also allows evaluation of patients with small bowel disease but a global assessment of acute small bowel

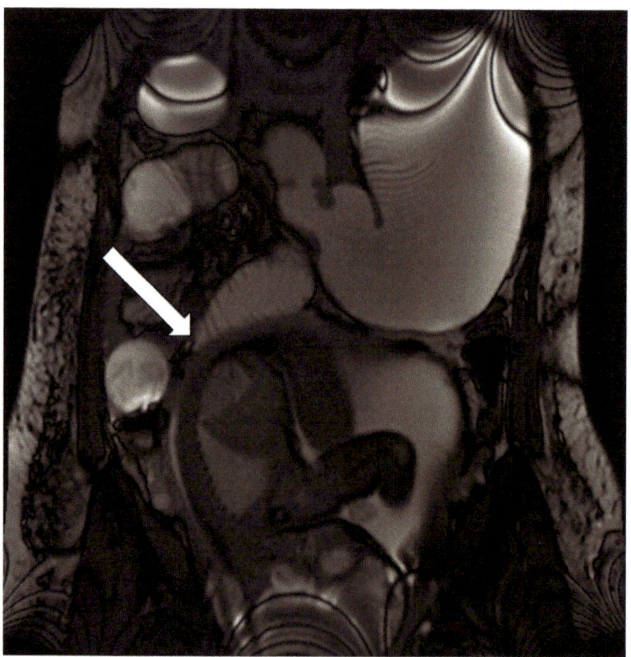

Fig. 19.1 Acute admission with vomiting at 34 weeks gestation and previous RYGB. MR abdomen with FISP coronal showing obstruction at the J-J anastomosis with dilatation and obstruction of the biliopancreatic limb (white arrow). Laparoscopic revision of the anastomosis post MRI with a healthy baby delivered 6 weeks later

diseases is challenging particularly in the setting of obstruction or in the presence of high volumes of bowel gas or intraperitoneal perforation. Its role is limited and may be in the incidental detection of important abnormalities when acute ultrasound is being performed for other reasons.

> **Key Point**
> - CT is the imaging technique of choice for acute abdomen emergency assessment of the small bowel. MR enterography is preferred to assess patients with Crohn's disease where this is feasible.

19.2.1.5 Relevant Diseases and Imaging Signs

Overt or Obscure GI Bleeding

Clinical Context
CT has an important role to detect the source of acute GI bleeding where an upper GI endoscopy has failed to detect the source. Overt denotes visible bleeding (usually melaena or hematochezia in proximal or distal small bowel bleeding, respectively), whereas obscure bleeding describes a bleeding source which is undetected after previous full assessment of the GI system with upper and lower GI endoscopy and small bowel [3]. The role of CT is to detect the source of haemorrhage and direct management to arrest bleeding using endovascular or endoscopic interventional therapies.

Upper GI bleeding is usually excluded by negative endoscopy to the second part of duodenum. Bleeding in the distal duodenum and rest of the small bowel makes up a minority of cases (around 10%). Video capsule endoscopy and double balloon enteroscopy both have a higher yield than CT for detection of the source of bleeding and should be the first line investigation, with CT reserved for unstable patients where there is active haemorrhage [3].

Since CT detection requires the identification of contrast extravasation then immediate access to scanning is the key.

Recommended CT Protocol
Triple phase CT protocol with weight-based iodinated contrast injection and non-contrast, late arterial and portal venous acquisition without oral contrast.

Relevant Conditions and Imaging Signs
Inflammatory bowel disease and Meckel diverticulum are frequent causes of small bowel bleeding in younger patients and NSAID enteropathy (Fig. 19.2) and angioectasia (Fig. 19.3) in older patients, while small bowel neoplasia is seen in both groups including benign polyposis syndromes (e.g., Peutz-Jeghers), lymphoma, neuroendocrine tumours, and adenocarcinoma [3, 4].

Acute bleeding is best appreciated by careful evaluation for contrast leak from vessels or tumours into the bowel lumen on thin slice reconstructions. Underlying structural lesions causing bleeding like tumours and benign small bowel strictures are better appreciated on enteric and portal venous phase imaging. Tumours and polyps typically enhance uniformly and maximally in the enteric and portal venous phase, while neuroendocrine tumours tend to hyper enhance in late arterial phase and wash out. Malignant tumours are indicated by transmural abnormalities extending into the perienteric fat and presence of metastatic disease in enlarged local lymph nodes or elsewhere on the scan [5]. Layered and homogenous enhancement patterns of diffuse or

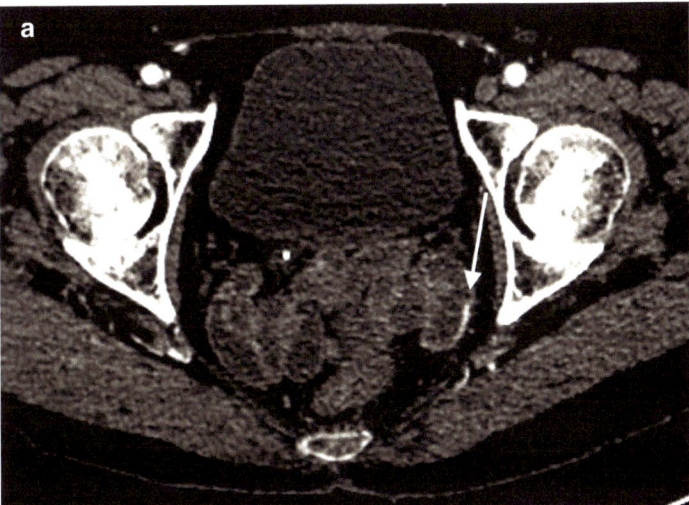
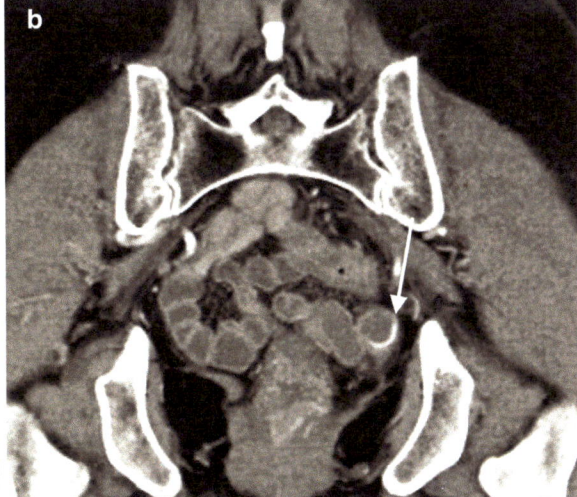

Fig. 19.2 (**a, b**) Axial arterial phase and coronal portal venous phase with contrast extravasation from a jejunal loop in the pelvis from NSAID-induced ulceration. The affected jejunal loop is not thickened

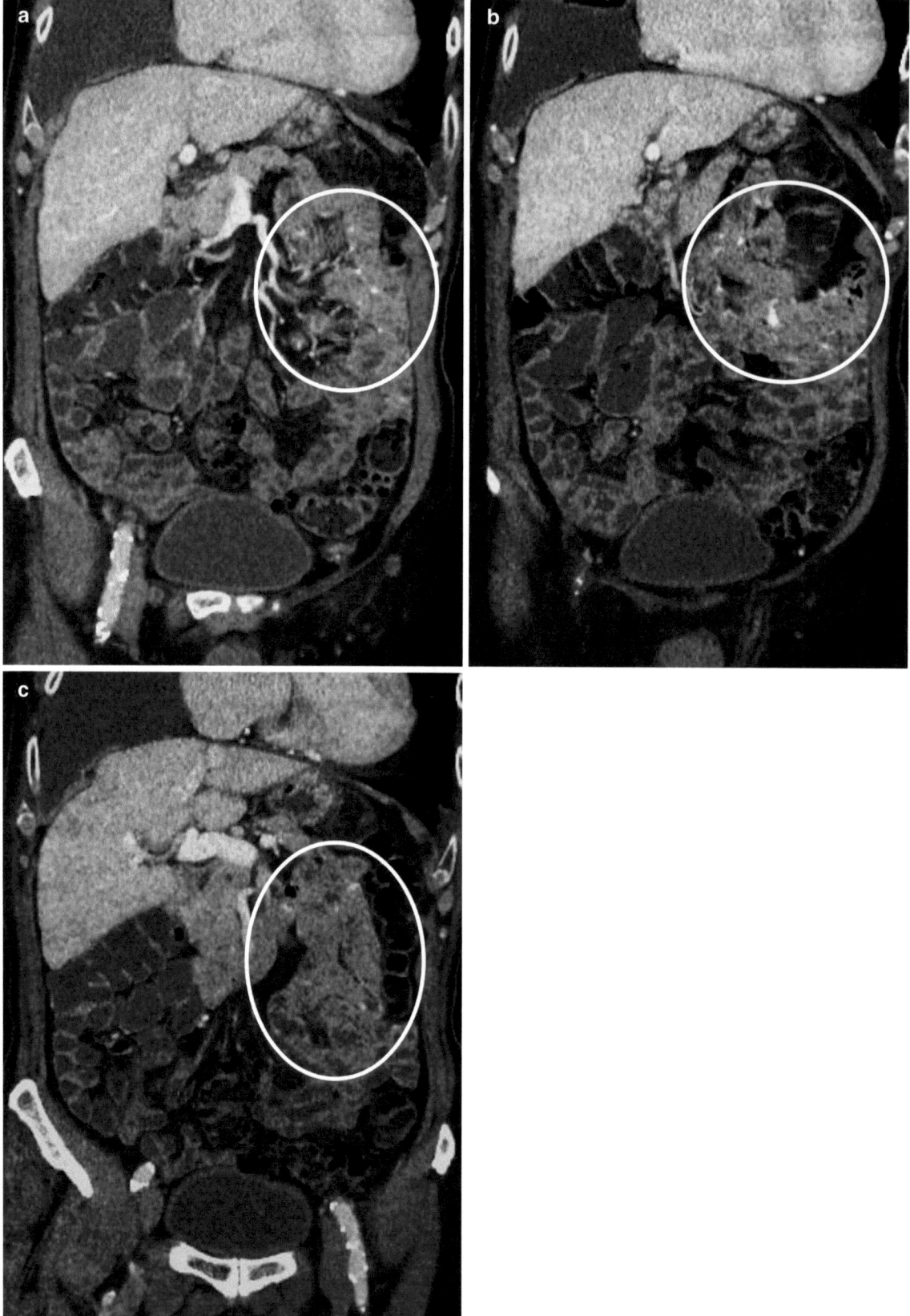

Fig. 19.3 (a–c) Coronal portal venous phase. A 50-year-old male on dialysis with obscure overt GI bleeding. Initial negative CT angiography and further bleeding. Characteristic multifocal angioectasia. Benefit of narrow windows for better visualization

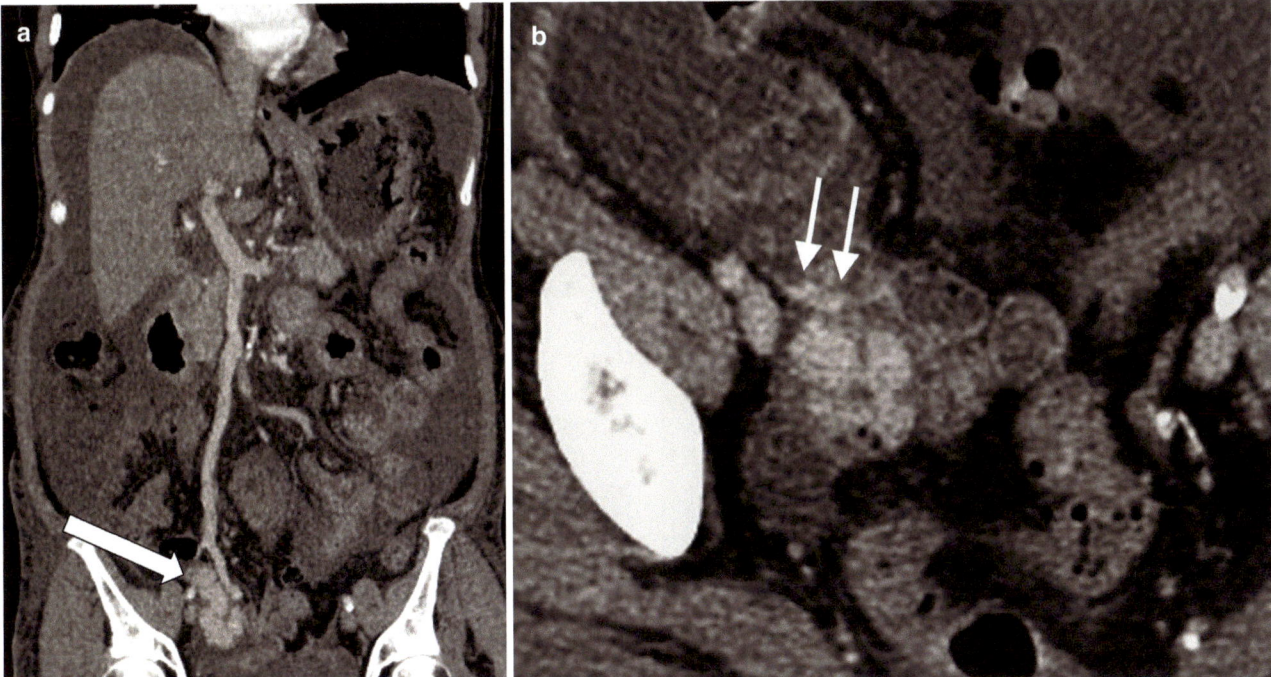

Fig. 19.4 (**a, b**) Coronal and axial CT in a 56-year-old male with occult overt bleeding. Ileal submucosal varices (arrows) and occult cryptogenic cirrhosis unsuspected clinically treated with TIPPS

multifocal small bowel thickening are recognised in Crohn's disease whereas in other forms of enteritis a multifocal 'skip' pattern is less likely.

Angioectasia is a common condition and associated with valvular heart disease in elderly patients. They are typically multiple and detected as a small 2–5 mm rounded enhancing lesion in the jejunum, best appreciated on a narrow abdominal window in an enteric or portal venous phase and detection may be aided with maximum intensity projection [2]. Varices may also be detected as a source of small bowel bleeding but are much less common (Fig. 19.4).

Suspicion of Bowel Obstruction

Clinical Context

CT is an accurate method for diagnosis of small bowel obstruction which is a common cause for acute abdominal presentation. Conservative management is favoured except where obstruction fails to resolve after a period of supportive care or where there are signs of strangulation and small bowel ischaemia. CT is an essential tool to confirm the diagnosis and underlying cause for small bowel obstruction and to search for signs that predict adverse outcomes such as ischaemia, warranting emergency surgery.

Recommended CT Protocol

A CT protocol with rapid weight-based iodinated contrast injection and portal venous acquisition without oral contrast. Where there is pre-scan concern for strangulation/ischaemia

or perforation a non-contrast assessment can assist in detection of intramural haemorrhage [6]. Thin slice acquisition and multiplanar reformation are required to assess for the site and cause of obstruction.

Relevant Conditions and Imaging Signs

'Open loop' obstruction describes a single transition point (Fig. 19.5), whereas a 'closed loop' is formed by a double transition point and leads to increased pressure in a localised small bowel segment which leads to ischaemia and necrosis. Adhesions are the commonest cause by far, from either focal bands or diffuse adhesions. Other causes include hernias (abdominal wall or internal), intrinsic small bowel diseases (Crohn's disease or tumour), obstructing intraluminal body (gallstone or bezoar), or peritoneal infiltration from tumour.

Assessment of the transition point requires a careful thin slice multiplanar assessment to look for an abrupt transition from dilated obstructed bowel to collapsed distal small bowel. Finding the transition point can be challenging when there are multiple dilated loops. The 'small bowel faeces sign' can be helpful when it is present to give a clue of the relevant bowel section to focus on [7].

Adhesions are indicated by absence of other findings, since a 'mass' or wall thickening at the transition points to an alternate pathology such as a tumour or inflammatory stricture which is unlikely to resolve with conservative management. Particular signs of a band adhesion are a 'fat notch sign' at the point of obstruction, whereas more diffuse

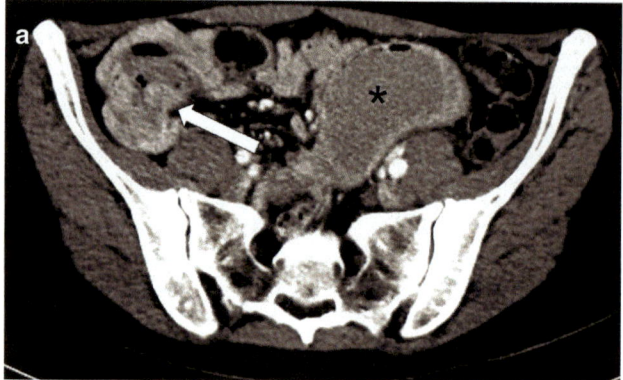

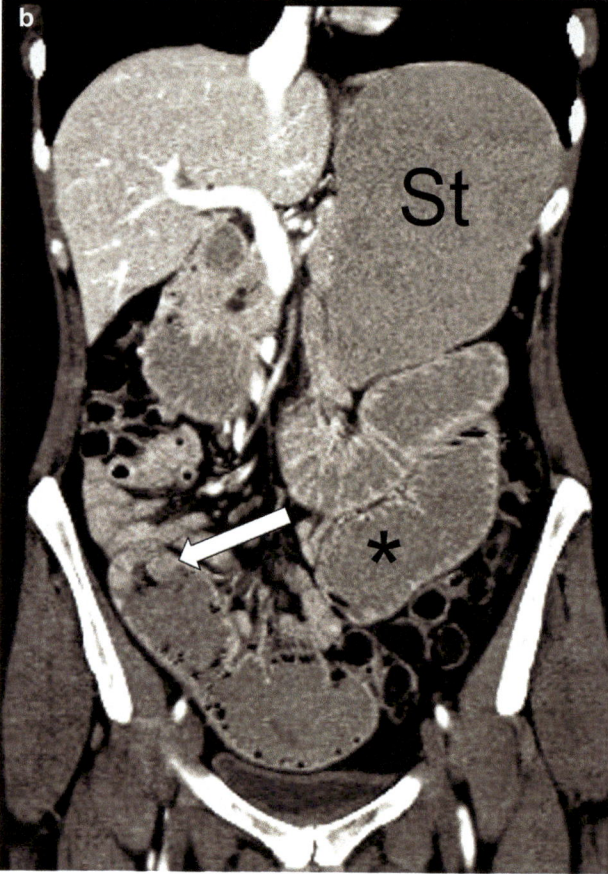

Fig. 19.5 (**a, b**) Axial and coronal portal venous phase CT with obstructing mid jejunal adenocarcinoma with focal annular tumour (arrow) at the transition of dilated small bowel (asterisk). Note grossly distended stomach (St)

adhesions cause generalised angulation and kinking of bowel loops from fixation instead of the expected unimpeded natural looping in the peritoneal cavity. An open loop adhesive obstruction has a single transition while the two transition points forming a closed loop are typically very close, leading to a C or U-shaped dilated segment. The closed loop is most commonly dilated, along with dilatation of the upstream small bowel; however other patterns are recognised with isolated dilatation of the closed loop alone and normal upstream

small bowel (flat belly closed loop obstruction); or a non-dilated closed loop and upstream dilatation [6].

Critical ancillary features predicting ischaemia in closed loop should be specifically searched for and consist of decreased bowel enhancement and diffuse mesenteric haziness (Fig. 19.6). Increased unenhanced bowel wall attenuation on non-contrast CT is also highly predictive of ischaemia in closed loop obstruction from intramural haemorrhage, and this is a potential benefit for including it in routine assessment of bowel ischaemia [6].

> **Key Point**
> • Closed loop obstruction has an increased risk of ischaemia. A double transition should be sought in any small bowel obstruction, along with decreased bowel enhancement and diffuse mesenteric haziness or increased unenhanced bowel wall attenuation on non-contrast CT.

Unexplained Acute Abdominal Pain with or Without Signs of Sepsis

Clinical Context

Small bowel disease can present acutely without obstruction. The main aetiologies relate to diseases causing perforation or ischaemia. Localised or free perforation may present with pain and sepsis and result from intrinsic small bowel diseases, such as Crohn's disease or diverticular disease, or from foreign bodies or trauma. Ischaemia (unrelated to closed loop obstruction) is another important cause and may be related to occlusion of arterial inflow (Fig. 19.7) or venous outflow or diseases of smaller vessels, such as vasculitis and typically presents with sudden onset symptoms. Non-obstructive mesenteric ischaemia is another explanation which is often multifactorial and related to hypoperfusion from cardiovascular disease producing reduced inflow. This can be exacerbated by other factors such as small or large vessel disease (e.g. related to diabetes or atherosclerosis) or medications causing vasoconstriction in critical care environments [8, 9].

Positive oral contrast is not advised as it delays the scan, it is not necessary for the diagnosis of perforation and it interferes with the assessment of bowel enhancement which is critical for the diagnosis of ischaemia [9].

Recommended CT Protocol

Unexplained acute abdominal pain with or without signs of sepsis: weight-based iodinated contrast injection without oral contrast and portal venous acquisition.

High clinical suspicion of ischaemia: weight-based iodinated contrast injection without oral contrast. A triple phase

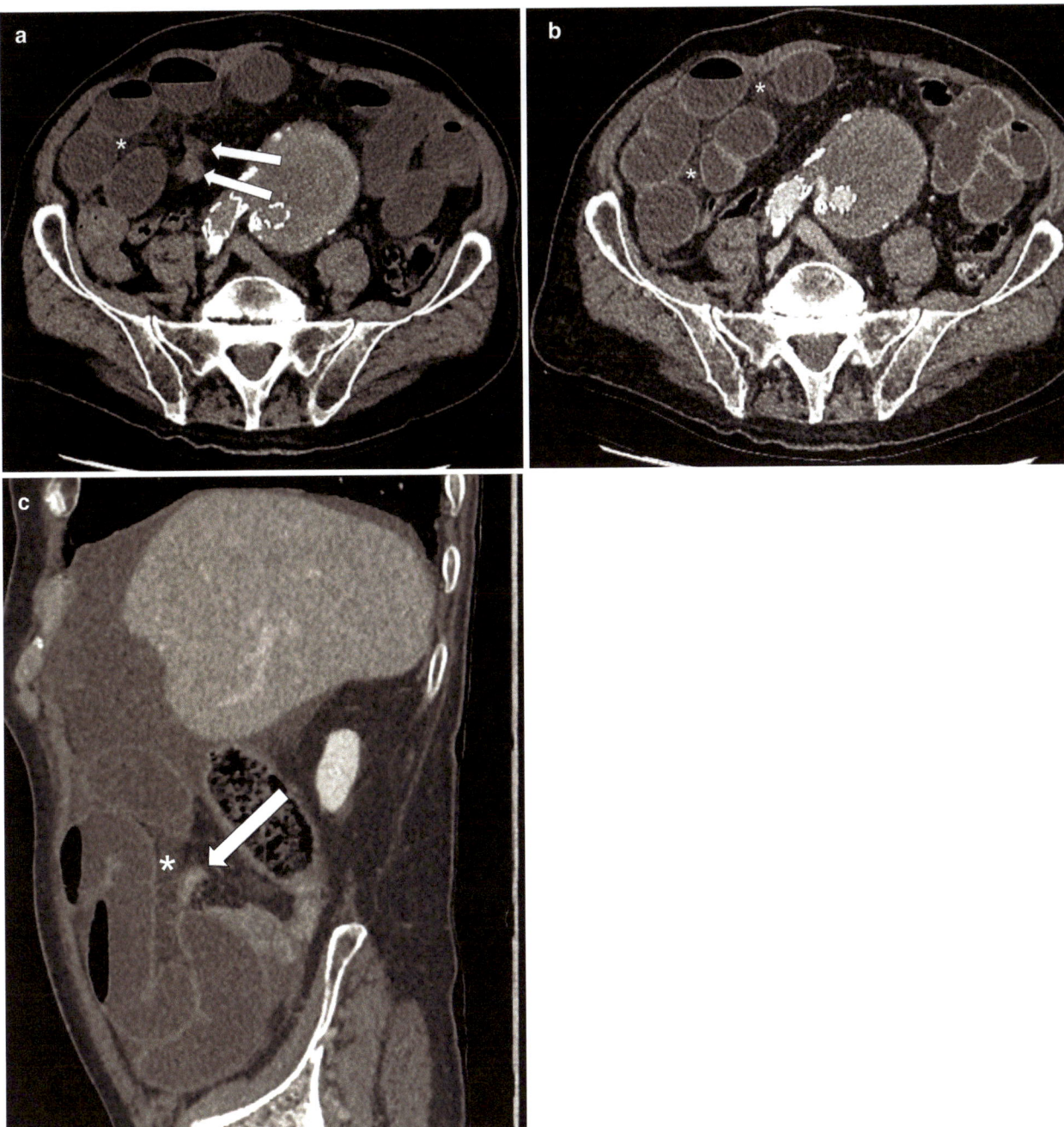

Fig. 19.6 (a) Closed loop small bowel obstruction from band adhesions. Previous EVAR for aortic aneurysm. Non-contrast CT with small bowel obstruction and two adjacent transition points (arrows) as well as stranding in the ileal mesentery (asterisks) in the right side of the abdomen from closed loop obstruction. No hyper density to indicate intramural haemorrhage. (b) axial and (c) sagittal portal venous phase images showing preserved small bowel enhancement

assessment is recommended with non-contrast, early arterial and portal venous acquisition without oral contrast.

Relevant Conditions and Imaging Signs
Perforation is accompanied by localised or free gas, with or without accompanying fluid, peritoneal thickening and enhancement and increased attenuation of mesenteric fat.

While the features or Crohn's disease and bowel tumours are well known, diverticular disease of the jejunum and ileum are a diagnostic challenge. These diverticula can be large and very diffuse and initially appear as additional gas and fluid-filled bowel loops. However, careful inspection reveals diverticula along the mesenteric border of the bowel which may solve an unexplained localised small bowel perforation

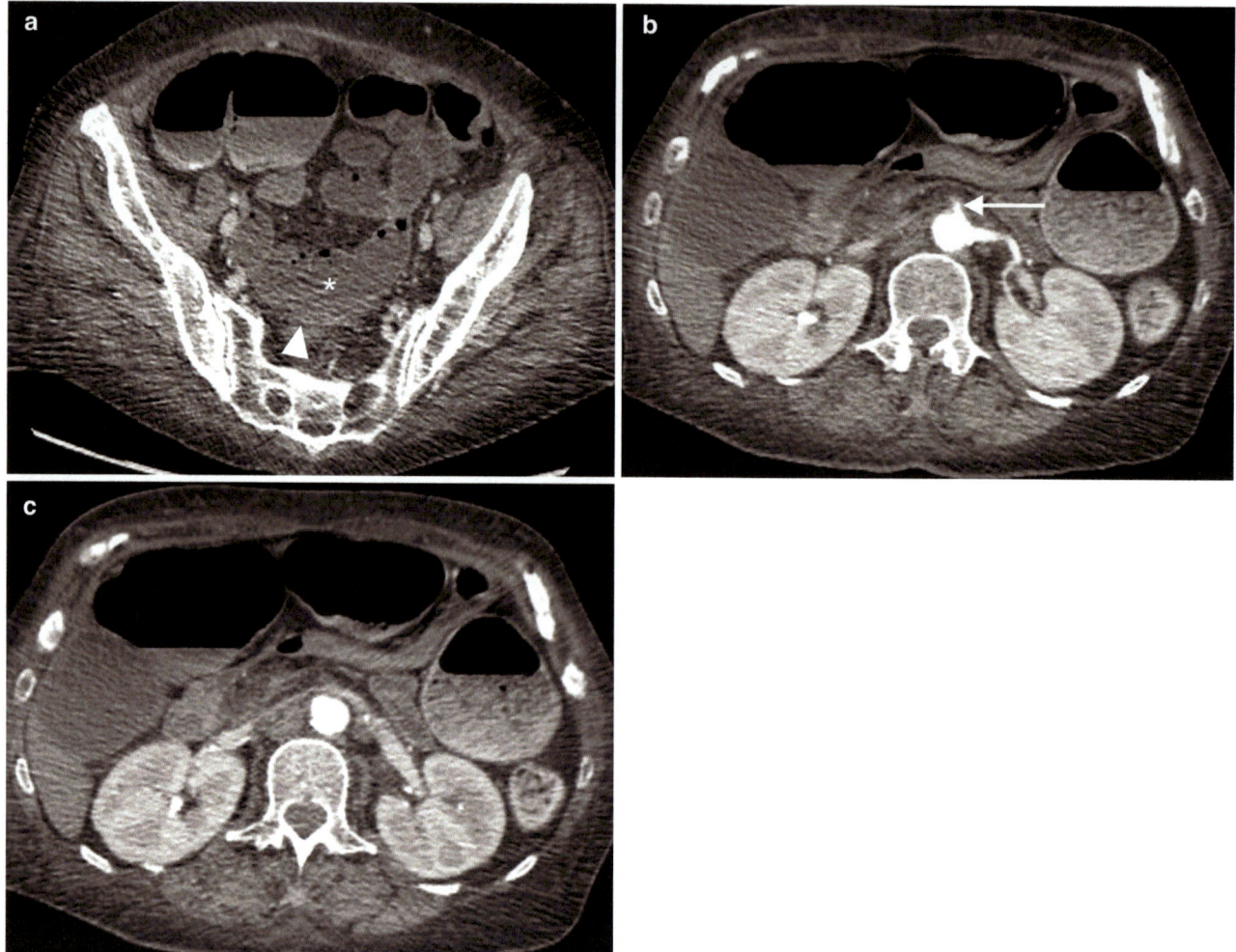

Fig. 19.7 (**a**) axial CT with dilated pelvic small bowel (asterisk) with lack of enhancement of the wall (arrowhead). (**b, c**) axial images of the SMA origin showing thrombosis with lack of contrast opacification (arrows)

(Fig. 19.8). Typically, these are elderly patients and managed conservatively with a confident diagnosis [10].

Foreign bodies present a challenge and difficult to detect without close evaluation of thin slice CT. Short linear densities protrude through the small bowel (most often fish bones or wood fragments) (Fig. 19.9). These are not expected clinically and patients can have recurrent admissions with relatively little related accompanying changes in bowel wall around the foreign body [11].

> **Key Point**
> • Foreign bodies including fish bones can be challenging to detect without thin slice evaluation and jejunal diverticulitis and perforation requires careful assessment for other diverticula on the mesenteric border of the small bowel to make the diagnosis.

Mesenteric arteries and veins need careful inspection on any CT performed for acute abdominal pain. Occlusive vascular diseases require thin slice reconstruction and multiplanar reformation to accurately detect and characterise arterial emboli from a cardiac source (atrial fibrillation or left ventricular mural thrombus) or thrombosis or vascular occlusion from atherosclerotic stenosis. This can be a challenging diagnosis as an unexpected finding on a portal venous phase study. Venous thrombosis may be accompanied by a primary condition or acute inflammatory processes elsewhere (such sigmoid diverticulitis). However, a pitfall for false-positive diagnosis relates to uneven mixing of contrast in the portal venous system, for example, caused by heart failure. Conversely non-occlusive mesenteric ischaemia shows vascular patency but has the other imaging features associated with ischaemia.

Small bowel ischaemia is accompanied by various additional signs including; bowel wall thickening; thinning of the bowel (which may be associated with dilatation); alteration

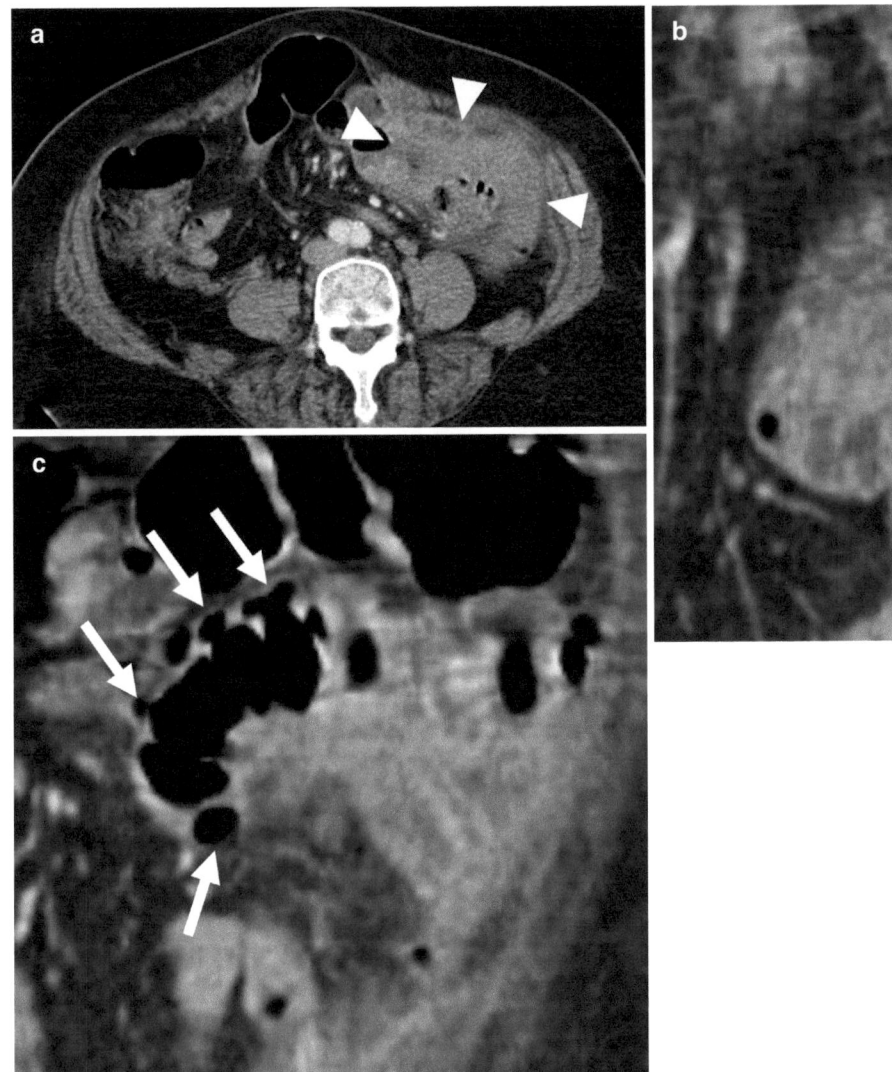

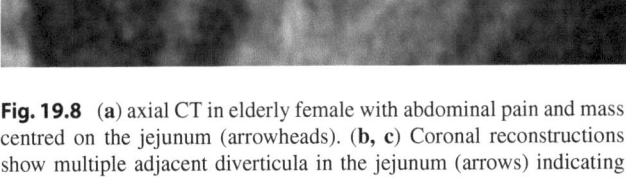

Fig. 19.8 (**a**) axial CT in elderly female with abdominal pain and mass centred on the jejunum (arrowheads). (**b, c**) Coronal reconstructions show multiple adjacent diverticula in the jejunum (arrows) indicating that this is inflammation from jejunal diverticulitis which resolved with antibiotics

of enhancement with hypo or absent perfusion or conversely hyper enhancement in acute ischaemia from reflex dilatation of small vessels; localised dilatation from ileus; pneumatosis intestinalis and portal venous gas (which is not specific to ischaemia); and inflammatory changes in the mesenteric fat and ascites in the peritoneum [8]. Signs of ischaemia may also be present in other organs such as the spleen and kidneys. Acute intramural haemorrhage is seen in ischaemia as well as close loop obstruction, caused from reperfusion in arterial occlusion or venous occlusion with vascular engorgement. If this is not appreciated, then haemorrhage

may be mistaken for preserved enhancement in the bowel wall when it is in fact ischaemic or infarcted [8].

19.2.2 Outpatient Presentation: Common Clinical Presentations

CT is a common tool for the investigation of patients with unexplained symptoms with suspicion of GI tract origin. These symptoms are often non-specific, which once again presents difficulties when deciding the optimal protocol as

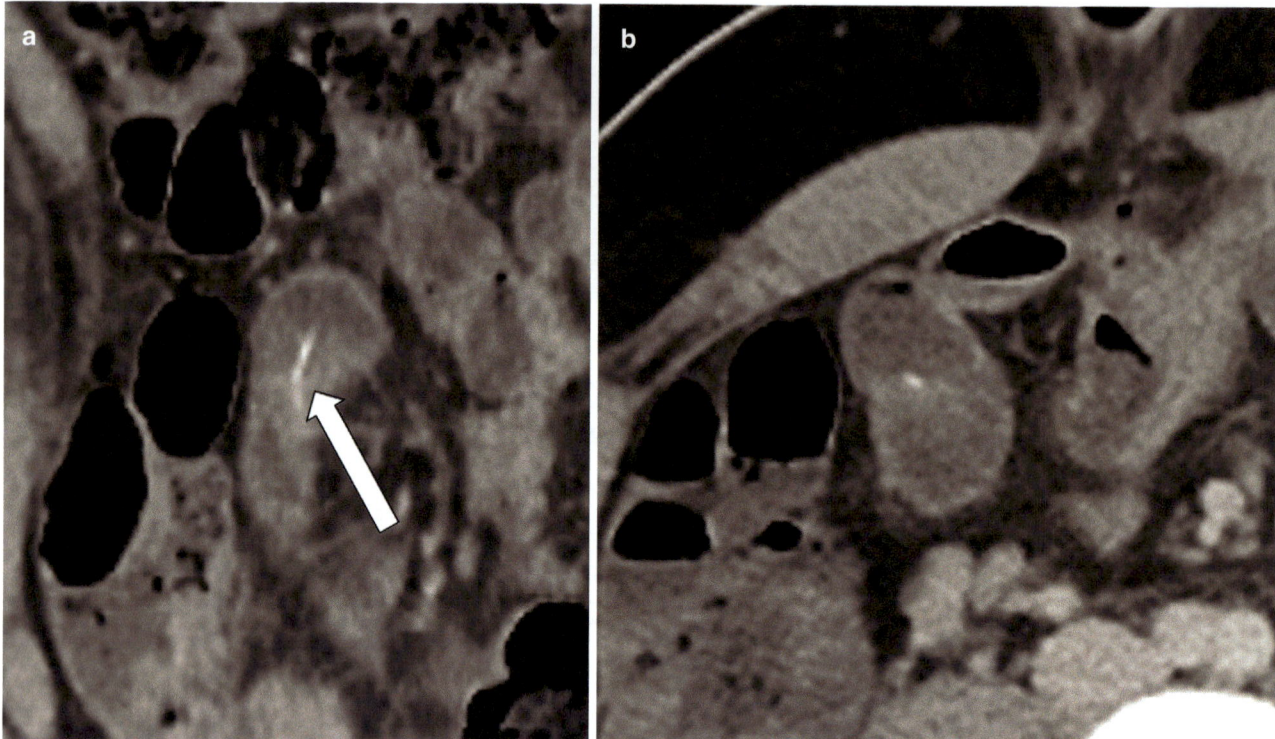

Fig. 19.9 (**a, b**) Axial and coronal CT in male with pyrexia post appendicectomy. The appendix was normal and faecal material was seen at peritoneal washout. Linear foreign body in the wall of the ileum (arrow) which was a wooden toothpick at repeat surgery

the clinical differential diagnosis is wide and an optimal imaging approach balances excessive radiation against an accurate diagnosis for a majority of patients.

19.2.2.1 CT Intravenous Contrast Considerations

CT Scan Phase Choices for Acquisition
- **Non-contrast CT** not indicated because of a low likelihood of haemorrhage being present and tumour calcification is easily detected on contrast enhanced scans.
- **Late arterial phase CT** (10 s post-peak aortic enhancement) may assist in the diagnosis of arterialised tumours (e.g. NET and metastases).
- **Enteric phase CT** (45–50 s post injection) for optimal evaluation of small bowel enhancement and detection of focal bowel lesions.
- **Portal venous phase CT** (65–75 s post injection) for global assessment of the viscera in the abdomen and pelvis.

19.2.2.2 CT Luminal Contrast: What Role?

Optimal small bowel assessment requires luminal distension with neutral contrast. Enteroclysis is advocated by some authors but this is invasive, challenging for patients and clinicians as it requires placement of a nasojejunal tube and a dedicated contrast pump for even delivery of contrast for dis-

tension. Enterography is more attractive requiring 1–1.5 L of Mannitol or PEG orally over 40–60 min. While luminal distension is less than enteroclysis, it is an effective and more practical diagnostic tool particularly if used for problem-solving in combination with prior video capsule endoscopy. Intravenous contrast is essential in combination.

> **Key Point**
> - CT enterography requires 1–1.5 L of neutral contrast over 40–60 mins prior to scanning and an enteric phase of contrast enhancement between 45–50 s after injection.

19.2.2.3 Weight Loss, Abdominal Pain, and Altered Bowel Habit? Malignancy? Inflammatory Bowel Disease

Clinical Context
Patients with an established diagnosis of Crohn's disease should have MR enterography assessment. However, some patients will have this diagnosis proposed after a CT scan for non-specific abdominal symptoms. Likewise, small bowel tumours may be detected when investigating these symptoms.

Recommended CT Protocol

CT protocol with rapid weight-based iodinated contrast injection and portal venous acquisition with water oral contrast (for prehydration).

High clinical suspicion of small bowel disease: CT enterography with 1–1.5 L Mannitol or PEG over 40–60 min and rapid (4 mL/s) weight-based iodinated contrast injection and enteric phase acquisition.

Relevant Conditions and Imaging Signs

The imaging features of Crohn's disease are well known [12]. The length and distribution of abnormal bowel segments should be reported in addition to complications such as fistula, abscess, or obstruction [12, 13]. Note that Crohn's disease has a bimodal age distribution with a significant proportion presenting over 60 years.

Small bowel tumours are rare. Patients with polyposis are often detected after screening but sporadic cases occur, and these can be very difficult to detect without optimal distension as they have similar post contrast enhancement to normal small bowel folds. Malignant tumours will usually appear as focal bowel thickening, as a large mass, as a transition point in incomplete small bowel obstruction or as a smaller abnormality related to a much more obvious abnormality, such as extensive lymphadenopathy in lymphoma or NET. Few signs are specific. Nodes are uncommon in GIST and metastasis should be considered particularly with a history of melanoma, breast, and lung cancer [5] (Fig. 19.10).

19.2.2.4 Iron Deficiency Anaemia with Occult Obscure GI Bleeding

Clinical Context

Radiological assessment is reserved for problem-solving after indeterminate video capsule endoscopy or where there is high suspicion of abnormality after negative capsule [3] (Fig. 19.10). Occasionally, CT is requested for 'road mapping' to plan the optimal route for double balloon enteroscopy (antegrade or retrograde via the colon) or where DBE is not possible because of adhesions and an operative approach is being considered. Active bleeding is highly unlikely and the detection is focused on optimal contrast enhancement.

Recommended CT Protocol

CT enterography with 1–1.5 L Mannitol or PEG over 40–60 min and rapid (4 mL/s) weight-based iodinated contrast injection and enteric phase acquisition (± portal venous phase).

Ct enteroclysis (selected cases: 2–3 L (Mannitol or PEG) pump infused via NJ tube (100–150 mL/min) and rapid

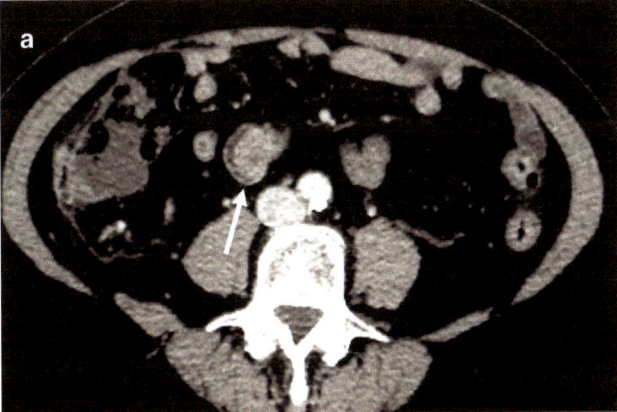
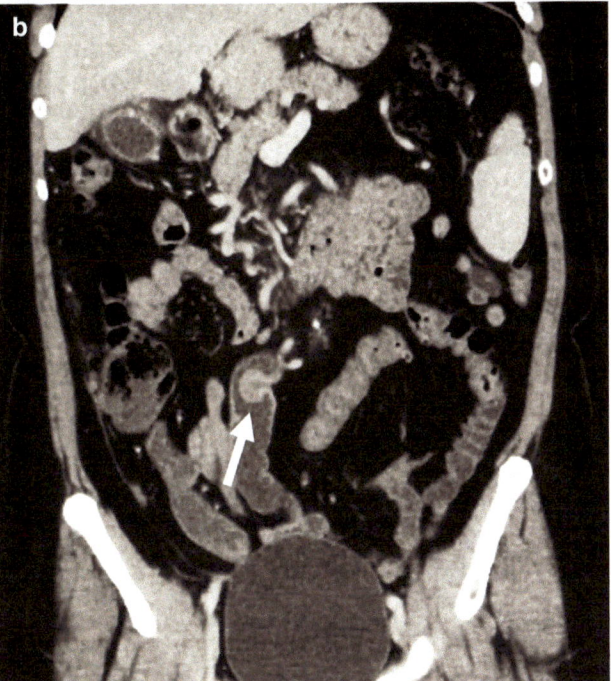

Fig. 19.10 (**a, b**) Abdominal pain and anaemia. Axial and coronal reconstructions showing polypoid enhancing tumour in the mid small bowel (arrows). Prior history of melanoma resection 2 years previously with metastasis confirmed at small bowel resection

(4 mL/s) weight-based iodinated contrast injection and enteric phase acquisition (± portal venous phase).

Relevant Conditions and Imaging Signs

Most tumours and vascular lesions are best detected with an enteric phase assessment and optimal distension [2, 5].

19.2.2.5 Small Bowel Intussusception

Intussusception is a common observation on CT performed for abdominal symptoms and is related to normal physiology from bowel contraction. Most cases can be dismissed where

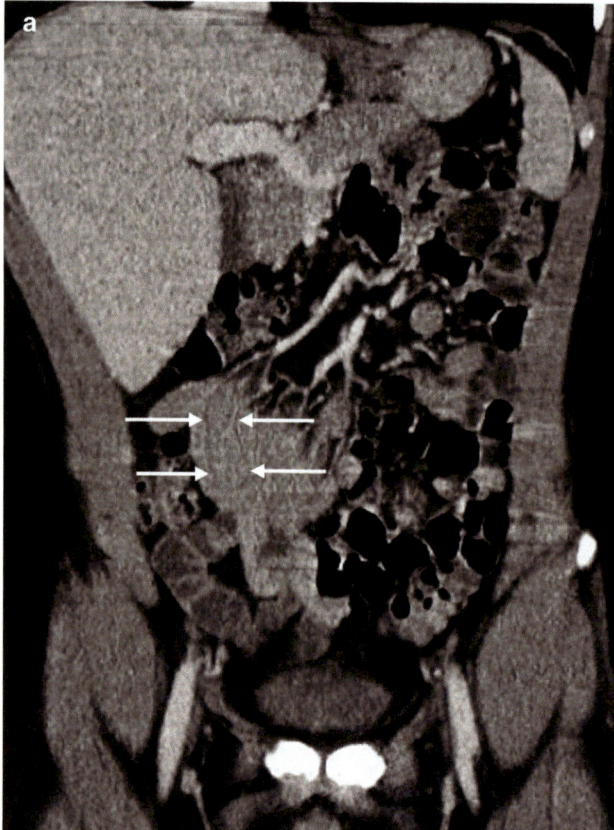

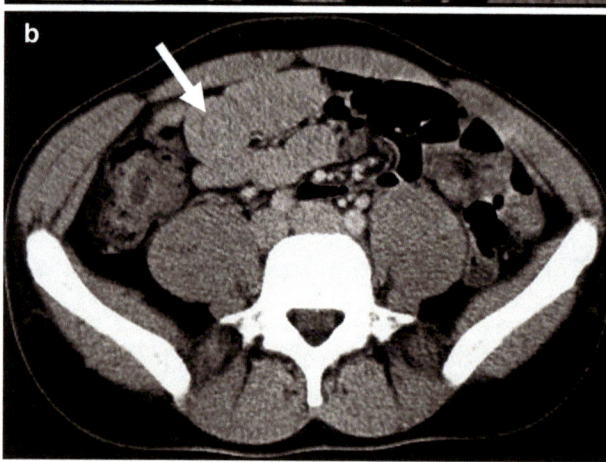

Fig. 19.11 (**a, b**) CT for intermittent abdominal pain in a 34-year-old male with short mid small bowel intussusception. There is no pathological lead point and the intussusception is short, consistent with an incidental physiological event rather than abnormality

there is no visible mass as a lead point, where the length of intussusception is less than 5 cm and there is no associated obstruction [14, 15] (Fig. 19.11).

Key Point
- Small bowel intussusception detected by CT does not require additional tests unless there is a pathological lead point, signs of associated obstruction or it is greater than 5 cm in length.

19.3 Concluding Remarks

Optimal CT technique tailored to the clinical situation is essential to detect the imaging signs that influence patient care and requires appropriate pre-selection of scan phases and adequate iodinated contrast rate and volume. The most important emergency considerations relate to the effective detection of active bleeding, the diagnosis of small bowel ischaemia and reliable identification of closed loop obstruction while outpatient assessment particularly requires detection of inflammatory bowel disease and malignancy with a minor role in the evaluation of obscure GI bleeding to supplement endoscopic techniques.

Take Home Messages
- Consider non-contrast CT before contrast administration for ischaemia to look for intramural haemorrhage.
- Remember enteric phase CT is optimal for small bowel assessment and is earlier than standard portal venous phase.
- Remember luminal contrast should not delay emergency CT, but neutral contrast is important for outpatient evaluation.

References

1. https://www.ranzcr.com/college/document-library/ranzcr-iodinated-contrast-guidelines. Accessed 25 Oct 2022.
2. Guglielmo FF, Wells ML, Bruining DH, et al. Gastrointestinal bleeding at CT angiography and CT Enterography: imaging atlas and glossary of terms. Radiographics. 2021;41:1632–56.
3. Pennazio M, Spada C, Eliakim R, et al. Small-bowel capsule endoscopy and device-assisted enteroscopy for diagnosis and treatment of small-bowel disorders: European Society of Gastrointestinal Endoscopy (ESGE) clinical guideline. Endoscopy. 2015;47:352–76.
4. Wells ML, Hansel SL, Bruining DH, et al. CT for evaluation of acute gastrointestinal bleeding. Radiographics. 2018;38:1089–107.
5. Jasti R, Carucci LR. Small bowel neoplasms: a pictorial review. Radiographics. 2020;40:1020–38.
6. Zins M, Millet I, Taourel P. Adhesive small bowel obstruction: predictive radiology to improve patient management. Radiology. 2020;296:480–92.
7. Khaled W, Millet I, Corno L, et al. Clinical relevance of the feces sign in small-bowel obstruction due to adhesions depends on its location. AJR Am J Roentgenol. 2018;210:78–84.
8. Copin P, Zins M, Nuzzo A, et al. Acute mesenteric ischemia: a critical role for the radiologist. Diagn Interv Imaging. 2018;99:123–34.
9. Garzelli L, Nuzzo A, Copin P, et al. Contrast-enhanced CT for the diagnosis of acute mesenteric ischemia. AJR Am J Roentgenol. 2020;215:29–38.
10. Lebert P, Ernst O, Zins M. Acquired diverticular disease of the jejunum and ileum: imaging features and pitfalls. Abdom Radiol. 2019;44:1734–43.
11. E Sliva GS, Gomes NBN, Pacheco EO, et al. Emergency CT of abdominal complications of ingested fish bones: what not to miss. Emerg Radiol. 2021;28:165–70.

12. Kucharzik T, Tielbeek J, Carter D, et al. ECCO-ESGAR topical review on optimizing reporting for cross-sectional imaging in inflammatory bowel disease. J Crohns Colitis. 2022;16: 523–43.

13. Maaser C, Sturm A, Vavricka SR, European Crohn's and colitis organisation [ECCO] and the European Society of Gastrointestinal and Abdominal Radiology [ESGAR], et al. ECCO-ESGAR guideline for diagnostic assessment in IBD part 1: initial diagnosis, monitoring of known IBD, detection of complications. J Crohns Colitis. 2019;13:144–64.

14. Olasky J, Moazzez A, Barrera K, et al. In the era of routine use of CT scan for acute abdominal pain, should all adults with small bowel intussusception undergo surgery? Am Surg. 2009;75:958–61.

15. Rea JD, Lockhart ME, Yarbrough DE, et al. Approach to management of intussusception in adults: a new paradigm in the computed tomography era. Am Surg. 2007;73:1098–105.

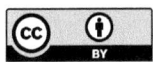

Congenital and Acquired Pathologies of the Pediatric Gastrointestinal Tract

Laura S. Kox, Anne M. J. B. Smets, and Thierry A. G. M. Huisman

Learning Objectives
- To understand the strengths and limitations of the different imaging modalities used for examining the pediatric gastrointestinal tract.
- To become familiar with the most frequent congenital and acquired pediatric gastrointestinal pathologies in which imaging plays an important role.

20.1 Introduction

Age is a key factor in the differential diagnosis of gastrointestinal (GI) pathology in children. In a variety of pediatric GI pathologies, imaging plays a major role.

In term neonates, congenital anomalies of the GI tract causing obstruction are at the forefront: atresia, intestinal malrotation with or without midgut volvulus, Hirschsprung's disease, meconium plug syndrome, and meconium ileus. In the premature neonate, necrotizing enterocolitis can be a life-threatening complication.

Intussusception is the most common cause of obstruction in infants and young children. In older children and adolescents, focus lies on inflammatory bowel disease. Appendicitis can occur at any age although most frequently in children older than 5. Duplication cysts of the GI tract are most commonly situated at the distal ileum. They are usually detected on prenatal ultrasound and sometimes only later in life when causing obstruction.

Different imaging modalities can be used to image the GI tract. Plain films, ultrasound, and contrast studies are the principal imaging tools. CT and MRI are problem solvers and are used in a specific context, such as trauma, inflammatory bowel disease (IBD), diseases of the biliary tree, and tumoral pathology.

20.2 Imaging Techniques

20.2.1 Conventional Radiography

In children with GI disorders, conventional abdominal radiographs still play a significant role, frequently in conjunction with ultrasound. Delineation of bowel gas is extremely helpful in abdominal pathology. Calcifications can easily be detected. In neonates and young children, abdominal radiographs are typically performed in a supine position. Horizontal beam examination in supine or left side down decubitus position can be added to detect small quantities of free intraperitoneal air.

Air is visible in the newborn stomach after the first swallow. After 12 h, most of the small bowel should be filled with air and by 24 h, air should appear in the rectum.

Small children typically have air throughout the entire GI tract and small and large bowel are usually not distinguishable from each other, especially when distended.

20.2.2 Ultrasound

Ultrasound is the first-choice imaging modality for the initial evaluation of the GI tract in children. With high frequency transducers, a detailed view of the abdominal contents can be obtained. One can evaluate peristalsis in real-time and vascularization of the bowel wall and the mesentery can be assessed. The graded compression technique is used to eliminate overlying gas and to reduce the distance between the GI

L. S. Kox · Anne M. J. B. Smets (✉)
Department of Radiology and Nuclear Medicine, Amsterdam UMC, University of Amsterdam, Amsterdam, The Netherlands
e-mail: l.s.kox@amsterdamumc.nl; a.m.smets@amsterdamumc.nl

Thierry A. G. M. Huisman
Department of Radiology, Texas Children's Hospital and Baylor College of Medicine, Houston, TX, USA
e-mail: huisman@texaschildrens.org

© The Author(s) 2023
J. Hodler et al. (eds.), *Diseases of the Abdomen and Pelvis 2023-2026*, IDKD Springer Series,
https://doi.org/10.1007/978-3-031-27355-1_20

tract and the transducer. In infants with a painful belly, most of the abdomen can be visualized from the flanks.

20.2.3 Fluoroscopy with Contrast Agents

In practice, in most pediatric radiology departments, water-soluble, low-osmolar, isotonic contrast agents at body temperature are used for the evaluation of the anatomy of the upper and lower GI tract in small children. Hyperosmolar contrast agents can cause pulmonary edema when aspirated and should be avoided at all times for upper GI series.

20.2.4 Computed Tomography (CT)

CT is reserved for emergent indications such as blunt or penetrating trauma, in cases when neither ultrasound or MRI can be used to assess the abdomen or when findings are inconclusive. The use of CT should be limited as much as possible because of the deleterious effect of radiation exposure, especially in young children.

20.2.5 Magnetic Resonance Imaging

MRI is indicated in non-acute situations when ultrasound is inadequate and for mapping of IBD, anomalies and diseases of the biliary tree and tumoral pathology. In addition, MRI can also be used in the fetal period. For example, gastroschisis, omphalocele, congenital diaphragmatic hernia and multiple other abdominal abnormalities can be easily differentiated by fetal MRI.

> **Key Point**
> Conventional radiographs and ultrasound are the modalities of choice for initial imaging of the gastrointestinal tract in children.

20.3 Obstruction of the Upper Gastrointestinal Tract

20.3.1 Hypertrophic Pyloric Stenosis

The etiology of hypertrophic pyloric stenosis is unknown. It occurs in about 2–5 per 1000 infants in a male-to-female ratio of approximately 4:1 [1]. Children typically present at an age of 2–8 weeks, classically with frequent forceful ("projectile") non-bilious vomiting, failure to thrive and even weight loss and dehydration. Ultrasound is the modality of

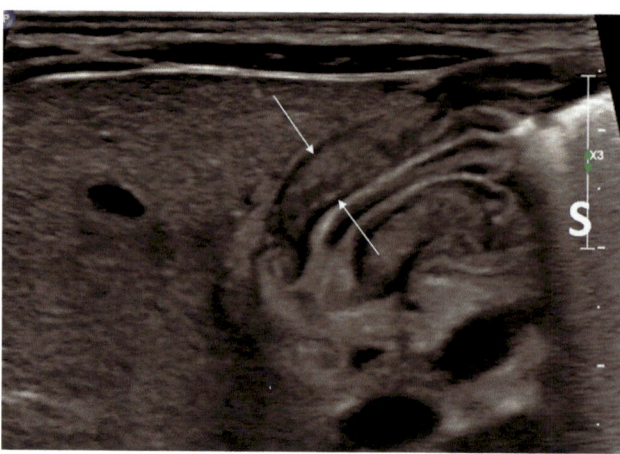

Fig. 20.1 Hypertrophic pyloric stenosis in a 5-week-old infant presenting with projectile vomiting: Thickening of the pyloric muscle (>3 mm) between the arrows and an elongated pyloric canal

choice to confirm the diagnosis of a hypertrophic pyloric muscle. Typical sonographic findings are [2] (Fig. 20.1):

1. Muscle thickness of >3 mm
2. Pyloric length of >15 mm
3. Protrusion of the mucosa into the distended gastric antrum

Pylorospasm, a transient contraction of the pyloric channel can mimic pyloric stenosis but the change in aspect of the pylorus during the examination is the key differentiating finding [3].

Foveolar hyperplasia, usually prostaglandin-induced, also shows a thickened pyloric wall, however, here the mucosa is thickened and not the muscular layer [4].

20.3.2 Duodenal Atresia and Stenosis

The most common cause of complete duodenal obstruction in neonates is duodenal atresia, which is thought to be caused by incomplete recanalization during gestation. It occurs in about 1 in 10.000 newborns and is associated with Down syndrome as well as with numerous congenital anomalies [5]. In most cases, the atresia is distal to the ampulla of Vater and the main symptom is biliary vomiting, which usually occurs within the first 24 h after birth. If the atresia is proximal to the ampulla, children present with non-biliary vomiting.

Plain films classically show a "double bubble" sign, in which the largest bubble on the left represents the stomach, and the smaller bubble to its right represents air in the dilated duodenum proximal to the atresia (Fig. 20.2a, b). Distal to the obstruction, no or minimal intestinal gas is visible [6]. No further radiological examination is required, and treatment is surgical.

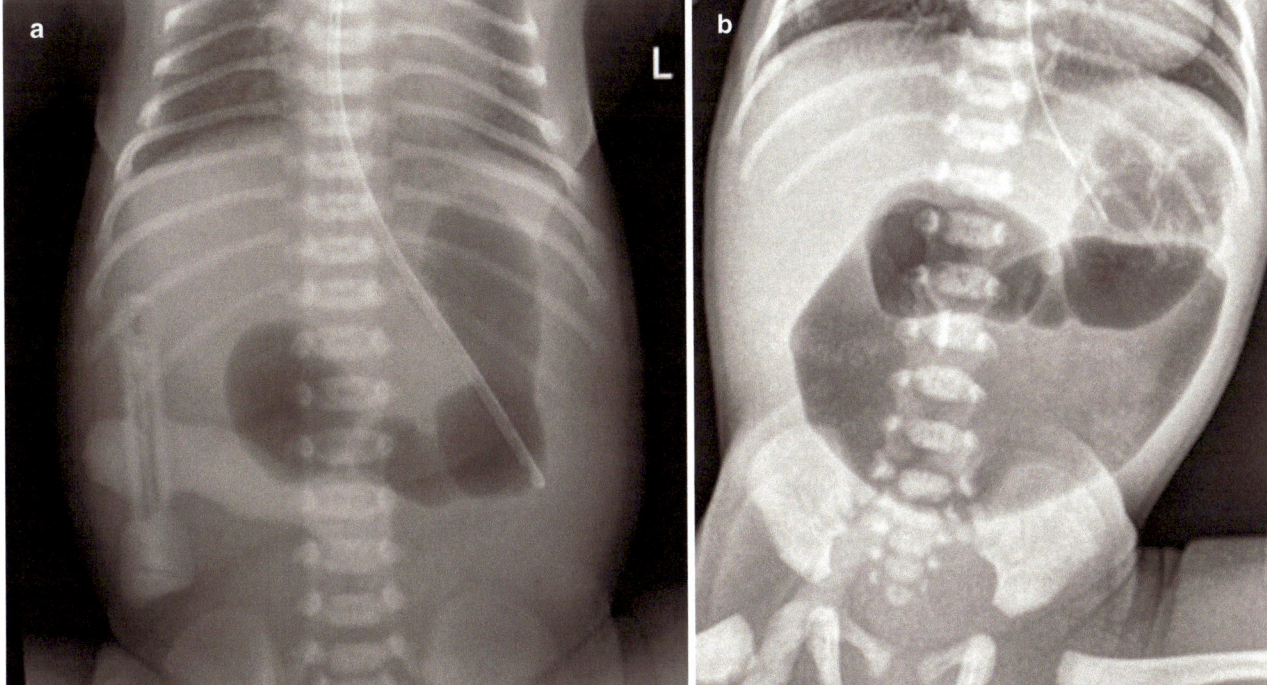

Fig. 20.2 (**a**) Duodenal atresia in a newborn: abdominal radiograph showing a classic double bubble sign of an air-distended stomach and proximal duodenum. No intestinal gas is visible more distally. (**b**) Small bowel atresia in a newborn: abdominal radiograph showing a triple bubble appearance, suggestive of a jejunal atresia

Potential causes of incomplete duodenal obstruction include duodenal stenosis, duodenal web, annular pancreas, midgut volvulus, and duplication cysts. Duodenal stenosis and duodenal web are radiologically difficult to differentiate. Radiography shows a distended stomach and duodenum filled with air, and little to normal amounts of air in the distal bowel. On fluoroscopy, duodenal web can exhibit the "windsock sign," produced by intraluminal ballooning of a duodenal diverticulum, surrounded by a mucosal web [7].

> **Key Point**
> Hypertrophic pyloric stenosis is a common cause of gastric outlet obstruction in neonates and can be diagnosed using ultrasound. Duodenal obstruction in neonates is most commonly caused by duodenal atresia, which is seen as a "double bubble sign" on conventional radiography.

20.3.3 Malrotation and Midgut Volvulus

Malrotation is a spectrum of disorders regarding the embryological intestinal rotation and fixation. It is always present in congenital diaphragmatic hernia and anterior bowel wall defects, i.e., omphalocele and gastroschisis. It is found more frequently in combination with intestinal atresia and is 25 times more frequent in patients with trisomy 13, 18, and 21 [8]. Midgut volvulus is a life-threatening complication of malrotation and a surgical emergency occurring most frequently in neonates and young infants. Due to an abnormal fixation and a short mesenteric root, the small bowel rotates around the axis of the superior mesenteric artery (SMA). This volvulus leads to varying degrees of bowel obstruction, lymphatic and venous drainage obstruction, and may eventually compromise the arterial supply. Bilious vomiting should prompt emergent exclusion of malrotation, with or without midgut volvulus. Imaging is crucial, primarily ultrasound and upper GI series [9].

In case of volvulus, the visualization of the whirlpool sign (Fig. 20.3a) showing the clockwise rotation of the bowel and the superior mesenteric vein around the SMA, has a 100% sensitivity and specificity in symptomatic children. In the absence of volvulus, malrotation should be excluded because of the associated risk of volvulus. An abnormal position of the superior mesenteric vessels (in a normal situation, the artery lies left and posteriorly to the vein) can be found; however, it is neither strongly sensitive nor specific. A retroperitoneal position of the third part of the duodenum, on ultrasound identified between the SMA and the aorta, is a sign of normal rotation [9].

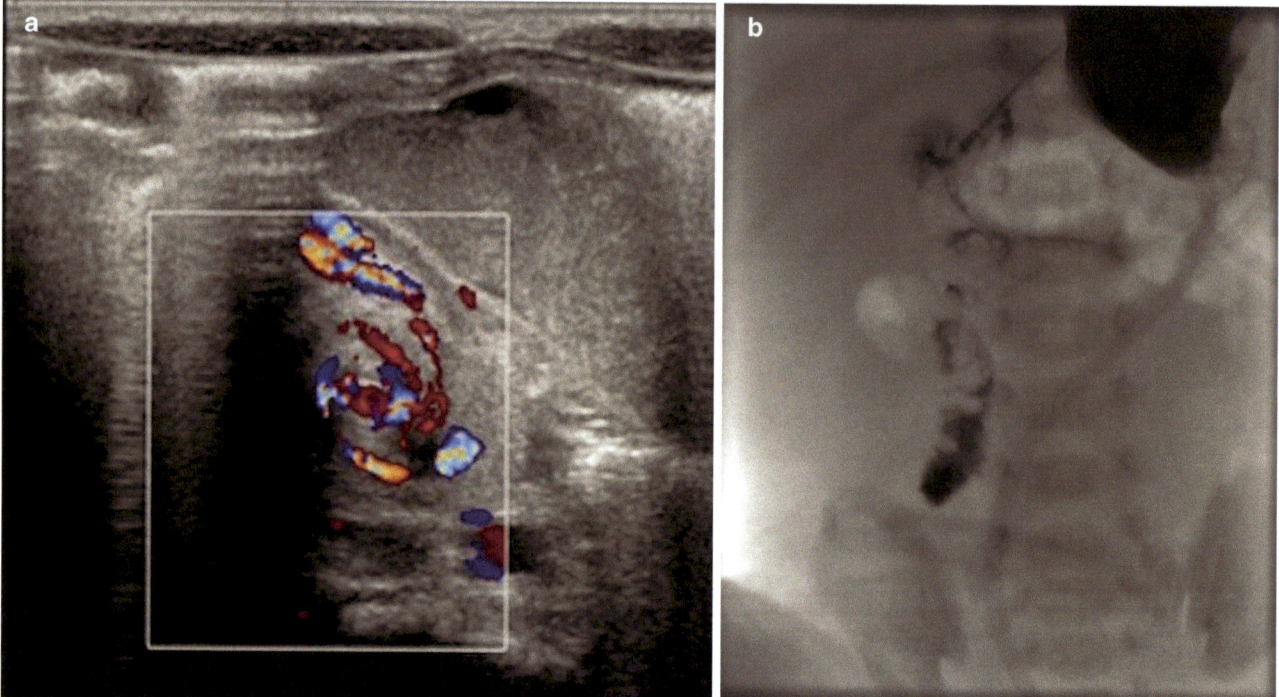

Fig. 20.3 (**a**) Malrotation with midgut volvulus in an infant: color Doppler shows a whirlpool-sign, the superior mesenteric vein and bowel rotating around the superior mesenteric artery. (**b**) Malrotation with midgut volvulus in another infant: on upper GI series, the typical corkscrew configuration of the twisted small bowel

Detection of the position of the caecum is not helpful as it is normal in 30% of patients with malrotation and can be located in a high position in normal neonates [10].

With an upper GI series, midgut volvulus is seen as a spiral twisting of the duodenum in a corkscrew appearance (Fig. 20.3b) or a beak-like configuration in case of complete obstruction. In malrotation without volvulus, there is an abnormal position of the duodenum and the duodeno-jejunal junction. Obstruction can also be caused by ligaments (Ladd bands) crossing the duodenum.

> **Key Point**
>
> Malrotation is a congenital abnormality of the intestinal anatomy, with midgut volvulus as a life-threatening complication. The sonographic "whirlpool sign" confirms the diagnosis of volvulus, and retroperitoneal position of the duodenum is highly indicative of the absence of malrotation.

20.4 Obstruction of the Lower Intestinal Tract

20.4.1 Meconium Ileus and Ileal Atresia

Atresia is most common in the jejunum and ileum. It is thought to be due to a vascular accident in utero. Meconium ileus is an obstruction in the distal ileum due to thickened meconium. It is a frequent initial presentation of cystic fibrosis (CF) but is also seen in very low birth weight premature infants, infants of diabetic mothers, and babies born via cesarean section. It may be complicated by in utero bowel perforation. Meconium may then be free in the peritoneal cavity or become walled off in a rim-calcified meconium pseudocyst which can be delineated on conventional radiography and may also be seen with ultrasound.

Meconium peritonitis is not specific to meconium ileus: it occurs in any newborn with intrauterine intestinal perforation with intraperitoneal spillage of meconium for any reason, causing a sterile peritonitis and formation of dystrophic calcifications (Fig. 20.4a) [11].

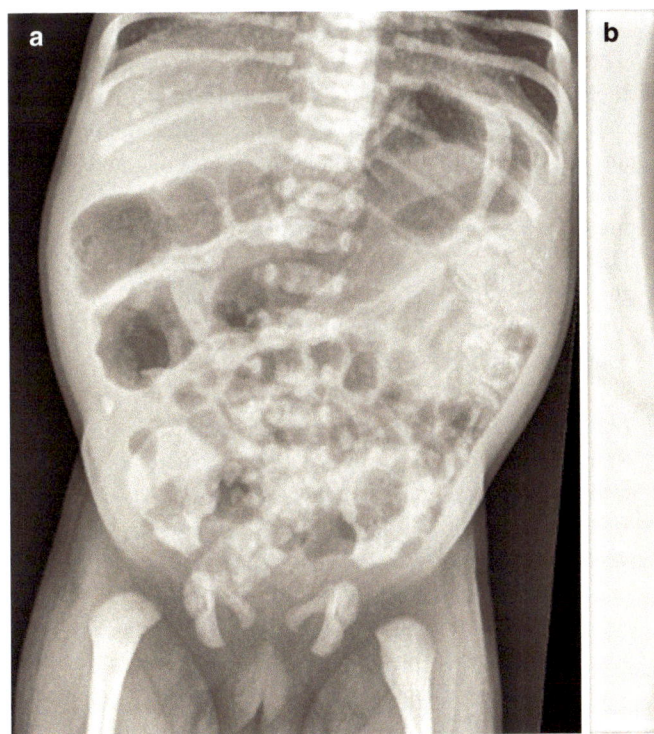
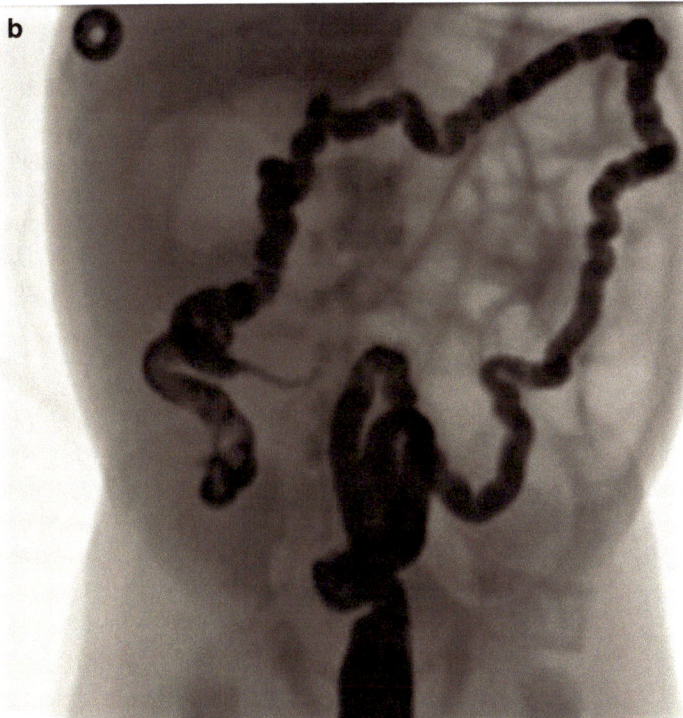

Fig. 20.4 (**a**) Meconium peritonitis: multiple intraperitoneal calcifications after perforation in utero in a newborn with cystic fibrosis and meconium ileus. (**b**) Uncomplicated meconium ileus: contrast enema shows an unused microcolon and delineation of multiple meconium plugs in the terminal ileum

In patients with distal intestinal obstruction, abdominal radiography will show gas-filled dilated bowel loops without gas in the rectum. In meconium ileus, the packed meconium can show a bubble soap appearance and intra-abdominal calcifications if in utero perforation has occurred. On contrast, enema a microcolon is seen, like in other causes of ileal obstruction, i.e., meconium ileus or long segment Hirschsprung's disease (Fig. 20.4b).

In meconium ileus, a water-soluble moderately hyper-osmolar contrast enema may be therapeutic by helping to evacuate the thickened meconium. Barium should be avoided to prevent a barium peritonitis in case of an intestinal perforation.

20.4.2 Meconium Plug Syndrome

This condition most often occurs in premature neonates and is sometimes described as small left colon or microcolon syndrome. It is associated with maternal diabetes, Hirschsprung's disease and cystic fibrosis [12]. Clinically, distension of the abdomen and failure to pass meconium in the first weeks of life are the presenting symptoms and are caused by impacted meconium obstructing the left colon [13].

Conventional radiography is usually non-specific, showing mild to moderately dilated bowel loops with few to no fluid levels. Fluoroscopy is diagnostic for meconium plug syndrome, showing a small caliber of the left-sided colon and sometimes contrast filling defects due to the retained meconium. The rectum is commonly normal in size, unlike Hirschsprung's disease, and the ascending and transverse colon also show a normal diameter with colonic haustrations. The iodine contrast administered during fluoroscopy often has additional therapeutic value as the laxative properties of the contrast medium can cause the patient to pass the meconium during or after the examination.

20.4.3 Hirschsprung's Disease

In Hirschsprung's disease, a variable length of distal bowel lacks ganglion cells and is unable to participate in normal peristaltic waves, resulting in a functional obstruction. The clinical presentation in neonates is one of distal obstruction, and failure to pass meconium in the first 24 h. Older children with Hirschsprung's disease present with constipation, abdominal distension, vomiting, and failure to thrive in more severe cases.

In neonates, abdominal radiography demonstrates evidence of distal bowel obstruction, but there is usually gas in the rectum. The length of the aganglionic segment is variable, most commonly the transition between abnormal and normal bowel is at the rectosigmoid junction, but the distal part of the GI tract is always affected. Diagnosis is made by biopsy and contrast enema may help indicate the zone of transition.

> **Key Point**
>
> In obstructing conditions of the lower intestine such as ileal atresia, meconium ileus or plug, and Hirschsprung's disease, conventional radiography can give an indication of obstruction location. Fluoroscopy as a next step has both diagnostic and therapeutic properties in meconium obstruction.

20.5 Necrotizing Enterocolitis

Necrotizing enterocolitis (NEC) is an inflammation of the GI tract in neonates, particularly of preterm infants. The incidence varies between 0.3 and 2.4 infants/1000 births and between 3.9 and 22.4% among infants weighing less than 1500 g. It is the most common newborn surgical emergency. The pathogenesis of NEC is not completely understood, but there are strong suggestions that it is multifactorial: a combination of a genetic predisposition, intestinal immaturity, and an imbalance in microvascular tone, accompanied by a strong likelihood of abnormal microbial colonization in the intestine and a highly immunoreactive intestinal mucosa [14]. The risk factors are very low birth weight, prematurity, formula feeding, hypoxic–ischemic insults and infection. Term neonates with structural congenital heart defects asphyxia and babies from mothers using recreational drugs are also at risk. NEC can affect the intestines diffusely, but it typically affects segments of bowel and most frequently the terminal ileum and the proximal ascending colon. Abdominal radiography and ultrasound are used to diagnose NEC. Dilated bowel loops, focal intramural gas, portal venous gas, fixed bowel loops, paucity of bowel gas and pneumoperitoneum can be seen on abdominal radiography (Fig. 20.5a, b). With ultrasound, one can detect lack of peristalsis, bowel wall thickening or thinning, degree of bowel wall perfusion, intramural gas, ascites, and pneumoperitoneum [15, 16].

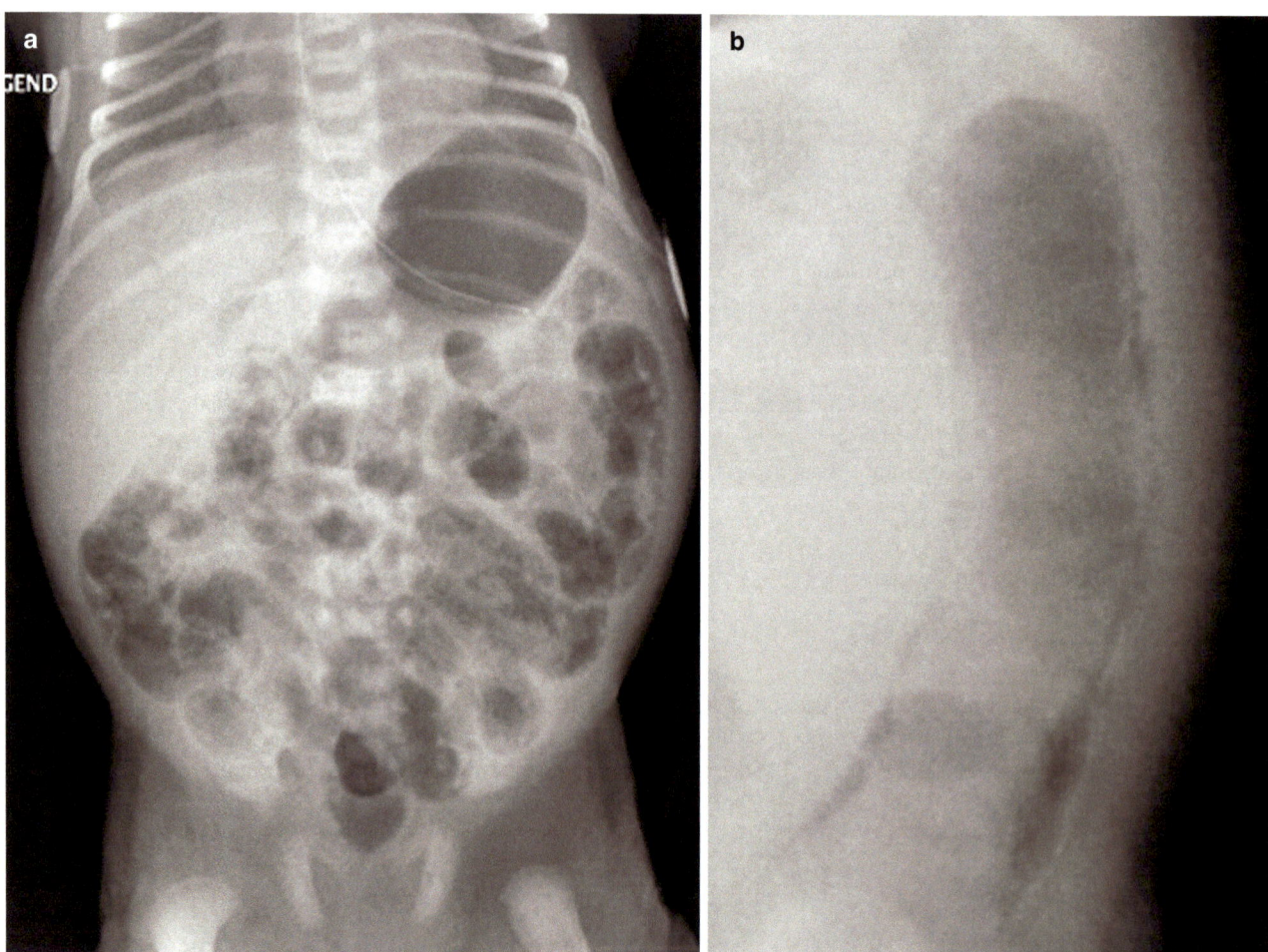

Fig. 20.5 (a) Premature infant with necrotizing enterocolitis: abdominal radiograph shows extensive intramural gas as well as portal venous gas. (b) Premature infant with necrotizing enterocolitis: left colon on an abdominal radiograph with intramural gas

20.6 Duplication Cysts

Intestinal duplication cysts are a rare entity, occurring in 0.2% of all children [17]. The etiology is unknown. Duplication cysts are associated with the presence of various other congenital anomalies. They can occur anywhere in the gastrointestinal tract. However, the most common location is in the distal ileum. The epithelial lining consists of gastric mucosa in up to one third of cases, which can sometimes lead to bleeding within the cyst. Most duplication cysts are detected prenatally or in the first year, after patients present with symptoms of gastrointestinal obstruction, and sometimes as a palpable mass or even as an intussusception.

Ultrasound is the preferred initial imaging technique. The imaging appearance of the cystic wall is usually thick compared to the bowel, and within the cyst often fluid-mucus level or blood after hemorrhage can be seen. Ultrasound characteristics that define a duplication cyst are the hyperechoic inner epithelial lining and a hypoechoic layer of smooth muscle within the wall. This typical double-layered appearance produces the classic "gut signature sign" (Fig. 20.6). The smooth muscle layer can also produce peristalsis within the cyst, which can be appreciated on ultrasound. Using the currently available high-resolution linear probes, the "five-layered cyst wall sign" can even be visualized, representing all wall layers normally seen in the gastro-

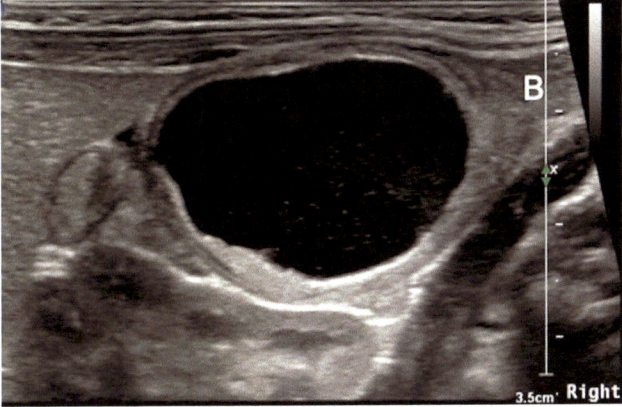

Fig. 20.6 Prenatally detected abdominal cyst in a newborn: typical hypo-hyperechoic double layered wall of a duplication cyst, gut signature. The cyst contains echogenic debris and shares a wall with the bowel (B)

intestinal tract. Finally, duplication cysts always demonstrate a close relation with any part of the gastrointestinal tract, even when actual communication with the bowel cannot be visualized. On ultrasound, the "Y configuration" demonstrating a shared wall between the cyst and the intestine, is indicative of a duplication cyst. Subsequent MRI can provide more information on the anatomical relations in the workup for surgery, with the cyst usually showing a low T1 signal intensity and a high T2 signal intensity.

The differential diagnoses include ovarian cyst, urachus cyst, mesenteric cyst, and lymphatic malformation. Treatment is surgical resection.

20.7 Intussusception

In ileo-colic intussusception, the terminal ileum invaginates through the ileocecal valve into the cecum. This is the most common cause of small bowel obstruction in children and occurs most often in the first year of life, with a 2:1 male-to-female ratio [18, 19]. In most cases, the cause is idiopathic. This means that the lead point is hypertrophied lymphoid tissue which cannot clearly be visualized. In a minority of cases, usually older children, possible lead points include enlarged lymph nodes, Meckel's diverticulum, duplication cyst, polyp, or diffuse bowel wall thickening caused by lymphoma or Henoch Schönlein purpura. The classic presentation of patients with intussusception is acute abdominal pain, vomiting, and bright red bloody or jelly-like stools although this triad is only present in less than 25% of patients [20].

Early diagnosis is essential to prevent bowel ischemia and perforation. The imaging method of choice in suspected intussusception is ultrasound. Typical ultrasound findings include the "donut sign" or "target sign" on transverse images of the bowel, and the "pseudo-kidney sign" on longitudinal images [21].

In patients with no signs of perforation, reduction of the intussusception can be done by an image-guided enema, pushing back the intussuscepted bowel segment with increasing intraluminal pressure. The most commonly used reduction methods are fluoroscopy-guided (with barium, water soluble contrast, or air) and ultrasound-guided (with water), the latter having the advantage that no ionizing radiation is used [20]. On ultrasound, the presence of dilated bowel loops indicating small bowel obstruction, and the presence of peritoneal fluid trapped between the intussuscepted bowel loops have been found to be predictors of unsuccessful outcome of reduction [22].

> **Key Point**
>
> In young infants, ileo-colic intussusception is mostly idiopathic, while in older children, a lead point is often the cause. The diagnosis is made by ultrasound, and fluoroscopy-guided or ultrasound-guided enema are the most commonly used methods for reduction of the intussusception.

20.8 Appendicitis

Appendicitis usually presents with abdominal pain, migrating from the periumbilical region to the right lower quadrant accompanied by fever and leukocytosis. However, one third of the children have atypical symptoms [23]. Ultrasound with graded compression is the preferred imaging modality for diagnosing pediatric appendicitis because of its high diagnostic accuracy and its noninvasive and nonradiating nature [24]. When ultrasound is not conclusive, MRI may be considered as an alternative modality.

An inflamed appendix is typically seen as a fluid-filled, non-compressible, blind-ending tubular structure with a diameter of 6 mm or more on longitudinal view and as a target image on transverse scan.

There may or may not be an appendicolith, pericecal, or periappendiceal fluid and enlarged mesenteric lymph nodes. Increased echogenicity of the periappendiceal fat is a useful sign. Differentiating perforated appendicitis from acute appendicitis prior to abscess formation is important: in the latter, management could be conservative. The constellation of dilated bowel, right lower quadrant echogenic fat, and complex fluid has a high specificity for perforated appendicitis.

Ruptured appendicitis can appear as a rounded structure with multiple rings that can very closely mimic the sonographic findings of intussusception [25]. Younger children and especially infants are at increased risk for perforation [26].

> **Key Point**
>
> Ultrasound is the imaging modality of choice in suspected appendicitis, showing an inflamed appendix, periappendiceal fluid, and inflamed fat. MRI may be an alternative imaging modality if ultrasound is non-conclusive. Infants are at increased risk for appendiceal perforation.

20.9 Inflammatory Bowel Disease

20.9.1 Crohn Disease

Crohn disease (CD) is the most common inflammatory small bowel disease. Presentation is usually above 10 years of age, with systemic symptoms such as weight loss, anorexia, malaise, and gastrointestinal symptoms like diarrhea and stools with blood and/or mucus. Any part of the GI tract can be involved, usually in a segmented distribution, but the terminal ileum and proximal colon are almost always affected. In children, there may be an isolated colonic involvement. Ultrasound and magnetic resonance enterography (MRE) are the preferred imaging methods [27–29].

In an early stage, the bowel wall is hypervascular and thickened in a concentric way with preservation of the wall stratification on ultrasound. The echogenicity of the surrounding mesentery is usually increased and also may show hyperemia. Mesenteric lymph nodes are typically increased in size and number. As the disease progresses, bowel wall stratification is lost and fibrosis develops. Fistula formation may occur, most commonly between cecum and terminal ileum.

20.9.2 Ulcerative Colitis

Ulcerative colitis is a less common idiopathic inflammatory bowel disease characteristically beginning in the rectum and extending proximally in a contiguous pattern, in contrast to CD. Bloody diarrhea and abdominal pain are frequent presenting features. Bowel wall is thickened, usually with preservation of the stratification [30].

> **Key Point**
>
> In children, Crohn disease is more common than ulcerative colitis. Ultrasound and MRE can display thickened bowel wall, hyperemic mesentery, and enlarged lymph nodes, followed by fibrosis in a later stage.

20.10 Concluding Remarks

There is a variety of GI pathology in the pediatric age group, and most of them are age-related. Several conditions can be live-threatening and need urgent action by the radiologist.

Take Home Messages

- Conventional radiographs and ultrasound are the modalities of choice for initial imaging of the gastrointestinal tract in children.
- Hypertrophic pyloric is diagnosed with ultrasound.
- A "double bubble sign" on conventional radiography is seen in duodenal atresia.
- The sonographic "whirlpool sign" confirms the diagnosis of volvulus, and a retroperitoneal position of the duodenum is highly indicative of the absence of malrotation.
- In obstructing conditions of the lower intestine, conventional radiography can give an indication of the obstruction location.
- Conventional radiography and ultrasound are the imaging modalities for necrotizing enterocolitis.
- Intestinal duplication cysts are characterized by their close relation with the gastrointestinal tract and their layered appearance.
- In older children with ileo-colic intussusception, a lead point has to be searched for.
- Ultrasound is the imaging modality of choice in suspected appendicitis. Infants are at increased risk for appendiceal perforation.
- Ultrasound and MRE are the modalities of choice to diagnose and monitor IBD in children.

References

1. Hernanz-Schulman M. Infantile hypertrophic pyloric stenosis. Radiology. 2003;227:319–31. https://doi.org/10.1148/radiol.2272011329.
2. Blumhagen JD, Maclin L, Krauter D, Rosenbaum DM, Weinberger E. Sonographic diagnosis of hypertrophic pyloric stenosis. Am J Roentgenol. 1988;150:1367–70. https://doi.org/10.2214/ajr.150.6.1367.
3. Cohen HL, Blumer SL, Zucconi WB. The sonographic double-track sign: not pathognomonic for hypertrophic pyloric stenosis; can be seen in pylorospasm. J Ultrasound Med. 2004;23:641–6. https://doi.org/10.7863/jum.2004.23.5.641.
4. Epifanio M, Baldisserotto M, Spolidoro JV, Ferreira S. Focal foveolar hyperplasia in an infant: color Doppler sonographic findings. J Ultrasound Med. 2009;28:81–4. https://doi.org/10.7863/jum.2009.28.1.81.
5. Berrocal T, Torres I, Gutiérrez J, Prieto C, Hoyo ML, Lamas M. Congenital anomalies of the upper gastrointestinal tract. Radiographics. 1999;19:855–72. https://doi.org/10.1148/radiographics.19.4.g99jl05855.
6. Traubici J. The double bubble sign. Radiology. 2001;220:463–4. https://doi.org/10.1148/radiology.220.2.r01au11463.
7. Gaio RCS, Vítor LMB. Intraluminal duodenal diverticulum: the windsock sign. Radiology. 2021;300:513–4. https://doi.org/10.1148/radiol.2021204576.
8. Applegate KE, Anderson JM, Klatte EC. Intestinal malrotation in children: a problem-solving approach to the upper gastrointestinal

series. Radiographics. 2006;26:1485–500. https://doi.org/10.1148/rg.265055167.
9. Nguyen HN, Navarro OM, Bloom DA, et al. Ultrasound for Midgut Malrotation and Midgut volvulus: AJR expert panel narrative review. AJR Am J Roentgenol. 2022;218:931–9. https://doi.org/10.2214/ajr.21.27242.
10. Berdon WE, Baker DH, Bull S, Santulli TV. Midgut malrotation and volvulus. Which films are most helpful? Radiology. 1970;96:375–84. https://doi.org/10.1148/96.2.375.
11. Douglas D. Meconium pseudocyst. Pediatr Radiol. 2010;40(Suppl 1):S105. https://doi.org/10.1007/s00247-010-1748-x.
12. Keckler SJ, St Peter SD, Spilde TL, et al. Current significance of meconium plug syndrome. J Pediatr Surg. 2008;43:896–8. https://doi.org/10.1016/j.jpedsurg.2007.12.035.
13. Siddiqui MM, Drewett M, Burge DM. Meconium obstruction of prematurity. Arch Dis Child Fetal Neonatal Ed. 2012;97:F147–50. https://doi.org/10.1136/adc.2010.190157.
14. Neu J, Walker WA. Necrotizing enterocolitis. N Engl J Med. 2011;364:255–64. https://doi.org/10.1056/NEJMra1005408.
15. Epelman M, Daneman A, Navarro OM, et al. Necrotizing enterocolitis: review of state-of-the-art imaging findings with pathologic correlation. Radiographics. 2007;27:285–305. https://doi.org/10.1148/rg.272055098.
16. Hwang M, Tierradentro-García LO, Dennis RA, Anupindi SA. The role of ultrasound in necrotizing enterocolitis. Pediatr Radiol. 2022;52:702–15. https://doi.org/10.1007/s00247-021-05187-5.
17. Sangüesa Nebot C, Llorens Salvador R, Carazo Palacios E, Picó Aliaga S, Ibañez Pradas V. Enteric duplication cysts in children: varied presentations, varied imaging findings. Insights Imaging. 2018;9:1097–106. https://doi.org/10.1007/s13244-018-0660-z.
18. Applegate KE. Intussusception in children: evidence-based diagnosis and treatment. Pediatr Radiol. 2009;39:140–3. https://doi.org/10.1007/s00247-009-1178-9.
19. Edwards EA, Pigg N, Courtier J, Zapala MA, MacKenzie JD, Phelps AS. Intussusception: past, present and future. Pediatr Radiol. 2017;47:1101–8. https://doi.org/10.1007/s00247-017-3878-x.
20. Plut D, Phillips GS, Johnston PR, Lee EY. Practical imaging strategies for intussusception in children. Am J Roentgenol. 2020;215:1449–63. https://doi.org/10.2214/AJR.19.22445.
21. Swischuk LE, Hayden CK, Boulden T. Intussusception: indications for ultrasonography and an explanation of the doughnut and pseudokidney signs. Pediatr Radiol. 1985;15:388–91. https://doi.org/10.1007/bf02388356.
22. Britton I, Wilkinson AG. Ultrasound features of intussusception predicting outcome of air enema. Pediatr Radiol. 1999;29:705–10. https://doi.org/10.1007/s002470050679.
23. Sivit CJ, Siegel MJ, Applegate KE, Newman KD. When appendicitis is suspected in children. Radiographics. 2001;21:247–62.; questionnaire 288–294. https://doi.org/10.1148/radiographics.21.1.g01ja17247.
24. Carpenter JL, Orth RC, Zhang W, Lopez ME, Mangona KL, Guillerman RP. Diagnostic performance of US for differentiating perforated from nonperforated pediatric appendicitis: a prospective cohort study. Radiology. 2017;282:835–41. https://doi.org/10.1148/radiol.2016160175.
25. Newman B, Schmitz M, Gawande R, Vasanawala S, Barth R. Perforated appendicitis: an underappreciated mimic of intussusception on ultrasound. Pediatr Radiol. 2014;44:535–41. https://doi.org/10.1007/s00247-014-2873-8.
26. Howell EC, Dubina ED, Lee SL. Perforation risk in pediatric appendicitis: assessment and management. Pediatric Health Med Ther. 2018;9:135–45. https://doi.org/10.2147/phmt.S155302.
27. Dillman JR, Smith EA, Sanchez RJ, et al. Pediatric small bowel Crohn disease: correlation of US and MR Enterography. Radiographics. 2015;35:835–48. https://doi.org/10.1148/rg.2015140002.

28. Gonzalez-Montpetit E, Ripollés T, Martinez-Pérez MJ, Vizuete J, Martín G, Blanc E. Ultrasound findings of Crohn's disease: correlation with MR enterography. Abdom Radiol. 2021;46:156–67. https://doi.org/10.1007/s00261-020-02622-3.

29. Schooler GR, Hull NC, Mavis A, Lee EY. MR imaging evaluation of inflammatory bowel disease in children: where are we now in 2019. Magn Reson Imaging Clin N Am. 2019;27:291–300. https://doi.org/10.1016/j.mric.2019.01.007.

30. Baud C, Saguintaah M, Veyrac C, et al. Sonographic diagnosis of colitis in children. Eur Radiol. 2004;14:2105–19. https://doi.org/10.1007/s00330-004-2358-5.

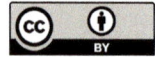

Congenital and Acquired Pathologies of the Pediatric Urogenital Tract

Erich Sorantin and Damien Grattan-Smith

Learning Objects
- Challenges and rational use of imaging modalities in congenital and acquired urinary tract pathologies.
- Imaging algorithms for most important clinical queries including incontinence.
- Get familiar with tumors of the urogenital tract.
- Learn about cardiovascular consequences of kidney diseases.

Key Point

Children are mirrors of the environment. Therefore for a successful investigation, a child friendly environment as well as staff is mandatory. Therefore, children should be imaged in dedicated Pediatric Radiology units and not mixed up with adults.

21.1 Introduction

Imaging of the urinary tract (UT) contributes considerably to the workload in Pediatric Radiology due to numerous diseases.

The purpose of this contribution is to present a short overview about most important CAKUT and acquired UT diseases.

21.2 Imaging Modalities

Due the many, physiologic, differences between children and adults it can be stated that "smallest children need the biggest machines" [1]. In order to avoid fear and uncooperative patients, Pediatric Radiology has to ensure an adequate environment for them as well as an appropriate set up of imaging modalities.

Ultrasound (US): US is the most important and starting modality of choice. US enables not only UT morphological assessment but quantitative parameters like bladder volume, residual void, and renal volumes [2]. Using the ellipsoid formula for bladder volumetry, it has to be considered that if the 3D baldder shape deviates from an ellipsoid the volume estimation getting less reliable.

Moreover, Doppler ultrasound and all its variants allow noninvasive assessment of blood flow, for example, thrombosis and vessel stenosis. Doppler tracings depict information about peripheral vessel resistance, and much more. Intravasal US contrast injection enables to visualize organ perfusion at almost no risk. Contrast-enhanced Sono Voiding Cysto-Urethrography (ceVUS) has already an established place in the diagnostic workup of urinary tract infection and suspected vesicoureteral reflux (VUR).

Due to the huge variation of body size in Pediatric Radiology, several transducers must be available including high resolution linear transducers, in order to ensure appropriate scanning an image quality for all children—regardless of age and size. It should not be forgotten that it can be performed bed-side.

Voiding Cysto-Urethrography (VCU): For decades VCU was the imaging modality of choice for VUR detection. Urine testing should be done before the procedure in order to avoid catheterization during urinary tract infection. In boys, appropriate imaging of the urethra during voiding is a must in order not to overlook posterior urethral valves

E. Sorantin (✉)
Division of Pediatric Radiology, Department of Radiology, Medical University Graz, Graz, Styria, Austria
e-mail: erich.sorantin@medunigraz.at

D. Grattan-Smith
Pediatric Radiologist, Atlanta, GA, USA

© The Author(s) 2023

J. Hodler et al. (eds.), *Diseases of the Abdomen and Pelvis 2023-2026*, IDKD Springer Series,
https://doi.org/10.1007/978-3-031-27355-1_21

(PUV). Modifications of the standard technique enable to assess also lower urinary tract dysfunction [3].

Intravenous Pyelography: It does not play a role anymore since ultrasound and Doppler ultrasound can deliver almost the same information. One exception of the rule might be ureteral stones in low resource countries.

Magnetic Resonance Imaging (MRI): MRI is second-line diagnostics and delivers high resolution anatomic details for almost all referrals. Using dedicated imaging sequences as well as free available post-processing techniques functional data like in Nuclear Medicine can be obtained including split renal function [4, 5].

Computed Tomography (CT): CT is rarely used, and there is almost no indication in pediatrics except for emergency situations like septic patients due to renal abscess, therapeutic interventions if ultrasound cannot be used as a navigational modality as well as in some cases of UT stone formation. There should be sized adapted protocols available on the CT machine in order to keep radiation exposure "as low as reasonable achievable (ALARA)." Furthermore, dual energy CT can help to characterize urinary tract stones for further patient management [6].

Nuclear Medicine: It enables to assess side-related functional renal parenchyma as well as in isotope renography the quantitative study of urine flow and in particular differentiation between obstructive and non-obstructive situation in PCD. It should be noted, that response to Furosemid can be missing due to kidney immaturity within the first 2–3 months of life and therefore can be misinterpreted as obstructed urinary flow.

> **Key Point**
> US and VCU represent the "workhorses" of UT imaging in children.

21.3 Normal Variations

It is difficult to make a distinct border line between normal variants and variants predisposing to illness. Persistent fetal lobulation, hypertrophied column of Bertin, and dromedary hump belong to the first group. It is already more complicated, for example, kidney hypoplasia (normal, configured but smaller kidney, hypertrophy of the contralateral one) since smaller kidneys are vascularized by smaller arteries thus increasing the risk of later hypertension. Double kidneys are frequently associated with double ureters and can predispose to hydronephrosis and VUR—see section antenatal hydronephrosis. Same applies to ectopic kidneys or crossed or fused kidneys (Fig. 21.1). The malposition itself is not the problem but associations with VUR or obstructed uri-

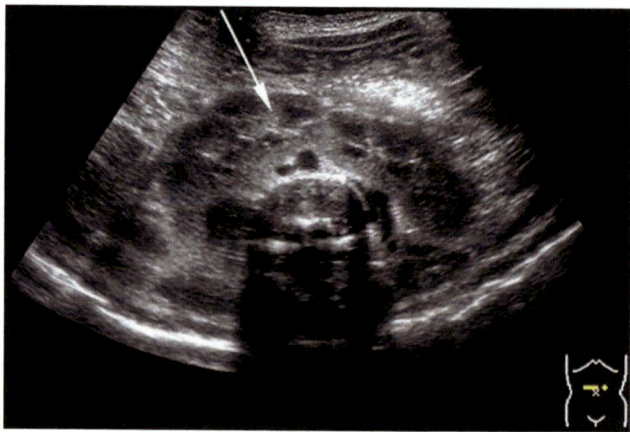

Fig. 21.1 US image from a horseshoe kidney, transverse cut of the abdomen. White arrow marks the kidney parenchymal bridge ventral to spine

nary flow. It is noteworthy to memorize that dysplastic or displaced kidneys usually have abnormal shaped calyces too.

21.4 Antenatal Hydronephrosis and CAKUT

Fetal antenatal hydronephrosis is a frequent finding on prenatal imaging in the order of 1.0–2.0% [7]. In order to ensure an adequate diagnostic algorithm, grading of the pelvicalyceal dilatation (PCD) can be graded according to a modified score of the "Society for Fetal Urology"(Fig. 21.2). According to literature, this is 50–70% transient/physiologic, due to ureteropelvic junction obstruction in 10–30%, vesicoureteral reflux 10–40%, ureterovesical junction obstruction/megaureter in 5–15%, multicystic dysplastic kidney disease 2–5%, posterior urethral valves 1–5%, and more uncommon ureterocele, ectopic ureter, duplex system, urethral atresia, Prune belly syndrome, and polycystic kidney diseases [7].

Furthermore, normal values according to gestational age were defined as listed in Table 21.1 [7]. Based on those ultrasounds, three patients' groups with different risk levels were defined as well as the appropriate imaging follow-up on these patients [8]. An isolated finding of an ampulla-shaped renal pelvis without PCD does not require further diagnostic workup.

An important point to remember is, that due to neonatal,physiologic oliguria PCD can be missed in US scans in the first days of life (Fig. 21.3).

In double kidneys with double ureters, both moieties can show PCD—due to the Weigert-Meyer law the ureter belonging to the upper moiety enters the bladder within the urinary bladder basal plate and thus leading to obstruction of urinary

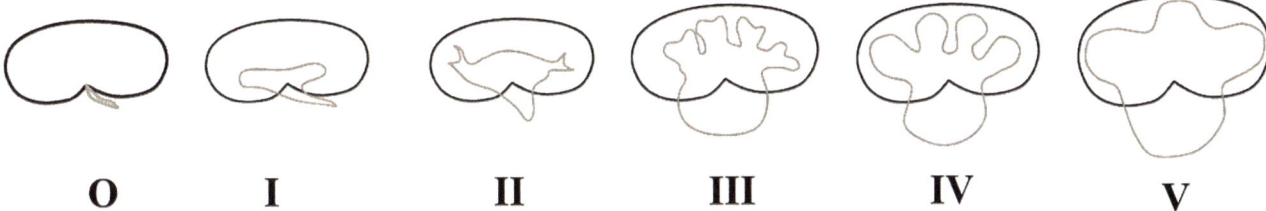

Fig. 21.2 schema of PCD dilatation. Numbers below the individual parts of the schema indicates type: O = no dilatation, I: only renal pelvis visible, II: renal pelvis and normaly shaped calyces are recognizeable, III: marked dilatation of renal pelvis (>10.0 mm), calyx fornix angles are rounded and papillary impression just reduced, no parenchymal narrowing, IV: same as III but parenchymal thickness is reduced, V: used in some instutions for the situation where parenchyma ist only a rim - modified after [2]

Table 21.1 normal sonography values for fetal UT [7]

Ultrasound findings		Time at presentation		
		16–27 weeks	>28 weeks	Postnatal (>48 h)
Renal pelvis anterior—Posterior diameter		<4 mm	<7 mm	<10 mm
Calyceal dilatation	Central	No	No	No
	Peripheral	No	No	No
Parenchymal thickness	Thickness	Normal	Normal	Normal
	Appearance	Normal	Normal	Normal
Ureter(s)		Normal	Normal	Normal
Bladder		Normal	Normal	Normal
Unexplained oligohydramnions		No	No	NA

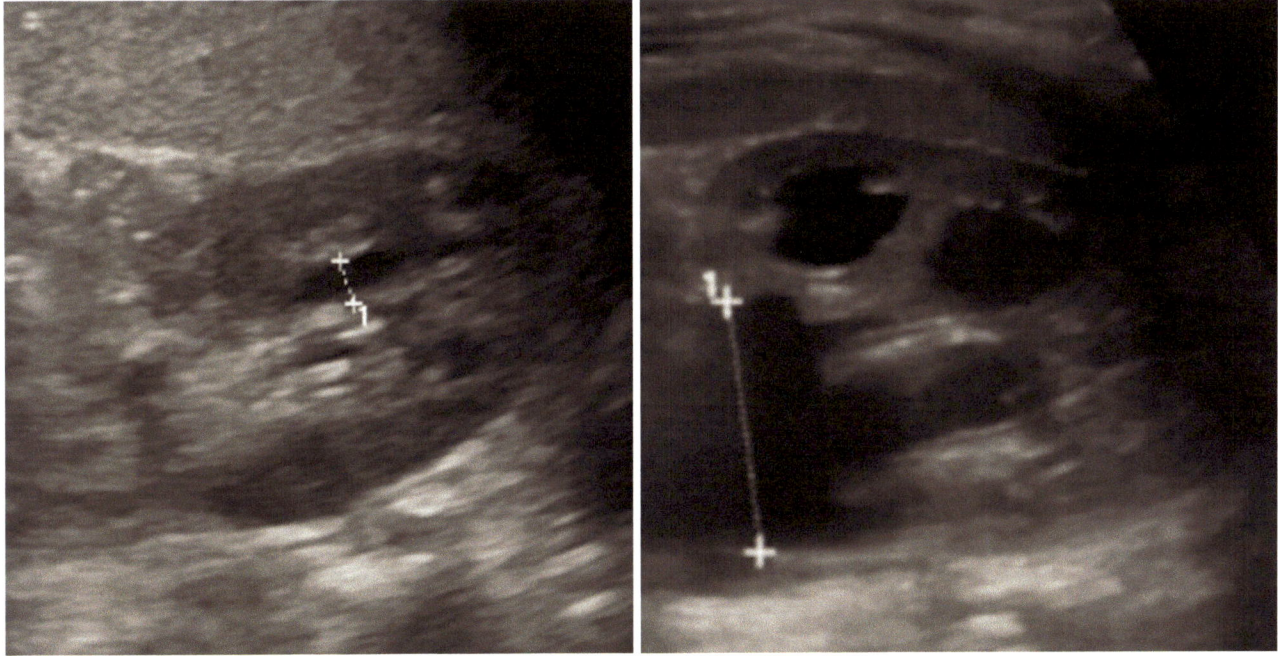

Fig. 21.3 influence on PCD by hydration. Neonate with known antenatal PCD. Left part: US on second day of life, no dilatation due to physiologic oliguria during first days of life, right part: US after a week PCD type IV

flow whereas the ureter draining the lower moiety enters the bladder in abnormal high position and therefore VUR is common [9].

> **Key Point**
> US scans in babies with antenatal diagnosed hydrone-phrosis should be taken after the third day of life in order to avoid false normal findings.
>
> In double kidneys, remember the Weigert-Meyer law.

Congenital anomalies of kidneys and urinary tract (CAKUT) are defined as "any structural and functional abnormalities of kidney, collecting system, bladder, and urethra" are frequent findings in 20–50% of fetal congenital abnormalities imaging [10] and up to 1 in 500 live births [11]. A list of those anomalies is given in Table 21.2. CAKUT pathogenesis is based on the disturbance of normal nephrogenesis, secondary to environmental or genetic causes (Capone et al. 2017). As environmental causes maternal diabetes as well as intrauterine exposure to ACE

Table 21.2 CAKUT spectrum of anomalies

Kidney anomalies	Renal agenesis
	Renal hypoplasia
	Duplication anomalies (duplex kidneys—only one collecting system
	Fusion anomalies (fused kidneys—One or more collecting systems, horseshoe kidney)
	Ectopic kidney (pelvic kidney, crossed ectopis)
	Renal dysplasia and multicystic kidney
	Cystic kidney disease (simply renal cyst, adult polycystic kidney disease, infantile polycystic kidney disease, medullary sponge kidney (MSK)
Abnormalities of the ureter and ureteropelvic junction	Ureteral atresia
	Obstruction of the ureteric junction obstructionDuplication of the ureter
	Ureterocele
	Ectopic ureter
	Prune belly syndrome (PBS)
	Obstructed mega-ureter
Abnormalities of the bladder	Bladder exstrophy
	Persistent urachus
	Vesicoureteral reflux
Anomalies of the penis and urethra in males	Males: Posterior urethral valves, double urethra
Anomalies of the testis	
Female genital anomalies	
Gonadal dysgenesis	
Disorders of sex development	

inhibitors were detected. In non-syndromic cases, mutations on HNF1B order PAX2 genes may be responsible [12].

Moreover, CAKUTs are responsible for 30–60% of chronic kidney disease starting already in childhood thus leading to renal replacement therapy already with 31 years as compared to others (61 years) [10].

21.5 Urinary Tract Infection (UTI)

UTI affects during first year of life about 0.7% of girls and 2.7% of uncircumcised boys [13]. There is bimodal age distribution with a peak within the first year of life and another between 2 and 4 years [13]. Diagnosis seems easy with urine testing but since there the used urine bag collection leads quite often to false-positive results. Differentiation between cystitis and pyelonephritis is not possible clinically. Any kidney parenchymal scar will increase the likelihood of hypertension later in life.

An imaging algorithm was published by the Taskforce Abdomen [14]. US is used as imaging modality of choice and should always include urinary bladder. In pyelonephritis, the nephritis part can be diagnosed swelling of kidney, loss of cortical differentiation, areas of reduced echogenicity (representing edema) or increased one due to hemorrhage. Pyelitis causes wall thickening as well as pus, free flowing particles, or sedimentation levels (Fig. 21.4)—but the latter needs time to happen, so patience is needed before scanning the child.

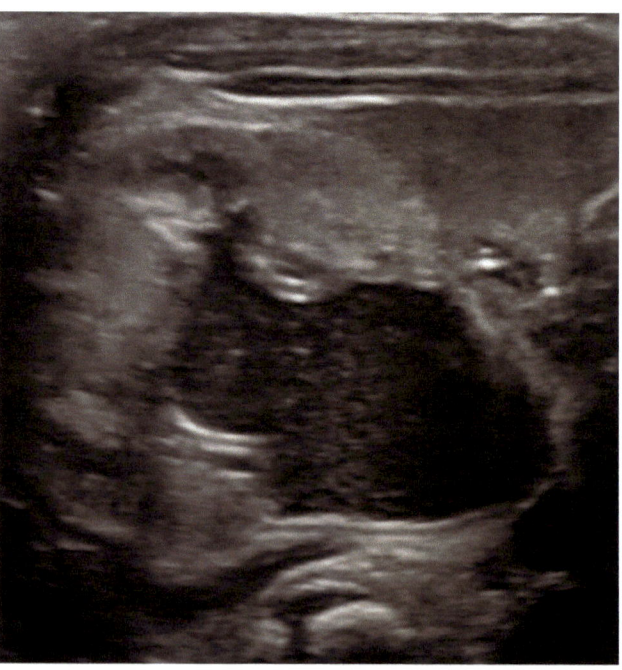

Fig. 21.4 child with urosepsis, kidney US, transverse section. There is massive dilated renal pelvis with free, flowing, echogenic particles corresponding to pus

Pyelonephritis can be diagnosed with equal accuracy by CT, MRI, and DMSA scan and ultrasound was reported to be less performant [15] Recently, it was published that contrast-enhanced US (ceUS) proves to be a valuable tool with almost comparable performance in regard to CT and DMSA scan but avoiding radiation exposure and sedation in small children [16].

> **Key Point**
> As in UTI, US is the starting modality of choice. ceUS enables to diagnose pyelonephritis with high confidence in doubtful cases.

21.6 Incontinence/Enuresis

Incontinence must be separated from enuresis. Incontinence represents an incomplete micturition at the wrong time point (e.g., urge) whereas enuresis is a complete micturition at the wrong time, being further divided in enuresis during night (enuresis nocturna) and/or during daytime (enuresis diurna),. Unfortunately, many cases of enuresis are labeled incorrectly as incontinence, especially many cases enuresis diurna are belonging to the group of incontinence (urge incontinence). Due to incorrect use of both terms, the problem is a wetting child. This could be due to anatomy (e.g., an ectopic ureter entering perineum or vagina in girls from a double system) or functional (e.g., urge incontinence) or a combination (enuresis nocturna due to small bladder volume, high fluid intake in evenings together with late wake up in nights), and there is also a family factor, where all relatives, for example, were suffering from enuresis nocturna. An overview about these entities can be found in [17].

> **Key Point**
> Do not mix terms incontinence and enuresis—these are different entities.

As usual starting imaging with US represents a good choice. Double systems can be ruled out and during full bladder scanning opening and closure the bladder sphincter can be observed—thus indicating urge incontinence. Moreover, an open bladder neck also points to bladder instability [18].

As mentioned already in the imaging modality section Fotter's VCU modification (only the procedure and no additional hardware needed) allows to analyze lower urinary tract dysfunctions with a performance almost comparable to bladder urodynamics.

21.7 Renal Masses

Kidney angiomyolipomas (fat content) are known to be in associated in 20% with tuberous sclerosis complex and pulmonary lymphangioleiomyomatosis [19]. Cystic renal masses include simply renal cysts, multicystic dysplastic kidneys, hereditary cystic renal diseases (autosomal dominant or recessive polycystic kidney disease) to cysts in renal dysplasia [20].

Cystic nephroma and cystic partially differentiated nephroblastoma cannot be distinguished by imaging, and it is believed that they represent the benign end of tumors originating from metamorphose, whereas Wilms tumor being on the malignant end of the spectrum. Another tumor originating from nephrogenic rests is the "Ossifying renal tumor of infancy (ORTI)." It appears like a staghorn calculus but enhances after contrast injection. Mesoblastic nephroma is the most common renal tumors in neonates and descend from mesenchyma. "Clear Cell Carcinoma of the kidney (CCSK)" is a solid tumor with cystic components and metastasizes in bones, which would be uncommon in Wilms tumor. Renal rhabdoid tumor is a solid tumor of toddlers which also shows subcapsular hemorrhage. Furthermore in 15%, it is associated with primary or secondary brain tumors.

"Renal Cell Carcinoma ("RCC" is similar to adults but occurs in children with Hippel Lindau disease.

Wilms tumor (nephroblastoma) represents the most common renal neoplasm in infancy (90%) and arises from nephrogenic rests (or nephroblastomatosis) [21]. Peak incidence is about 2–3 years of age and appears sold but can also be heterogenous due to hemorrhage. Calcifications can be seen up to 15% in CT [21]. In addition, renal vein invasion can be found. In 2%, there is a familial predisposition and several associations due to mutations of WT1 (WAGR syndrome, Denys-Drash syndrome, Frasier syndrome, Bloom syndrome) and WT2 (Beckwith-Wiedemann syndrome, Perlman syndrome, Simpson-Golabi-Behmel syndrome, Sotos syndrome) genes. Moreover, isolated abnormalities can be found like isolated abnormalities: cryptorchidism in 3%, hemihypertrophy in 3%, hypospadias in 2%, sporadic aniridia, and renal fusion (https://radiopaedia.org/articles/wilms-tumour).

> **Key Point**
> Wilms tumor most frequent renal tumor in childhood. Renal tumors in children may have several important associations.

21.8 Hematuria and Renal Calculi

Hematuria is a relatively common finding in children. It may be found incidentally by urine analysis (microscopic hematuria) or when gross hematuria is evident. Ultrasound is the primary imaging modality looking for structural abnormalities such as renal anomalies, ureteric calculi, and renal or bladder masses. The most common causes of gross hematuria are inflammatory processes in the bladder and glomerulonephritis. Other considerations include renal calculi and bladder rhabdomyosarcoma.

Adolescents and school aged children with renal colic present in the typical way, but infants may present with irritability and inconsolable crying. Ultrasound and radiography are the initial imaging modalities of choice with low dose CT being the most definitive. The goal is to identify the presence, position, number, and size of the renal calculi. Stones can be seen in the pelvicalyceal systems, ureters, or bladder. On ultrasound, signs of renal calculi include shadowing echogenic foci, dilatation of the urinary tract, and increased parenchymal echogenicity. Color Doppler ultrasound can be used to elicit the twinkle artifact. Low dose CT is used if the ultrasound is normal or if further anatomic details are needed for surgical planning. CT is complementary to US and is used for problem solving. When properly performed radiation doses are minimized and optimally adapted to the child's size.

Renal stones are unusual in children and their presence may indicate an underlying metabolic abnormality. In those with a metabolic abnormality, there can be repeated episodes over the years so judicious use of imaging is important.

> **Key Point**
> Hematuria is common in childhood. The common causes are renal calculi as well as inflammatory and neoplastic conditions.

21.9 Trauma

The kidney is the most commonly injured organ of the urinary tract in children and can occur in up to 20% of all blunt injury cases [21]. Most children are treated conservatively, but if they are hemodynamically unstable operative management may be required. Injuries to the ureter, bladder or urethra are usually seen in the setting of polytrauma [22]. The pediatric kidney is relatively mobile within Gerota's fascia so lacerations and contusions are caused by crushing of the kidneys against the spine or ribs. Undiagnosed pre-existing renal abnormalities are found incidentally in up to 20% of children who are imaged in the setting of acute trauma [23].

Imaging has a pivotal role in managing blunt or penetrating trauma to the genitourinary tract. In many places, ultrasound is first modality used especially if the patient has minimal symptoms. In cases of urinary tract injury, multiphase post-contrast CT of the urinary tract is recommended including delayed post-contrast scans (Fig. 21.5) [22].

In children with renal trauma, imaging is used to classify any injury to the kidney, to identify underlying congenital abnormalities and demonstrate the extent of any other injury. Initial ultrasound helps to identify patients needing more extensive investigation and is particularly useful for follow-up of renal injuries, hematomas, and urinomas. It must be remembered that ultrasound is insensitive for detecting renal lacerations. Most urinomas are asymptomatic and will resolve spontaneously.

CECT with delayed urographic phase is the gold standard for grading renal injuries. It allows accurate evaluation of injuries to the renal parenchyma, the renal vessels, and collecting systems. CT is recommended in children with high energy or penetrating trauma and/or when there is a drop in hematocrit associated with any degree of hematuria [24].

Renal injuries are graded based on CT findings using the AAST Organ Injury Scale [25]. It describes a scale of progressively more severe injury with Grade I representing parenchymal contusion and subcapsular hematoma to Grade V which represents a completely shattered kidney. Most renal injuries in children are Grade I–III while only about 20% are Grade IV or V. Most children are treated conservatively and surgical intervention is required only in clinically unstable patients. Ureteral injuries are uncommon in children [26]. Bladder rupture can be either intra-peritoneal or extra-peritoneal and is usually associated with fractures of the pelvis. Urethral injuries are rare and most often seen in boys with blunt perineal trauma. Retrograde urethrogram is performed to evaluate urethral trauma. In children being evaluated for trauma, if they have normal genitourinary examination, normal voiding and without gross hematuria, no imaging of the lower GU tract is required.

Contrast-enhanced US has emerged as a promising tool to assess renal injuries [27].

> **Key Point**
> The kidney is the most commonly injured organ of the urinary tract. Most children are treated conservatively. Underlying congenital abnormalities are commonly found.

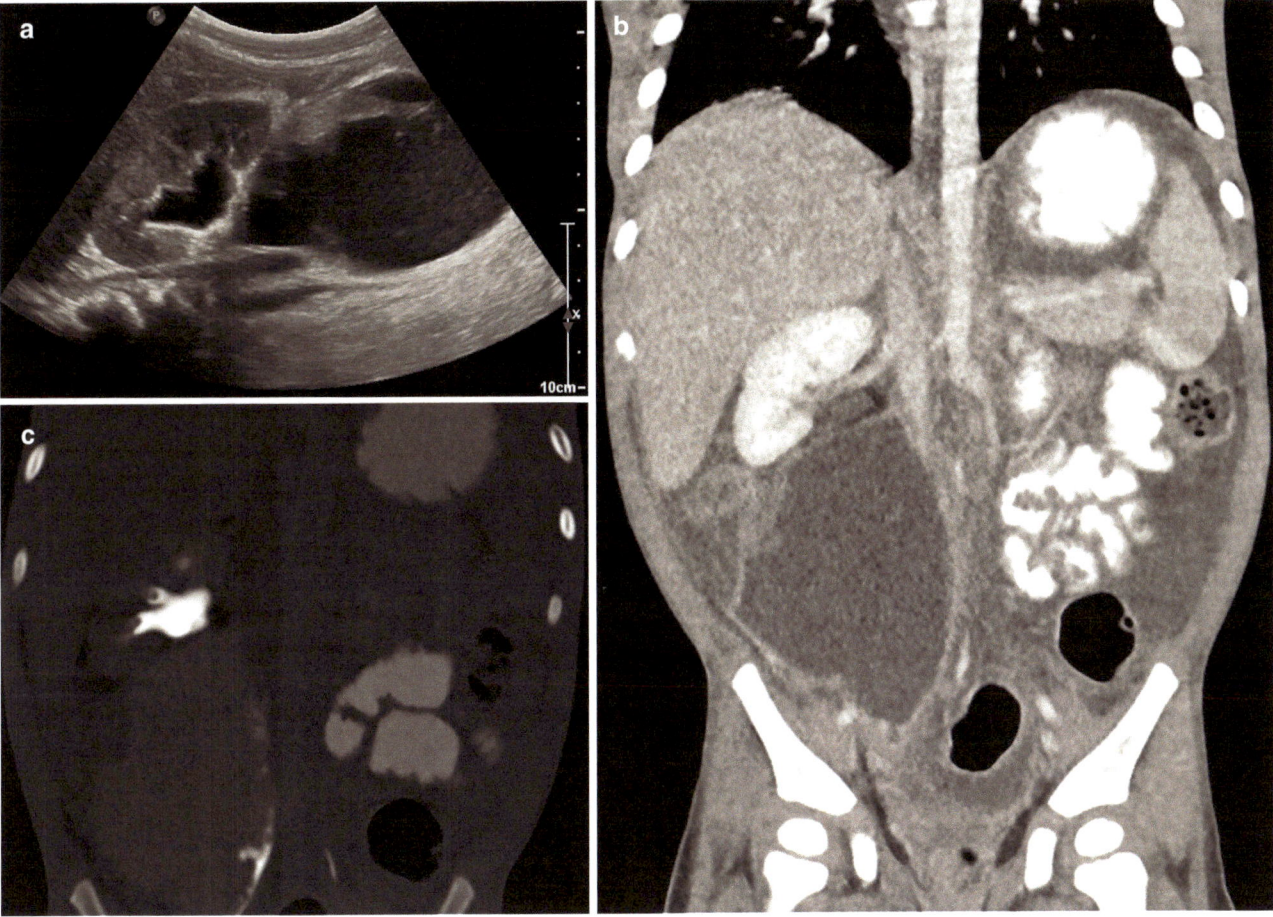

Fig. 21.5 6 year old boy involved in motor vehicle accident (**a**) Sagittal ultrasound image through the right kidney shows mild right-sided hydronephrosis with an inferior fluid collection with moderate low level echos (**b**) nephrogenic phase CT demonstrates homogeneous enhance-ment of the right kidney with inferior fluid collection. (**c**) delayed phase CT with wide windowing showing contrast collecting in the inferior fluid collection indicating a urinoma

21.10 Acute Kidney Injury (AKI) and Chronic Renal Failure (CRF)

Renal failure in infants and children may be acute or chronic, reversible, or irreversible and may lead to dialysis or renal transplantation. Pathophysiologically, there are three major causes:

- Intrinsic renal disease
- Obstructive uropathy
- Pre-renal disease secondary to a systemic or extra-renal disease

Acute kidney injury is characterized by an abrupt deterioration of kidney function and is commonly seen in critically ill children. It can be seen in 30% of children in intensive care units. Clinically, there is usually increased blood pressure with oliguria or anuria. The diagnosis is based on laboratory findings with elevated serum creatine, electrolyte disturbances, low protein, and often metabolic acidosis. US plays a central role in evaluating the etiologies of renal failure and helping to differentiate acute from chronic failure. The imaging findings must be correlated with biological and clinical data.

Neonatal AKI may be suggested prenatally, but the diagnosis is often only established after birth. The most common renal causes are ARPKD, congenital nephrotic syndromes (CNS), or neonatal glomerulonephritis (GN). In children with ARPCKD, the kidneys are large, echogenic and have a salt and pepper appearance of the parenchyma. Neonatal CNS and GN present with large kidneys and non-specific echo pattern, often with loss of the normal corticomedullary differentiation. Colour Doppler findings are also non-specific. Corticomedullary differentiation depends on whether the cortex, medulla, or both are affected. Medullary and cortical necrosis in the neonate results from lack of renal perfusion. On US, the cortex in cortical necrosis first appears hyperechoic, then shrinks and finally calcifies. In medullary necrosis, calcifications develop within the medulla. The value of ultrasound is not to be specific, but to rule out other causes of AKI.

Renal vein thrombosis (RVT) is most often seen in neonates with adrenal gland hemorrhage, dehydration, or thrombotic syndromes. RVT can occur in utero and unilateral RVT usually presents with hypertension and hematuria. In the acute phase on US, the kidney is enlarged, echogenic and with loss of the CMD. On CDS, the color signals from the affected renal veins are missing. The kidney may atrophy with calcification in the vessels.

The three most common causes of ARF in children in developing countries are hemolytic uremic syndrome (HUS), glomerulonephritis, and postoperative sepsis/pre-renal ischemia. In industrialized countries, the three commonest causes are intrinsic renal disease, postoperative septic shock, and organ/bone marrow transplantation [28]. Hemolytic uremic syndrome is comprised of hemolytic microangiopathic anemia, thrombocytopenia, and AKI and is caused by toxins released from certain strains of *E coli*. The patients often have a history of hemorrhagic enterocolitis. In the acute phase, the renal cortex becomes markedly hyperechoic bilaterally with increase corticomedullary differentiation. On Doppler analysis, the RI is markedly elevated with diffuse decreased cortical perfusion on CDS. Proximal tubular necrosis may follow toxic ingestions or medication. Tubular and vascular obstruction causing prolonged renal ischemia can follow renal parenchymal uric acid accumulation, sickle cell crisis, myoglobulinemia, and renal vein thrombosis. Cortical and tubular necrosis may occur following hemorrhagic shock, severe dehydration, crush injuries, thermal burns, and septic shock.

The incidence of ESRD has been stable over the past 30 years worldwide, but prevalence has increased [29]. The most common cause of pediatric CRF is CAKUT accounting for up to 50% of cases. The next most common causes are the hereditary nephropathies and glomerulonephritis. Infants of low birth weight and have an increased risk of developing ESRD in adolescence. Chronic renal failure is defined as a GFR <50 ml/min per 1.73 m/kidney. On ultrasound, the kidneys are small with loss of CMD and small cysts.

Congenital nephrotic syndromes (CNS) encompass diseases in which there is massive proteinuria occurring after birth. The most common form of CNS is the Finnish type. On US, at birth, the kidneys are large and hyperechoic. The CMD is present but the pyramids are irregular and within weeks will no longer be visible. Other causes of CNS include diffuse mesangial sclerosis which can be part of Denys-Drash syndrome.

Renal diseases that include primary and secondary tubulopathy are numerous. Hypercalciuria is a constant finding and may lead to nephrocalcinosis which is easily seen on US (Fig. 21.6). Secondary hyperparathyroidism may develop leading to renal osteodystrophy which can result in abnormalities affecting the growth plates, epiphyseal displacement, and fractures.

> **Key Point**
> US is the key imaging examination in children with AKI or CRF. Ultrasound is key to differentiating pre-, post-, and intrarenal causes. Most nephropathies have a similar appearance with large kidneys usually indicating acute disease and small kidneys in chronic diseases.

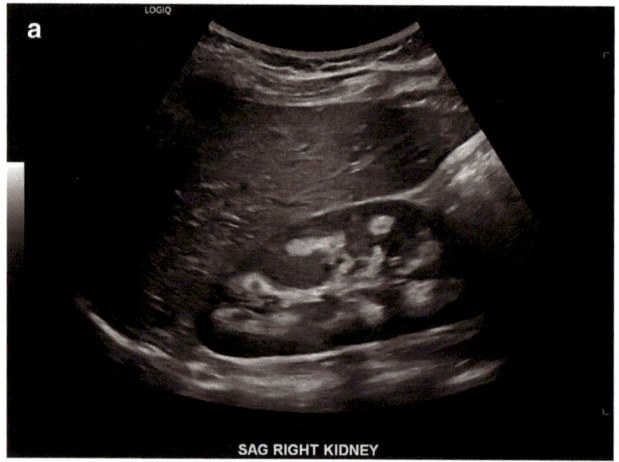
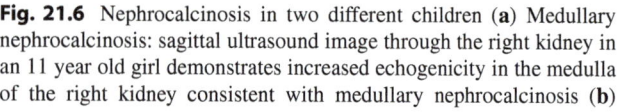
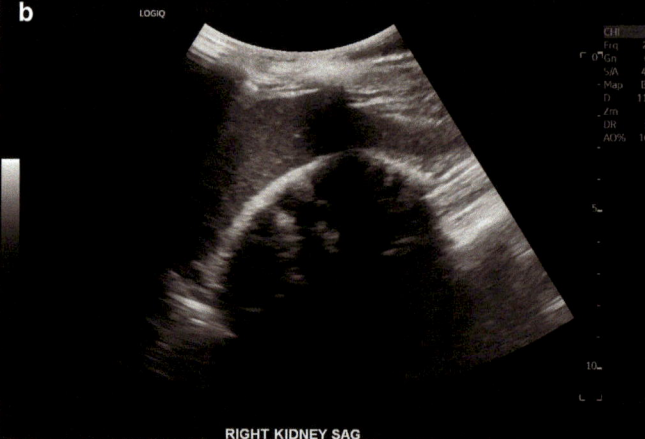

Fig. 21.6 Nephrocalcinosis in two different children (**a**) Medullary nephrocalcinosis: sagittal ultrasound image through the right kidney in an 11 year old girl demonstrates increased echogenicity in the medulla of the right kidney consistent with medullary nephrocalcinosis (**b**) Cortical nephrocalcinosis: sagittal image through the right kidney in a 7 year old boy demonstrates increased echogenicity and shadowing from the renal cortex

21.11 Renal Causes of Hypertension

A renal cause for hypertension is suspected when hypertension is severe or refractory to multiple drugs. Renovascular hypertension is responsible for 5–25% of hypertension in children [30]. There are numerous causes of aortic and renal artery narrowing leading to renal hypertension. These are often syndromic and include idiopathic/fibromuscular dysplasia, NF1, Williams syndrome, mid-aortic syndrome, inflammatory arteritis as well as extrinsic compression.

Ultrasound is the initial modality to assess for renal anomalies or scarring as well as non-renal lesions such as pheochromocytoma. Doppler evaluation can be used to assess for renal artery stenosis by showing a tardus parvus pattern of the spectral waveform with slow systolic acceleration. Pathologic flow parameters include peak systolic flow >180 cm/s, acceleration time > 80 ms, renal artery to aortic flow velocity ratio >3 and difference in RI more than 0.05 [30]. Renal Doppler ultrasound is reasonably specific but not sensitive enough to exclude renal vascular abnormalities [31].

CT angiography or MR angiography can verify a renovascular cause for hypertension by demonstrating one or more areas of stenosis or if there are collateral vessels present. CTA and MRA are excellent for evaluating the aorta and main renal arteries, but for smaller intraparenchymal branches visualization is limited [32]. Children are referred for catheter renal angiography if no abnormality has been identified on noninvasive techniques and there is persistent failure of medical therapy. Angiography is considered the gold standard in establishing the diagnosis of renovascular disease as no noninvasive technique can exclude renovascular disease [32].

> **Key Point**
> Renal causes of hypertension are common in children. Ultrasound is the initial modality used to identify underlying renal abnormalities. However, only catheter angiography can exclude renovascular disease.

21.12 Disorders of Sexual Differentiation

Disorders of sexual development (DSD) are defined as conditions in which chromosomal sex is not consistent with phenotypic sex or in which the phenotype is not classifiable as either male or female [33]. DSD can be divided into three categories: those with 46 XX karyotype, those with a 46XY karyotype, and those relating to sex chromosomes [34]. Disorders of sex development occur when the male hormone (androgens and anti-Mullerian hormone) secretion or action

is insufficient in the 46 XY fetus or when there is androgen excess in the 46 XX fetus. DSD with ambiguous genitalia are typically diagnosed clinically in the newborn period, whereas those associated with male and female phenotypes may not present until adolescence. Patients with pure gonadal dysgenesis or complete androgen insensitivity usually are phenotypic females who present at puberty with primary amenorrhea.

Diagnosis and classification of these disorders is complex and the role of imaging in infants is to identify a uterus and or cervix, to locate the gonads, and to define the anatomy of cloacal malformations, Mullerian duct anomalies, urinary tract anomalies as well as anorectal and spine malformations. Ultrasound has been the primary modality to identify the internal organs, and occasionally fluoroscopic genitography and VCUG are used to assess the vagina, urethra, and any fistulas or complex tracts. Contrast-enhanced ultrasound and MR genitography are being used more often in the evaluation of these anomalies especially in defining the anatomy of the urogenital tract, anorectal malformations, and to identify otherwise occult gonad [35, 36]. Both techniques are similar to traditional fluoroscopic genitography in that contrast material is used to demonstrate the anatomy of the various cavities.

When performing a genitogram, it is important to ensure that all perineal orifices are examined [37]. It is also important to preserve the morphological appearance by only inserting the catheters a short distance. The goal is to define a male or female urethral configuration and identify any fistulous communication with the vagina or rectum [38]. Demonstration of the level at which the vagina opens into a urogenital sinus and its relationship to the external sphincter is important in surgical planning. The vagina is evaluated to determine its presence or absence, its relationship to the urethra and to identify the uterus. The presence of hydrocolpos associated with ambiguous genitalia and two perineal orifices confirms the presence of a urogenital sinus. In the presence of a large hydrocolpos, the bladder may be displaced anteriorly making it difficult to see so care is needed to make sure a fluid filled vagina is not confused with the urinary bladder. The uterus often is identified capping the vagina and the distended vagina often contains a fluid-debris level.

In cloacal malformations, the genital, urinary, and gastrointestinal tracts open into a single common channel classically located at the expected site of the urethra [39]. It is almost exclusively seen in girls. Cloacal malformations are divided into two groups depending on the length of the common channel. A common channel less than 3 cm is more easily repaired and has a lower incidence of associated anomalies.

Mullerian duct anomalies are a broad and complex spectrum of anomalies that often present with primary amenorrhea in adolescents. MR is the imaging method of choice in defining these anomalies [40]. Uterus, fallopian tubes, cervix, and upper two thirds of the vagina are derived from the Mullerian ducts. The ovaries are embryologically separate and not typically involved in Mullerian duct anomalies. In patients with Mullerian duct anomalies, renal and ureteric anomalies are common. In addition to the well-known association with renal agenesis which is found in up to 30%, there is also a high incidence of ectopic, malrotated, or dysplastic kidneys. Additionally, 25% of patients with renal agenesis have distal ureteric remnants or ectopic ureteric insertion. These ureteric remnants may become distended by menstrual blood leading to abdominal pain, infection or present with urinary incontinence and recurrent UTI. All patients with Mullerian duct anomalies need assessment of the urinary tract to identify renal agenesis, ectopic ureters, or ureteric stumps.

Mayer-Rokitansky-Kuster-Hauser syndrome is a heterogeneous disorder characterized by ureterovaginal atresia in 46XX girls. Abnormalities of the genital tract may range from upper vaginal atresia to total Mullerian agenesis with associated urinary tract anomalies.

The external genitalia are normal. Cyclical abdominal pain due to endometrial tissue or even hematometra in the rudimentary uterus may be a cause of clinical confusion. The ovaries are ectopic in 40% of cases and are readily identified on pre-operative MR imaging. Herlyn-Werner-Wunderlich syndrome is characterized by uterus didelphys and unilateral hematocolpos related to an obstructed hemivagina with unilateral renal agenesis. They are often diagnosed early in infancy but may present in adolescence with hematocolpos, hematometra, or hematosalpinx. The diagnostic dilemma in these patients is that most have regular menstruation because one uterus is not obstructed.

> **Key Point**
> Disorders of sexual differentiation are complex disorders that often present at birth but may not become apparent until puberty.

21.13 Testicular and Ovarian Pathology

21.13.1 Cryptorchidism

Cryptorchidism or undescended testis is one of the most common congenital malformations on infant males seen in up to 5% of full-term and 45% of preterm neonates. In most cases, there is spontaneous descent within the first few months of life. Undescended testis is initially evaluated with ultrasound which can easily detect testes in the inguinal canal. However, ultrasound cannot reliably detect intra-abdominal testes which represent 20% non-palpable testes. MRI cannot diagnose monorchidism. Both the American Urologic Association and the European Association of Urology guidelines recommend against imaging for the routine management of patients with non-palpable testes. However, if there is associated ambiguous genitalia or hypospadias, there is a higher likelihood of an underlying disorder of sexual development. In this instance, ultrasound or MR is recommended to look for internal female pelvic organs specifically the uterus.

21.13.2 Scrotal Masses

A palpable scrotal mass should be characterized as intra- or extratesticular, solid or cystic, and characterized by its vascularity. Testicular tumors account for approximately 1–2% of all pediatric solid tumors. Most testicular tumors present as a painless scrotal mass. Hydroceles are often also present. The first line of evaluation is high resolution ultrasound (7.5–12.5 MHz) with Doppler interrogation. Testicular tumors in prepubertal boys differ in several aspects to testicular tumors after puberty: they have a lower incidence, they have a different histologic distribution (teratomas and yolk sac tumors are more common and germ cell tumors are less common), and they are more often benign. Testicular tumors can generally be classified as germ cell or stromal tumors.

Teratomas are usually benign in prepubertal children and represent about 40% of testicular tumors. They present at a median age of 13 months. Yolk sac tumors are the predominant prepubertal malignant germ cell tumor. Epidermoid cysts are of ectodermal origin and are always benign. Keratin-producing epithelium is responsible for the keratinized squamous epithelial deposits which appear hyperechogenic on US. Juvenile granulosa cell tumors usually occur in first year of life. Leydig cell tumors arising from the testosterone producing Leydig cells should be suspected in boys with premature puberty, with high testosterone and low gonadotropin levels. Patients are typically 6–10 years old. One specific tumor type is the gonadoblastoma which contains germ cell and stromal cell types and occurs almost exclusively in the setting of DSDs.

Paratesticular tumors are less common than testicular tumors and may be benign or malignant. Benign tumors include leiomyoma, fibroma, lipoma, hemangioma, and lymphangioma. The most common malignant tumor is the paratesticular rhabdomyosarcoma and the rare melanotic neuroectodermal tumor of infancy.

Testicular microlithiasis is increasingly seen in prepubertal boys and represents multiple tiny calcification in the testes. Microlithiasis appears as small non-shadowing hyperechoic foci ranging in diameter from 1–3 mm.

Microlithiasis is usually seen bilaterally. A recent metanalysis showed only 4 out of 296 boys with microlithiasis <19 developed a testicular tumor [41]. However, there is ongoing debate about the relationship to developing germ cell tumors but at present, there is no compelling evidence that regular sonographic follow-up is useful.

Up to a third of boys with congenital adrenal hyperplasia (CAH) will have testicular adrenal rest tumors (TARTS). These are thought to be ectopic adrenal cells with are growing under pathological stimulation from ACTH. They have no malignant potential but may be associated with impaired fertility.

21.13.3 Acute Scrotal Pain

The most common causes of acute scrotal pain are torsion of the testis or appendix testis, and epididymitis/epididymo-orchitis. Other causes of acute scrotal pain include mumps orchitis, varicocele, scrotal hematoma, incarcerated hernia, or appendicitis. Trauma can cause hematomas, testicular contusion, rupture, dislocation, or torsion.

Torsion of the testis most often occurs in the neonatal period and around puberty, whereas torsion of appendix testis occurs over a wider age range. Epididymitis affects two age groups: less than 1 year and 12–15 years. Perinatal testicular torsion most often occurs prenatally. Most cases of perinatal torsion are extravaginal, in contrast to the usual intravaginal torsion which occurs during puberty.

In general, the duration of symptoms is shorter in testicular torsion, and torsion of the appendix testis is compared to epididymitis. Prepubertal males are more likely to present with atypical symptoms and delayed diagnosis. Testicular torsion is a spectrum ranging from partial to complete. The torsed testis becomes enlarged and develops heterogeneous echogenicity. In partial torsion, there is asymmetric decreased flow to the affected testis. On Doppler ultrasound, there is absence of flow to the testis with complete torsion. With partial torsion, there may be absent or reversed diastolic flow or tardus parvus waveforms.

With torsion of the testicular appendages, there is focal pain over the superior aspect of the testis. Ultrasound demonstrates an extratesticular avascular nodule of varying echogenicity. Retrograde infection is frequently the source of epididymo-orchitis. Sexually transmitted infections are usually seen in adolescents. In acute cases, the epididymis is enlarged and hypervascular.

21.13.4 Ovarian Neoplasms

Ovarian neoplasms can be divided according to their cell of origin into three groups: germ cell, sex cord-stromal, and epithelial.

Most ovarian tumors in children are benign but 10–30% will be malignant. They usually present with pain or a palpable abdominal mass and may be associated with ovarian torsion. If the tumor secretes sex hormones, they may present with precocious puberty or virilization. The tumors are usually identified on ultrasound and more definitively evaluated with MR imaging. If the mass is malignant, FDG-PDT/CT has been shown to improve accuracy when detecting metastases [42].

Germ cell tumors are most common ovarian tumor in girls. Unlike adults, up to 30% of GCT in girls are malignant. Mature cystic teratomas are the most common benign ovarian neoplasm and are commonly known as dermoid cysts. Dysgerminomas are the most common malignant ovarian tumor. Their imaging appearance is determined by their content which is usually a mix of cyst, calcifications, fat, and sometimes hair. In contrast to epithelial neoplasms, which spread through peritoneal dissemination, GCTs usually disseminate through the lymphatic system. The prognosis for GCTs is excellent.

Sex-cord stroma tumors can be either benign or malignant. The two most common tumors in children are the granulosa cell tumor and the Sertoli-Leydig cell tumor. These tumors usually present with endocrine dysfunction and are usually confined to the ovary. The appearance is variable and includes both cystic and solid masses.

Epithelial tumors can also be benign or malignant and represent up to 15% of ovarian tumors in children. Most are benign and include serous, mucinous, and mixed cystadenomas. Carcinomas are very rare. Epithelial tumors usually appear as unilocular or multilocular cystic masses with numerous septations.

Adnexal torsion can involve the ovary and/or the fallopian tube. It occurs equally in pre- and post-menarchal girls and may be associated with a lead point such as a teratoma. The clinical presentation can be confusing with intermittent pain due to torsion/detorsion complex. On ultrasound, there is an enlarged, heterogenous pelvic mass with several peripherally dilated cysts and absent Doppler flow. Increased volume is the most common finding. It should be remembered that the presence of flow on Doppler US does not exclude torsion as the ovaries have dual arterial supply. In some cases, CT is the initial modality performed and recognition of the characteristic findings is important for prompt diagnosis (Fig. 21.7).

> **Key Point**
> The most common tumors of the testis and ovary in childhood are germ cell tumors. In prepubertal boys, most intratesticular tumors are benign, whereas after puberty they are malignant. Ovarian and testicular torsion may be intermittent leading to a confusing clinical presentation.

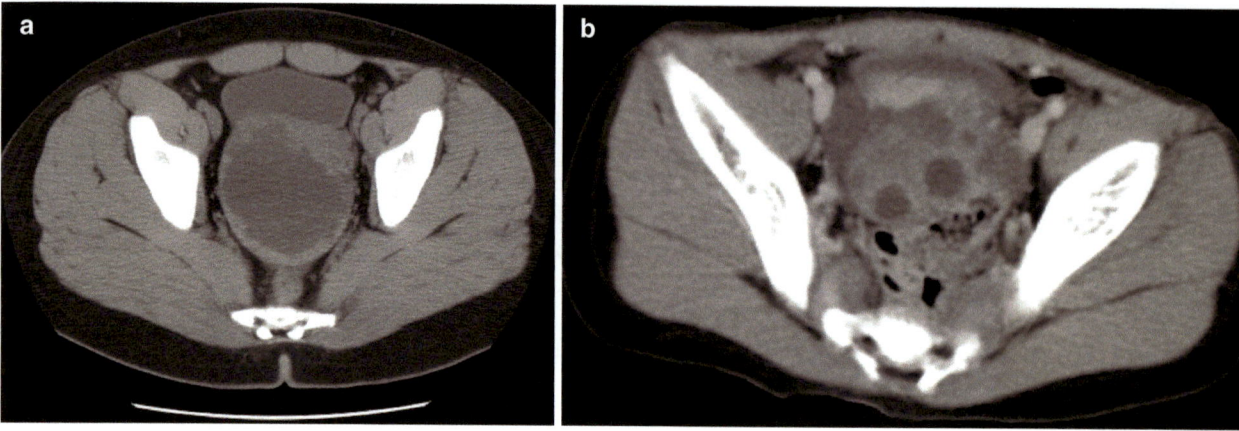

Fig. 21.7 14 year old girl with severe abdominal pain secondary to ovarian torsion (**a**) axial post contrast CT shows a large necrotic mass in the pelvis (**b**) inferior image through the pelvis demonstrates the peripheral cysts typical for ovarian torsion

21.14 Concluding Remarks

Most imaging evaluations in the infant or child begin with ultrasound. The next imaging steps are determined by the initial differential diagnosis obtained by integrating the clinical presentation with the ultrasound findings. It is important to be aware of the unique challenges involved in the imaging of children. Congenital abnormalities, urinary tract infection`, and tumors of the genitourinary tract represent a majority of indications for imaging in a pediatric radiology practice.

> **Take Home Points**
> 1. Ultrasound is the workhorse of imaging the genito-urinary tract.
> 2. Congenital abnormalities are very common.
> 3. Awareness of common normal variants is important.
> 4. Pediatric urological conditions are diverse with many different approaches to imaging and management.

References

1. Sorantin E, Coradello H, Wiltgen M. Computer-assisted mechanical ventilation of newborns. Anaesthesist. 1992;41(6):342–5.
2. Riccabona M, Avni FE, Blickman JG, Dacher JN, Darge K, Lobo ML. Imaging recommendations in paediatric uroradiology: minutes of the ESPR workgroup session on urinary tract infection, fetal hydronephrosis, urinary tract ultrasonography and voiding cystourethrography, Barcelona, Spain, June 2007. Pediatr Radiol. 2008;38(2):138–45.
3. Fotter R, Kopp W, Klein E, Höllwarth M, Uray E. Unstable bladder in children: functional evaluation by modified voiding cystourethrography. Radiology. 1986;161(3):811–3. https://doi.org/10.1148/radiology.161.3.3786739.
4. Khrichenko D, Darge K. Functional analysis in MR urography—made simple. Pediatr Radiol. 2010;40(2):182–99.
5. McDaniel BB, Jones RA, Scherz H, Kirsch AJ, Little SB, Grattan-Smith JD. Dynamic contrast-enhanced MR urography in the evaluation of pediatric Hydronephrosis: part 2, anatomic and functional assessment of Uteropelvic junction obstruction. Am J Roentgenol. 2005;185(6):1608–14.
6. Siegel MJ, Ramirez-Giraldo JC. Dual-energy CT in children: imaging algorithms and clinical applications. Radiology. 2019;291(2):286–97.
7. Nguyen HT, Benson CB, Bromley B, Campbell JB, Chow J, Coleman B, u. a. Multidisciplinary consensus on the classification of prenatal and postnatal urinary tract dilation (UTD classification system). J Pediatr Urol. 2014;10(6):982–98.
8. Pelliccia P, Sferrazza Papa S, Cavallo F, Tagi VM, Di Serafino M, Esposito F, u. a. Prenatal and postnatal urinary tract dilation: advantages of a standardized ultrasound definition and classification. J Ultrasound. 2019;22(1):5–12.
9. Sudhamani SSS, Kumar SH, Bhalekar S. The Weigert–Meyer law of ureteral duplication. Ann Pathol lab med. 2019;6(7):C80–2.
10. Tain YL, Luh H, Lin CY, Hsu CN. Incidence and risks of congenital anomalies of kidney and urinary tract in newborns. Medicine (Baltimore). 2016;95(5):e2659.
11. Rodriguez MM. Congenital anomalies of the kidney and the urinary tract (CAKUT). Fetal Pediatr Pathol. 2014;33(5–6):293–320.
12. Capone VP, Morello W, Taroni F, Montini G. Genetics of congenital anomalies of the kidney and urinary tract: the current state of play. Int J Mol Sci. 2017;18(4):796.
13. Leung AKC, Wong AHC, Leung AAM, Hon KL. Urinary tract infection in children Recent Patents. Inflamm Allergy Drug Discov. 2019;13(1):2–18.
14. Imaging Algorithm in childhood UTI [Internet]. 2022. Verfügbar unter. https://www.espr.org/app/uploads/Imaging-algorithm-in-childhood-UTI.pdf
15. Majd M, Nussbaum Blask AR, Markle BM, Shalaby-Rana E, Pohl HG, Park JS. Acute pyelonephritis: comparison of diagnosis with 99m Tc-DMSA SPECT, spiral CT, MR imaging, and power Doppler US in an experimental pig model. Radiology. 2001;218(1):101–8.
16. Jung HJ, Choi MH, Pai KS, Kim HG. Diagnostic performance of contrast-enhanced ultrasound for acute pyelonephritis in children. Sci Rep. 2020;10(1):10715.
17. Sorantin E, Lindbichler F, Richard F. Lower urinary tract dysfunction. In: Carty H, Brunelle F, Stringer DA, SCS K, editors. Herausgeber. Imaging Children. New York: Springer; 2005. p. 863–71.
18. Hausegger KA, Fotter R, Sorantin E, Schmidt P. Urethral morphology and bladder instability. Pediatr Radiol. 1991;21(4):278–80.

19. Vos N, Oyen R. Renal Angiomyolipoma: the good, the bad, and the ugly. J Belg Soc Radiol. 2018;102(1):41.

20. Ferro F, Vezzali N, Comploj E, Pedron E, Di Serafino M, Esposito F. Pediatric cystic diseases of the kidney. J Ultrasound. 2019;22(3):381–93.

21. Chung EM, Graeber AR, Conran RM. Renal tumors of childhood: radiologic-pathologic correlation part 1. The 1st decade: from the radiologic pathology archives. Radiographics. 2016;36(2):499–522.

22. Riccabona M, Lobo ML, Papadopoulou F, Avni FE, Blickman JG, Dacher JN, Damasio B, Darge K, Ording-Müller LS, Vivier PH, Willi U. ESPR uroradiology task force and ESUR paediatric working group: imaging recommendations in paediatric uroradiology, part IV: minutes of the ESPR uroradiology task force mini-symposium on imaging in childhood renal hypertension and imaging of renal trauma in children. Pediatr Radiol. 2011;41:939–44.

23. Schmidlin FR, Iselin CE, Naimi A, Rohner S, Borst F, Farshad M, Niederer P, Graber P. The higher injury risk of abnormal kidneys in blunt renal trauma. Scand J Urol Nephrol. 1998;32:388–92.

24. Coccolini F, Moore EE, Kluger Y, et al. Kidney and uro-trauma: WSES-AAST guidelines. World J Emerg Surg. 2019;14:54.

25. Kozar RA, Crandall M, Shanmuganathan K, Zarzaur BL, Coburn M, Cribari C, Kaups K, Schuster K, Tominaga GT. AAST PAC organ injury scaling 2018 update: spleen, liver, and kidney. J Trauma Acute Care Surg. 2018;85:1119–22.

26. Singer G, Arneitz C, Tschauner S, Castellani C, Till H. Trauma in pediatric urology. Semin Pediatr Surg. 2021;30:151085.

27. Di Serafino M, Iacobellis F, Schillirò ML, Ronza R, Verde F, Grimaldi D, Dell Aversano Orabona G, Caruso M, Sabatino V, Rinaldo C, Romano L. The technique and advantages of contrast-enhanced ultrasound in the diagnosis and follow-up of traumatic abdomen solid organ injuries. Diagnostics (Basel). 2022;12:435.

28. Chan JC, Williams DM, Roth KS. Kidney failure in infants and children. Pediatr Rev. 2002;23:47–60.

29. Kaspar CD, Bholah R, Bunchman TE. A review of pediatric chronic kidney disease. Blood Purif. 2016;41:211–7.

30. Patel PA, Cahill AM. Renovascular hypertension in children CVIR Endovasc. 2021;4:10.

31. Chhadia S, Cohn RA, Vural G, Donaldson JS. Renal Doppler evaluation in the child with hypertension: a reasonable screening discriminator. Pediatr Radiol. 2013;43:1549–56.

32. Trautmann A, Roebuck DJ, McLaren CA, Brennan E, Marks SD, Tullus K. Non-invasive imaging cannot replace formal angiography in the diagnosis of renovascular hypertension. Pediatr Nephrol. 2017;32:495–502.

33. Mansour SM, Hamed ST, Adel L, Kamal RM, Ahmed DM. Does MRI add to ultrasound in the assessment of disorders of sex development? Eur J Radiol. 2012;81:2403–10.

34. Profeta G, Micangeli G, Tarani F, Paparella R, Ferraguti G, Spaziani M, Isidori AM, Menghi M, Ceccanti M, Fiore M, Tarani L. Sexual developmental disorders in pediatrics. Clin Ter. 2022;173:475–88.

35. Chow JS, Bellah RD, Darge K, Ntoulia A, Phelps AS, Riccabona M, Back SJ. Contrast-enhanced genitosonography and colosonography: emerging alternatives to fluoroscopy. Pediatr Radiol. 2021;51:2387–95.

36. Baughman SM, Richardson RR, Podberesky DJ, Dalrymple NC, Yerkes EB. 3-dimensional magnetic resonance genitography: a different look at cloacal malformations. J Urol. 2007;178:1675–8. discussion 1678

37. Shopfner CE. Genitography in intersexual states. Radiology. 1964;82:664–74.

38. Wright NB, Smith C, Rickwood AM, Carty HM. Imaging children with ambiguous genitalia and intersex states. Clin Radiol. 1995;50:823–9.

39. Jaramillo D, Lebowitz RL, Hendren WH. The cloacal malformation: radiologic findings and imaging recommendations. Radiology. 1990;177:441–8.

40. Hall-Craggs MA, Kirkham A, Creighton SM. Renal and urological abnormalities occurring with Mullerian anomalies. J Pediatr Urol. 2013;9:27–32.

41. Yu CJ, Lu JD, Zhao J, Wei Y, Zhao TX, Lin T, He DW, Wu SD, Wei GH. Incidence characteristics of testicular microlithiasis and its association with risk of primary testicular tumors in children: a systematic review and meta-analysis. World J Pediatr. 2020;16:585–97.

42. Hart A, Vali R, Marie E, Shaikh F, Shammas A. The clinical impact of ^{18}F-FDG PET/CT in extracranial pediatric germ cell tumors. Pediatr Radiol. 2017;47:1508–13.

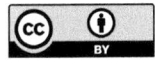

Correction to: Diseases of the Pancreas

Thomas K. Helmberger and Riccardo Manfredi

Correction to:
J. Hodler et al. (eds.), *Diseases of the Abdomen and Pelvis 2023-2026*,
https://doi.org/10.1007/978-3-031-27355-1_9

The original version of this chapter was published with German letters in Table 9.3 which has been removed now, and we have retained the value "0.9/100.000" in the "Incidence" row.

The updated original version of this chapter can be found at https://doi.org/10.1007/978-3-031-27355-1_9

© The Author(s) 2023
J. Hodler et al. (eds.), *Diseases of the Abdomen and Pelvis 2023-2026*, IDKD Springer Series,
https://doi.org/10.1007/978-3-031-27355-1_22